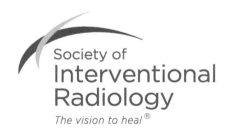

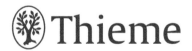

Vertebral Augmentation

The Comprehensive Guide to Vertebroplasty, Kyphoplasty, and Implant Augmentation

Douglas P. Beall, MD
Chief of Services
The Spine Fracture Institute at Summit Medical Center Oklahoma
Oklahoma City, Oklahoma, USA

Associate Editors:
Allan L. Brook
M. R. Chambers
Joshua A. Hirsch
Alexios Kelekis
Yong-Chul Kim
Scott Kreiner
Kieran Murphy

524 illustrations

Thieme
New York • Stuttgart • Delhi • Rio de Janeiro

Library of Congress Cataloging-in-Publication Data is available from the publisher

Important note: Medicine is an ever-changing science undergoing continual development. Research and clinical experience are continually expanding our knowledge, in particular our knowledge of proper treatment and drug therapy. Insofar as this book mentions any dosage or application, readers may rest assured that the authors, editors, and publishers have made every effort to ensure that such references are in accordance with **the state of knowledge at the time of production of the book.**

Nevertheless, this does not involve, imply, or express any guarantee or responsibility on the part of the publishers in respect to any dosage instructions and forms of applications stated in the book. **Every user is requested to examine carefully** the manufacturers' leaflets accompanying each drug and to check, if necessary in consultation with a physician or specialist, whether the dosage schedules mentioned therein or the contraindications stated by the manufacturers differ from the statements made in the present book. Such examination is particularly important with drugs that are either rarely used or have been newly released on the market. Every dosage schedule or every form of application used is entirely at the user's own risk and responsibility. The authors and publishers request every user to report to the publishers any discrepancies or inaccuracies noticed. If errors in this work are found after publication, errata will be posted at www.thieme.com on the product description page.

Some of the product names, patents, and registered designs referred to in this book are in fact registered trademarks or proprietary names even though specific reference to this fact is not always made in the text. Therefore, the appearance of a name without designation as proprietary is not to be construed as a representation by the publisher that it is in the public domain.

Thieme Publishers New York
333 Seventh Avenue, New York, NY 10001 USA
+1 800 782 3488, customerservice@thieme.com

Georg Thieme Verlag KG
Rüdigerstrasse 14, 70469 Stuttgart, Germany
+49 [0]711 8931 421, customerservice@thieme.de

Thieme Publishers Delhi
A-12, Second Floor, Sector-2, Noida-201301
Uttar Pradesh, India
+91 120 45 566 00, customerservice@thieme.in

Thieme Publishers Rio de Janeiro,
Thieme Publicações Ltda.
Edifício Rodolpho de Paoli, 25º andar
Av. Nilo Peçanha, 50 – Sala 2508
Rio de Janeiro 20020-906 Brasil
+55 21 3172 2297

Cover design: Thieme Publishing Group
Typesetting by DiTech Process Solutions, India

Printed in USA by King Printing Company, Inc.   5 4 3 2 1

ISBN 978-1-68420-015-3

Also available as an e-book:
eISBN 978-1-68420-016-0

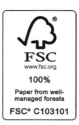

FSC
www.fsc.org
100%
Paper from well-managed forests
FSC® C103101

Contents

9   Sacroplasty: Management of Sacral Insufficiency Fractures   73
Kieran Murphy

10   Cervical and Posterior Arch Augmentation   82
Luigi Manfre, Nicole S. Carter, Joshua A. Hirsch, and Ronil V. Chandra

11   Balloon Kyphoplasty   88
James Mooney, John W. Amburgy, D. Mitchell Self, Leah J. Schoel, and M.R. Chambers

12   Vertebral Augmentation with Implants   99
Dimitrios K. Filippiadis, Stefano Marcia, and Alexios Kelekis

Contents

35 Miscellaneous Tips by the Masters of Vertebral Augmentation

Videos

Video 21.1   Lateral thoracic fluoroscopic video of the thoracic spine showing a needle entering the posterior vertebral body of T9 and previous vertebral augmentation with PMMA at the T10 and T11 levels. The VCF at T9 is mobile and the superior end plate can be seen to move superoinferiorly with respiration.

Video 21.2   Lateral thoracic fluoroscopic video of the thoracic spine taken after vertebral augmentation with PMMA at the T9 level shows two cannulas and bone fillers within the T9 vertebral body that is now stable. No movement of the superior end plate is seen with respiration.

Preface

Vertebral augmentation has been one of my favorite spine treatments since I performed my first case in 1994 and saw the incredibly good and immediate results. This was done under the aegis of Dr. John Mathis, who published the last comprehensive work on vertebral augmentation in 2006. Fourteen years later, we have seen significant advancements in techniques, literature, and augmentation devices and all of these topics have been covered in this book.

What we know now about the treatment of vertebral compression fractures (VCFs) that we didn't know a decade ago is that treating these fractures with augmentation is demonstrably life-saving and life-prolonging and is one of the very few things we do in medicine that attains this benchmark. To break it down to a personal level for those practitioners performing vertebral augmentation, the number of patients needed to treat (statistically called the NNT) to save 1 life at 1 year is only 15 patients and, on the average, additional life expectancy of each treated patient will be between 2 and 7 years.

In my own practice centered on the treatment of painful spine conditions, vertebral augmentation produces the best results of anything we do with an average pain score that decreased from 9/10 to 1.4/10 in our patients at the first post-treatment visit in the largest post-market trial done to date. The transition of technologies from vertebroplasty to intravertebral implants has given new dimensions and made significant improvements in pain as well as greater anatomic restoration and fewer subsequent fractures.

This book is designed to be a comprehensive guide and has certainly accomplished that by discussing all aspects of vertebral augmentation including the history, techniques, approaches, troubleshooting, implant augmentation, pre-procedure and post-procedure assessments, osteoporosis treatment, fill material, and augmentation outside of the spine. One of the chapters is written by the global masters of vertebral augmentation that includes personal tips, tricks, and pearls they use in their own practices. We have also included conditions and concepts that were never before described in the medical literature. It has been a pleasure and a privilege to be involved in the writing of this book. I would like to thank all the associate editors, contributors, and all others who have made this work possible. From an amazing beginning of a transoral injection of bone cement into a painful benign tumor affecting the C2 vertebral body to today's incredible advancements, vertebral augmentation just keeps getting better and better.

Douglas P. Beall, MD

Contributors

John W. Amburgy, MD
Department of Neurological Surgery
University of Alabama at Birmingham
Birmingham, Alabama, USA

Thomas Guido Andreshak, MD
Physician
Consulting Orthopaedic Associates, Inc
Toledo, Ohio, USA

Hamed Asadi, PhD, FRANZCR, CCINR, EBIR
Interventional Radiology Service
Department of Radiology
Northern Hospital
Melbourne, Victoria, Australia

Luigi La Barbera, PhD
Postdoctoral Research Fellow
Laboratory of Biological Structure Mechanics
Department of Chemistry, Materials and Chemical
    Engineering "Giulio Natta"
Politecnico di Milano
Milan, Lombardy, Italy

John D. Barr, MD, FACR, FAHA, FSIR, FSNIS
Professor
Departments of Radiology and Neurological Surgery
University of Texas Southwestern Medical Center
Dallas, Texas, USA

Stephan Becker, MD
Orthopaedic Surgeon, Spine Surgeon, Sports Medicine,
    Chirotherapy
Fellow of the European Board of Orthopaedics and
    Traumatology
Fellow New Westminster College
New Westminster, British Columbia, Canada
Professor
Associé Université de Sherbrooke
Sherbrooke, Quebec, Canada

Andrew Brook
Bachelor of Sciences
University of Chicago
Chicago, Illinois, USA

Allan L. Brook, MD, FSIR, FACR
Director of Interventional Neuroradiology
Professor of Radiology and Neurosurgery
Montefiore Medical Center
The University Hospital for Albert Einstein College of
Medicine
Bronx, New York, USA

Nicole S. Carter, MBBS
Medical Doctor
Alfred Hospital
Research Fellow
Interventional Neuroradiology
Monash Health
Melbourne, Victoria, Australia

M. R. Chambers, DVM, MD
Professor
Department of Neurological Surgery
University of Alabama at Birmingham
Birmingham, Alabama, USA

Ronil V. Chandra, MMed, FRANZCR, CCINR
Associate Professor
Head of Interventional Neuroradiology Unit
Monash Imaging
Monash University
Melbourne, Victoria, Australia

Alessandro Cianfoni, MD
Head of Diagnostic and Interventional Neuroradiology
Neurocenter of Southern Switzerland- NSI-EOC
Lugano, Ticino, Switzerland

Olivier Clerk-Lamalice, MD-MSc, FRCPC, FIPP
President and Founder
Beam Interventional and Diagnostic Imaging
Calgary, Alberta, Canada

Tyler M. Coupal, MD
Vancouver General Hospital
The University of British Columbia
Vancouver, British Columbia, Canada

Aaron L. Cross, DO
Resident
University of Miami/ Jackson Memorial Hospital
Miami, Florida, USA

Timothy Deer, MD, DABPM, FIPP
President and CEO
The Spine and Nerve Center of the Virginias
Charleston, West Virginia, USA

Michael J. DePalma, MD
President and Medical Director
Virginia iSpine Physicians
President
Director of Research
Virginia Spine Research Institute, Inc
Richmond, Virginia, USA

J. Dana Dunleavy, MD
CEO and Co-founder
Imaging Law
Boca Raton, Florida, USA

Murray Echt, MD
Neurosurgery Resident
Leo M. Davidoff Department of Neurosurgery
Montefiore Medical Center
The University Hospital for Albert Einstein College of Medicine
Bronx, New York, USA

Dimitrios K. Filippiadis, MD, PhD
Assistant Professor
Diagnostic and Interventional Radiology 2nd Department of Radiology
University General Hospital "ATTIKON" Medical School
National and Kapodistrian University of Athens
Haidari, Athens, Greece

Bassem Georgy, MD
Assistant Clinical Professor
Department of Radiology
University of California at San Diego
La Jolla, California, USA

Andrew I. Gitkind, MD, MHA
Vice Chairman and Medical Director
Montefiore Spine Center
Assistant Professor
Department of Physical Medicine and Rehabilitation
Montefiore Medical Center
The University Hospital for Albert Einstein College of Medicine
Bronx, New York, USA

Bassam Hamze, MD
Department of Radiology
Lariboisière Hospital
Public Assistance of Paris Hospitals
Paris-Diderot University
Paris, France

Steven M. Henick
Medical Student
Albert Einstein College of Medicine
Bronx, New York, USA

Joshua A. Hirsch, MD
Vice Chair
Procedural Services and Service Line Chief of Neurointerventional Radiology
Chief of Interventional Spine Service
Massachusetts General Hospital
Boston, Massachusetts, USA

Alexios Kelekis, MD, PhD, EBIR
Associate Professor
Diagnostic and Interventional Radiology 2nd Radiology Department
University General Hospital "ATTIKON" Medical School
National and Kapodistrian University of Athens
Haidari, Athens, Greece

Danyal Khan
Medical Student
Royal College of Surgeons in Ireland
Dublin, Ireland

Majid Khan, MD
Director
Non Vascular Spine Intervention
Associate Professor
Radiology and Radiological Science
Johns Hopkins University Hospital
Baltimore. Maryland, USA

Young Hoon Kim, MD, PhD
Assistant Professor of Anesthesiology and Pain Medicine
Catholic University of
Seoul ST. Mary's Hospital
Seoul, Korea

Yong-Chul Kim, MD, PhD
Professor of Anesthesiology and Pain Medicine
Seoul National University School of Medicine
Director
Pain Management Center
Seoul National University Hospital
Seoul, Korea

Jae Hun Kim, MD, PhD
Associate Professor of Anesthesiology and Pain Medicine
Director
Pain Management Center
Konkuk University Medical Center
Seoul, Korea

Kyung-Hoon Kim, MD, PhD
Professor of Anesthesiology and Pain Medicine
Pusan National University College of Medicine
Director
Pain Management Center
Pusan National University Yangsan Hospital
Yangsan, Korea

Hong Kuan Kok, MB BCh, BAO, MRCPI, FFRRCSI, FRCR, EBIR
Interventional Radiology Service
Department of Radiology
Northern Hospital
Melbourne, Victoria, Australia

David Kramer, MD
Associate Professor of Anesthesiology
Albert Einstein College of Medicine
Bronx, New York, USA

Scott Kreiner, MD
Director of Interventional Spine and Sports Medicine
Barrow Brain and Spine
Phoenix, Arizona, USA

Marie-Constance Lacasse, MD, CM, FRCPC
Neuroradiology Fellow
University of Toronto
Toronto, Ontario, Canada

Jean-Denis Laredo, MD
Senior Radiologist and Past Chairman
Department of Radiology
Lariboisière Hospital
Assistance Publique des Hôpitaux de Paris
Paris University
Paris, France

Pyung-Bok Lee, MD, PhD
Associate Professor of Anesthesiology and Pain Medicine
Seoul National University College of Medicine
Director
Pain Management Center
Seoul National University Bundang Hospital
Bundang, Gyeonggi-do, Korea

Thabele Leslie-Mazwi, MD
Interventional Neuroradiology Service
Department of Radiology
Austin Hospital
Melbourne, Victoria, Australia

Julian Maingard, BMedSci
Faculty of Health
School of Medicine
Deakin University
Waurn Ponds, Victoria, Australia

Paul I. Mallinson, MD
Radiologist
Vancouver General Hospital
The University of British Columbia
Vancouver, British Columbia, Canada

Grace Maloney, MD
Interventional Spine and Sports Physician
Barrow Brain and Spine
Phoenix, Arizona, USA

Laxmaiah Manchikanti, MD
Co-Director
Pain Management Centers of America
Medical Director
Pain Management Centers of Paducah and Marion
Ambulatory Surgery Center and Pain Care Surgery Center
Clinical Professor
Anesthesiology and Perioperative Medicine
University of Louisville
Professor of Anesthesiology-Research
Department of Anesthesiology School of Medicine
LSU Health Sciences Center
Paducah, Kentucky, USA

Luigi Manfre, MD
Chairperson
Diagnostic and Interventional Spine - European Society of Neuroradiology ESNR
Director
Department of Minimal Invasive Spine Therapy
Institute of Oncology for Mediterranean I.O.M
Viagrande (Catania), Sicily, Italy

Stefano Marcia, MD
Chairman
Department of Radiology
SS. Trinità Hospital
Cagliari, Sardinia, Italy

James Mooney, MD
Department of Neurological Surgery
University of Alabama at Birmingham
Birmingham, Alabama, USA

Sarah Morgan, MD, RD, CCD
Professor of Nutrition Sciences and Medicine
Department of Medicine
Division of Clinical Immunology and Rheumatology
University of Alabama at Birmingham
Birmingham, Alabama, USA

Peter L. Munk, MD
Director of Musculoskeletal Imaging
Vancouver General Hospital
The University of British Columbia
Vancouver, British Columbia, Canada

Kieran Murphy, MB, FRCPC, FSIR
Professor of Radiology
Director of Clinical Faculty
Techna Research Institute
University of Toronto
Toronto, Ontario, Canada

David Nussbaum, MD
Neuroradiology Specialist
Union Hospital
Elkton, Maryland, USA

Wayne J. Olan, MD
Director
Minimally Invasive and Endovascular Neurosurgery
The George Washington University Medical Center
Washington, DC, USA

Gregory Parnes, MD
Radiology Resident
Albert Einstein College of Medicine
Bronx, New York, USA

Marco C. Pinho, MD
Assistant Professor
Department of Radiology and Center for Advanced Imaging
   Research
University of Texas Southwestern Medical Center
Dallas, Texas, USA

Patrick R. Pritchard, MD
Associate Professor
Department of Neurological Surgery
University of Alabama at Birmingham
Birmingham, Alabama, USA

Susannah Ryan
Medical Student
Royal College of Surgeons in Ireland
Dublin, Ireland

Amanda Schnell, MD
Assistant Professor
Division of Clinical Immunology and Rheumatology
Department of Medicine
University of Alabama at Birmingham
Birmingham, Alabama, USA

Leah J. Schoel, MD
School of Medicine
University of Alabama at Birmingham
Birmingham, Alabama, USA

D. Mitchell Self, MD, MS IV
School of Medicine
University of Alabama at Birmingham
Birmingham, Alabama, USA

Andrew L. Sherman, MD
Professor and Vice Chair
Department of Physical Medicine and Rehabilitation
University of Miami Miller School of Medicine
Miami, Florida, USA

Neal H. Shonnard, MD
Orthopedic Surgeon
Proliance Surgeons, Inc
Seattle, Washington, USA

Lee-Anne Slater, FRANZCR, CCINR
Interventional Neuroradiologist
Monash Health
Melbourne, Victoria, Australia

Adam Thakore
Neuroscience Student
Trinity College
Dublin, Ireland

Steven M. Theiss MD
Professor
Department of Orthopedic Surgery
University of Alabama at Birmingham
Birmingham, Alabama, USA

Deborah H. Tracy, MD, MBA
Interventional Pain Physician
Institute of Interventional Pain Management
Brooksville, Florida, USA

Derrick D. Wagoner, DO
Interventional Pain Physician
Gershon Pain Specialists
Virginia Beach, Virginia, USA

James R. Webb, MD
Chief of Staff
Dr. James Webb and Associates
Tulsa, Oklahoma, USA

Edward Yoon, MD
Assistant Professor
Department of Radiology
Hospital for Special Surgery
New York, USA

1 History and Introduction to Vertebral Augmentation

M.R. Chambers

Summary

Vertebral augmentation is a category of minimally invasive procedures that have become central in the treatment of pathologic and painful vertebral compression fractures (VCFs) due to osteoporosis, trauma, and neoplasia. Osteoporotic VCFs are the most common indication for vertebral augmentation, which has also been used to treat fractures in patients with benign tumors such as hemangiomas or Langerhans cell vertebral histiocytosis (LCVH) and in genetic disorders that give rise to weak vertebrae such as osteogenesis imperfecta. In theory, near immediate anterior column stability and pain relief follows an intravertebral injection of bone cement that stabilizes the osseous fractures and eliminates osseous and periosteal movements, while thermal polymerization of the cement ablates pain receptors in the basivertebral plexus, trabecular bone, and subjacent to the vertebral end plates. Over three decades of innovation and advancements have produced treatment options with improved safety and efficacy. Results of numerous studies have demonstrated reduction of pain, and improved function and quality of life. Responses have been significant and durable across a wide range of etiologies.

Keywords: vertebral compression fracture, vertebral augmentation, vertebroplasty, balloon kyphoplasty, osteoporosis, spinal metastasis, multiple myeloma, bone cement, vertebral implants

1.1 Introduction

Acrylic cements have been used for augmentation of weakened or partially destroyed bones for decades. The first use of methyl methacrylate as an adjunct to internal fixation of malignant neoplastic fractures was reported in 1972.[1] Vertebral augmentation has since become central in the treatment of pathologic vertebral compression fractures (VCFs) due to osteoporosis, trauma, and neoplasia. The procedure has also been used to treat fractures in patients with benign tumors such as hemangiomas or LCVH and in genetic disorders that give rise to weak vertebrae such as osteogenesis imperfecta.[2–7]

Osteoporotic VCFs (OVCFs) are the most common indication for vertebral augmentation. As with any fracture, principles of fixation for VCFs include vertebral body (VB) reduction to restore normal anatomical relationships, fixation to provide absolute or relative stability, preservation of blood supply to soft tissues and bone, and early safe mobilization of the injured part and the patient (▶Fig. 1.1).

Before the availability of vertebral augmentation, the principal surgical option for compression fractures was decompression and instrumented fusion. Outcomes were often dismal in elderly osteoporotic patients.[8] Nonoperative management options were equally disappointing. Initial management included bed rest and immobilization in an external orthotic

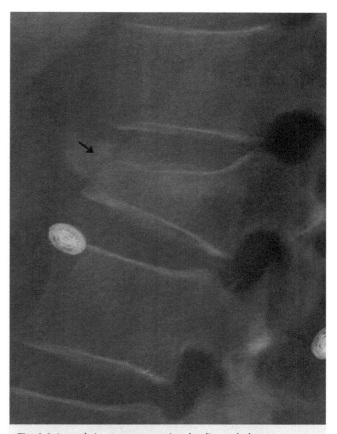

Fig. 1.1 Lateral view on a conventional radiograph demonstrates a vertebral compression fracture (*black arrow*).

if feasible and tolerable, depending on the degree of kyphosis and pain. Narcotics were prescribed for analgesia and nasal calcitonin for antiresorptive and analgesic effects. Bed rest and immobilization, however, led to accelerated osteoporotic bone loss and many elderly patients were at risk of polypharmacy and narcotic side effects including constipation, confusion, and respiratory depression as well as the many unappreciated consequences of social isolation.[9,10] Patients treated with nonsurgical management (NSM) were also at an increased risk of mortality primarily from pneumonia due to their deconditioned status.[11]

1.2 Mechanisms of Pain Relief

Two general hypotheses prevail regarding the mechanism of pain relief offered by augmentation of VCFs: (1) an intravertebral injection of polymethyl methacrylate (PMMA) cement stabilizes micro-fractures and eliminates periosteal micro-movements and pain; (2) thermal polymerization of

PMMA following injection ablates pain receptors in the trabecular bone, vertebral periosteum, and vascular structures. This combination leads to near immediate postoperative anterior column stability and pain relief.[12] Although ablation of the basivertebral nerve within the VB does produce significant pain relief in patients with diskogenic back pain, degenerative end plate changes, and an intact VB,[13] low exothermic or nonexothermic bone cements can produce equivalent pain relief in patients with VCFs to that of cements with thermal neuroablation capability.[14] The pain relief in patients with VCFs, therefore, is much more likely or completely due to the reestablishment of the mechanical stability of the VB rather than the ablative effects of the fill material on the VB innervation.

1.3 Procedures

1.3.1 Vertebroplasty

Vertebroplasty was first performed in 1984 but not reported until 1987. In the first known image-guided percutaneous vertebral augmentation, Galibert et al successfully injected PMMA into a C2 vertebra that had been partially destroyed by an aggressive hemangioma.[15]

Vertebroplasty involves the percutaneous injection of cement such as PMMA directly into the cancellous bone of a fractured VB to alleviate pain and prevent further loss of VB height or progression of kyphotic deformity. Although the procedure does not improve spinal deformity, it stabilizes the vertebra and improves the function of individuals debilitated by painful VCFs (▶Fig. 1.2).

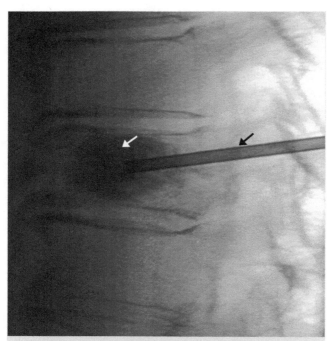

Fig. 1.2 A vertebroplasty procedure is demonstrated with the cannula of the needle (*black arrow*) placed in the vertebral body and the polymethylmethacrylate is shown within the vertebral body (*white arrow*).

1.3.2 Kyphoplasty

Kyphoplasty was first performed in 1998 as a modification of vertebroplasty with the intent of restoring vertebral height and reducing kyphotic angulation for improved outcomes and reduced procedural risks. VCFs cause debilitating pain and may also be associated with significant kyphosis. Kyphosis reduces compartment sizes of the chest, abdomen, and pelvis, which results in pulmonary restriction, decreased appetite, and urinary incontinence. These processes can lead to life-altering deconditioning, weight loss, social isolation, and depression.

During kyphoplasty, a balloon tamp is inflated within the VB to compress and displace cancellous bone prior to the injection of cement. This creates a cavity that can reduce the vertebral fracture and after removal of the balloon allows the injection of cement directly into the cavity that is the path of least resistance. This injection of cement into the cavity allows for greater control of the cement and reduces the risk of cement leakage (▶Fig. 1.3).

Inflation of the tamp restores VB height and reduces kyphotic angulation to improve sagittal alignment, attenuating the risk of progressive deformity by reducing the bending moment (M).[16,17] Illustrating the importance of the moment arm, Archimedes said, "Give me a lever long enough and a place to stand and I will move the earth." VB failure is believed to result from an excessive bending moment, which is the product of the moment arm (the distance between the mid VB and the plumb line representing the center of gravity, D) and the force (gravity, F) applied to the moment arm[18] (▶Fig. 1.4). The moment arm, and therefore the bending moment and risk of VB failure, increases as kyphosis progresses.

1.3.3 Radiofrequency Kyphoplasty

A novel technique approved for use in the United States in 2008 (StabiliT Vertebral Augmentation System, Merit Medical, Jordan, UT, United States) is radiofrequency kyphoplasty (RFK). RFK uses radiofrequency heat to control the viscosity of the PMMA that is injected into the VB. Rather than using inflatable bone tamps, a small navigational cannula is inserted unilaterally into the vertebra. The cannula creates pathways for the cement and preserves more of the existing cancellous bone. The pathways are filled with ultra–high viscosity bone cement, which permeates into the surrounding bone, stabilizes the fracture, and restores vertebral height (▶Fig. 1.5). The infusion of ultra–high viscosity cement in a slower and more controlled fashion is designed to reduce the risk of cement leakage.[19-23]

1.3.4 Percutaneous Radiofrequency Ablation

Radiofrequency ablation (RFA) is a modified electrocautery technique for use in select patients with painful spinal metastases.[24] RFA and vertebral augmentation is a combination therapy for painful osseous metastases that cannot be or are incompletely palliated with radiation therapy. Combined treatment with RFA and vertebral augmentation has been successful in reducing pain and in improving function and quality of life.[24-28] Using image guidance, a partially insulated electrode attached to a radiofrequency generator is passed into the vertebra.[29,30] The heat generated by radiofrequency

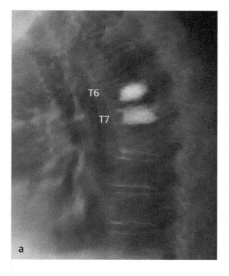
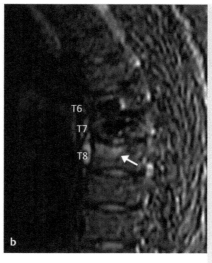
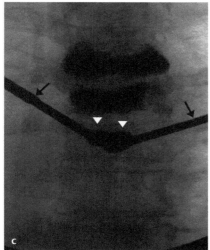
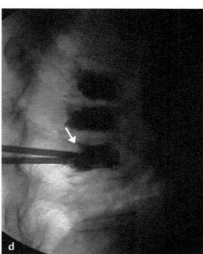

Fig. 1.3 (a) Kyphoplasty in a patient with two previous vertebral augmentation procedures at T6 and T7. (b) The patient had recurrence of pain and adjacent level vertebral fracture at T8 (*white arrow*). (c) An anteroposterior fluoroscopic view of the mid-thoracic spine with balloons (*white arrowheads*) placed through two needle cannulas (*black arrows*). (d) The lateral fluoroscopic view shows cement injected into the vertebral body (*white arrow*).

energy (50–90°C) causes destruction of the malignant tissue and creates a small cavity in the VB[31,32] (▶ Fig. 1.6). Additionally, percutaneous radiofrequency ablation destroys sensory nerve fibers, and tumor cells that release nerve-stimulating factors. There is also evidence to show that RFA carried out before percutaneous vertebral augmentation reduces the risk of cement leakage.[33]

Examples of devices for RFA include STAR Tumor Ablation System (Merit Medical, Jordan, UT, United States), CAVITY SpineWand (ArthroCare, Austin, TX, United States), and OsteoCool RF Ablation system (Medtronic, Dublin, Ireland). The OsteoCool ablation probe is internally cooled with circulating water. The RF energy heats the tissue, while circulating water moderates the temperature. The system automatically moderates power to keep RF heating within the desired treatment range. This combination creates large-volume lesions without excessive heating, thereby reducing risks of potential thermal damage to adjacent tissue.

1.3.5 Vertebral Augmentation with Implants

Significant and lasting pain relief has been achieved with both vertebroplasty and kyphoplasty. Restoration of height does not appear requisite for pain relief, but height restoration and reduction of kyphotic angulation are important components in the reestablishment of normal sagittal balance and protection from future fractures.[17,34] Recovery of VB height during kyphoplasty may be partially lost over time. Newer next-generation vertebral augmentation systems have been introduced to improve fracture reduction, indefinitely restore the height of the VB, and further reduce risks of cement leakage.[35,36]

SpineJack (Stryker, Kalamazoo, MI, United States) is a titanium implant inserted using a bilateral transpedicular approach to treat fractures between and including T5 and L5. A direct lift mechanism expands vertically like a car jack and allows for progressive controlled reduction of the fracture prior to cement injection (▶ Fig. 1.7).[32]

The *OsseoFix Spinal Fracture Reduction System* (Alphatec Spine, 2009) is a titanium mesh device that expands into the VB and acts as a scaffold to facilitate reduction and stabilization of fractures between and including T6 and L5. There is no direct lift mechanism, but the foreshortening of the titanium tube reduces the end plate by direct superior and inferior pressure from the center of the tube as it expands during the implant's deployment. The mesh expands to compact the trabecular bone and increase the VB height, allowing cement interdigitation.[37]

The device was introduced as an alternative to vertebroplasty and kyphoplasty to reduce cement leakage (▶Fig. 1.8).

The *Vertebral Body Stenting System* (VBS) consists of an expandable cobalt–chromium alloy stent mounted on a balloon catheter. The device is typically inserted via a bilateral transpedicular approach and inflated to maximum of 30 atm to symmetrically expand both stents. The stent is optimally expanded to a maximum diameter of 17 mm and balloons are deflated and removed, leaving both stents to maintain the restored height prior to injection of the cement (▶Fig. 1.9).[32]

The *Kiva VCF Treatment System*, indicated for use in the treatment of spinal fractures in the thoracic and/or lumbar spine from T6 to L5, received clearance from the U.S. Food and Drug Administration on January 24, 2014. The Kiva implant is a percutaneous uniportal vertebral augmentation device that is designed to restore VB height and reduce cement leakage. The polyether ether ketone flexible implant (PEEK-OPTIMA) is inserted over a removable, fully coiled nitinol guidewire.[38] The coil is inserted into the VB and acts as a scaffold for the implant. The Kiva implant is then inserted around the coil, the coil is removed, and cement is injected through the perforated implant for controlled delivery (▶Fig. 1.10).

1.4 Indications and Contraindications

Primary indications for vertebral augmentation include osteoporotic compression fractures, vertebral metastasis, multiple myeloma, vertebral hemangioma, vertebral osteonecrosis, traumatic VCFs, and reinforcement of a pathologically weak VB before and during surgical stabilization procedures. In clinical practice, the most common indication is a painful osteoporotic vertebral fracture that has not responded to NSM including rest, immobilization in an orthotic brace, narcotic analgesic medications, and nasal calcitonin for antiresorptive and analgesic effects.

In 2018, a multidisciplinary expert panel of orthopaedic and neurosurgeons, interventional radiologists, and pain specialists, using the RAND/UCLA Appropriateness Method (RUAM), developed the Clinical Care Pathway (CCP), defining patient-specific

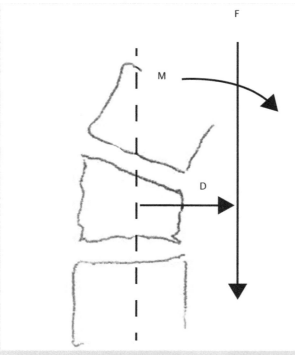

Fig. 1.4 The bending moment (M) is the product of moment arm (D) and gravity (F). As kyphosis progresses, the moment arm increases, thereby increasing the risk of vertebral failure. (This image is provided courtesy of Dr. M.R. Chambers.)

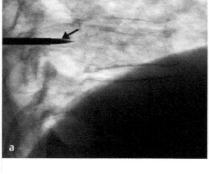
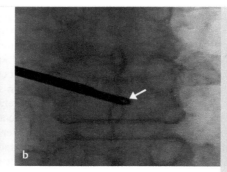
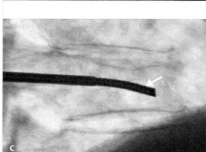
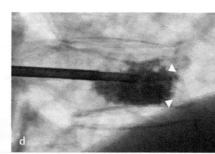

Fig. 1.5 Radiofrequency kyphoplasty. **(a)** Lateral fluoroscopic view shows the needle just proximal to the posterior vertebral body wall (*black arrow*) entering via a transpedicular approach. **(b, c)** Posteroanterior and lateral fluoroscopic views show the channel creation device (*white arrow*) just across the midline in the anterior portion of the vertebral body. **(d)** Lateral fluoroscopic view shows cement being injected into the vertebral body (*white arrowheads*) after having just been heated with radiofrequency energy.

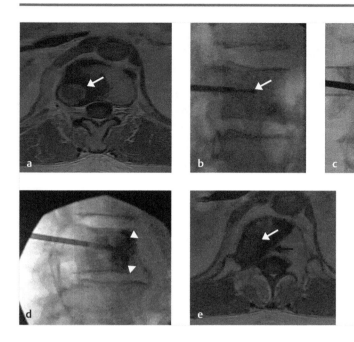

Fig. 1.6 Radiofrequency ablation. **(a)** Axial T1-weighted MR image shows a metastasis (*white arrow*) in a 55-year-old man with metastatic lung cancer. **(b, c)** Lateral and posteroanterior fluoroscopic views show the STAR radiofrequency device in the posterolateral portion of the L2 vertebral body (*white arrows*). **(d)** Lateral fluoroscopic view shows cement being injected into the vertebral body (*white arrowheads*). **(e)** Axial T1-weighted MR image obtained 3 months after radiofrequency ablation shows the cement within the vertebral body (*black arrow*) but no further evidence of the metastasis seen in **a** (*white arrow*).

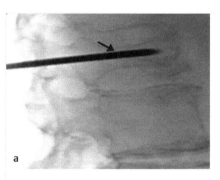
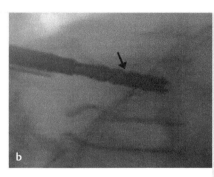
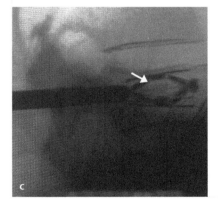
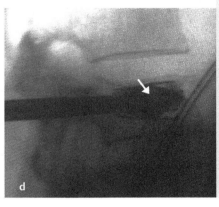

Fig. 1.7 SpineJack. Lateral fluoroscopic views obtained during a vertebral augmentation with the SpineJack shows the initial needle access into the vertebral body (*black arrow* in **a**), followed by a template to clean the site after drilling (*black arrow* in **b**). The SpineJack is then placed and expanded (*white arrow* in **c**) and then cement is injected around the implant (*white arrow* in **d**).

recommendations for vertebral fragility fractures (VFF). The panel assessed the relative importance of signs and symptoms for the suspicion of VFF, the relevance of diagnostic procedures, and the appropriateness of vertebral augmentation versus NSM for a variety of clinical scenarios. Their report included the following guidelines for relative and absolute contraindications.[39]

Absolute contraindications include active infection at the surgical site and untreated blood-borne infections, and a nonpainful osteoporotic vertebral fracture that is completely healed or is clearly responding to conservative management. Strong contraindications include osteomyelitis, pregnancy, allergy to fill material, coagulopathy, spinal instability, myelopathy from the fracture, the presence of a neurologic deficit, and neural impingement.

Relative contraindications include cardiorespiratory compromise such that safe sedation or anesthesia cannot be achieved, breach of the posterior vertebral cortex by a tumor, and/or tumor extension into the spinal canal. It was

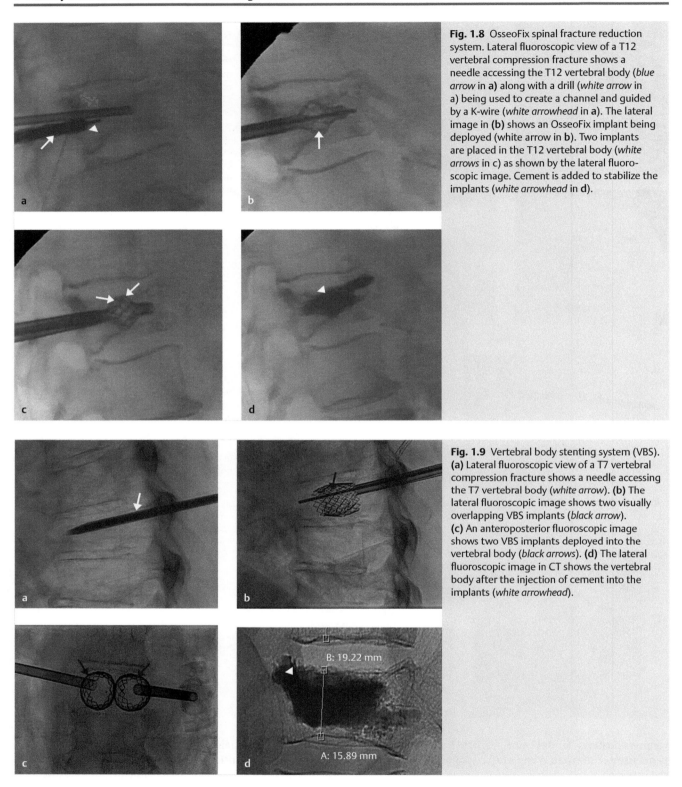

Fig. 1.8 OsseoFix spinal fracture reduction system. Lateral fluoroscopic view of a T12 vertebral compression fracture shows a needle accessing the T12 vertebral body (*blue arrow* in **a**) along with a drill (*white arrow* in **a**) being used to create a channel and guided by a K-wire (*white arrowhead* in **a**). The lateral image in (**b**) shows an OsseoFix implant being deployed (*white arrow* in **b**). Two implants are placed in the T12 vertebral body (*white arrows* in **c**) as shown by the lateral fluoroscopic image. Cement is added to stabilize the implants (*white arrowhead* in **d**).

Fig. 1.9 Vertebral body stenting system (VBS). (**a**) Lateral fluoroscopic view of a T7 vertebral compression fracture shows a needle accessing the T7 vertebral body (*white arrow*). (**b**) The lateral fluoroscopic image shows two visually overlapping VBS implants (*black arrow*). (**c**) An anteroposterior fluoroscopic image shows two VBS implants deployed into the vertebral body (*black arrows*). (**d**) The lateral fluoroscopic image in CT shows the vertebral body after the injection of cement into the implants (*white arrowhead*).

determined that fracture repulsion and canal compromise per se is not generally a contraindication, provided the fracture fragment is not causing neural impingement or clinical symptoms related to this compromise. Significant fracture retropulsion with canal compromise is a relative contraindication. A CT scan may be used to determine integrity of posterior wall in patients with mild retropulsion of fracture fragment(s). Vertebra plana has been previously mentioned as a relative contraindication as it renders the procedure technically difficult but the RUAM group determined that vertebra plana was not a relative contraindication to performing vertebral augmentation.

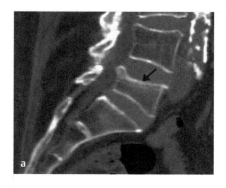
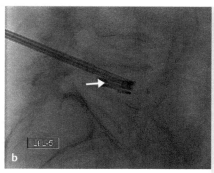
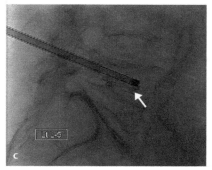
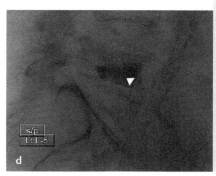

Fig. 1.10 Kiva implant. Sagittal CT image shows a vertebral compression fracture of L5 (*black arrow* in **a**). Lateral fluoroscopic view shows the nitinol coil within the vertebral body (*white arrow* in **b**). Lateral fluoroscopic view shows the PEEK (polyether ether ketone) implant coiled in the vertebral body (*white arrow* in **c**) and image (**d**) shows the implant after the injection of cement (*white arrowhead*).

1.5 Risks and Complications

Complications are few but, as with any surgical procedure, may include infection, bleeding, cardiac or respiratory complications of anesthesia, injury, and failure to achieve intended goals. Potential complications specific to percutaneous augmentation include cement leakage, pulmonary embolism, radiculopathies, rib fractures, subsequent vertebral fractures, and spinal cord or neural compression.[40–42]

1.6 Clinical Applications and Evidence

A comprehensive literature review is presented in Chapter 15. Numerous randomized controlled trials, systematic reviews, and meta-analyses have been employed to study and compare vertebral augmentation treatment options.[43–45] Although we consider results from randomized controlled trials, it is important to remember that these were developed to evaluate drug therapies, not devices and surgical procedures.[46] Given their relatively recent introduction, there are limited data available with sufficient power for decision-making with respect to newer vertebral augmentation implants and devices. Future trials with additional observations and longer follow-ups are anticipated.

1.6.1 Osteoporosis

VCFs are the most common type of fracture related to osteoporosis and are associated with significant rates of morbidity and mortality. Annual direct medical expenditures exceed $1 billion in the United States.[47] Contemporary natural history data suggest that more than 70% of patients with moderate or severe pain may fail to achieve significant pain relief within 12 months of symptom onset.[48] Physicians in the Neuroradiology Department at the University Hospital in Lyon, France, began to treat osteoporotic vertebral fractures with vertebroplasty in 1989. They used an 18-gauge needle to inject bone cement into seven patients, four of whom had OVCFs and the other three VCFs attributed to spinal metastases.[49] They reported that seven of the eight patients had an excellent pain reduction response to the vertebroplasty and that the eighth patient had a good response.

Vertebroplasty

Vertebroplasty was introduced to the United States when, in the early 1990s, clinicians from the University of Virginia performed the procedure using the technique introduced by the French clinicians.[50] The use of vertebroplasty then dramatically increased, primarily for the treatment of OVCFs, until the advent of balloon kyphoplasty (BKP) in the late 1990s.

In 2009, a great deal of controversy followed the publication of two randomized trials comparing vertebroplasty and sham procedures to treat osteoporotic vertebral fractures. The studies were intended to account for placebo effect in the setting of vertebroplasty. The authors reported that, although there were substantial reductions in overall pain in both study groups, there was no statistically significant benefit offered by vertebroplasty. Critics pointed out many flaws in design, patient selection, power, and generalization of inferences of both trials.

The first study randomized 75 participants with one or two painful osteoporotic vertebral fractures confirmed by MRI and less than 1 year's duration to vertebroplasty or a sham procedure. Participants were stratified according to treatment center, sex, and duration of symptoms. The primary outcome was "overall pain" at 3 months. There were substantial reductions in overall pain in both study groups, but vertebroplasty was not better in any measured outcome compared to controls, regardless of duration of symptoms. This trial by Buchbinder et al was to include 200 patients, but only 78 were enrolled over 4 years. Two of the four study hospitals withdrew after including only five patients each. As a result, 68% of the procedures were performed in one hospital by one radiologist. Only 32% of patients received treatment within 6 weeks of onset of pain, suggesting that many fractures being treated were already healed with expected persistent edema on MR imaging.

The second trial randomly assigned 131 patients with one to three painful OVCFs to undergo either vertebroplasty or a simulated procedure without cement. The primary outcomes were disability and the patients' ratings of average pain intensity during the preceding 24 hours at 1 month. This study involved only outpatients; inpatients hospitalized with acute fracture pain were excluded. The protocol required 4 weeks of medical therapy before enrollment was possible and fractures were present for up to 1 year. Only 44% of patients had pain of less than 6 weeks' duration; 56% of patients had pain for over 3 months. The minimum pain score for enrollment was 3/10 and the average pain score was 6.9. As patients with maximal back pain tend to have the greatest improvement on pain score, bias was presumably introduced, as those patients with the greatest pain likely did not agree to participate in a trial that might randomize them to a nontreatment arm. Finally, a significantly greater crossover from the control group versus the vertebroplasty group could indicate dissatisfaction with the sham procedure that was not captured by pain scales.[51]

Kyphoplasty

In 2001, Garfin et al reported on new technologies in the spine for the treatment of painful OVCF and noted a 95% improvement in pain and significant improvement in function following BKP. Vertebral height and kyphosis were improved by over 50% when kyphoplasty was performed within 3 months of the onset of pain, less so if treatment was delayed more than 3 months. Both vertebroplasty and kyphoplasty were described as "safe and effective" in the treatment of painful OVCF that did not respond to conventional treatments. Kyphoplasty was noted to facilitate realignment of the spinal column and regain VB height—morphologic improvements thought to decrease pulmonary, gastrointestinal, and early morbidity consequences of fractures.[52] Numerous prospective and retrospective studies have since demonstrated the safety and efficacy of kyphoplasty in the treatment of pain and deformity of OVCF.[53]

Results of the FREE trial, a randomized controlled trial comparing the efficacy and safety of BKP to nonsurgical care for VCFs were published in 2009.[54] Adults with one to three acute painful vertebral fractures from T5 to L5 due to primary or secondary osteoporosis, multiple myeloma, or osteolytic metastatic tumors were enrolled at 21 sites in eight countries. Participants were randomized and the primary outcome, the change from baseline to 1 month in the short-form 36 (SF-36) physical component summary (PCS) score, was evaluated at 1 month. Patients in the kyphoplasty group had statistically significant improvement in mean SF-36 PCS scores at 1 month when compared to the control group.

Next, Van Meirhaeghe et al performed a multicenter randomized controlled trial comparing BKP to NSM with a focus on surgical aspects and radiographic vertebral deformity. Adults with one to three VCFs were randomized within 3 months of onset of pain to undergo bilateral BKP or NSM. Compared to NSM, the BKP group had greater improvements in SF-36 PCS scores at 1 month and greater functionality assessed with "timed up and go." At 24 months, BKP improved quality of life, decreased the pain averaged during 24 months, and resulted in better improvement of index VB kyphotic angulation.[53]

The EVOLVE trial, a large prospective, clinical study of kyphoplasty, investigating 12-month disability, quality of life, and safety outcomes specifically in a Medicare-eligible population, published in 2017, represented characteristic patients seen in routine clinical practice. A total of 354 patients with painful VCFs were enrolled at 24 U.S. sites with 350 undergoing kyphoplasty. Four co-primary endpoints included back pain, disability, function, and quality of life. With all endpoints demonstrating statistically significant improvement at every time point, kyphoplasty was deemed a safe, effective, and durable procedure for treating patients with painful VCF due to osteoporosis or cancer.[55]

SpineJack

A cadaveric study of 24 VB fractures comparing SpineJack to BKP showed height restoration was better in the SpineJack group. Clinical implications included better sagittal balance restoration and reduction of kyphotic deformity with the potential for fewer adjacent level vertebral fractures with the SpineJack.[56]

A single prospective randomized post-market clinical study compared the safety and effectiveness of SpineJack to the KyphX Xpander Inflatable Bone Tamp to treat 30 patients with painful OVCFs. Reduction of pain and disability was greater in the SpineJack group immediately following and at 12 months after the procedure. Quality of life showed distinct improvements in both groups. Patients in the SpineJack cohort had fewer adjacent level fractures (ALFs) at 1 year, while the additional VCF rate was approximately the same between the two groups. SpineJack produced a larger restoration of the VB angle, which was still evident 12 months after implantation.[57]

Preliminary data available at the time of this writing from the 151-patient randomized placebo-controlled SAKOS trial comparing the SpineJack to the KyphX Xpander Inflatable Bone Tamp also suggests that both SpineJack and BKP have comparable effects on functional improvement and quality of life, but SpineJack appears to be significantly better than BKP for pain relief and VB height restoration with a decreased rate of adjacent fractures.[58]

In terms of pain relief measured by the Visual Analog Scale (VAS), 5 days after surgery, there was a marked reduction in pain in both patient groups. The mean reduction was around 50 mm, but there was no significant difference between the two groups. The pain progressively improved over the first 6 months in the SpineJack group only resulting in a significantly improved pain score in the SpineJack group as compared to the BKP group at 1 month ($p = 0.029$) and at 6 months ($p = 0.021$) after surgery.

When evaluating ALFs, the responder rate at month 6 in the intention to treat (ITT) population was significantly higher following the SpineJack procedure compared to BKP (88.1 vs. 59.7%; *p* < 0.0001) and superiority for ALF reduction for the SpineJack procedure was confirmed at 12 months with a responder rate of 73.5 versus 42.9% with BKP (*p* < 0.0001).

In the ITT population, the mean restoration of midline height was significantly more following the SpineJack procedure than after BKP (1.14 ± 2.61 vs. 0.24 ± 2.21 mm; median: 0.90 vs. 0.45 mm; *p* = 0.0163). This result was confirmed in the per protocol (PP) population as well (*p* = 0.0060).

OsseoFix

A prospective consecutive cohort study determined OsseoFix to be a successful and safe minimally invasive therapy for OVCFs, even those with posterior wall involvement. Twenty-four patients with 32 OVCFs from T6 to L4 were treated with OsseoFix. After 12 months, there were significant improvements in mean Oswestry Disability Index (ODI; 70.6 to 30.1%), VAS pain (7.7 to 1.4), and mean kyphotic angle (11.7 degrees). There was only one case of loss of height in a stabilized VB, one pronounced postoperative hematoma, and no changes in the posterior vertebral wall or adjacent fractures. There were no cases of cement leakage.[37]

Vertebral Body Stenting System

In a 2014 randomized controlled trial comparing BKP to the VBS, the primary outcome was the kyphotic angle measurement on radiographic imaging. Secondary outcomes included radiation exposure time, complications, and cement extravasation. The mean kyphotic angle correction was 4.5 degrees with BKP and 4.7 degrees with VBS. This difference was not significant. There was also no significant difference in radiation exposure times and the rate of cement leakage. It was concluded that, given the fact that VBS was associated with a slightly higher balloon pressures and more material-related complications (one complication in BKP vs. nine complications with VBS), VBS offered no benefit over BKP.[38,59]

Kiva

In 2013, Korovessis et al prospectively and randomly compared BKP and KIVA vertebral augmentation for treating osteoporotic VB fractures.[60] Although pain, disability and function outcomes were similar in both groups, the authors reported significant restoration of the Gardner angle in patients treated with Kiva, whereas BKP did not meet significance. Lower cement volumes used and decreased extravasation rates were reported for Kiva.

In the same year, Otten et al prospectively compared the Kiva VCF treatment system and the KyphX Systems (Kyphon Inc., Sunnyvale, CA, United States) for BKP specifically evaluating clinical efficacy and safety.[61] Patient-reported outcomes were measured preoperatively before device implantation and 6 months after treatment. Back pain severity was evaluated with the standard 10-cm VAS for the Kiva VCF treatment system and a numeric rating scale (0–100, steps of 10) for BKP. Condition-specific functional impairment was evaluated with the ODI score. During surgery, the operation time was recorded. All adverse events, which could be attributed to the treatment and further complications, such as new fractures, were documented. Cement extravasations and their location were confirmed by intraoperative fluoroscopy and postoperative radiography. New fractures were evaluated by radiographic controls. The anterior vertebral body and the mid vertebral heights were measured radiological in the digital system by caliper preoperatively, postoperatively, 3 months, and 6 months postoperatively. The authors described the KIVA system as safe and effective for the treatment of VCFs with pain and function improved as effectively by Kiva as by BKP. Pain was reportedly better controlled by Kiva at the 6-month comparison. The operation time needed to complete the procedure with the Kiva treatment system was shorter, cement volume was lower, and subsequent fractures were less frequent following treatment with KIVA. The authors acknowledged the relatively small study population and 6 months to be only an intermediate follow-up period.

Kiva was shown to be noninferior to kyphoplasty for the treatment of OVCFs based on reduction in pain, improvement in function, and absence of device-related serious adverse events at 12 months in the KAST study. Published in 2015, this large randomized trial of 300 subjects with OVCFs randomly selected to receive either Kiva or BKP had as its primary endpoint a composite of a reduction in pain, improvement in function, and absence of device-related serious adverse events at 12 months. Secondary endpoints included cement usage, cement extravasation, and ALFs. The primary endpoint demonstrated noninferiority of KIVA to BKP and there were no device-related serious adverse events that occurred. Analysis of secondary endpoints revealed statistical superiority of Kiva with respect to cement use and cement extravasation. There was a reduced rate of ALFs in the group treated with Kiva, but this fell just short of statistical significance.[62]

Given evidence of relative risk reduction rate in ALF with Kiva (31.6% [95% confidence interval (CI): −22.5%, 61.9%]) demonstrated in KAST, Beall et al used clinical data from KAST as well as unit cost data from the published literature to predict a direct medical cost savings of $1,118 per patient and $280,876 per representative U.S. hospital when comparing Kiva to BKP.[63]

1.6.2 Trauma

Controversies exist regarding the appropriate imaging and indications, timing, and choice of surgical management of traumatic injuries to the thoracolumbar spine. Sixty-five percent of thoracolumbar fractures occur due to motor vehicle injuries or falls from a height, with the remainder contributed by sports injuries and violence. Since these are high-velocity injuries, thoracolumbar fractures are commonly associated with other injuries like rib fractures, pneumohemothorax, and, rarely, great vessel injuries, hemopericardium, and diaphragmatic rupture.[64,65] Seatbelt (Chance) fractures and flexion–distraction injuries are often associated with intra-abdominal visceral injuries.[66] A careful history regarding the injury mechanism, pain, and neurological symptoms is essential. Axial, nonradiating back pain of stabbing or aching quality is the most common symptom. Patients with neurological injury may complain of weakness, paresthesia, or anesthesia below the injury level and urinary retention. Thorough inspection of the spine should be performed after a careful log roll maneuver to look for abrasions, tenderness, local kyphosis, and a palpable gap in between spinous processes. Neurological assessment should follow the standard American Spinal Injury Association (ASIA) guidelines (see Chapter 2).

Vertebroplasty and Kyphoplasty

In 2002, using a human cadaveric model, Verlaan et al posited that failure after short-segment pedicle screw fixation for the treatment of vertebral fractures was the result of a redistribution of disk material through the fractured end plate into the VB, causing a decrease in anterior column support. This lack of support could lead to instrument breakage and recurrent kyphosis after removal of the instrumentation. They reported "balloon vertebroplasty" (kyphoplasty) to be a safe and feasible procedure for the restoration of traumatic thoracolumbar vertebral fractures.[67]

In 2003, the Society of Interventional Radiology (SIR) Standards of Practice Committee published "Quality Improvement Guidelines for Percutaneous Vertebroplasty." Indications for vertebroplasty at that time included the following: (1) painful primary and secondary OVCFs refractory to medical therapy; (2) painful vertebrae with extensive osteolysis or invasion secondary to benign or malignant tumor (i.e., hemangioma, multiple myeloma, or metastatic disease); and (3) painful vertebral fracture associated with osteonecrosis (Kummel's disease).[68]

Since then, many cases of nonosteoporotic vertebral fractures have been treated with vertebral augmentation. In 2004, Chen et al successfully treated a 33-year-old man with L1, L2, and L5 burst fractures with vertebroplasty. The authors proposed the procedure as a useful intervention in select patients with lumbar burst fractures.[69] In a 2015 prospective cohort study, Elnoamany demonstrated vertebroplasty to be an effective first-line treatment to decrease pain, increase mobility, and decrease narcotic administration in patients with nonosteoporotic compression fractures.[70]

Kiva

In 2014, Korovessis et al retrospectively compared two procedures and two cements: BKP with calcium phosphate (Group A) and KIVA implant with PMMA (Group B). Vertebral augmentation was used to reinforce three-vertebra pedicle screw constructs for A2 and A3 single fresh nonosteoporotic lumbar (L1–L4) fractures in 38 consecutive age- and diagnosis-matched patients. Both groups had diminished pain and improved function as well as improved anterior VB height, segmental kyphosis, and spinal canal encroachment. The Kiva implant/PMMA group had significantly improved posterior VB height; however, short-segment construct restoration had no impact on functional outcomes. The authors advised the use of PMMA in fresh traumatic lumbar fractures.[71]

SpineJack

More recently, in a case report by Polis et al, percutaneous extrapedicular vertebral augmentation with the SpineJack implant was used to treat a traumatic T8 vertebral fracture in a 15-year-old adolescent boy. CT scans demonstrated an A2.2 (AO/Magerl) fracture of T8. After 6 months of conservative management, severe pain persisted and angle of thoracic kyphosis progressed. The procedure eliminated clinical symptoms and resulted in partial reduction and rebalance of the VCF without limiting motion.[72]

1.6.3 Bone Disease, Cancer, Metastases, and Multiple Myeloma

Benign conditions such as vertebral hemangiomas and giant cell tumors may cause severe intractable pain. More than 30% of patients with advanced cancer have been reported to develop spinal metastases. The rate is higher (70%) in those with cancers of the breast, lung, or prostate.[73] Metastatic lesions often cause bone lysis, weaken the vertebrae, and result in painful pathologic fractures with significant morbidity. Multiple myeloma, a cancer that typically starts in the bone marrow, also has a substantial rate of spinal involvement.[74,75] Open surgical decompression and instrumented stabilization may not be feasible and failure may lead to catastrophic consequences. Pain management is often inadequate and radiation therapy may be slow to become effective.

Vertebroplasty and Kyphoplasty

In 1987, Nicola and Lins described "a new method, intraoperative retrograde embolization with a methyl methacrylate polymer," which was injected into a vertebral hemangioma with no further stabilization or radiation required.[76]

Giant cell tumors of the spine are rare and benign but can be aggressive and exhibit a high local recurrence rate with VB and neural arch destruction. Total spondylectomy with appropriate reconstruction for preservation of spinal integrity is the treatment of choice but is not always feasible. In 1997, Chui reported treatment of a giant cell tumor extending into the spinal canal. Decompressive laminectomy and posterolateral fusion followed by an injection of PMMA into a giant cell tumor resulted in radiological improvement with no tumor recurrence at 7 years.[77]

In 2003, Fourney et al reported that vertebroplasty and kyphoplasty were safe and feasible to treat painful VCFs in well-selected patients with refractory spinal pain due to myeloma bone disease or metastases in cancer patients. The authors noted at that time that precise indications for the techniques were evolving, with the current North American experience largely limited to osteoporotic compression fractures. This was the only study to date to directly compare vertebroplasty and kyphoplasty in patients with cancer (multiple myeloma and metastatic spinal lesions) and equivalent results in relieving pain were reported. Both procedures provided significant pain relief in a high percentage of patients, and this appeared durable over time.[78]

In 2007, Shaibani et al reviewed the indications and contraindications of vertebroplasty and kyphoplasty, appropriate patient selection and evaluation, techniques, outcomes, and potential complications when performed for the alleviation of pain for osteolytic tumors of the spine. The authors pointed out that, although both vertebroplasty and kyphoplasty were highly effective in reducing pain from osteoporotic or pathological VCFs and osteolytic tumors, supporting data were based on individual experiences and published case series rather than prospective randomized trials.

Numerous studies have since demonstrated the efficacy and safety of vertebroplasty and kyphoplasty in the treatment of spinal metastasis with rapid, significant, and sustained reductions in pain, disability, and analgesic usage, and improved quality of life.

The Cancer Patient Fracture Evaluation (CAFÉ) trial was the first randomized controlled trial designed to compare the safety and efficacy of BKP with NSM for the treatment of painful VCFs in patients with cancer.[79] Patients were from 22 sites in Europe, the United States, Canada, and Australia. Primary outcome measure was back-specific functional status at 1 month. The results supported the beneficial effects and safety of BKP compared with NSM for treating painful VCFs in patients with cancer.

To establish whether the CAFÉ trial findings were consistent with those of other published studies in patients with cancer and VCFs, a systematic review of the literature was performed by Bastian in 2012. A review of 22 published studies (12 prospective, including the CAFÉ trial, and 10 retrospective) extended the findings from the CAFÉ trial and confirmed BKP to be a safe and effective treatment that quickly reduces pain, stabilizes VB height and kyphosis, and improves physical function and quality of life in patients with cancer and painful VCFs.[78–100]

Astur and Avanzi performed a systematic review to assess the efficacy of kyphoplasty in controlling pain and improving quality of life in oncologic patients with pathologic compression fractures due to spinal metastasis or multiple myeloma. Based on moderate evidence that patients treated with BKP displayed better scores for pain, disability, quality of life, and Karnofsky Performance Status compared with those undergoing the conventional treatment, the study concluded that BKP could be considered an early treatment option for patients with symptomatic neoplastic spinal disease.[101]

Radiofrequency Ablation

Combination treatment with RFA and vertebral augmentation has been successful in reducing pain and in improving function and quality of life.[24–28] Early intervention with RFA and vertebral augmentation may improve the remaining quality of life in cancer patients with pathologic VCFs.[25] Although no comparative clinical trials have been performed, there is evidence to show that RFA carried out before percutaneous vertebral augmentation reduces the risk of cement leakage.[33]

In a retrospective study of 26 patients with 38 vertebral metastases treated between 2005 and 2009, Zheng et al reported image-guided RFA with kyphoplasty to be safe and effective when used with careful consideration of bone cement volume/viscosity, injection location, and temperature to treat thoracolumbar vertebral metastases.[30]

Wallace et al performed a retrospective review of 72 patients with 110 spinal metastases treated with RFA and vertebral augmentation for pain palliation between April 2012 and July 2014. Eighty-one percent (89/110) of metastases involved the posterior VB, while 45% (49/110) involved the pedicles. Patients reported clinically significant decreased pain scores at both 1- and 4-week follow-ups. No major complications occurred related to RFA and there were no instances of symptomatic cement extravasation. The combination therapy was shown to be a safe and effective therapy for palliation of painful spinal metastases, including tumor involving the posterior VB and/or pedicles.[102]

Kiva

Anselmetti et al, in a 2012 case report, described the Kiva system as "a novel and effective minimally invasive treatment option for patients suffering from severe pain due to osteolytic vertebral metastasis."[103] This finding was subsequently supported by data as 40 patients with a painful spine malignancy involving the vertebral wall, not responding to conventional therapies and without surgical indications, underwent vertebral augmentation with the Kiva intravertebral implant for pain palliation. All patients experienced functional improvement and clinically relevant reduction of pain at 1 month. All patients on opiates switched to NSAIDs or no treatment at all. All patients were able to discontinue use of an external orthotic following treatment. Seven of 43 (16.3%) treated vertebrae showed imaging evidence of a bone cement leakage.[104]

In a controlled, comparative randomized study, kyphoplasty and the KIVA implant provided equally significant pain relief in cancer patients with osteolytic metastasis. Anterior, posterior, and middle VB height ratio and Gardner's angle improved insignificantly in both groups. Pain and disability improved postoperatively similarly in both groups. Low-viscosity PMMA cement was used and there were no cases of cement leakage in the Kiva group. Safety of both augmentation techniques was demonstrated, even with significant osteolysis.[105]

1.6.4 Langerhans Cell Vertebral Histiocytosis

LCVH is a benign disease and extremely rare in the lumbar spine of adults.[106] Although uncommon, a variety of treatment modalities have been reported for management, including systemic chemotherapy, curettage with and without bone grafting, internal fixation and fusion, intralesional corticosteroid injection, and radiotherapy.[106,107] In 1994, Cardon et al reported the first known case of LCVH treated with percutaneous vertebroplasty and described it as a suitable alternative when conservative and open surgical treatments were not feasible, providing pain relief, fracture stabilization, rapid recovery, and early weight bearing.[108]

1.6.5 Osteogenesis Imperfecta

In 2002, Rami et al extended the indications for vertebral augmentation when they reported the first case of vertebroplasty used to treat a VCF secondary to osteogenesis imperfecta.[109]

1.7 Conclusion

Vertebral augmentation is a category of minimally invasive procedures that have become central in the treatment of VCFs. Many clinical trials, systematic reviews, and meta-analyses have studied and compared the growing number of vertebral augmentation modalities.[43–45] Results confirm significant and durable responses to treatment across a wide range of etiologies, including osteoporosis, trauma, and primary and metastatic cancer. Augmentation relieves pain and, in the case of kyphoplasty and implants, restores vertebral height and corrects kyphotic angulation in select patients, thereby decreasing the risk of future adjacent fractures. Appropriate patient selection is essential for successful outcomes.

As Albers and Latchaw noted in an editorial in Pain Physician:[110]

> *"...what of the active 78-year-old woman who suffers an osteoporotic vertebral compression fracture that significantly alters her lifestyle? If she only undergoes medical therapy, she is at risk for isolation, deconditioning, dependency, depression, thrombophlebitis, stroke, and pulmonary diseases such as emboli and infection. The opioids may make her nauseated and constipated so she may not eat. This is not an uncommon story. Morbidity and mortality risks are real life issues, not just statistics."*

Vertebral augmentation has been shown to offer statistically significant benefits to patients with painful and pathologic VCFs associated with osteoporosis, trauma, and malignancy. There have been many innovative advancements since the first vertebroplasty was performed in 1984. Numerous options are now available, each with its own advantages and disadvantages, and criteria for appropriateness. As physicians and clinical investigators, we have a responsibility to limit bias and ensure that appropriate treatments are made available, especially to vulnerable populations.[111] The example of the elderly osteoporotic woman is a poignant reminder of our mission to provide our patients with the safest, evidence-based, effective, and affordable health care available.[112-114]

References

[1] Harrington KD, Johnston JO, Turner RH, Green DL. The use of methylmethacrylate as an adjunct in the internal fixation of malignant neoplastic fractures. J Bone Joint Surg Am 1972;54(8):1665–1676

[2] McGraw JK, Lippert JA, Minkus KD, Rami PM, Davis TM, Budzik RF. Prospective evaluation of pain relief in 100 patients undergoing percutaneous vertebroplasty: results and follow-up. J Vasc Interv Radiol 2002; 13(9, Pt 1):883–886

[3] Zoarski GH, Snow P, Olan WJ, et al. Percutaneous vertebroplasty for osteoporotic compression fractures: quantitative prospective evaluation of long-term outcomes. J Vasc Interv Radiol 2002;13(2, Pt 1):139–148

[4] Atalay B, Caner H, Gokce C, Altinors N. Kyphoplasty: 2 years of experience in a neurosurgery department. Surg Neurol 2005;64(Suppl 2):S72–S76

[5] Burton AW, Mendel E. Vertebroplasty and kyphoplasty. Pain Physician 2003;6(3):335–341

[6] Kaemmerlen P, Thiesse P, Jonas P, et al. Percutaneous injection of orthopedic cement in metastatic vertebral lesions. N Engl J Med 1989;321(2):121

[7] Tschirhart CE, Finkelstein JA, Whyne CM. Optimization of tumor volume reduction and cement augmentation in percutaneous vertebroplasty for prophylactic treatment of spinal metastases. J Spinal Disord Tech 2006;19 (8):584–590

[8] Dickman CA, Fessler RG, MacMillan M, Haid RW. Transpedicular screw-rod fixation of the lumbar spine: operative technique and outcome in 104 cases. J Neurosurg 1992;77(6):860–870

[9] Kim HJ, Yi JM, Cho HG, et al. Comparative study of the treatment outcomes of osteoporotic compression fractures without neurologic injury using a rigid brace, a soft brace, and no brace: a prospective randomized controlled non-inferiority trial. J Bone Joint Surg Am 2014;96(23):1959–1966

[10] Rzewuska M, Ferreira M, McLachlan AJ, Machado GC, Maher CG. The efficacy of conservative treatment of osteoporotic compression fractures on acute pain relief: a systematic review with meta-analysis. Eur Spine J 2015;24(4):702–714

[11] Cauley JA, Thompson DE, Ensrud KC, Scott JC, Black D. Risk of mortality following clinical fractures. Osteoporos Int 2000;11(7):556–561

[12] Levine SA, Perin LA, Hayes D, Hayes WS. An evidence-based evaluation of percutaneous vertebroplasty. Manag Care 2000;9(3):56–60, 63

[13] Fischgrund JS, Rhyne A, Franke J, et al. Intraosseous basivertebral nerve ablation for the treatment of chronic low back pain: a prospective

[14] Bae H, Hatten HP Jr, Linovitz R, et al. A prospective randomized FDA-IDE trial comparing Cortoss with PMMA for vertebroplasty: a comparative effectiveness research study with 24-month follow-up. Spine 2012;37(7):544–550

[15] Galibert P, Deramond H, Rosat P, Le Gars D. Preliminary note on the treatment of vertebral angioma by percutaneous acrylic vertebroplasty Neurochirurgie 1987;33(2):166–168

[16] Lieberman IH, Dudeney S, Reinhardt MK, Bell G. Initial outcome and efficacy of "kyphoplasty" in the treatment of painful osteoporotic vertebral compression fractures. Spine 2001;26(14):1631–1638

[17] Feltes C, Fountas KN, Machinis T, et al. Immediate and early postoperative pain relief after kyphoplasty without significant restoration of vertebral body height in acute osteoporotic vertebral fractures. Neurosurg Focus 2005;18(3):e5

[18] Benzel E. Physical Principles and Kinematics. Biomechanics of Spine Stabilization. New York, NY: Thieme Publishers; 2001:19–28

[19] Bornemann R, Kabir K, Otten LA, et al. [Radiofrequency kyphoplasty - an innovative method for the treatment of vertebral compression fractures - comparison with conservative treatment]. Z Orthop Unfall 2012;150(4):392–396

[20] Dalton BE, Kohm AC, Miller LE, Block JE, Poser RD. Radiofrequency-targeted vertebral augmentation versus traditional balloon kyphoplasty: radiographic and morphologic outcomes of an ex vivo biomechanical pilot study. Clin Interv Aging 2012;7:525–531

[21] Erdem E, Akdol S, Amole A, Fryar K, Eberle RW. Radiofrequency-targeted vertebral augmentation for the treatment of vertebral compression fractures as a result of multiple myeloma. Spine 2013;38(15):1275–1281

[22] Robertson SC. Percutaneous vertebral augmentation: StabilitiT a new delivery system for vertebral fractures. Acta Neurochir Suppl (Wien) 2011;108: 191–195

[23] Moser FG, Maya MM, Blaszkiewicz L, Scicli A, Miller LE, Block JE. Prospective single-site experience with radiofrequency-targeted vertebral augmentation for osteoporotic vertebral compression fracture. J Osteoporos 2013;2013:791397

[24] Goldberg SN, Gazelle GS, Dawson SL, Rittman WJ, Mueller PR, Rosenthal DI. Tissue ablation with radiofrequency using multiprobe arrays. Acad Radiol 1995;2(8):670–674

[25] Kam NM, Maingard J, Kok HK, et al. Combined vertebral augmentation and radiofrequency ablation in the management of spinal metastases: an update. Curr Treat Options Oncol 2017;18(12):74

[26] Lencioni R, Goletti O, Armillotta N, et al. Radio-frequency thermal ablation of liver metastases with a cooled-tip electrode needle: results of a pilot clinical trial. Eur Radiol 1998;8(7):1205–1211

[27] Miao Y, Ni Y, Yu J, Zhang H, Baert A, Marchal G. An ex vivo study on radiofrequency tissue ablation: increased lesion size by using an "expandable-wet" electrode. Eur Radiol 2001;11(9):1841–1847

[28] Livraghi T, Goldberg SN, Monti F, et al. Saline-enhanced radio-frequency tissue ablation in the treatment of liver metastases. Radiology 1997;202(1): 205–210

[29] Schaefer O, Lohrmann C, Herling M, Uhrmeister P, Langer M. Combined radiofrequency thermal ablation and percutaneous cementoplasty treatment of a pathologic fracture. J Vasc Interv Radiol 2002;13(10):1047–1050

[30] Zheng L, Chen Z, Sun M, et al. A preliminary study of the safety and efficacy of radiofrequency ablation with percutaneous kyphoplasty for thoracolumbar vertebral metastatic tumor treatment. Med Sci Monit 2014;20:556–563

[31] Munk PL, Murphy KJ, Gangi A, Liu DM. Fire and ice: percutaneous ablative therapies and cement injection in management of metastatic disease of the spine. Semin Musculoskelet Radiol 2011;15(2):125–134

[32] Goetz MP, Callstrom MR, Charboneau JW, et al. Percutaneous image-guided radiofrequency ablation of painful metastases involving bone: a multicenter study. J Clin Oncol 2004;22(2):300–306

[33] Kassamali RH, Ganeshan A, Hoey ET, Crowe PM, Douis H, Henderson J. Pain management in spinal metastases: the role of percutaneous vertebral augmentation. Ann Oncol 2011;22(4):782–786

[34] Mooney J, Amburgy J, Self D, Agee B, Pritchard P, Chambers M. Vertebral Height Restoration Following Kyphoplasty. Unpublished Data

[35] Fields AJ, Lee GL, Keaveny TM. Mechanisms of initial endplate failure in the human vertebral body. J Biomech 2010;43(16):3126–3131

[36] Noriega D, Krüger A, Ardura F, et al. Clinical outcome after the use of a new craniocaudal expandable implant for vertebral compression fracture treatment: one year results from a prospective multicentric study. BioMed Res Int;2015:927813

[37] Ender SA, Gradl G, Ender M, Langner S, Merk HR, Kayser R. OsseoFix system for percutaneous stabilization of osteoporotic and tumorous vertebral compression fractures - clinical and radiological results after 12 months. RoFo Fortschr Geb Rontgenstr Nuklearmed 2014;186(4):380–387

[38] Vanni D, Galzio R, Kazakova A, et al. Third-generation percutaneous vertebral augmentation systems. J Spine Surg 2016;2(1):13–20

[39] Hirsch J, Chambers M, Beall DP. Management of Vertebral Fragility Fractures: A Clinical Care Pathway Developed by a Multispecialty Panel Using the RAND/UCLA Appropriateness Method. Unpublished Data

[40] Padovani B, Kasriel O, Brunner P, Peretti-Viton P. Pulmonary embolism caused by acrylic cement: a rare complication of percutaneous vertebroplasty. AJNR Am J Neuroradiol 1999;20(3):375–377

[41] Deramond H, Depriester C, Galibert P, Le Gars D. Percutaneous vertebroplasty with polymethylmethacrylate. Technique, indications, and results. Radiol Clin North Am 1998;36(3):533–546

[42] Mika A, Unnithan VB, Mika P. Differences in thoracic kyphosis and in back muscle strength in women with bone loss due to osteoporosis. Spine 2005;30(2):241–246

[43] Goldstein CL, Chutkan NB, Choma TJ, Orr RD. Management of the Elderly With Vertebral Compression Fractures. Neurosurgery 2015;77(Suppl 4):S33–S45

[44] Hadjipavlou AG, Tzermiadianos MN, Katonis PG, Szpalski M. Percutaneous vertebroplasty and balloon kyphoplasty for the treatment of osteoporotic vertebral compression fractures and osteolytic tumours. J Bone Joint Surg Br 2005;87(12):1595–1604

[45] Bouza C, López T, Magro A, Navalpotro L, Amate JM. Efficacy and safety of balloon kyphoplasty in the treatment of vertebral compression fractures: a systematic review. Eur Spine J 2006;15(7):1050–1067

[46] Manchikanti L, Singh V, Caraway DL, Benyamin RM, Hirsch JA. Medicare physician payment systems: impact of 2011 schedule on interventional pain management. Pain Physician 2011;14(1):E5–E33

[47] Burge R, Dawson-Hughes B, Solomon DH, Wong JB, King A, Tosteson A. Incidence and economic burden of osteoporosis-related fractures in the United States, 2005–2025. J Bone Miner Res 2007;22(3):465–475

[48] Suzuki N, Ogikubo O, Hansson T. The course of the acute vertebral body fragility fracture: its effect on pain, disability and quality of life during 12 months. Eur Spine J 2008;17(10):1380–1390

[49] Lapras C, Mottolese C, Deruty R, Lapras C Jr, Remond J, Duquesnel J. Percutaneous injection of methyl-metacrylate in osteoporosis and severe vertebral osteolysis (Galibert's technic). Ann Chir 1989;43(5):371–376

[50] Jensen ME, Evans AJ, Mathis JM, Kallmes DF, Cloft HJ, Dion JE. Percutaneous polymethylmethacrylate vertebroplasty in the treatment of osteoporotic vertebral body compression fractures: technical aspects. AJNR Am J Neuroradiol 1997;18(10):1897–1904

[51] Kallmes DF, Comstock BA, Heagerty PJ, et al. A randomized trial of vertebroplasty for osteoporotic spinal fractures. N Engl J Med 2009;361:569–579

[52] Garfin SR, Yuan HA, Reiley MA. New technologies in spine: kyphoplasty and vertebroplasty for the treatment of painful osteoporotic compression fractures. Spine 2001;26(14):1511–1515

[53] Van Meirhaeg, he J, Bastian L, Boonen S, Ranstam J, Tillman JB, Wardlaw D; FREE investigators. A randomized trial of balloon kyphoplasty and nonsurgical management for treating acute vertebral compression fractures: vertebral body kyphosis correction and surgical parameters. Spine 2013;38(12):971–983

[54] Wardlaw D, Cummings SR, Van Meirhaeghe J, et al. Efficacy and safety of balloon kyphoplasty compared with non-surgical care for vertebral compression fracture (FREE): a randomised controlled trial. Lancet 2009;373(9668):1016–1024

[55] Beall DP, Chambers MR, Thomas S, et al. Prospective and multicenter evaluation of outcomes for quality of life and activities of daily living for balloon kyphoplasty in the treatment of vertebral compression fractures: the EVOLVE trial. Neurosurgery 2019;84(1):169–178

[56] Krüger A, Oberkircher L, Figiel J, et al. Height restoration of osteoporotic vertebral compression fractures using different intravertebral reduction devices: a cadaveric study. Spine J 2015;15(5):1092–1098

[57] A Prospective, Multicenter, Randomized, Comparative Clinical Study to Compare the Safety and Effectiveness of Two Vertebral Compression Fracture (VCF) Reduction Techniques: the SpineJack and the KyphX Xpander Inflatable Bone Tamp. Identification No NCT02461810; 2015

[58] Interim clinical study report for: Prospective A. Multicenter, Randomized, Comparative Clinical Study to Compare the Safety and Effectiveness of Two Vertebral Compression Fracture (VCF) Reduction Techniques: The SpineJack

[59] and the KyphX Xpander Inflatable Bone Tamp. The U.S. National Library of Medicine and Clinical Trials.gov Web site. https://clinicaltrials.gov/ct2/show/NCT02461810. Published May 1, 2018. Accessed June 17, 2018

[59] Werner CM, Osterhoff G, Schlickeiser J, et al. Vertebral body stenting versus kyphoplasty for the treatment of osteoporotic vertebral compression fractures: a randomized trial. J Bone Joint Surg Am 2013;95(7):577–584

[60] Korovessis P, Vardakastanis K, Repantis T, Vitsas V. Balloon kyphoplasty versus KIVA vertebral augmentation: comparison of 2 techniques for osteoporotic vertebral body fractures: a prospective randomized study. Spine 2013;38(4):292–299

[61] Otten LA, Bornemnn R, Jansen TR, et al. Comparison of balloon kyphoplasty with the new VCF system for the treatment of vertebral compression fractures. Pain Physician 2013;16(5):E505–E512

[62] Tutton SM, Pflugmacher R, Davidian M, Beall DP, Facchini FR, Garfin SR. KAST Study: the Kiva System as a vertebral augmentation treatment-a safety and effectiveness trial: a randomized, noninferiority, trial comparing the Kiva System with Balloon Kyphoplasty in treatment of osteoporotic vertebral compression fractures. Spine 2015;40(12):865–875

[63] Beall DP, Olan WJ, Kakad P, Li Q, Hornberger J. Economic analysis of Kiva VCF treatment system compared to balloon kyphoplasty using randomized Kiva Safety and Effectiveness Trial (KAST) data. Pain Physician 2015;18(3):E299–E306

[64] Benson DR, Burkus JK, Montesano PX, Sutherland TB, McLain RF. Unstable thoracolumbar and lumbar burst fractures treated with the AO fixateur interne. J Spinal Disord 1992;5(3):335–343

[65] McLain RF, Sparling E, Benson DR. Early failure of short-segment pedicle instrumentation for thoracolumbar fractures. A preliminary report. J Bone Joint Surg Am 1993;75(2):162–167

[66] Chance GQ. Note on a type of flexion fracture of the spine. Br J Radiol 1948;21(249):452

[67] Verlaan JJ, van Helden WH, Oner FC, Verbout AJ, Dhert WJ. Balloon vertebroplasty with calcium phosphate cement augmentation for direct restoration of traumatic thoracolumbar vertebral fractures. Spine 2002;27(5):543–548

[68] Sacks D, McClenny TE, Cardella JF, Lewis CA. Society of Interventional Radiology clinical practice guidelines. J Vasc Interv Radiol 2003;14(9, Pt 2):S199–S202

[69] Chen JF, Wu CT, Lee ST. Percutaneous vertebroplasty for the treatment of burst fractures. Case report. J Neurosurg Spine 2004;1(2):228–231

[70] Elnoamany H. Percutaneous vertebroplasty: a first line treatment in traumatic non-osteoporotic vertebral compression fractures. Asian Spine J 2015;9(2):178–184

[71] Korovessis P, Vardakastanis K, Repantis T, Vitsas V. Transpedicular vertebral body augmentation reinforced with pedicle screw fixation in fresh traumatic A2 and A3 lumbar fractures: comparison between two devices and two bone cements. Eur J Orthop Surg Traumatol 2014;24(Suppl 1):S183–S191

[72] Polis B, Krawczyk J, Polis L, Nowosławska E. Percutaneous extrapedicular vertebroplasty with expandable intravertebral implant in compression vertebral body fracture in pediatric patient-technical note. Childs Nerv Syst 2016;32(11):2225–2231

[73] Wibmer C, Leithner A, Hofmann G, et al. Survival analysis of 254 patients after manifestation of spinal metastases: evaluation of seven preoperative scoring systems. Spine 2011;36(23):1977–1986

[74] Callander NS, Roodman GD. Myeloma bone disease. Semin Hematol 2001;38(3):276–285

[75] Lecouvet FE, Malghem J, Michaux L, et al. Vertebral compression fractures in multiple myeloma. Part II. Assessment of fracture risk with MR imaging of spinal bone marrow. Radiology 1997;204(1):201–205

[76] Nicola N, Lins E. Vertebral hemangioma: retrograde embolization-stabilization with methyl methacrylate. Surg Neurol 1987;27(5):481–486

[77] Lee CG, Kim SH, Kim DM, Kim SW. Giant cell tumor of upper thoracic spine. J Korean Neurosurg Soc 2014;55(3):167–169

[78] Fourney DR, Schomer DF, Nader R, et al. Percutaneous vertebroplasty and kyphoplasty for painful vertebral body fractures in cancer patients. J Neurosurg 2003;98(1, Suppl):21–30

[79] Berenson J, Pflugmacher R, Jarzem P, et al; Cancer Patient Fracture Evaluation (CAFE) Investigators. Balloon kyphoplasty versus non-surgical fracture management for treatment of painful vertebral body compression fractures in patients with cancer: a multicentre, randomised controlled trial. Lancet Oncol 2011;12(3):225–235

[80] Chen F, Xia YH, Cao WZ, et al. Percutaneous kyphoplasty for the treatment of spinal metastases. Oncol Lett 2016;11(3):1799–1806

[81] Pflugmacher R, Taylor R, Agarwal A, et al. Balloon kyphoplasty in the treatment of metastatic disease of the spine: a 2-year prospective evaluation. Eur Spine J 2008;17(8):1042–1048

[82] Eleraky M, Papanastassiou I, Setzer M, Baaj AA, Tran ND, Vrionis FD. Balloon kyphoplasty in the treatment of metastatic tumors of the upper thoracic spine. J Neurosurg Spine 2011;14(3):372–376

[83] Dalbayrak S, Onen MR, Yilmaz M, Naderi S. Clinical and radiographic results of balloon kyphoplasty for treatment of vertebral body metastases and multiple myelomas. J Clin Neurosci 2010;17(2):219–224

[84] Gerszten PC, Germanwala A, Burton SA, Welch WC, Ozhasoglu C, Vogel WJ. Combination kyphoplasty and spinal radiosurgery: a new treatment paradigm for pathological fractures. J Neurosurg Spine 2005;3(4):296–301

[85] Sandri A, Carbognin G, Regis D, et al. Combined radiofrequency and kyphoplasty in painful osteolytic metastases to vertebral bodies. Radiol Med (Torino) 2010;115(2):261–271

[86] Gerszten PC, Monaco EA III. Complete percutaneous treatment of vertebral body tumors causing spinal canal compromise using a transpedicular cavitation, cement augmentation, and radiosurgical technique. Neurosurg Focus 2009;27(6):E9

[87] Khanna AJ, Reinhardt MK, Togawa D, Lieberman IH. Functional outcomes of kyphoplasty for the treatment of osteoporotic and osteolytic vertebral compression fractures. Osteoporos Int 2006;17(6):817–826

[88] Köse KC, Cebesoy O, Akan B, Altinel L, Dinçer D, Yazar T. Functional results of vertebral augmentation techniques in pathological vertebral fractures of myelomatous patients. J Natl Med Assoc 2006;98(10):1654–1658

[89] Lane JM, Hong R, Koob J, et al. Kyphoplasty enhances function and structural alignment in multiple myeloma. Clin Orthop Relat Res 2004(426):49–53

[90] Huber FX, McArthur N, Tanner M, et al. Kyphoplasty for patients with multiple myeloma is a safe surgical procedure: results from a large patient cohort. Clin Lymphoma Myeloma 2009;9(5):375–380

[91] Zou J, Mei X, Gan M, Yang H. Kyphoplasty for spinal fractures from multiple myeloma. J Surg Oncol 2010;102(1):43–47

[92] Qian Z, Sun Z, Yang H, Gu Y, Chen K, Wu G. Kyphoplasty for the treatment of malignant vertebral compression fractures caused by metastases. J Clin Neurosci 2011;18(6):763–767

[93] Dudeney S, Lieberman IH, Reinhardt MK, Hussein M. Kyphoplasty in the treatment of osteolytic vertebral compression fractures as a result of multiple myeloma. J Clin Oncol 2002;20(9):2382–2387

[94] Astolfi S, Scaramuzzo L, Logroscino CA. A minimally invasive surgical treatment possibility of osteolytic vertebral collapse in multiple myeloma. Eur Spine J 2009;18(Suppl 1):115–121

[95] Cardoso ER, Ashamalla H, Weng L, et al. Percutaneous tumor curettage and interstitial delivery of samarium-153 coupled with kyphoplasty for treatment of vertebral metastases. J Neurosurg Spine 2009;10(4):336–342

[96] Ashamalla H, Cardoso E, Macedon M, et al. Phase I trial of vertebral intracavitary cement and samarium (VICS): novel technique for treatment of painful vertebral metastasis. Int J Radiat Oncol Biol Phys 2009;75(3):836–842

[97] Pflugmacher R, Schulz A, Schroeder RJ, Schaser KD, Klostermann CK, Melcher I. A prospective two-year follow-up of thoracic and lumbar osteolytic vertebral fractures caused by multiple myeloma treated with balloon kyphoplasty. Z Orthop Ihre Grenzgeb 2007;145(1):39–47

[98] Lieberman I, Reinhardt MK. Vertebroplasty and kyphoplasty for osteolytic vertebral collapse. Clin Orthop Relat Res 2003(415, Suppl):S176–S186

[99] Bastian L. Balloon Kyphoplasty in the Treatment of Vertebral Compression Fractures in Cancer Patients. Eur Oncol Haematol 2012;8(3):144–147

[100] Vrionis FD et al., Tech Reg Anesth Pain Manag, 2005;9:39

[101] Astur N, Avanzi O. Balloon kyphoplasty in the treatment of neoplastic spine lesions: a systematic review. Global Spine J 2019;9(3):348–356

[102] Wallace AN, Greenwood TJ, Jennings JW. Radiofrequency ablation and vertebral augmentation for palliation of painful spinal metastases. J Neurooncol 2015;124(1):111–118

[103] Anselmetti GC, Tutton SM, Facchini FR, Miller LE, Block JE. Percutaneous vertebral augmentation for painful osteolytic vertebral metastasis: a case report. Int Med Case Rep J 2012;5:13–17

[104] Anselmetti GC, Manca A, Tutton S, et al. Percutaneous vertebral augmentation assisted by PEEK implant in painful osteolytic vertebral metastasis involving the vertebral wall: experience on 40 patients. Pain Physician 2013;16(4):E397–E404

[105] Korovessis P, Vardakastanis K, Vitsas V, Syrimpeis V. Is Kiva implant advantageous to balloon kyphoplasty in treating osteolytic metastasis to the spine? Comparison of 2 percutaneous minimal invasive spine techniques: a prospective randomized controlled short-term study. Spine 2014;39(4):E231–E239

[106] Cheyne C. Histiocytosis X. J Bone Joint Surg Br 1971;53(3):366–382

[107] Zhong WQ, Jiang L, Ma QJ, et al. Langerhans cell histiocytosis of the atlas in an adult. Eur Spine J 2010;19(1):19–22

[108] Cardon T, Hachulla E, Flipo RM, et al. Percutaneous vertebroplasty with acrylic cement in the treatment of a Langerhans cell vertebral histiocytosis. Clin Rheumatol 1994;13(3):518–521

[109] Rami PM, McGraw JK, Heatwole EV, Boorstein JM. Percutaneous vertebroplasty in the treatment of vertebral body compression fracture secondary to osteogenesis imperfecta. Skeletal Radiol 2002;31(3):162–165

[110] Albers SL, Latchaw RE. The effects of randomized controlled trials on vertebroplasty and kyphoplasty: a square PEG in a round hole. Pain Physician 2013;16(4):E331–E348

[111] Beall DP, Tutton SM, Murphy K, Olan W, Warner C, Test JB. Analysis of Reporting Bias in Vertebral Augmentation. Pain Physician 2017;20(7):E1081–E1090

[112] Wilson DC, Connolly RJ, Zhu Q, et al. An ex vivo biomechanical comparison of a novel vertebral compression fracture treatment system to kyphoplasty. Clin Biomech (Bristol, Avon) 2012;27(4):346–353

[113] Olivarez LM, Dipp JM, Escamilla RF, et al. Vertebral augmentation treatment of painful osteoporotic compression fractures with the Kiva VCF Treatment System. SAS J 2011;5(4):114–119

[114] Korovessis P, Repantis T, Miller LE, Block JE. Initial clinical experience with a novel vertebral augmentation system for treatment of symptomatic vertebral compression fractures: a case series of 26 consecutive patients. BMC Musculoskelet Disord 2011;12:206

2 Vertebral Compression Fractures

Amanda Schnell, Sarah Morgan, James Mooney, D. Mitchell Self, John W. Amburgy, and M.R. Chambers

Summary

Vertebral compression fractures (VCFs) result from either trauma or pathologic weakening of the bone by conditions such as osteoporosis or malignancy. They often cause severe pain, physical limitation, and disability, and lead to increased morbidity and mortality with considerable heath care expenditures. Fracture classification systems have been designed to identify spinal instability and guide treatment. The public health and economic impact is considerable. Regardless of etiology, timely and accurate diagnosis will assist in determining the appropriate treatment.

Keywords: vertebral compression fracture, vertebral fracture classification system, vertebral augmentation, osteoporosis, bone mineral density, trauma, multiple myeloma, malignancy, kyphoplasty

2.1 Introduction

Vertebral compression fractures (VCF) result from either trauma or pathologic weakening of the bone by conditions such as osteoporosis or malignancy. They often cause severe pain, physical limitation, and disability, and lead to increased morbidity and mortality.[1-6] Vertebral fractures, whether they are symptomatic or asymptomatic, are associated with increased morbidity and mortality, and patients with osteoporotic vertebral fragility fractures have an increased risk of mortality compared to age-matched controls.[7-9] Annual health care expenditures to diagnose and treat vertebral fractures are considerable and are on the rise.[10]

The thoracolumbar region is the most common location for fractures of the vertebral column.[11-13] The thoracic spine is functionally rigid due to coronally oriented facet joints, thin intervertebral disks, and stabilization offered by the rib cage, so significant trauma is required for fracture or dislocation unless the vertebrae are pathologically weakened by disease (▶Fig. 2.1). The presence of the spinal cord in this region predisposes the patient to neurological injury if the canal is compromised causing significant impingement on indwelling the neural tissue. The lumbar spine, on the other hand, is relatively flexible due to the thicker intervertebral disks, sagittally orientated facet joints, and absence of the rib cage (▶Fig. 2.2). The relatively lesser incidence of neurological injury in lumbar fractures can be attributed to the large size of the neural canal and the greater resilience of the cauda equina nerve roots. The thoracolumbar junction (T10–L2) is uniquely positioned between the rigid thoracic spine and the mobile lumbar spine. This transition from the less mobile thoracic spine with its associated ribs and sternum to the more dynamic lumbar spine subjects the region to significant biomechanical stress.[12,13] Among thoracolumbar injuries, 50 to 60% affect the transitional zone (T11–L2), 25 to 40% affect the thoracic spine, and 10 to 14% involve the lower lumbar spine and sacrum.[14]

2.2 Presentation and Diagnosis

Vertebral fractures may have a profound and untoward effect on quality of life. The presentation of patients with VCFs varies depending on etiology, severity, and the level or levels affected. Discrete onset axial back pain after lifting or bending is often reported and may or may not be associated with sciatica. Pain is typically positional, worsened by weight-bearing activities, transition from one position to another, and by lying supine. Patients without significant trauma rarely have neurologic deficits, but elderly osteoporotic patients, in particular, have marked functional impairment with activity reduced by postural changes and pain. Multiple thoracic fractures can result in severe kyphosis, which may lead to restrictive lung disease.[15] Lumbar fractures may alter abdominal anatomy, leading to constipation, abdominal pain and distention, reduced appetite, premature satiety, and urinary incontinence.[16] These restrictions increase the risk of losing independence, social isolation, and clinical depression.

2.3 Epidemiology

2.3.1 Osteoporosis

Osteoporosis is the most common condition associated with VCFs and affects approximately 700,000 individuals each year in the United States and 30 to 50% of people older than 50 years worldwide.[17-20] Osteoporosis or "porous bone" is a systemic bone disorder resulting from an imbalance between bone formation and bone loss and is characterized by diminished bone strength. Bone strength is dependent on both the quality of the bone and the bone mineral density (BMD). Bone quality refers to architecture, mineralization, accumulation of damage (microfractures), and turnover. Bone density is determined by peak bone mass, which is usually attained by age 30 and subsequent bone loss.[21]

Osteoporosis can occur in both sexes, but is more common in women following menopause.[21] Both men and women have age-related decline in BMD in middle age due to increased bone resorption as compared to bone formation. This is especially common in women as they experience more rapid bone loss in the early years after menopause.[21] Peak bone mass is achieved only after linear bone growth has ceased. Therefore, bone mass attained early in life may be the most important determinant of skeletal strength later in life.[21,22] Factors that affect achievement of peak bone mass include lifetime calcium and vitamin D intake, physical activity, smoking, alcohol, eating disorders, and endocrine disorders.[22] Characteristics associated with low bone mass later in life include female sex, increased age, estrogen deficiency, white race, low body mass index (BMI), and a family history of fractures.[21]

As a complication of osteoporosis, VCFs are associated with significant morbidity and mortality and are an increasing public health risk as the population continues to age (▶Fig. 2.3). Vertebral

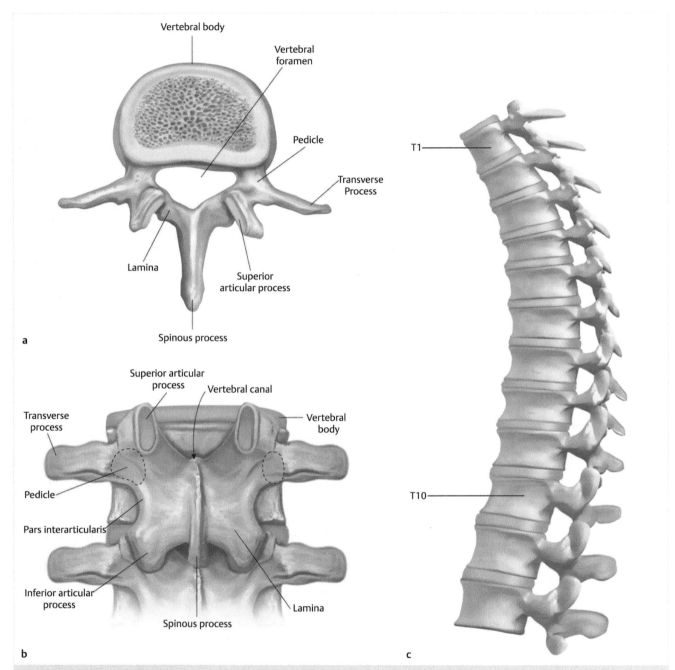

Fig. 2.1 (a–c) Anatomy of the thoracic spine. (Source: An H, Singh K, ed. Surgical anatomy. In: Synopsis of Spine Surgery. 3rd ed. New York, NY: Thieme; 2016.)

fracture incidence increases substantially with age in both males and females. The annual incidence of vertebral fractures increases from 0.9% among middle-aged women in their 50s to 60s to an incidence of 1.7% among those 80 years and older.[10,17,23] The mere presence of a vertebral fracture is associated with increased risk of future fractures. If the patient presents with one VCF, the risk of having another one within the first year is increased by fivefold.[17] If the patient has two fractures, the risk increases to 12-fold and if three or more fractures are present, the risk is 75 times increased for having another vertebral fracture.

BMD as measured in gram per square centimeter (g/cm²) and its related T-score are used to screen for the objective presence of osteoporosis. The T-score is the number of standard deviations above or below the mean BMD for a healthy 30-year-old reference patient. The U.S. standard is to use data for a 30-year-old of the same sex and ethnicity, but the World Health Organization (WHO) recommends using data for a 30-year-old white female for everyone. Values for 30-year-olds are used in postmenopausal women and men older than 50 years because they better predict risk of future fracture. The criteria of the WHO are as follows: Normal is a T-score of -1.0 or higher. Osteopenia is defined as between -1.0 and -2.5. Osteoporosis is defined as -2.5 or lower, meaning a bone density that is 2.5 standard deviations below the mean of the reference.[24]

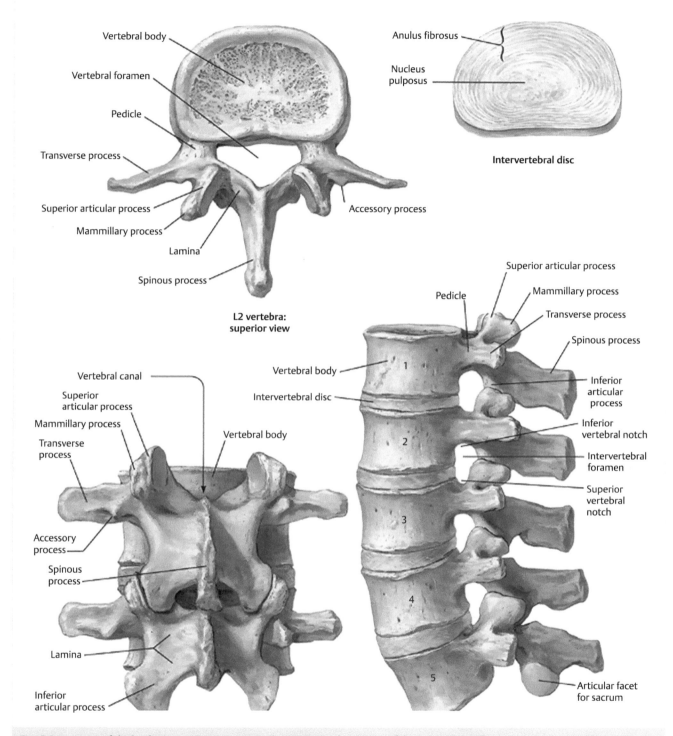

Fig. 2.2 Anatomy of the lumbar spine. (Source: Kim D, Choi G, Lee S, ed. Anatomy of the intervertebral foramen. In: Endoscopic Spine Procedures. 1st Edition. New York, NY: Thieme; 2011.)

It should be noted that while bone density scanning and determination of the patient's BMD and T-score are valuable from a screening and treatment monitoring perspective, it does not determine which vertebral fractures are osteoporotic VCFs as a greater proportion of vertebral fragility fractures occurs in patients with either a normal bone density or with osteopenia as compared to patients whose T-score shows osteoporosis. The

clinical scenario and amount of force required to produce that VCF is a far better determination of whether the patient's fracture is traumatic or the result of osteoporosis than their T-score.

Using data from the National Health and Nutrition Examination Survey (NHANES), an estimated 16% of U.S. men and almost 30% of U.S. women aged 50 and over have osteoporosis as defined by their bone BMD.[25] An estimated 50% of

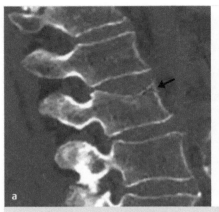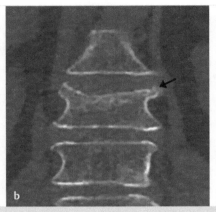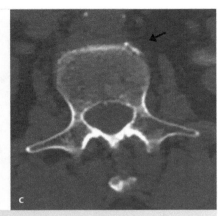

Fig. 2.3 Vertebral compression fracture is illustrated by the *black arrows* and shown in the sagittal plane **(a)**, coronal plane **(b)**, and axial plane **(c)**. (These images are provided courtesy of Dr. M. R. Chambers.)

women and 20% of men in the United States will sustain an osteoporotic fracture at some point in their lifetime.[16] The prevalence of vertebral fracture is similar in men and women and increases with age from less than 5% in those younger than 60 years of age to 11% in those age 70 to 79 years to 18% in those aged 80 years or older.[26] The age-correlated prevalence rates in the United States are very similar to those in Europe, as published by the European Vertebral Osteoporosis Study.[18,27–31]

More than 2 million osteoporotic fractures including 700,000 VCFs were diagnosed in 2005 and that number of osteoporotic fractures is projected to increase to over 3 million fractures by 2025, an increase of 52%.[32] Importantly, this calculation may be an underestimate as it has been projected that less than one-third of all vertebral fractures are clinically diagnosed (see Chapter 34: Treatment of Osteoporosis after Vertebral Augmentation).[33]

2.3.2 Cancer

Metastases

The spine is the most frequent site of bone metastasis.[34] In patients with cancer, the risk for pathologic VCF results from bone involvement, with fracture incidence estimated to be 24, 14, 6, and 8% among patients with multiple myeloma (MM) and cancers of the breast, prostate, and lung, respectively.[35,36] These fractures are most often of the compression or burst type and may result in axial or radicular pain, and sometimes neurologic and/or motor/sensory deficits. The incidence of symptomatic metastatic spinal tumors in the United States is estimated to be approximately 160,000 per year[37] and between 6 and 24% of these patients are predicted to have a VCF at some point over the course of their disease.[35] Unfortunately, pathologic fractures of the spine are often the initial manifestation of a metastatic malignancy (▶Fig. 2.4).

Multiple Myeloma

Although often perceived as a rare disease, MM is in fact the second most commonly diagnosed hematologic malignancy in the Western world.[38] MM comprises 1.6% of all bone malignancies in the United States and occurs primarily in the elderly,

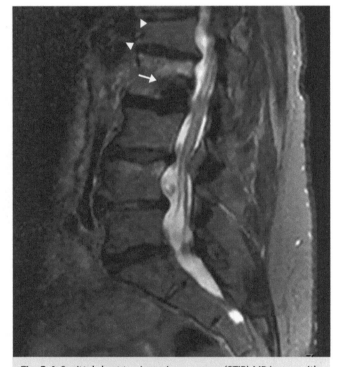

Fig. 2.4 Sagittal short tau inversion recovery (STIR) MR image with a region of decreased signal present within the posteroinferior portion of the L2 vertebral body consistent with a blastic metastasis (*white arrow*). Decreased height and normal marrow signal is noted in the L1 vertebral body (*white arrowheads*) consistent with a chronic osteoporotic vertebral compression fracture vertebral body. (This image is provided courtesy of Dr. M. R. Chambers.)

with a median age at diagnosis of 69 years.[39] The 5-year survival rate is less than 50%.[40] VCFs are the most common type of fractures in patients with MM, occurring at the onset of the disease in 34 to 64% of patients.[41,42]

Unlike osteoporosis, which causes weakening of trabecular bone structure and lower bone mass, the mechanisms of MM leading to significant structural weakness are varied and remain incompletely understood. There is increased osteoclast precursor differentiation and, consequently, enhanced bone resorption.[43] Early diagnosis and treatment are critical in slowing the disease progression and the corresponding deterioration of the patient's quality of life.[44]

Most MM patients report back pain at the time of initial diagnosis.[45] Up to 80% of patients with MM are diagnosed during routine imaging.[46] Radiological findings include diffuse bone loss, focal osteolytic bone lesions, bone marrow edema, and fragility fractures of the axial skeleton.[47] Bone marrow edema is a common MR imaging finding of acute VCFs but may be difficult to see due to bone marrow signal abnormalities seen in patients with MM.[48] Diffuse bone loss alone is often misdiagnosed as osteoporosis until more symptoms associated with MM develop.[49] When focal osteolytic lesions or significant diffuse bone loss is evident, risk for vertebral fractures is high.[50]

The patient's osteoporosis status could be an indicator of disease progression to MM.[51] Twenty percent of osteoporotic patients presenting with vertebral fractures may have either monoclonal gammopathy of undetermined significance or MM.[50] Almost 80% of MM patients are diagnosed with osteoporosis and the level of BMD has a major impact on survival.[52,53] However, there are several problems with the use of BMD as a diagnostic tool of MM. First, the decline in BMD as a result of aging and/or osteoporosis is well understood; it declines 0.1 to 0.2% per year due to aging while after menopause and onset of osteoporosis, it peaks to 1 to 2% and then slows back to the decline seen in normal aging.[47] The decline in BMD in MM-induced osteoporosis is less well understood and unpredictable. In a recent study, Borggrefe et al found that BMD of fracture cases in MM patients were significantly reduced in men, but not in women.[54] Second, as has been mentioned previously, BMD and T-score as determined by dual X-ray absorptiometry (DXA) has been challenged as a limited tool for the diagnosis of osteoporosis itself as it only partially estimates fracture risk. The use of DXA as a diagnostic evaluation tool in MM is even less valid.[55] Also, routine assessment of BMD in MM patients is not recommended due to methodological difficulties in these patients and the frequent use of bisphosphonates in all symptomatic MM patients.[56] Finally, there are no established and well-defined clinical criteria to differentiate osteoporotic VCFs and MM-induced osteoporotic VCFs, but MR imaging can be helpful in patients who are suspected to have MM (▶Fig. 2.5).[57]

2.3.3 Trauma

The annual incidence of traumatic spinal injuries is greater than 160,000 in North America.[58] According to Hu et al, the incidence of traumatic spinal injuries was 64/100,000 population/y in Canada alone.[59] Of the injuries to the thoracolumbar region, around 50 to 60% affect the transitional zone (T11–T12), with another 25 to 40% affecting the thoracic spine, and the remainder affecting the lower lumbar spine and sacrum.[14] The peak incidence of thoracolumbar fractures is observed in patients who are between 20 and 40 years of age with these injuries being more common in men.[14,60] Thoracolumbar fractures are associated with neurologic injury in 20 to 36% of cases[61,62] and the type of fracture affects both the chances for and the extent of a neurological deficit. In a multicenter study, the incidence of neurological deficit ranged from 22 to 51% depending on the fracture type (AO Classification type A: 22%; type B: 28%; type C: 51%; ▶Table 2.1).[11,63]

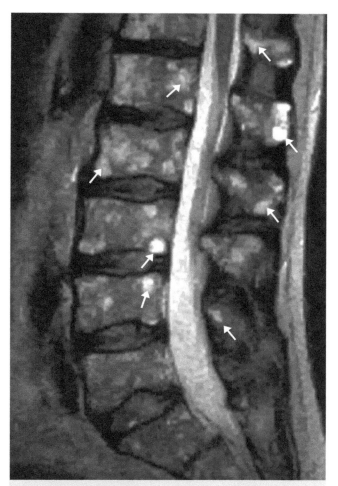

Fig. 2.5 Multiple myeloma. Mid-sagittal T2-weighted MR images of the lumbar spine show multiple, well-circumscribed, high-signal-intensity lesions throughout the lumbar spine (*white arrows*) consistent with plasma cell infiltration of the lumbar spine bone marrow. (Source: Khanna A, ed. Extradural tumors. In: MRI Essentials for the Spine Specialist. 1st ed. New York, NY: Thieme; 2014.)

Most thoracolumbar fractures are associated with trauma and 65% occur due to motor vehicle injuries or falls from a height, with a lesser portion of these fractures attributed to sports injuries or violence. Due to the high-velocity nature of these traumatic fractures, they are commonly associated with other injuries such as hemopneumothorax, rib fractures, vessel injuries, and diaphragmatic rupture.[64,65] Seatbelt (Chance) fractures and flexion–distraction injuries are other traumatic spinal fractures that are often associated with intra-abdominal visceral injuries. First described in 1948 by G.Q. Chance, the Chance fracture is a purely bony injury extending from posterior to anterior through the spinous process, pedicles, and vertebral body (VB), respectively. Seen most often in the upper lumbar spine in adults, it typically results from excessive flexion, as caused by a lap belt (without shoulder belt support) injury during a motor vehicle accident. Incidence has been reduced dramatically by the required use of shoulder belts in motor vehicles.

History and physical examination help guide the choice of the initial imaging modality. Many times, advanced and/or dynamic imaging will be needed to detect spinal instability. A careful

Table 2.1 AO classification system

Type A: Compression injuries
Failure of anterior structures under compression; posterior soft tissue is intact even with posterior element fractures
A1: Wedge fracture—fracture of a single end plate without involvement of the posterior wall

• A1.1: End plate impaction
  – Up to 5 degrees of end plate impaction
  – Posterior wall is intact

• A1.2: Wedge impaction
  – Greater than 5 degrees of end plate impaction
  – Posterior wall is intact

• A1.3: Biconcave (VB collapse)
  – Symmetric loss of VB height
  – Posterior wall is intact

A2: Split fracture—fracture of both end plates without involvement of the posterior wall

• A2.1: Sagittal
  – Extremely rare in the thoracolumbar spine
  – Posterior wall is intact

• A2.2: Coronal   – Posterior wall is intact

• A2.3: Multiple (pincer)
  – Central VB is crushed and filled with disk material
  – Posterior wall is intact

A3: Burst fracture—fracture with any involvement of the posterior wall; only a single end plate is fractured

• A3.1: Incomplete
  – Upper or lower half is burst
  – Posterior wall is NOT intact
  – Fracture fragments are retropulsed into the spinal canal to some degree
  – Posterior ligamentous complex remains intact

• A3.2: Burst split
  – One half of the VB is burst
  – The other half is has split sagittally
  – Posterior wall is NOT intact
  – Fracture fragments are retropulsed into the spinal canal to some degree

• A3.3 (and A4): complete—fracture with involvement of the posterior wall and both end plates
  – More frequently associated with neurologic injury
  – Posterior wall is NOT intact
  – Fracture fragments are retropulsed into the spinal canal to some degree

Type B: Distraction
Failure of the posterior or anterior tension band.
B1: Posterior soft tissues (subluxation with transosseous tension band disruption [chance fracture])
B2: Posterior tension band disruption together with a type A fracture (classified separately)
B3: Anterior disk (extension spondylolysis)B3: Anterior disk (extension spondylolysis)
Type C: Multidirectional with translation
Failure of all elements leading to dislocation or displacement
C1: Anterior posterior (dislocation)
C2: Lateral (lateral shear)
C3: Rotational (rotational burst)

history regarding vertebral fracture injury mechanism, pain, and the presence or absence of neurological symptoms is essential. The patient may report pain associated with movement and/or with prolonged positions and give-way weakness or a feeling of "instability." Axial, nonradiating back pain of stabbing or aching quality is the most common symptom. Patients with neurological injury may complain of weakness, paresthesia, or anesthesia below the injury level and may have urinary retention. Thorough inspection of the spine should be performed after a careful log roll maneuver to look for abrasions, tenderness, local kyphosis, and a palpable gap in between spinous processes. Neurological assessment should follow the standard American Spinal Injury Association (ASIA) guidelines (▶ Fig. 2.6).[66]

As the spinal cord normally ends between the L1 and L2 level and the cauda equina fills the distal canal, varied neurological injury patterns can be observed with thoracolumbar fractures. Neurological injuries at or above L1 can injure the spinal cord

and injuries below L2 typically affect only the nerve roots of the cauda equina. Conus medullaris syndrome, characterized by exclusive damage to sacral innervations to the bowel and bladder with intact lumbar nerve roots, is a unique feature of T12–L1 injuries.

2.4 Vertebral Fracture Classification Systems

Numerous classification systems have been proposed to describe thoracolumbar spinal fractures resulting from osteoporosis, neoplasia, or acute trauma. Each system was designed to improve upon the last as a reliable way to identify spinal instability and, ultimately, to guide treatment.

In 1938, Watson-Jones first described the concept of spinal instability and developed a system that integrated the posterior

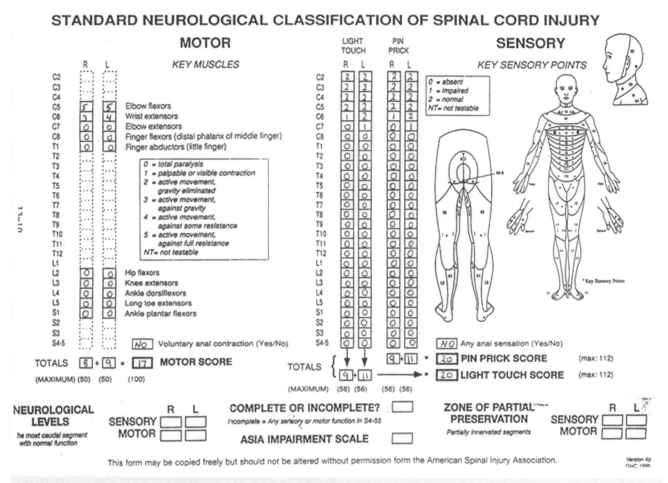

Fig. 2.6 American Spinal Injury Association (ASIA) Guidelines.

ligamentous complex to described seven fracture types in three major patterns: simple wedge fractures, comminuted fractures, and fracture-dislocations.[67]

Over a decade later in 1949, Nicoll improved the classification system by formally defining the anatomy that was responsible for spinal stability, including the VB, the disks, the intervertebral joints, and the interspinous ligament.[68] He emphasized the importance of the interspinous ligament as a crucial component of stability.

Holdsworth was the first to describe stability in terms of two columns.[69,70] In his two-column theory, compressing the anterior column causes distraction of the posterior column and vice versa. Holdsworth expanded on Nicoll's assumption that the interspinous ligament was paramount in determining stability. He described a posterior ligamentous complex (the posterior column) and believed that the entire posterior column was crucial for stability. Therefore, loss of integrity to this posterior ligamentous complex would define instability. Holdsworth also described mechanisms of spinal injuries and defined six groups: anterior wedge-compression fractures, dislocations, rotational fracture-dislocations, extension injuries, burst fractures, and shearing fractures. This classification system predates the modern imaging modalities and is now rarely used.

Panjabi[71] and White et al[72] described three conceptually separate but interdependent components responsible for stability:

(1) a passive subsystem consisting of the vertebrae, facets, intervertebral disks, spinal ligaments, and joint capsules; (2) an active subsystem of spinal muscles and tendons; and (3) a control subsystem for neural feedback, including the neural control centers and force transducers located in ligaments, tendons, and muscles.

Introduced in 1982, the Allen and Ferguson system, also rarely used, was a "mechanistic" system that classified spinal injuries based on three common mechanical modes of failure of the spine: compression–flexion, distraction–flexion, and compression–extension.[73]

Also introduced in 1982, the Denis three-column spinal stability classification system describes fracture types and included possible mechanisms of failure. The anterior column is defined as the anterior longitudinal ligament, the anterior half of the VB, and the anterior half of the annulus fibrosis. The posterior column consists of everything posterior to the posterior longitudinal ligament: the facet joints, pedicles, and supraspinous ligaments. The novel middle column contains a middle osteoligamentous complex formed by the posterior half of the VB, the posterior longitudinal ligament, and posterior annulus fibrosus (▶ Fig. 2.7).[74]

As this model has an additional column, novel mechanisms of injury are described. There are four major types: compression, burst, seatbelt type, and flexion–distraction. Compression fractures are classified according to whether they are caused

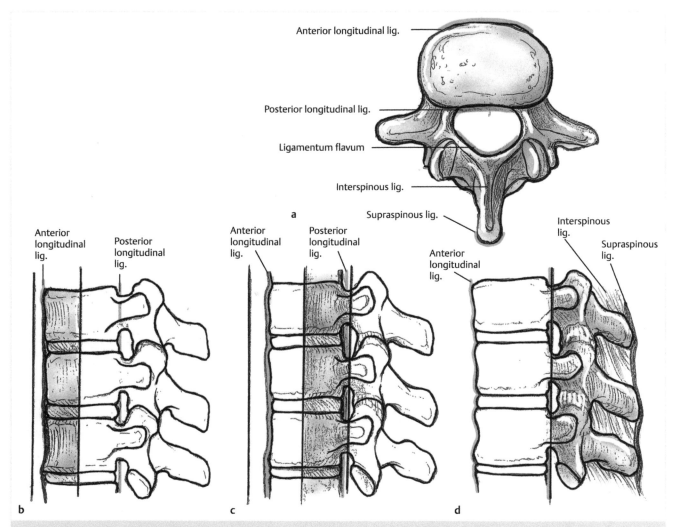

Fig. 2.7 Illustration of the three columns of the spine as described by Denis. **(a)** Axial view. The lateral views show the **(b)** anterior, **(c)** middle, and **(d)** posterior columns and their anatomic contents. (Source: Khanna A, ed. Traumatic conditions. In: MRI Essentials for the Spine Specialist. 1st ed. New York, NY: Thieme; 2014.)

by anterior or lateral flexion. These injuries cause anterior column compression sometimes associated with posterior column distraction. Burst fractures are classified according to whether an axial load alone caused the fractures or whether flexion, rotation, and/or lateral flexion are also involved. These injuries cause anterior and middle column compression, and may sometimes also produce associated posterior column distraction. Seatbelt fractures are defined by their distinctive flexion–disruption mechanism of injury. The anterior column may be intact or distracted, but the middle and posterior columns are distracted. Fracture-dislocations are classified according to whether the dislocation involves rotation, shear, or flexion–distraction. Each of these injuries is further subdivided and can produce any pattern of column involvement (▶Table 2.2 and ▶Fig. 2.8). Minor fractures—those of the transverse processes, articular processes, pars interarticularis, and spinous processes involve only a part of the posterior column and are not thought to lead to acute instability.[75]

Using this system, only compression fractures without involvement of the posterior wall would be amenable to treatment with vertebral augmentation. While low-velocity compression fractures were currently considered stable, Denis

Table 2.2 Denis' classification of spinal fracture

Type	Mechanism	Columns involved
Compression • Anterior • Lateral	Flexion Anterior flexion Lateral flexion	Anterior column compression with/without posterior column distraction
Burst • A • B • C • D • E	Axial load Axial load plus flexion Axial load plus flexion Axial load plus rotation Axial load plus lateral flexion	Anterior and middle column compression with/without posterior column distractionz
Seatbelt	Flexion–distraction	Anterior column intact or distracted; middle and posterior column distraction
Fracture-dislocation • Flexion–rotation • Shear • Flexion–distraction	Flexion–rotation Shear (anteroposterior or posteroanterior) Flexion–distraction	Any columns can be affected (alone or in combination)

Source: Adapted from Dr. B. Nurboja and Mr. D. Choi.

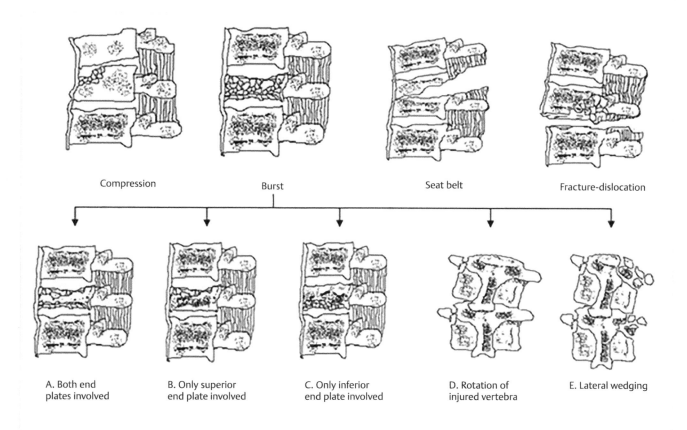

Compression   Burst   Seat belt   Fracture-dislocation

A. Both end plates involved   B. Only superior end plate involved   C. Only inferior end plate involved   D. Rotation of injured vertebra   E. Lateral wedging

Fig. 2.8 Denis' definitions of types of spinal fracture. (Adapted from Denis.[75])

felt that all burst fractures were unstable and required surgical instrumentation for stabilization. As every burst fracture required the same treatment, the five subdivisions were thought to be of little value.

The following year, McAfee et al simplified this system and was the first to describe a stable burst fracture: a fracture having anterior and middle column compression without posterior column disruption. The McAfee system of classifying acute traumatic spinal injuries is based on three forces (axial compression, axial distraction, and translation within the transverse plane) as they act to injure the middle column. Computed tomography can be used as a reliable method of identifying unstable burst fractures by illustrating facet joint subluxation or disruption of the neural arch.[76] With this system, vertebral augmentation would be appropriate for compression fractures, including stable burst fractures.

The AO (Arbeitsgemeinshaft fur Osteosynthesefragen) Classification is a highly detailed system published in 1994 by Magerl et al.[61] This Swiss system returns to a two-column model and remains the basis for modern fracture fixation. It classifies thoracolumbar fractures into three major groups based on the mechanism of injury: compression (type A), distraction (type B), and multidirectional with translation or torsion (type C). It takes into account the morphological appearance, the direction of the force or mechanism of injury, and increasing destruction of the injury.[77] Its comprehensive description includes the nature of injury, the degree of instability, and prognostic aspects that are important for choosing the most appropriate treatment.

The modified AO classification includes morphology of the fracture, neurological status, and description of relevant patient-specific modifiers (▶Fig. 2.9).[78] The fracture morphology is assessed based on three main injury patterns: type A0–A4 (compression injury to the VB without posterolateral ligamentous complex [PLC] involvement), type B1–B3 (tension band disruption—the failure of posterior [PLC] or anterior [anterior longitudinal ligament] constraints), and type C (translation injuries). Neurologic status is classified as follows: no neurologic injury (N0), transient (resolved) neurologic deficit (N1), radicular symptoms (N2), incomplete spinal cord injury or any degree of cauda equina injury (N3), complete spinal cord injury (N4), and unknown neurologic status (NX). Two modifiers were also included: M1 to indicate indeterminate posterolateral complex status and M2 to designate patient-specific comorbidity (that might preclude general anesthesia and surgery, such as ankylosing spondylitis or diffuse burns overlying the surgical approach).

Based on this classification, type A4 fractures (burst fracture or sagittal split involving both end plates) and B1–B3 and C injuries almost always require instrumented surgical stabilization for optimal outcome.[11] Vertebral augmentation may be indicated to treat type A injuries, specifically, A1.1, A1.2, A1.3, A2.1, A2.2, A2.3 and A3.1.

The Thoracolumbar Injury Classification and Severity Scale. (TLICS) was introduced in 2005 by the Spine Trauma Study Group (STSG; ▶Table 2.3). It has been validated and shown to have good reliability. It uses a composite scoring system based on the mechanism of injury (as determined by the morphology

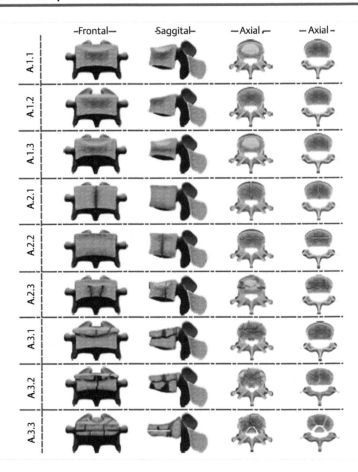

Fig. 2.9 AO classification system: type A fracture subclassifications.

Table 2.3 The Thoracolumbar Injury Classification System (TLICS)

Three independent predictors of TLICS				
1	Morphology Immediate stability	• Compression • Burst • Translation/rotation • Distraction	1 2 3 4	• Radiographs • CT
2	Integrity of PLC Long-term stability	• Intact • Suspected • Injured	0 2 3	• MRI
3	Neurological status	• Intact • Nerve root • Complete cord • Incomplete cord • Cauda equine	0 2 2 3 3	• Physical examination
Predicts		• Need for surgery	0–3 4 >4	• Nonsurgical • Surgeon's choice • Surgical

Abbreviations: CT, computed tomography; MRI, magnetic resonance imaging; PLC, posterior ligamentous complex.

on imaging), integrity of the posterior ligamentous complex, and neurological status of the patient.[79] Evaluation of the PLC requires MR imaging, a modality that has limited worldwide availability.[80] The TLICS is designed to assist in clinical management of thoracolumbar spine injuries and uses features important in predicting spinal stability, future deformity, and progressive neurologic compromise, as well as predicting appropriate treatment recommendations.[79,81] The three major morphologic descriptors are compression or burst, rotation/translation, and distraction. For compression injuries, the prefixes axial, flexion, or lateral more precisely describe the injury morphology.

A score of 3 or less, as with compression injuries, suggests a stable fracture, while a score of 5 or more suggests that surgical instrumentation for stabilization should be considered. This classification system also provides a guide for determining the optimal approach (anterior, posterior, and combined anteroposterior) for surgically treated patients based on the status of the posterior ligamentous complex and the patient's neurologic

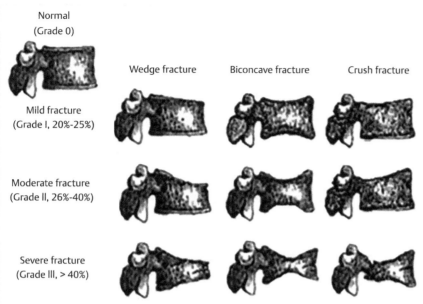

Normal
(Grade 0)

Wedge fracture   Biconcave fracture   Crush fracture

Mild fracture
(Grade I, 20%-25%)

Moderate fracture
(Grade II, 26%-40%)

Severe fracture
(Grade III, > 40%)

Fig. 2.10 Genant semiquantitative classification of osteoporotic vertebral fractures.

status. A score of 4 might be handled conservatively or surgically, according to the physician's judgment. A1, A2, and A3.1 fractures as classified by the AO system would be assigned 0 to 3 points using the TLICS system and vertebral augmentation would be included in the treatment options.

The systems described above were all designed to identify spinal instability and ultimately to guide treatment. The Genant semiquantitative method of classifying osteoporotic vertebral fractures was introduced in 1993 by Harry Genant, who noted[82]:

"Vertebral fractures are the most common consequence of osteoporosis, occurring in a substantial portion of the post-menopausal population. Most vertebral fractures, however, are not clinically recognized, and can accumulate silently. It is established that the presence of a vertebral fracture is a strong risk factor for subsequent osteoporotic fractures, and that those with low bone density and vertebral fractures are at highest risk."

Prior to the introduction of the Genant system, osteoporotic vertebral fractures were frequently underdiagnosed worldwide, with false-negative rates as high as 30% despite a strict radiographic protocol that provided an unambiguous vertebral fracture definition and minimized the influence of inadequate film quality. Failure was a global problem attributable to either the lack of radiographic detection or a use of ambiguous terminology in imaging reports. A standardized method for viewing and describing vertebral fractures was needed.[83]

The Genant classification system is based on height loss involving the anterior, posterior, and/or middle VB (▶ Fig. 2.10). In this semiquantitative assessment, each vertebra receives a severity grade based upon the degree of vertebral height loss. Unlike the other approaches, the type of the deformity (wedge, biconcavity, or compression) is not linked to grading. Thoracic and lumbar vertebrae from T4 to L4 are graded on visual inspection and without direct vertebral measurement as normal (grade 0), mildly deformed (grade 1: reduction of 20–25% of height over 10–20% of the vertebral area), moderately deformed (grade 2: reduction of 26–40% of height over 21–40%

of the vertebral area), or severely deformed (grade 3: reduction of >40% of height and vertebral area; grade 0.5 designates "borderline" vertebrae that show some deformation but cannot be clearly assigned as a grade 1 fracture.)

The Genant semiquantitative method has been tested and applied in a number of clinical drug trials and epidemiological studies.[82,84–87] The reproducibility of the method for the diagnosis of prevalent and incident vertebral fractures was found to be high, with intraobserver agreement of 93 to 99% and interobserver agreement of 90 to 99%. In experienced hands, the approach is both sensitive and specific.[87] A "spinal fracture index" can be calculated from this semiquantitative assessment as the sum of all grades assigned to the vertebrae divided by the number of the evaluated vertebrae. Loss of individual vertebral height can be assessed on serial imaging for a meaningful interpretation of follow-up radiographs.[7]

2.5 Treatment

The rationale for vertebral augmentation in stable vertebral fractures, regardless of etiology, is preservation or restoration of vertebral height, stabilization, or correction of kyphotic angulation and elimination of pain, allowing patients an early return to activity.

2.5.1 Osteoporotic Vertebral Compression Fractures

Prior to the introduction of vertebral augmentation procedures, management of patients with stable osteoporotic VCFs consisted primarily of rest, analgesic medications, and immobilization in an orthotic brace. Many of these patients develop disabling pain, deformity (kyphosis), and reduced pulmonary function. Additionally, bone loss in osteoporotic patients is accelerated by inactivity and may lead to continued and accelerated bone loss at a rate of up to 2% per week.[9]

Weight bearing is an important factor in preventing bone loss and is an important step toward halting or slowing progressive bone loss in the patients.[88–92] While medical management, including nonsteroidal anti-inflammatory drugs, calcitonin, teriparatide, abaloparatide, bisphosphonates, and parathyroid hormone have been shown to offer some benefit in pain control and function, medications do carry risks of side effects. For example, bisphosphonates have been associated with osteonecrosis of the jaw and atypical femoral fractures.

In geriatric patients with osteoporotic vertebral fractures, including those involving the posterior wall of the VB, kyphoplasty has been shown to be an effective procedure with only rare complications. Between 2002 and 2008, Krüger et al performed kyphoplasty on 97 patients, each with at least one AO classification A3.1 fracture. Ninety-seven patients (68 females; average age: 76.1 [59–98 years]) with involvement of the vertebra's posterior margin were treated by kyphoplasty. The fractures of 75 patients were caused by falls from little height, 5 patients had suffered traffic accidents, and in the case of 17 patients, no type of trauma was remembered. According to the AO classification, there were 109 A3.1.1 fractures and 1 A3.1.3 fracture. Prior to surgery, all patients were neurologically intact. Seventy-nine fractures were accompanied by a narrowing of the spinal canal with a mean degree of narrowing of 15% (10–40). Overall, 134 vertebrae were treated by balloon kyphoplasty (81 × 1 VB, 22 × 2 VB, 3 × 3 VB). Cement leakage was observed after surgery in 47.4% of patients but in every case, patients remained asymptomatic form the leakage. Using the Visual Analog Scale (VAS 1–10), patients stated that prior to surgery their pain averaged 8.1, whereas after surgery it significantly decreased and averaged 1.6 ($p < 0.001$).[93]

2.5.2 Pathologic Vertebral Fractures due to Neoplasia

In patients with pathologic fractures due to neoplasia, various types of medical, surgical, and radiologic oncology management are most often indicated for the primary disease. Treatment of pathologic fractures due to malignancy may include radiation, radiofrequency ablation, vertebral augmentation, and/or open surgical procedures to decompress neural elements, reduce tumor burden, and stabilize the spine.[94] Evidence has shown that vertebral augmentation dramatically reduces pain and improves quality of life.[95,96]

In a systematic review to assess the efficacy of kyphoplasty in controlling pain and improving quality of life in oncologic patients with metastatic spinal disease or MM and pathologic compression fractures of the spine, Astur and Avanzi found moderate evidence that patients treated with balloon kyphoplasty displayed better scores for pain (Numeric Pain Rating Scale), disability (Roland–Morris Disability Questionnaire), quality of life (Short Form 36 [SF-36] Health Survey), and functional status (Karnofsky Performance Status) compared with those undergoing the conventional treatment. Patients treated with kyphoplasty also have better recovery of vertebral height.

The control group was any other treatment modality. This study concluded that balloon kyphoplasty could be considered as an early treatment option for patients with symptomatic neoplastic spinal disease, and called for further randomized clinical trials (RCTs) to improve the quality of evidence.[97]

An earlier RCT compared balloon kyphoplasty with nonsurgical management (NSM) and allowed an optional crossover at 1 month after enrollment and included patients with various neoplastic disorders including MM and breast, lung, and prostate cancers. They found statistically significant improvements in the patients' pain, function, and quality of life as measured by the Numeric Rating Scale, the Roland–Morris Disability Questionnaire, and the SF-36 Health Survey, respectively. There was either no change in quality of life and activity or minimal change in back pain in the NSM patients. Seventy-three percent of the patients who initially received NSM crossed over to balloon kyphoplasty and 55% of these patients crossed over within on1 week of their 1-month follow-up visit. They concluded that balloon kyphoplasty provided better results than NSM at 1 month in all measures and these improvements seen at 1 month were generally sustained at 1 year. They also concluded the balloon kyphoplasty was safe for use in patients with neoplastic VB involvement as the number of patients with adverse events was similar between the balloon kyphoplasty and NSM groups.

2.5.3 Traumatic Vertebral Fractures

Importantly, no system used to classify traumatic vertebral fractures addresses sagittal balance or persistent clinical ailments. The most frequently used classifications in traumatic vertebral fracture assessment are AO and TLICS. Using the AO classification scale, injuries classified as A1, A2 (except for pincer fractures: A2.3), and A3.1 are stable and may be treated with vertebral augmentation. Specifically, A1.1, A1.2, A1.3, A2.1, A2.2, and A3.1 may be safely treated with vertebral augmentation. According to the TLICS system, these same fractures are estimated as 3 or less points, do not require surgical instrumentation for stabilization, and are amenable to treatment with vertebral augmentation.

In fractures amenable to vertebral augmentation, Chen et al. found significant reductions in hospitalization time and mortality in patients treated with vertebral augmentation as compared with those patients treated with NSM.[1] A more recent study showed slightly longer hospitalization but greater discharge to home for augmented patients as compared to much higher rates of discharge to long-term care facilities in the patients treated with NSM.[6] Recent Medicare claims–based analyses of over 1 million VCF patients with 5- to 10-year follow-up, performed with propensity score matching to account for selection bias, concluded that there was a highly statistically significant reduction of both morbidity and mortality in patients treated with vertebral augmentation as compared to those treated with NSM.[3,6] In these analyses comparing NSM to vertebral augmentation, NSM patients had significantly higher rates of pneumonia, deep venous thrombosis, cardiac complications, and urinary tract infections.[3,6]

Treatment of symptomatic VCFs with vertebral augmentation (vertebroplasty or kyphoplasty) has been shown in various studies to be a cost-effective intervention that both decreases pain and improves survival.[98–100]

2.6 Public Health and Economic Impact

2.6.1 Osteoporosis

Osteoporosis and associated osteoporotic fractures have a profound economic burden and public health impact. The number of osteoporotic fractures diagnosed annually may, in fact, be a gross underestimate given, as has been mentioned previously, that only an estimated one-third of all vertebral fractures are clinically diagnosed.[33] This impacts the reimbursement strategies of payers, influences policy makers in the public health sector, and encourages the pharmaceutical companies to conduct clinical trials for new agents to reduce fracture risk.[101]

More recent data suggest that osteoporotic VCFs affect up to one million persons in the United States annually, and 25% of woman in their lifetime.[20,102] A retrospective analysis using the Premier Perspective Database (now Premier Healthcare Database) revealed that among *all* osteoporosis-related fracture admissions for the years 2010 to 2013, the mean hospital cost was $12,839 (95% confidence interval [CI]) and the mean length of stay (LOS) was 5.1 days. During the admission, 7.4% of the patients were sent to the intensive care unit and the mortality rate was 1.5% with an additional or adjacent fracture occurring in 2.3% of the patients during the 60-day postdischarge period[103] The majority of costs are incurred by inpatient care, long-term care facilities, and then outpatient care in that order.[32] In the year following a fracture, medical and hospitalization costs were 1.6 to 6.2 times higher than prefracture costs and 2.2 to 3.5 times higher than those for matched controls with costs totaling up to $71,000 for a hip fracture and up to $68,000 for a vertebral fracture.[104] Medicare pays for approximately 80% of these costs.[32] In addition to the medical costs, there are other significant indirect costs that include reduced productivity due to disability, reduced earnings, and premature death.[105] The cost of care of osteoporosis, in part due to an aging population, is expected to rise to $25.3 billion by 2025.[32]

2.6.2 Cancer

Patients with bone metastasis secondary to prostate or breast cancer or MM are predisposed to skeletal-related events (SREs), including surgery or radiation to the spinal column, pathologic fractures, and spinal cord compression. Barlev et al examined costs from a payer perspective for SRE-associated hospitalizations among patients with MM or bone metastasis secondary to prostate or breast cancer.[106] Patients with SRE hospitalizations were selected from the MarketScan commercial and Medicare databases (from January 1, 2003, through June 30, 2009). Sampled patients had on the average at least two medical claims with primary or secondary ICD-9-CM diagnosis codes for prostate cancer, breast cancer, or MM, and at least one subsequent hospitalization with principal diagnosis or procedure codes indicating bone surgery, pathologic fracture, or spinal cord compression. A total of 555 patients had 572 hospitalizations. The mean age range was 61 to 72 years, and the range of mean LOS per admission was from 5.9 to 11.6 days. The range of

mean health plan payment per hospital admission across tumor types was $22,390 to 26,936 for pathologic fracture without spinal cord compression.[106]

2.6.3 Trauma

When considering the estimated costs of hospital care and outpatient visits for patients with traumatic thoracolumbar spine fractures, one must remember that, although the LOS for patients treated operatively may be shorter than those treated nonoperatively, the total costs, including surgical expenses, may be higher. Cost-effectiveness then becomes central. That is, surgery must offer a better outcome for the increased cost. Outcomes must be factored into the analysis for a reliable cost-effective value. Unstable fractures and those with neurologic impairment may require surgical treatment, extensive rehabilitative services, and these patients often develop long-term disability.[107]

Siebenga et al compared surgical versus nonsurgical treatment for management of individuals with traumatic thoracolumbar spine fractures. This study included direct costs, general-practitioner visit and absenteeism costs, and private health care expenditures. The study included individuals with traumatic thoracolumbar spine fractures (T10–L4 fractures without neurological deficit) treated between 1998 and 2003 in a single European institution. Mean direct costs during this time period for the surgical treatment (US$ 21,960) were significantly higher than those for the conservative management (US$ 11,880). However, the general-practitioner visit costs, private expenditures, and absenteeism costs for the surgical group (US$ 13, US$ 550, and US$ 6630, respectively) were significantly lower than those for the nonsurgical group (US$ 34, US$ 816, and US$ 10,329, respectively).[108]

The Nationwide Emergency Department Sample (NEDS) is a set of hospital-based emergency department databases included in the Healthcare Cost and Utilization Project (HCUP) family. These databases are created by the Agency for Healthcare Research and Quality (AHRQ) through a Federal-State-Industry partnership. Based on the HCUP Nationwide Inpatient Sample (NIS) and NEDS databases queried, there were an estimated 795,300 hospital discharges and emergency department visits for spinal fractures in the United States in 2010–2011. The great majority of spinal fracture patients (773,000, or 97%) were treated for osteoporotic or pathologic VCFs with little or no trauma. Nearly half of discharges and visits for VCFs were for patients 75 years and older and 58% were females.[107] Traumatic fractures were far less common, with 27,100 (3%) hospital discharges or outpatient visits reported. Numbers were too small for reliable reporting in the National Center for Health Statistics (NCHS) databases, which include outpatient and physician office visits. These fractures predominantly involved men (~60%) and were most likely to involve patients between the ages of 18 and 44 years.[107]

The average LOS for patients with a spine fracture diagnosis was 6.8 days and the average charge was $69,500. For patients with traumatic spinal fractures, the average hospital stay was more than twice as long as for osteoporotic/pathologic VCFs (14 vs. 6.6 days), and average charges three times as high ($197,700 vs. 65,700). Differences in LOS and charges were shown to be greater for those younger than 45 years (▶ Fig. 2.11).

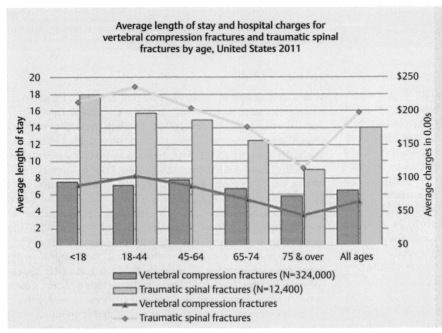

Fig. 2.11 Average length of stay and hospital charges for osteoporotic VCFs and traumatic spinal fractures by age in the United States, 2011. Source: United States Bone and Joint Initiative: The Burden of Musculoskeletal Diseases in the United States (BMUS), Third Edition, 2014. Rosemont, IL. Available at http://www.boneandjointburden.org. Accessed on [8/12/2018].

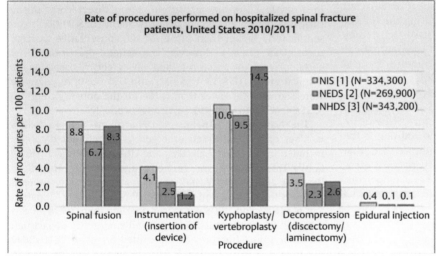

Fig. 2.12 Inpatient procedures for spinal fractures in the United States, 2010/2011. Source: United States Bone and Joint Initiative: The Burden of Musculoskeletal Diseases in the United States (BMUS), Third Edition, 2014. Rosemont, IL. Available at http://www.boneandjointburden.org. Accessed on [8/12/2018].

Only a small proportion of patients hospitalized with any spinal fracture undergo surgery (▶Fig. 2.12). According to the NIS database, fusion (8.8%) and vertebral augmentation (kyphoplasty or vertebroplasty, 10.6%) are the most common procedures performed. Similar rates of procedures were found in the NEDS hospitalized patients and National Hospital Discharge Survey (NHDS) databases. Of patients discharged with the diagnosis of VCF, only 12% were treated with kyphoplasty or vertebroplasty. These patients were twice as likely to be female, and were most likely to be 65 years or older. The majority of spinal fusion procedures were performed on patients younger than 44 years with traumatic fractures.[107]

2.6.4 Cost-Effectiveness

Cost-effectiveness analysis is a way of determining the value of an intervention.

Determining an acceptable cost-effectiveness threshold, that is, the amount we are willing to pay for an intervention, is a value judgment. Patients may have different thresholds than payers. Garber and Phelps suggest that "most, but not all, decision makers in the United States will conclude that interventions that cost less than $50,000 to $60,000 per quality-adjusted life year (QALY) gained are reasonably efficient."[109,110]

In 2013, Borse performed cost–utility analysis of balloon kyphoplasty and vertebroplasty, the two most commonly employed augmentation procedures used to treat osteoporotic VCFs. The cost–utility ratio for vertebroplasty was $34,688 per QALY gained and that for a balloon kyphoplasty was $32,767 per QALY gained. In an incremental comparison between kyphoplasty and vertebroplasty, balloon kyphoplasty was more cost-effective when compared to vertebroplasty.[111]

For additional information regarding the cost-effectiveness of vertebral augmentation refer to Chapter 16: Cost-Effectiveness of Vertebral Augmentation.

2.7 Conclusion

VCFs can lead to severe pain, physical limitation and disability, and increased morbidity and mortality. In patients with conditions such as osteoporosis or malignancy, pathologic weakening of the bone allows even the most minor trauma to result in fractures. These fractures are very common and the public health and economic impact is considerable. The most common causes of vertebral fractures are osteoporosis, metastatic disease, MM, and trauma. Regardless of etiology, timely and accurate diagnosis is essential to determine the appropriate treatments.

Trauma patients with injuries leading to an unstable spine must be treated rapidly and with great attention to mechanism of injury, the type of injury, and the treatment necessary to adequately protect the spine. It is equally important to provide an accurate and timely diagnosis in patients with metastatic malignancies to the spine and in elderly patients with osteoporotic VCFs. One must consider all safe treatment options and the implications and literature evidence supporting these options. Conservative therapy often consists simply of rest and optimal pain management, but care must be taken to avoid dismissing the effects of pain and the side effects or lack of efficacy of medical management. Importantly, bed rest in an osteoporotic patient may accelerate bone loss, worsen the patient's functional status, and significantly increase their chances of morbidity and mortality.

Given the social, public health, and economic impact of osteoporotic VCFs, it is imperative to understand the natural history of osteoporosis and invest not only in the interventional treatment of these fractures but also in the prevention of future fractures by treating the underlying condition of osteoporosis and in education of the patient of their underlying disease process that produced the osteoporotic fracture. When a compression fracture is secondary to osteoporosis, the physician should explain what osteoporosis is, why the patient likely has it, and how to best treat their condition, and to make sure that the patient receives treatment by either the physician that performs the vertebral augmentation or an osteoporosis specialty clinic. This is a treatment pathway that will optimize the patient's bone health and reduce or prevent future fragility fractures. In addition to optimizing treatment, it is important that the patient understand the importance of bone health and the benefits of lifestyle modification such as adequate intake of calcium and vitamin D as well as exercise and fall prevention.

Vertebral augmentation offers safe and durable pain relief and an opportunity to significantly improve quality of life with an excellent risk–benefit ratio across a wide range of etiologies.

References

[1] Chen AT, Cohen DB, Skolasky RL. Impact of nonoperative treatment, vertebroplasty, and kyphoplasty on survival and morbidity after vertebral compression fracture in the medicare population. J Bone Joint Surg Am 2013;95(19): 1729–1736

[2] Zampini JM, White AP, McGuire KJ. Comparison of 5766 vertebral compression fractures treated with or without kyphoplasty. Clin Orthop Relat Res 2010;468(7):1773–1780

[3] Edidin AA, Ong KL, Lau E, Kurtz SM. Morbidity and mortality after vertebral fractures: comparison of vertebral augmentation and nonoperative management in the Medicare population. Spine 2015;40(15):1228–1241

[4] Lange A, Kasperk C, Alvares L, Sauermann S, Braun S. Survival and cost comparison of kyphoplasty and percutaneous vertebroplasty using German claims data. Spine 2014;39(4):318–326

[5] Silverman SL. The clinical consequences of vertebral compression fracture. Bone 1992;13(Suppl 2):S27–S31

[6] Ong KL, Beall DP, Frohbergh M, Lau E, Hirsch JA. Were VCF patients at higher risk of mortality following the 2009 publication of the vertebroplasty "sham" trials? Osteoporos Int 2018;29(2):375–383

[7] Grigoryan M, Guermazi A, Roemer FW, Delmas PD, Genant HK. Recognizing and reporting osteoporotic vertebral fractures. Eur Spine J 2003;12(Suppl 2):S104–S112

[8] Assessment of fracture risk and its application to screening for postmenopausal osteoporosis. Report of a WHO Study Group. World Health Organ Tech Rep Ser 1994;843:1–129

[9] Kado DM, Browner WS, Palermo L, Nevitt MC, Genant HK, Cummings SR; Study of Osteoporotic Fractures Research Group. Vertebral fractures and mortality in older women: a prospective study. Arch Intern Med 1999;159(11):1215–1220

[10] Baaj AA, Downes K, Vaccaro AR, Uribe JS, Vale FL. Trends in the treatment of lumbar spine fractures in the United States: a socioeconomics perspective: clinical article. J Neurosurg Spine 2011;15(4):367–370

[11] Rajasekaran S, Kanna RM, Shetty AP. Management of thoracolumbar spine trauma: an overview. Indian J Orthop 2015;49(1):72–82

[12] Wood KB, Li W, Lebl DR, Ploumis A. Management of thoracolumbar spine fractures. Spine J 2014;14(1):145–164

[13] el-Khoury GY, Whitten CG. Trauma to the upper thoracic spine: anatomy, biomechanics, and unique imaging features. AJR Am J Roentgenol 1993;160(1):95–102

[14] Gertzbein SD. Scoliosis Research Society. Multicenter spine fracture study. Spine 1992;17(5):528–540

[15] Harrison RA, Siminoski K, Vethanayagam D, Majumdar SR. Osteoporosis-related kyphosis and impairments in pulmonary function: a systematic review. J Bone Miner Res 2007;22(3):447–457

[16] Cosman F, de Beur SJ, LeBoff MS, et al; National Osteoporosis Foundation. Clinician's guide to prevention and treatment of osteoporosis. Osteoporos Int 2014;25(10):2359–2381

[17] Lindsay R, Silverman SL, Cooper C, et al. Risk of new vertebral fracture in the year following a fracture. JAMA 2001;285(3):320–323

[18] Ensrud KE, Schousboe JT. Clinical practice. Vertebral fractures. N Engl J Med 2011;364(17):1634–1642

[19] Felsenberg D, Silman AJ, Lunt M, et al; European Prospective Osteoporosis Study (EPOS) Group. Incidence of vertebral fracture in europe: results from the European Prospective Osteoporosis Study (EPOS). J Bone Miner Res 2002;17(4):716–724

[20] Riggs BL, Melton LJ III. The worldwide problem of osteoporosis: insights afforded by epidemiology. Bone 1995;17(5, Suppl):505S–511S

[21] NIH Consensus Development Panel on Osteoporosis Prevention, Diagnosis, and Therapy, March 7–29, 2000: highlights of the conference. South Med J 2001;94(6):569–573

[22] Heaney RP, Abrams S, Dawson-Hughes B, et al. Peak bone mass. Osteoporos Int 2000;11(12):985–1009

[23] Ballane G, Cauley JA, Luckey MM, El-Hajj Fuleihan G. Worldwide prevalence and incidence of osteoporotic vertebral fractures. Osteoporos Int 2017;28(5):1531–1542

[24] Prevention and Management of Osteoporosis: report of a WHO Scientific Group. Paper presented at WHO Scientific Group on the Prevention and Management of Osteoporosis2000; Geneva, Switzerland

[25] Wright NC, Saag KG, Dawson-Hughes B, Khosla S, Siris ES. The impact of the new National Bone Health Alliance (NBHA) diagnostic criteria on the prevalence of osteoporosis in the United States: supplementary presentation. Osteoporos Int 2017;28(11):3283–3284

[26] Cosman F, Krege JH, Looker AC, et al. Spine fracture prevalence in a nationally representative sample of US women and men aged ≥40 years: results from the National Health and Nutrition Examination Survey (NHANES) 2013–2014. Osteoporos Int 2017;28(6):1857–1866

[27] Wong CC, McGirt MJ. Vertebral compression fractures: a review of current management and multimodal therapy. J Multidiscip Healthc 2013; 6:205–214

[28] Francis RM, Baillie SP, Chuck AJ, et al. Acute and long-term management of patients with vertebral fractures. QJM 2004;97(2):63–74

[29] Nevitt MC, Cummings SR, Stone KL, et al. Risk factors for a first-incident radiographic vertebral fracture in women > or = 65 years of age: the study of osteoporotic fractures. J Bone Miner Res 2005;20(1):131–140

[30] Melton LJ III, Lane AW, Cooper C, Eastell R, O'Fallon WM, Riggs BL. Prevalence and incidence of vertebral deformities. Osteoporos Int 1993;3(3):113–119

[31] O'Neill TW, Felsenberg D, Varlow J, Cooper C, Kanis JA, Silman AJ. The prevalence of vertebral deformity in european men and women: the European Vertebral Osteoporosis Study. J Bone Miner Res 1996;11(7):1010–1018

[32] Burge R, Dawson-Hughes B, Solomon DH, Wong JB, King A, Tosteson A. Incidence and economic burden of osteoporosis-related fractures in the United States, 2005–2025. J Bone Miner Res 2007;22(3):465–475

[33] Cooper C, Atkinson EJ, O'Fallon WM, Melton LJ III. Incidence of clinically diagnosed vertebral fractures: a population-based study in Rochester, Minnesota, 1985–1989. J Bone Miner Res 1992;7(2):221–227

[34] Cho JH, Ha JK, Hwang CJ, Lee DH, Lee CS. Patterns of treatment for metastatic pathological fractures of the spine: the efficacy of each treatment modality. Clin Orthop Surg 2015;7(4):476–482

[35] Saad F, Lipton A, Cook R, Chen YM, Smith M, Coleman R. Pathologic fractures correlate with reduced survival in patients with malignant bone disease. Cancer 2007;110(8):1860–1867

[36] Beall DP, Chambers MR, Thomas S, et al. Prospective and multicenter evaluation of outcomes for quality of life and activities of daily living for balloon kyphoplasty in the treatment of vertebral compression fractures: the EVOLVE Trial. Neurosurgery 2019;84(1):169–178

[37] Siegel RL, Miller KD, Jemal A. Cancer statistics, 2015. CA Cancer J Clin 2015;65(1):5–29

[38] Mitsiades CS, Mitsiades N, Munshi NC, Anderson KC. Focus on multiple myeloma. Cancer Cell 2004;6(5):439–444

[39] Anitha D, Baum T, Kirschke JS, Subburaj K. Risk of vertebral compression fractures in multiple myeloma patients: a finite-element study. Medicine (Baltimore) 2017;96(2):e5825

[40] Howlader N, Noone A, Krapcho M. SEER Cancer Statistics Review, 1975–2013. 2016. http://seer.cancer.gov/csr/1975_2013/

[41] Edwards BJ, Langman CB, Bunta AD, Vicuna M, Favus M. Secondary contributors to bone loss in osteoporosis related hip fractures. Osteoporos Int 2008;19(7):991–999

[42] Anselmetti GC, Manca A, Montemurro F, et al. Percutaneous vertebroplasty in multiple myeloma: prospective long-term follow-up in 106 consecutive patients. Cardiovasc Intervent Radiol 2012;35(1):139–145

[43] Mirza F, Canalis E. Management of endocrine disease: secondary osteoporosis: pathophysiology and management. Eur J Endocrinol 2015;173(3):R131–R151

[44] Pittari G, Costi D, Raballo M, Maulucci L, Baroni MC, Mangoni M. Intravenous neridronate for skeletal damage treatment in patients with multiple myeloma. Acta Biomed 2006;77(2):81–84

[45] Tipples K, Robinson A. Optimal management of cancer treatment-induced bone loss: considerations for elderly patients. Drugs Aging 2011;28(11):867–883

[46] Sezer O. Myeloma bone disease: recent advances in biology, diagnosis, and treatment. Oncologist 2009;14(3):276–283

[47] Faiman B, Licata AA. New tools for detecting occult monoclonal gammopathy, a cause of secondary osteoporosis. Cleve Clin J Med 2010;77(4):273–278

[48] Layton KF, Thielen KR, Cloft HJ, Kallmes DF. Acute vertebral compression fractures in patients with multiple myeloma: evaluation of vertebral body edema patterns on MR imaging and the implications for vertebroplasty. AJNR Am J Neuroradiol 2006;27(8):1732–1734

[49] Kanis JA. Diagnosis of osteoporosis and assessment of fracture risk. Lancet 2002;359(9321):1929–1936

[50] Golombick T, Diamond T. Prevalence of monoclonal gammopathy of undetermined significance/myeloma in patients with acute osteoporotic vertebral fractures. Acta Haematol 2008;120(2):87–90

[51] Weiss BM, Abadie J, Verma P, Howard RS, Kuehl WM. A monoclonal gammopathy precedes multiple myeloma in most patients. Blood 2009;113(22):5418–5422

[52] Tosi P. Diagnosis and treatment of bone disease in multiple myeloma: spotlight on spinal involvement. Scientifica (Cairo) 2013;2013:104546

[53] Coleman R. Skeletal Complications of Malignancy. Skeletal Complications of Malignancy Symposium, Bethesda, MD; 1997

[54] Borggrefe J, Giravent S, Thomsen F, et al. Association of QCT bone mineral density and bone structure with vertebral fractures in patients with multiple myeloma. J Bone Miner Res 2015;30(7):1329–1337

[55] Anitha D, Kim KJ, Lim SK, Lee T. Implications of local osteoporosis on the efficacy of anti-resorptive drug treatment: a 3-year follow-up finite element study in risedronate-treated women. Osteoporos Int 2013;24(12):3043–3051

[56] British Committee for Standards in Haematology in Conjunction with the UK Myeloma Forum(UKMF). Guidelines on the Diagnosis and Management of Multiple Myeloma. 2010. http://www.bcshguidelines.com/. Accessed May 1, 2018

[57] Mulligan M, Chirindel A, Karchevsky M. Characterizing and predicting pathologic spine fractures in myeloma patients with FDG PET/CT and MR imaging. Cancer Invest 2011;29(5):370–376

[58] Singh A, Tetreault L, Kalsi-Ryan S, Nouri A, Fehlings MG. Global prevalence and incidence of traumatic spinal cord injury. Clin Epidemiol 2014;6:309–331

[59] Hu R, Mustard CA, Burns C. Epidemiology of incident spinal fracture in a complete population. Spine 1996;21(4):492–499

[60] Gertzbein SD, Khoury D, Bullington A, St John TA, Larson AI. Thoracic and lumbar fractures associated with skiing and snowboarding injuries according to the AO comprehensive classification. Am J Sports Med 2012;40(8):1750–1754

[61] Magerl F, Aebi M, Gertzbein SD, Harms J, Nazarian S. A comprehensive classification of thoracic and lumbar injuries. Eur Spine J 1994;3(4):184–201

[62] Kraemer WJ, Schemitsch EH, Lever J, McBroom RJ, McKee MD, Waddell JP. Functional outcome of thoracolumbar burst fractures without neurological deficit. J Orthop Trauma 1996;10(8):541–544

[63] Knop C, Blauth M, Bühren V, et al. Surgical treatment of injuries of the thoracolumbar transition. 1: epidemiology Unfallchirurg 1999;102(12):924–935

[64] Benson DR, Burkus JK, Montesano PX, Sutherland TB, McLain RF. Unstable thoracolumbar and lumbar burst fractures treated with the AO fixateur interne. J Spinal Disord 1992;5(3):335–343

[65] McLain RF, Sparling E, Benson DR. Early failure of short-segment pedicle instrumentation for thoracolumbar fractures. A preliminary report. J Bone Joint Surg Am 1993;75(2):162–167

[66] Maynard FM Jr, Bracken MB, Creasey G, et al; American Spinal Injury Association. International Standards for Neurological and Functional Classification of Spinal Cord Injury. Spinal Cord 1997;35(5):266–274

[67] Watson-Jones R. The results of postural reduction of fractures of the spine. J Bone Joint Surg 1938;20:567–586

[68] Nicoll EA. Fractures of the dorso-lumbar spine. J Bone Joint Surg Br 1949;31B(3):376–394

[69] Holdsworth F. Fractures, dislocations, and fracture-dislocations of the spine. J Bone Joint Surg 1963;45:6

[70] Holdsworth F. Fractures, dislocations, and fracture-dislocations of the spine. J Bone Joint Surg Am 1970;52(8):1534–1551

[71] Panjabi MM. The stabilizing system of the spine. Part I. Function, dysfunction, adaptation, and enhancement. J Spinal Disord 1992;5(4):383–389, discussion 397

[72] White AA III, Johnson RM, Panjabi MM, Southwick WO. Biomechanical analysis of clinical stability in the cervical spine. Clin Orthop Relat Res 1975(109):85–96

[73] Allen BL Jr, Ferguson RL, Lehmann TR, O'Brien RP. A mechanistic classification of closed, indirect fractures and dislocations of the lower cervical spine. Spine 1982;7(1):1–27

[74] Denis F. Updated classification of thoracolumbar fractures. Orthopaedic Transactions 1982;6:8–9

[75] Denis F. The three column spine and its significance in the classification of acute thoracolumbar spinal injuries. Spine 1983;8(8):817–831

[76] McAfee PC, Yuan HA, Fredrickson BE, Lubicky JP. The value of computed tomography in thoracolumbar fractures. An analysis of one hundred consecutive cases and a new classification. J Bone Joint Surg Am 1983;65(4):461–473

[77] Gomleksiz C, Egemen E, Senturk S, et al. Thoracolumbar fractures: a review of classifications and surgical methods. J Spine 2015;4:250

[78] Vaccaro AR, Oner C, Kepler CK, et al; AOSpine Spinal Cord Injury & Trauma Knowledge Forum. AOSpine thoracolumbar spine injury classification system: fracture description, neurological status, and key modifiers. Spine 2013;38(23):2028–2037

[79] Lee JY, Vaccaro AR, Lim MR, et al. Thoracolumbar injury classification and severity score: a new paradigm for the treatment of thoracolumbar spine trauma. J Orthop Sci 2005;10(6):671–675

[80] Kepler CK, Vaccaro AR, Schroeder GD, et al. The Thoracolumbar AOSpine Injury Score. Global Spine J 2016;6(4):329–334

[81] West C, Roosendaal S, Bot J, Smithuis F. Spine Injury—TLICS Classification: Thoraco-Lumbar Injury Classification and Severity. http://www.radiologyassistant.nl/en

[82] Genant HK, Wu CY, van Kuijk C, Nevitt MC. Vertebral fracture assessment using a semiquantitative technique. J Bone Miner Res 1993;8(9):1137–1148

[83] Delmas PD, van de Langerijt L, Watts NB, et al; IMPACT Study Group. Under-diagnosis of vertebral fractures is a worldwide problem: the IMPACT study. J Bone Miner Res 2005;20(4):557–563

[84] Heuck AF, Block J, Glueer CC, Steiger P, Genant HK. Mild versus definite osteo-porosis: comparison of bone densitometry techniques using different statis-tical models. J Bone Miner Res 1989;4(6):891–900

[85] Storm T, Thamsborg G, Steiniche T, Genant HK, Sørensen OH. Effect of inter-mittent cyclical etidronate therapy on bone mass and fracture rate in women with postmenopausal osteoporosis. N Engl J Med 1990;322(18):1265–1271

[86] Watts NB, Harris ST, Genant HK, et al. Intermittent cyclical etidronate treat-ment of postmenopausal osteoporosis. N Engl J Med 1990;323(2):73–79

[87] Wu CY, Li J, Jergas M, Genant HK. Comparison of semiquantitative and quan-titative techniques for the assessment of prevalent and incident vertebral fractures. Osteoporos Int 1995;5(5):354–370

[88] Palombaro KM. Effects of walking-only interventions on bone miner-al density at various skeletal sites: a meta-analysis. J Geriatr Phys Ther 2005;28(3):102–107

[89] Brown CJ, Friedkin RJ, Inouye SK. Prevalence and outcomes of low mobility in hospitalized older patients. J Am Geriatr Soc 2004;52(8):1263–1270

[90] Creditor MC. Hazards of hospitalization of the elderly. Ann Intern Med 1993;118(3):219–223

[91] Hoenig HM, Rubenstein LZ. Hospital-associated deconditioning and dysfunc-tion. J Am Geriatr Soc 1991;39(2):220–222

[92] Harper CM, Lyles YM. Physiology and complications of bed rest. J Am Geriatr Soc 1988;36(11):1047–1054

[93] Krüger A, Zettl R, Ziring E, Mann D, Schnabel M, Ruchholtz S. Kyphoplasty for the treatment of incomplete osteoporotic burst fractures. Eur Spine J 2010;19(6):893–900

[94] Schuster JM, Grady MS. Medical management and adjuvant therapies in spi-nal metastatic disease. Neurosurg Focus 2001;11(6):e3

[95] Genev IK, Tobin MK, Zaidi SP, Khan SR, Amirouche FML, Mehta AI. Spinal com-pression fracture management: a review of current treatment strategies and possible future avenues. Global Spine J 2017;7(1):71–82

[96] Berenson J, Pflugmacher R, Jarzem P, et al; Cancer Patient Fracture Evalua-tion (CAFE) Investigators. Balloon kyphoplasty versus non-surgical fracture management for treatment of painful vertebral body compression fractures in patients with cancer: a multicentre, randomised controlled trial. Lancet Oncol 2011;12(3):225–235

[97] Astur N, Avanzi O. Balloon kyphoplasty in the treatment of neoplastic spne lesions: a systematic review. Global Spine J 2019;9(3):348–356

[98] Svedbom A, Alvares L, Cooper C, Marsh D, Ström O. Balloon kyphop-lasty compared to vertebroplasty and nonsurgical management in patients hospitalised with acute osteoporotic vertebral compression fracture: a UK cost-effectiveness analysis. Osteoporos Int 2013;24(1): 355–367

[99] Garfin SR, Reilley MA. Minimally invasive treatment of osteoporotic vertebral body compression fractures. Spine J 2002;2(1):76–80

[100] Edidin AA, Ong KL, Lau E, Kurtz SM. Mortality risk for operated and nonoper-ated vertebral fracture patients in the medicare population. J Bone Miner Res 2011;26(7):1617–1626

[101] Siris ES, Adler R, Bilezikian J, et al. The clinical diagnosis of osteoporosis: a position statement from the National Bone Health Alliance Working Group. Osteoporos Int 2014;25(5):1439–1443

[102] Edidin AA, Ong KL, Lau E, Kurtz SM. Life expectancy following diagnosis of a vertebral compression fracture. Osteoporos Int 2013;24(2):451–458

[103] Weycker D, Li X, Barron R, Bornheimer R, Chandler D. Hospitalizations for osteoporosis-related fractures: economic costs and clinical outcomes. Bone Rep 2016;5:186–191

[104] Budhia S, Mikyas Y, Tang M, Badamgarav E. Osteoporotic fractures: a system-atic review of U.S. healthcare costs and resource utilization. Pharmacoeco-nomics 2012;30(2):147–170

[105] Office of the Surgeon General. Bone Health and Osteoporosis: A Report of the Surgeon General. Rockville, MD: Office of the Surgeon General (US); 2004

[106] Barlev A, Song X, Ivanov B, Setty V, Chung K. Payer costs for inpatient treatment of pathologic fracture, surgery to bone, and spinal cord com-pression among patients with multiple myeloma or bone metastasis secondary to prostate or breast cancer. J Manag Care Pharm 2010;16(9): 693–702

[107] The Burden of Musculoskeletal Diseases in the United States(BMUS). Paper presented at United States Bone and Joint Initiative, Rosemont, IL; 2014

[108] Siebenga J, Segers MJ, Leferink VJ, et al. Cost-effectiveness of the treatment of traumatic thoracolumbar spine fractures: nonsurgical or surgical therapy? Indian J Orthop 2007;41(4):332–336

[109] Owens DK. Interpretation of cost-effectiveness analyses. J Gen Intern Med 1998;13(10):716–717

[110] Garber AM, Phelps CE. Economic foundations of cost-effectiveness analysis. J Health Econ 1997;16(1):1–31

[111] Borse MS. Cost utility analysis of balloon kyphoplasty and vertebroplasty in the treatment of vertebral compression fractures in the United States. Theses and Dissertations: University of Toledo: Toledo, OH; 2013

3 Preprocedure Assessment Prior to Vertebral Augmentation

Scott Kreiner and Grace Maloney

Summary

Vertebral compression fractures (VCFs) are common and are increasing in number with the aging of the population. Patients with VCFs are optimally treated by accurate and early diagnosis and treatment. The patients with asymptomatic fractures must be recognized to be different than those with fractures and moderate to severe pain or pain that is increasing as the latter patients typically are not effectively treated with nonsurgical management (NSM). Correct identification of VCFs via cross-sectional imaging is important and the preprocedure assessment includes such factors as risks, cost, and the patient's ability to tolerate NSM or percutaneous vertebral augmentation (PVA). If the patient is provisionally deemed to be a candidate for PVA, there should be an assessment of the indications and contraindications. The ideal candidate for vertebral augmentation is a patient with a symptomatic fracture seen on cross sectional imaging than cannot tolerate NSM and has positive physical examination signs and no absolute contraindication. The PVA procedure should be done with the appropriate equipment and personnel and in a facility designed to accommodate these procedures. After the augmentation procedure the patient should undergo the appropriate follow-up to ensure the optimal recovery from both the fracture and the procedure and they should also receive appropriate therapy for the underlying disorder that originally predisposed them to the vertebral fracture.

Keywords: vertebral compression fracture, percutaneous vertebral augmentation, contraindications, preprocedure assessment, sedation, postprocedure management

3.1 Introduction

Vertebral compression fractures are common and becoming more common as our population ages. Appropriate early diagnosis and management is key to obtaining optimal outcomes for these patients. While many patients have fractures that are only incidentally seen on imaging at some point after the fracture, the presence of a single compression fracture substantially increases the risk for future fractures. In addition to the commonly seen asymptomatic fracture, there is a prominent subset of patients that present with moderate to severe pain that does not resolve with NSM. For these reasons, early identification and optimal management of compression fractures improve outcomes in these patients.

3.2 Anatomy, Radiologic Imaging, Identification, and Interpretation of Vertebral Compression Fractures

Selection of appropriate patients for PVA is essential to obtaining optimal outcomes. Traditionally, the patient populations considered to benefit most from PVA generally fall into three categories as follows: elderly osteoporotic individuals with acute or subacute VCFs, individuals with compression fractures refractory to NSM, and individuals with compression fractures secondary to malignancy.

Chronicity of a VCF is an important factor to consider when considering PVA. While patients with older painful fractures commonly derive substantial benefit from PVA in terms of pain relief and improved functionality after failing conservative management, the best outcomes are seen in more acute fractures with evidence of bone marrow edema or fracture nonhealing.[1]

Identification of these fractures using current imaging technology is critical. The majority of osteoporotic VCFs occur at the thoracolumbar junction. Patient examination including palpation and percussion of the vertebral bodies can help identify the involved segment (see Chapter 4: Physical Examination Findings in Patients with Vertebral Compression Fractures). Imaging of the spine is ideally performed with magnetic resonance (MR) imaging. In cases of severe claustrophobia or MR imaging incompatibility (non-MRI compatible pacemaker, cochlear implant, etc.), imaging studies should include a computed tomography (CT) scan of the involved area. In order to distinguish between acute, subacute, and chronic fractures, the presence of edema on a sagittal T2 fat-saturated or short tau inversion recovery (STIR) sequence in combination with a sagittal T1-weighted sequence is the best indicator of an acute or subacute fracture. In cases of MR imaging incompatibility, CT scanning in combination with nuclear medicine bone scan or single-photon emission computed tomography (SPECT) imaging is usually required to distinguish between newer versus older fractures.[2] In cases of complex fractures, the imaging evaluation with MRI and/or CT of the spine optimizes visualization of the fracture and may allow for more specific and directed treatment.

3.3 Preprocedure Assessment

While individuals with acute or subacute compression fractures will likely achieve good outcomes after PVA, other factors for consideration include procedural risks, procedure cost, and the patient's functional ability and ability to tolerate NSM.

The elderly osteoporotic patients with compression fractures are a group who derives a substantial benefit from PVA. Pain from a VCF is significantly limiting to patients of all ages, but the deconditioning associated with patient immobility is especially detrimental to the elderly population. Immobility places these patients at greater risk for pneumonia, pulmonary embolism, skin breakdown, and many other complications. Muscle atrophy from disuse is compounded by bracing and leads to decline in activities of daily life (ADLs), which is associated with increased mortality.[3] Narcotic medications used for analgesia of the severe pain are more poorly tolerated by the elderly.[4] When considering the risks of PVA as compared to the risks of immobility in this elderly osteoporotic population, the benefits of the procedure usually outweigh

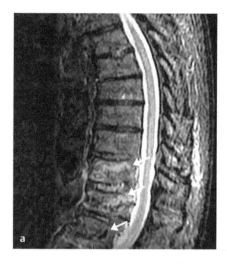
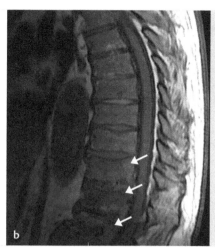

Fig. 3.1 Sagittal short tau inversion recovery (STIR; **a**) and T1-weighted (**b**) MR images show vertebral compression fractures with bone marrow edema (*white arrows* in **a** and **b**). The cause of these fractures was determined to be related to multiple myeloma following biopsy at the time of vertebral augmentation.

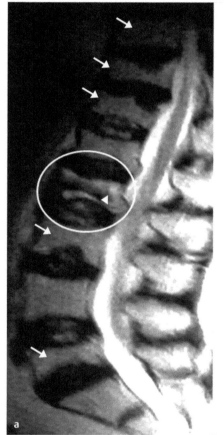
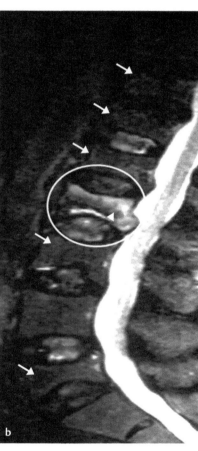

Fig. 3.2 Sagittal T2-weighted (**a**) and short tau inversion recovery (STIR; **b**) MR images show multiple vertebral compression fractures without significant bone marrow edema (*white arrows* in **a** and **b**) more typical of chronic vertebral fractures. The L2 vertebral body shows bone marrow edema (area within *white circles*) indicating an acute or subacute vertebral compression fracture. Intravertebral fluid-filled clefts are also seen in the L2 vertebral body (*white arrowheads*).

the risks and in elderly patients with moderate to severe pain the risks of NSM are usually greater than the risks of PVA.[5]

For the younger patient with a traumatic VCF, NSM is typically attempted first. Younger patients tend toward greater resilience in terms of functional decline, toleration of pain medications, and ability to heal bony injuries. However, in cases of severe or ongoing pain refractory to NSM, PVA may be reasonable provided that imaging findings correspond to the patient's clinical presentation and physical examination findings.

The third group who benefits significantly from PVA are patients with pathologic fractures due to neoplasia.[6] In cases of pathologic fractures (▶ Fig. 3.1), if there is no known preexisting malignancy, bone biopsy performed at the time of the PVA can assist with diagnosis of the neoplasm.

3.4 General Indications, Contraindications, and Procedure Complications

As mentioned previously, compression fractures may be identified incidentally on imaging and are not causing pain (▶ Fig. 3.2). However, in patients who present with substantial back pain and have a compression fracture, PVA may be appropriate. The major indications for vertebral augmentation are the presence of a symptomatic osteoporotic vertebral body fracture(s) that are refractory to medical therapy or that are too symptomatic for the patient to tolerate NSM and in vertebral bodies weakness or fracture due to neoplastic involvement.[7] These fractures include symptomatic nondisplaced vertebral body fractures (seen on MR imaging or nuclear bone scan but has no obvious loss of vertebral body height) and patients with fracture progression and progressive loss of vertebral body height. In patients with mild pain, no functional impairment, or pain that is managed well with NSM such as oral medications and bracing, PVA may be performed later or not at all.

Absolute contraindications to PVA are infection at this site of the vertebral augmentation and an untreated blood-borne infection.[8] A strong contraindication is osteomyelitis of the vertebral column.[8] A contraindication that is usually contraindicated is for women who are pregnant.[8] Relative contraindications that may or may not result in the discontinuation of the planned vertebral augmentation procedure include allergy to fill material, coagulopathy, spinal instability, myelopathy from the vertebral fracture, neurologic deficit, neural impingement, and fracture retropulsion with canal compromise.[8]

Overall, PVA is a very safe and well-tolerated procedure. Despite its optimal safety profile, there have been a few case reports of procedural complications. These include infections of the soft tissues, disk (diskitis), and/or bone[9–14] (osteomyelitis), bleeding, and symptomatic extravasation of polymethyl methacrylate (PMMA).[15–21] Intradiskal leakage of PMMA has also been shown to increase the risk of adjacent-level fractures.[22]

3.5 Equipment and Room Setup

Room setup and equipment used for the procedure will vary based on physician preference and availability (►Fig. 3.3 and ►Fig. 3.4). This section will provide minimum safe requirements for the performance of vertebral augmentation.

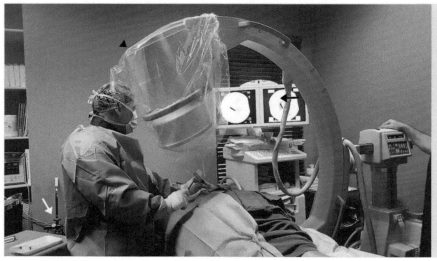

Fig. 3.3 Office-based procedure suite. Nurse (not shown) is to the left; note the monitor (*black arrow*), C-arm (*black arrowhead*), and oxygen (*white arrow*) available. Strict sterile technique is necessary for the performance of vertebral augmentation.

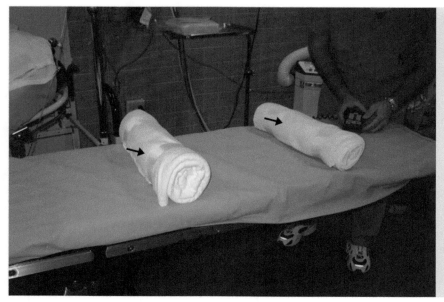

Fig. 3.4 The patient is placed in a prone position with towel rolls (*black arrows*) or gel pads under their shoulders and pelvis to put the spine in extension and facilitate vertebral fracture reduction.

As with any procedure, it is of utmost importance that the physician performing this procedure has been trained in the performance of vertebral augmentation and is prepared to manage any complications that may arise during the procedure. It is also important that appropriately trained personnel including nurse, and radiologic technology and other appropriate procedural or operating room personnel are present to assist the interventionalist/surgeon during this procedure.

Patients undergoing PVA should have intravenous access in place for the administration of fluids and medications as needed. Sedation may be beneficial in vertebral augmentation cases, as these patients typically have moderate to severe pain associated with their fractures, and the process of obtaining access to the vertebral body and reducing the fractured bone can be painful. The judicious use of local anesthetics is important and can help minimize the degree of sedation required to successfully perform this procedure. The decision to use sedation should be made on a case-by-case basis. If the physician performing the procedure decides to administer and supervise the sedation, they should be trained and qualified to do so. In these situations, a separate health care provider (registered nurse or other appropriately trained personnel) is required to assist with the administration of the medications and monitoring of the patient. Vital signs should be recorded at regular intervals and, if sedation is administered, pulse oximetry and cardiac monitoring must be used.

Because of the nature of the fracture and the frailty of patients who typically develop fractures that require treatment, antibiotic prophylaxis is recommended to decrease the risk of perioperative infection. Cephalosporins (cefazolin or cefuroxime) are the preferred drug due to their low toxicity, though Vancomycin and clindamycin are alternatives in patients with an allergy to cephalosporins or penicillin. These antibiotics cover primarily gram-positive organisms and may be combined with gentamycin, which covers primarily gram-negative organisms, and has been shown to penetrate into the intervertebral disk much more readily than other perioperative antibiotics.[23]

Strict sterile technique should be followed at all times as they pertain to the facilities, materials, patient preparation, physician preparation, and PVA materials preparation. Examples include, but are not limited to, the following:
- Skin overlying the target region should be prepared for an aseptic procedure, preferably using chlorhexidine-alcohol or povidone-iodine. The area should then be draped to create a sterile field.
- Barriers including sterile gloves, sterile gown, hat, and masks should be utilized during the procedure.
- Sterile equipment should be utilized, including a sterile C-arm cover.
- Single-use syringes/needles and single-dose vials should be employed.

3.6 Procedure

- The patient is typically placed in a prone position on the table. Pillows should be placed under the upper chest and pelvis to promote thoracic and lumbar extension, which will assist in the reduction of the compressed vertebrae.

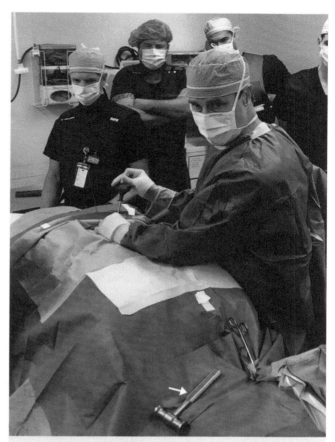

Fig. 3.5 The patient is sterilely prepped and draped and gowns, gloves, and masks are worn for this sterile image-guided procedure. The needles are placed into the vertebral body with a mallet (*white arrow*) typically using fluoroscopic guidance.

- CT or fluoroscopic viewing should be utilized to guide the entry to the vertebral body (▶Fig. 3.5). See Chapter 6: Approaches to the Vertebral Body, for the various approaches to achieve optimal outcomes.
- It is desirable to achieve as much fracture reduction as possible. This reduces the risk of adjacent-level fracture and minimizes the kyphotic deformity.
- The cement, once prepared, may then be injected into the vertebral body. Volumes of cement ranging from 15 to 25% of the noncompressed vertebral body volume at the same level is necessary to adequately treat the fracture and to restore the vertebral body strength and stiffness as well as to relieve pain.[24] Extravasation of cement from overfilling the vertebral cavity should be avoided.
- Incisions should receive some type of closure via a simple stitch, Dermabond, or Steri-strip-type closure bandage. In addition, if there is wound drainage, an appropriate dressing should be applied.
- The patient should be maintained in the prone immobile position while the cement sets. Setting time is temperature and cement specific though typically in the range of 10 to 20 minutes. Refer to product recommendations for the working time of the specific PMMA used.

3.7 Postprocedure Management

Most commonly, vertebral augmentation is performed as an outpatient procedure. It is appropriate to discharge the patient home following appropriate postanesthesia care. Neurological assessments should occur frequently during the immediate postprocedure recovery. Initiation of ambulation postprocedure must be carefully supervised.

As these patients are being treated for a fracture, at discharge, the patient should be instructed to avoid activities that may lead to additional or adjacent-level fracture. This includes activities that substantial increase the axial load on the spine such as lifting heavy objects, jumping from a height, or pulling objects against considerable resistance. Patients should also receive the usual postinterventional procedure instructions to minimize infection. These include keeping the incision clean and dry and no soaking in a bath, hot tub, pool, or lake for at least 48 hours after the procedure.

Finally, the cause of the fractures should be determined and treated. While not within the scope of this text, this includes diagnosis and management of osteoporosis and/or referral for malignancy workup.

References

[1] Tanigawa N, Komemushi A, Kariya S, et al. Percutaneous vertebroplasty: relationship between vertebral body bone marrow edema pattern on MR images and initial clinical response. Radiology 2006;239(1):195–200

[2] Maynard AS, Jensen ME, Schweickert PA, Marx WF, Short JG, Kallmes DF. Value of bone scan imaging in predicting pain relief from percutaneous vertebroplasty in osteoporotic vertebral fractures. AJNR Am J Neuroradiol 2000;21(10):1807–1812

[3] Brown CJ, Friedkin RJ, Inouye SK. Prevalence and outcomes of low mobility in hospitalized older patients. J Am Geriatr Soc 2004;52(8):1263–1270

[4] Cherasse A, Muller G, Ornetti P, Piroth C, Tavernier C, Maillefert JF. Tolerability of opioids in patients with acute pain due to nonmalignant musculoskeletal disease. A hospital-based observational study. Joint Bone Spine 2004;71(6):572–576

[5] Wardlaw D, Cummings SR, Van Meirhaeghe J, et al. Efficacy and safety of balloon kyphoplasty compared with non-surgical care for vertebral compression fracture (FREE): a randomised controlled trial. Lancet 2009;373(9668): 1016–1024

[6] Berenson J, Pflugmacher R, Jarzem P, et al; Cancer Patient Fracture Evaluation (CAFE) Investigators. Balloon kyphoplasty versus non-surgical fracture management for treatment of painful vertebral body compression fractures in patients with cancer: a multicentre, randomised controlled trial. Lancet Oncol 2011;12(3):225–235

[7] ACR. ACR–ASNR–ASSR–SIR–SNIS Practice parameter for the performance of vertebral augmentation. 2017

[8] Hirsch JA, Beall DP, Chambers MR, et al. Management of vertebral fragility fractures: a clinical care pathway developed by a multispecialty panel using the RAND/UCLA Appropriateness Method. Spine J 2018;18(11):2152–2161

[9] Abdelrahman H, Siam AE, Shawky A, Ezzati A, Boehm H. Infection after vertebroplasty or kyphoplasty. A series of nine cases and review of literature. Spine J 2013;13(12):1809–1817

[10] Alfonso Olmos M, Silva González A, Duart Clemente J, Villas Tomé C. Infected vertebroplasty due to uncommon bacteria solved surgically: a rare and threatening life complication of a common procedure: report of a case and a review of the literature. Spine 2006;31(20):E770–E773

[11] Mummaneni PV, Walker DH, Mizuno J, Rodts GE. Infected vertebroplasty requiring 360 degrees spinal reconstruction: long-term follow-up review. Report of two cases. J Neurosurg Spine 2006;5(1):86–89

[12] Park JW, Park SM, Lee HJ, Lee CK, Chang BS, Kim H. Infection following percutaneous vertebral augmentation with polymethylmethacrylate. Arch Osteoporos 2018;13(1):47

[13] Syed MI, Avutu B, Shaikh A, Sparks H, Mohammed MI, Morar K. Vertebral osteomyelitis following vertebroplasty: is acne a potential contraindication and are prophylactic antibiotics mandatory prior to vertebroplasty? Pain Physician 2009;12(4):E285–E290

[14] Walker DH, Mummaneni P, Rodts GE Jr. Infected vertebroplasty. Report of two cases and review of the literature. Neurosurg Focus 2004;17(6):E6

[15] Chen JK, Lee HM, Shih JT, Hung ST. Combined extraforaminal and intradiscal cement leakage following percutaneous vertebroplasty. Spine 2007;32(12):E358–E362

[16] Chen YJ, Tan TS, Chen WH, Chen CC, Lee TS. Intradural cement leakage: a devastatingly rare complication of vertebroplasty. Spine 2006;31(12): E379–E382

[17] Esmende SM, Daniels AH, Palumbo MA. Spinal cord compression after percutaneous kyphoplasty for metastatic compression fracture. Spine J 2013;13(7):831–832

[18] Grelat M, Le Van T, Fahed E, Beaurain J, Madkouri R. Rare complication of percutaneous technique: intradural cement leakage and its surgical treatment. World Neurosurg 2018;118:97

[19] Kulkarni AG, Shah SP, Deopujari CE. Epidural and intradural cement leakage following percutaneous vertebroplasty: a case report. J Orthop Surg (Hong Kong) 2013;21(3):365–368

[20] Teng MM, Cheng H, Ho DM, Chang CY. Intraspinal leakage of bone cement after vertebroplasty: a report of 3 cases. AJNR Am J Neuroradiol 2006;27(1):224–229

[21] Wu CC, Lin MH, Yang SH, Chen PQ, Shih TT. Surgical removal of extravasated epidural and neuroforaminal polymethylmethacrylate after percutaneous vertebroplasty in the thoracic spine. Eur Spine J 2007;16 (Suppl 3):326–331

[22] Jesse MK, Petersen B, Glueck D, Kriedler S. Effect of the location of endplate cement extravasation on adjacent level fracture in osteoporotic patients undergoing vertebroplasty and kyphoplasty. Pain Physician 2015;18(5): E805–E814

[23] Jackson AR, Eismont A, Yu L, et al. Diffusion of antibiotics in intervertebral disc. J Biomech 2018;76:259–262

[24] Martinčič D, Brojan M, Kosel F, et al. Minimum cement volume for vertebroplasty. Int Orthop 2015;39(4):727–733

4 Physical Examination Findings in Patients with Vertebral Compression Fractures

Scott Kreiner

Summary

Certain painful spine conditions justify a more prompt approach to imaging evaluation and the most common of these conditions is a painful vertebral compression fracture. Although some fractures heal and are not painful, others are persistently very painful and cause a substantial amount of discomfort and debilitation. Due to the significant increase in morbidity and permanent loss of function, appropriate management of vertebral compression fractures (VCFs) is critically important. VCFs typically involve the anterior column and cause pain with transition from one position to another. In patients with profound osteoporosis VCFs can occur with very little force and the presence of one or more fractures progressively and dramatically increases the risk of sustaining additional VCFs. The signs and symptoms of fractures or back pain due to tumor or infections are called red flag conditions and must be recognized early to ensure prompt and appropriate treatment. Additionally the typical presentation of an osteoporotic VCF should be known to facilitate prompt fracture diagnosis. The patients usually present with transitional pain when moving from one position to another and reliable physical examination signs of a painful VCF include pain with closed fist percussion and pain when lying supine.

Keywords: vertebral compression fracture, physical examination, osteoporosis, closed-fist percussion, post-procedure management

4.1 Introduction

It is known that the majority of spine pain is benign and will improve fairly rapidly. For this reason, most guidelines on the treatment of back pain generally recommend avoiding advanced imaging to reduce unnecessary expenditures and patient exposure to ionizing radiation. However, certain conditions justify more rapid utilization of advanced imaging and early treatment. The most prevalent of these conditions is compression fractures of the spine. These fractures occur when the bone is not of sufficient strength to handle the axial load applied to the vertebral body. The most common causes of loss of vertebral strength are osteoporosis and neoplasms involving the spine. Other conditions including infection of the vertebrae and high-velocity trauma can also predispose to vertebral fractures by weakening the vertebral body or by overwhelming the vertebral strength by force, respectively.

The incidence of VCFs has been rising over the last few decades, due to the rising age of our population. Many VCFs are asymptomatic and heal only to be identified incidentally on imaging studies. However, many of these fractures can cause severe pain and often become chronically painful, leading to substantial disability.[1] In addition, the presence of multiple fractures, occurring over the course of months or years, may lead to hyperkyphosis with secondary decrease in pulmonary function, abdominal distention with early satiety leading to malnutrition, as well as increased mortality.[2–5] For these reasons, diagnosis of VCFs, along with appropriate management, can improve health outcomes.

4.2 Presentation of Vertebral Compression Fractures

Compression fractures of the thoracolumbar spine typically result from a flexion-type injury. This results in a fracture of the anterior column (involving the anterior vertebral body and anterior longitudinal ligament), most commonly with a wedge-type appearance (▶Fig. 4.1). The primary symptom of a compression fracture is pain in the area of the fracture and pain with movement or transition from one position to another. Neurologic deficits are very unusual in patients with osteoporotic VCFs. The transitional pain usually manifests itself when patients go from a sitting to standing position or from a lying to sitting position and VCF-related pain also often causes difficulty with standing and walking.[6]

As mentioned earlier, these fractures occur when the compressive strength of the vertebral body is insufficient to tolerate

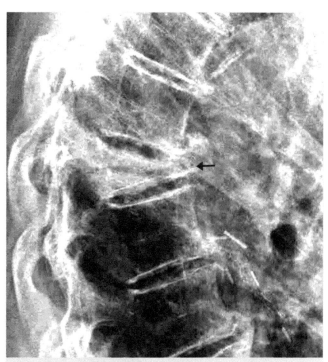

Fig. 4.1 Lateral conventional radiograph of the thoracic spine shows a wedge-type vertebral compression fracture of the T7 vertebral body (*black arrow*).

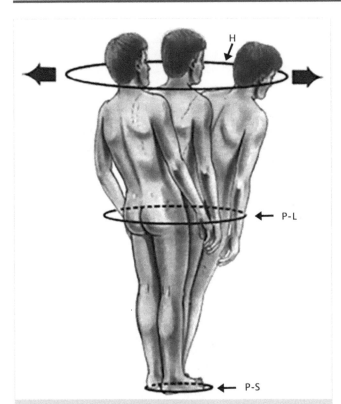

Fig. 4.2 The cone of economy. The figure outlines the "stable" zone surrounding the individual that is conical in shape from the feet to the head. Deviation from the center within the zone results in greater muscular effort and energy expenditure to maintain an upright posture. Deviation of the body outside the cone results in falling or requiring support. H, head; P-L, pelvic level; P-S, polygon of sustentation.

Table 4.1 Risk factors of vertebral compression fractures[16–19]

Modifiable	Nonmodifiable
Osteoporosis	History of prior compression fracture
Smoking (tobacco use)	Age (>55 y)
Alcohol consumption	Female gender
Inadequate physical activity	Race (Caucasian, Asian)
Low body weight	History of fractures in adulthood
Impaired eyesight	History of compression fractures in first-degree relative
Frailty	Dementia
Dietary calcium deficiency	Susceptibility to falling
Dietary vitamin D deficiency	
Estrogen deficiency	
Early menopause	
Bilateral salpingo-oophorectomy	
Postmenopausal amenorrhea for more than 1 y	

4.3 Risk Factors

Certain health conditions increase the risk of VCF. Osteoporosis is the biggest risk factor. In fact, if bone mineral density is decreased by 2 standard deviations, then fracture risk is increased by four to six times.[15] Of the remaining risk factors, many are also risk factors for osteoporosis. Certain risk factors represent activities and behaviors that the patient has control over and are therefore modifiable (▶Table 4.1). These include alcohol consumption, smoking, estrogen deficiency, frailty, low body weight, insufficient physical activity, dietary calcium deficiency, and dietary vitamin D deficiency. Nonmodifiable risk factors (▶Table 4.1) include advanced age, race (Caucasian or Asian), female gender, susceptibility of falling, history of fractures in adulthood, first-generation family history of fractures, and previous steroid treatment.[16–19]

Certain other historical features are also predictive of new compression fractures. The biggest is a history of prior compression fracture, which has been shown to result in a fivefold increase in the risk of a new compression fracture.[20,21] In addition, patients with a history of two prior compression fractures have shown a 12-fold increase in fracture risk and patients with three or more vertebral fractures have a 75-fold increased risk of additional vertebral fractures.[19–21] These new fractures are most likely to be adjacent to or near the prior fractures and are most common in the mid-thoracic or thoracolumbar area.[22]

4.4 Red Flags

Primary care physicians are frequently taught in training to identify "red flag" conditions to assess the need for advanced imaging in patients presenting with back pain. There have been a number of studies looking at these red flags[23–33] in patients with back pain. While these findings are similar to risk factors for osteoporotic compression fractures, the presence or absence of certain factors has been used to direct care. The most common red flags associated with compression fracture are the

the axial load applied to the vertebral body. In patients with osteoporosis or severe osteoporosis, even minor trauma such as a vigorous cough or sneeze, or even turning over in bed can cause a fracture. In fact, it has been reported that approximately 30% of vertebral fractures in severely osteoporotic patients occur when the patient is in bed.[7,8] It has been hypothesized that the load in these cases results from paraspinal muscle contraction.[9–11] In patients with only moderate weakening of the vertebral body usually from osteoporosis, fractures typically occur with activities such as lifting, pulling, stepping down from an elevated height, or falling. In the absence of osteoporosis, a severe axial load is typically required for fracture, typically as a result of a motor vehicle collision or a fall from substantial height. When compression fractures occur in patients younger than 55 years, or in an isolated vertebral body where fractures are uncommon (L5 or above T5), neoplastic involvement must be ruled out.[12]

VCFs are not always painful and are commonly detected only incidentally on imaging for other reasons. On occasion, multiple compression fractures can result in a kyphotic deformity, which impacts the sagittal balance of the patient, causing them to fall outside of the cone of economy (▶Fig. 4.2).[13] When this occurs, patients experience fatigue and pain resulting from biomechanical stresses and paraspinal spasm as a result of the increased work required to maintain an erect posture.[14]

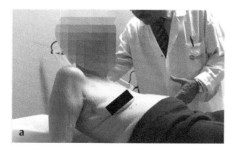
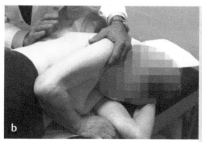
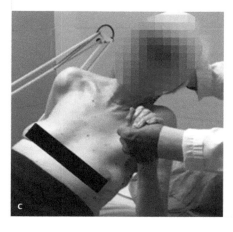
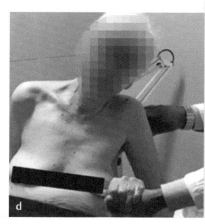

Fig. 4.3 A 76-year-old woman who had a T8 fracture 14 days before the examination. **(a)** Images showing the patient while trying to take a supine position, **(b)** lying on the left flank, **(c)** standing up to sit, and **(d)** almost seated. (Reproduced with permission of Postacchini R, Paolino M, Faraglia S, Cinotti G, Postacchini F. Assessment of patient's pain-related behavior at physical examination may allow diagnosis of recent osteoporotic vertebral fracture. Spine J 2013;13:1126–1133.)

following: advanced age (>70), female gender, night pain, low bone mineral density, recent weight loss, immunosuppression, chronic steroid use, and history of trauma.

4.5 Observational Findings Suggesting Compression Fracture

There are few studies evaluating patients who have a fracture and what findings are evident on physical examination. Postacchini et al[34] evaluated pain-related behavior to determine if there were certain behavioral features that were prognostic of the presence of a painful compression fracture. In this study, patients with back pain were recorded on video and asked to take six consecutive positions on the examination table: to sit on the edge of the bed, to lie supine, to turn on the flank, to take the prone position, to turn again on the flank, and then to sit on the edge of the bed again. The evaluators then used six parameters to evaluate the patient's behavior: grimacing, sighing, clenching or blocking their eyelids, gaping or strongly tightening their lips, asking for help by the examiner to take positions, and refusal, or extreme difficulty in turning to the prone position. In this study, they found that demonstration of at least two out of six pain behaviors while performing the six consecutive position changes was highly sensitive and specific for the presence of a VCF (▶ Fig. 4.3).

Langdon et al[35] evaluated two physical examination findings to determine if they were helpful in diagnosing the presence of an acute compression fracture. The first sign was the closed-fist percussion sign in which the examiner percusses the length of the spine while examining the patient's face in a mirror. The test is positive when the patient complains of severe or sharp pain. In this series of 83 patients, closed-fist percussion had a sensitivity of 88% and a specificity of 90%.

Additionally, Langdon et al evaluated the ability (or inability) of the patient to lie supine on the examination table. The test was positive when the patient was unable to lie on the table because of severe pain. This test showed a sensitivity of 81% and a specificity of 93%.

References

[1] Phillips FM. Minimally invasive treatments of osteoporotic vertebral compression fractures. Spine 2003;28(15, Suppl):S45–S53

[2] Leech JA, Dulberg C, Kellie S, Pattee L, Gay J. Relationship of lung function to severity of osteoporosis in women. Am Rev Respir Dis 1990;141(1):68–71

[3] Lyles KW, Gold DT, Shipp KM, Pieper CF, Martinez S, Mulhausen PL. Association of osteoporotic vertebral compression fractures with impaired functional status. Am J Med 1993;94(6):595–601

[4] Schlaich C, Minne HW, Bruckner T, et al. Reduced pulmonary function in patients with spinal osteoporotic fractures. Osteoporos Int 1998;8(3):261–267

[5] Leidig-Bruckner G, Minne HW, Schlaich C, et al. Clinical grading of spinal osteoporosis: quality of life components and spinal deformity in women with chronic low back pain and women with vertebral osteoporosis. J Bone Miner Res 1997;12(4):663–675

[6] Lad SP, Patil CG, Lad EM, Boakye M. Trends in pathological vertebral fractures in the United States: 1993 to 2004. J Neurosurg Spine 2007;7(3):305–310

[7] Bostrom MP, Lane JM. Future directions. Augmentation of osteoporotic vertebral bodies. Spine 1997;22(24, Suppl):38S–42S

[8] Garfin SR, Yuan HA, Reiley MA. New technologies in spine: kyphoplasty and vertebroplasty for the treatment of painful osteoporotic compression fractures. Spine 2001;26(14):1511–1515

[9] Kim DH, Vaccaro AR. Osteoporotic compression fractures of the spine; current options and considerations for treatment. Spine J 2006;6(5):479–487

[10] Leblanc AD, Schneider VS, Evans HJ, Engelbretson DA, Krebs JM. Bone mineral loss and recovery after 17 weeks of bed rest. J Bone Miner Res 1990;5(8):843–850

[11] Shen MS, Kim YH. Vertebroplasty and kyphoplasty: treatment techniques for managing osteoporotic vertebral compression fractures. Bull NYU Hosp Jt Dis 2006;64(3–4):106–113

[12] Lieberman IH, Dudeney S, Reinhardt MK, Bell G. Initial outcome and efficacy of "kyphoplasty" in the treatment of painful osteoporotic vertebral compression fractures. Spine 2001;26(14):1631–1638

[13] Schwab F, Patel A, Ungar B, Farcy JP, Lafage V. Adult spinal deformity-postoperative standing imbalance: how much can you tolerate? An overview of key parameters in assessing alignment and planning corrective surgery. Spine 2010;35(25):2224–2231

[14] Wu SS, Lachmann E, Nagler W. Current medical, rehabilitation, and surgical management of vertebral compression fractures. J Womens Health (Larchmt) 2003;12(1):17–26

[15] Marshall D, Johnell O, Wedel H. Meta-analysis of how well measures of bone mineral density predict occurrence of osteoporotic fractures. BMJ 1996;312(7041):1254–1259

[16] Alexandru D, So W. Evaluation and management of vertebral compression fractures. Perm J 2012;16(4):46–51

[17] Cummings SR, Melton LJ. Epidemiology and outcomes of osteoporotic fractures. Lancet 2002;359(9319):1761–1767

[18] Lindsay R, Burge RT, Strauss DM. One year outcomes and costs following a vertebral fracture. Osteoporos Int 2005;16(1):78–85

[19] Meunier PJ, Delmas PD, Eastell R, et al; International Committee for Osteoporosis Clinical Guidelines. Diagnosis and management of osteoporosis in postmenopausal women: clinical guidelines. Clin Ther 1999;21(6):1025–1044

[20] Lindsay R, Silverman SL, Cooper C, et al. Risk of new vertebral fracture in the year following a fracture. JAMA 2001;285(3):320–323

[21] Ross PD, Davis JW, Epstein RS, Wasnich RD. Pre-existing fractures and bone mass predict vertebral fracture incidence in women. Ann Intern Med 1991;114(11):919–923

[22] Melton LJ III, Kallmes DF. Epidemiology of vertebral fractures: implications for vertebral augmentation. Acad Radiol 2006;13(5):538–545

[23] Downie A, Williams CM, Henschke N, et al. Red flags to screen for malignancy and fracture in patients with low back pain: systematic review. BMJ 2013;347:f7095

[24] Downie A, Williams CM, Henschke N, et al. Red flags to screen for malignancy and fracture in patients with low back pain. Br J Sports Med 2014;48(20):1518

[25] Enthoven WT, Geuze J, Scheele J, et al. Prevalence and "red flags" regarding specified causes of back pain in older adults presenting in general practice. Phys Ther 2016;96(3):305–312

[26] Ferrari R. Imaging studies in patients with spinal pain: practice audit evaluation of Choosing Wisely Canada recommendations. Can Fam Physician 2016;62(3):e129–e137

[27] Greene G. "Red flags": essential factors in recognizing serious spinal pathology. Man Ther 2001;6(4):253–255

[28] Henschke N, Maher CG, Refshauge KM. A systematic review identifies five "red flags" to screen for vertebral fracture in patients with low back pain. J Clin Epidemiol 2008;61(2):110–118

[29] Henschke N, Maher CG, Refshauge KM, et al. Prevalence of and screening for serious spinal pathology in patients presenting to primary care settings with acute low back pain. Arthritis Rheum 2009;60(10):3072–3080

[30] Premkumar A, Godfrey W, Gottschalk MB, Boden SD. Red flags for low back pain are not always really red: a prospective evaluation of the clinical utility of commonly used screening questions for low back pain. J Bone Joint Surg Am 2018;100(5):368–374

[31] Underwood M, Buchbinder R. Red flags for back pain. BMJ 2013;347:f7432

[32] Verhagen AP, Downie A, Popal N, Maher C, Koes BW. Red flags presented in current low back pain guidelines: a review. Eur Spine J 2016;25(9):2788–2802

[33] Williams CM, Henschke N, Maher CG, et al. Red flags to screen for vertebral fracture in patients presenting with low-back pain. Cochrane Database Syst Rev 2013(1):CD008643

[34] Postacchini R, Paolino M, Faraglia S, Cinotti G, Postacchini F. Assessment of patient's pain-related behavior at physical examination may allow diagnosis of recent osteoporotic vertebral fracture. Spine J 2013;13(9):1126–1133

[35] Langdon J, Way A, Heaton S, Bernard J, Molloy S. Vertebral compression fractures--new clinical signs to aid diagnosis. Ann R Coll Surg Engl 2010;92(2):163–166

5 Medical Pain Management in Patients with Vertebral Compression Fractures

Young Hoon Kim and Yong-Chul Kim

Summary

Vertebral compression fractures (VCFs) can result from osteoporosis, trauma, or neoplasm. Among these causes, the osteoporotic compression fracture is the most commonly encountered. Patients with compression fractures manifest a wide range of symptoms from being asymptomatic to having excruciating pain. In general, if VCFs heal, the symptoms will improve in approximately 6 to 12 weeks; however, during this time, the health-related quality of life can deteriorate. Therefore, management of the patient's symptoms including adequate pain control is needed. Nonsurgical treatment is the traditional first-line management for VCFs and medications may also be prescribed to maximize patient comfort along with other procedures such as vertebroplasty or kyphoplasty. Although relatively little data on the medical management of nonoperative management of osteoporotic VCF have been reported, experts recommend that the pain management should initially begin with acetaminophen and/or nonsteroidal anti-inflammatory drugs. Analgesics (including narcotics and tramadol), muscle relaxants, and transdermal lidocaine can also be used for pain control. Additionally, medications to control neuropathic pain can be used in patients with VCFs and accompanying foraminal stenosis or tumor invasion. Finally, VCFs occur predominantly in older patients, and physicians must be aware of the pharmacological properties of the medications and their effects on elderly patients.

Keywords: acetaminophen, analgesics, medical management, nonsteroidal anti-inflammatory drug, nonsurgical management, vertebral compression fracture

5.1 Introduction

Osteoporosis, trauma, or neoplasm can all lead to vertebral compression fractures (VCFs). The osteoporotic compression fracture is the most commonly encountered type of fracture and the spectrum of symptoms vary widely from being asymptomatic to having excruciating pain. Nonsurgical management is the traditional first-line management for VCFs. The goals of nonsurgical management are pain control, early mobilization, prevention of deformity, and functional restoration. In spite of the nonsurgical management of VCFs being fairly common, there are relatively little data on the clinical outcomes of nonoperative management of osteoporotic VCF that have been reported.[1-3] Additionally, the studies related to the cost-effectiveness of nonsurgical management have also been sparse. In a retrospective, propensity score-matched study of vertebroplasty, kyphoplasty, and nonsurgical management for the treatment of VCFs in 2,740 patients, vertebroplasty and kyphoplasty were identified to be significantly costlier at 1-year follow-up, but at 2- and 4-year follow-ups, no significant difference in cost was found.[4] Moreover, the American Academy of Orthopaedic Surgeons determined that the strength of recommendation

Table 5.1 Commonly used medications for the management of the vertebral compression fracture

Medication	Acute stage	Subacute to chronic stage
Acetaminophen	+	+
NSAID	+	–
Muscle relaxant	+	–
Tramadol	+	+
Transdermal lidocaine	+	+
Opioid	–	+
Anticonvulsant	–	+

Abbreviations: NSAID, nonsteroidal anti-inflammatory drug; +, available; –, not available.

of the opioids/analgesics for patients who have VCFs is inconclusive due to a lack of data.[1] In practice, however, the medical management with or without bracing is usually recommended as the initial conventional treatment of VCFs.[2] Although medications are often used with other therapies for the treatment of back pain, they remain the mainstay in the management of moderate to severe fracture pain.

VCFs usually manifest with nociceptive pain. However, when there is concomitant foraminal stenosis, severe spinal canal stenosis, or tumor invasion, they may present with accompanying neuropathic pain. Neuropathic pain is a direct consequence of a lesion or a compressive irritation affecting the nervous system.[5] It is not easy to treat and the information available from randomized controlled trials upon which to base treatment in this matter is scarce. The management decisions may therefore be based on the individual physician's perspectives and experience with this condition. The medications to manage pain include acetaminophen, nonsteroidal anti-inflammatory drugs (NSAIDs), analgesics (including narcotics and tramadol), muscle relaxants, transdermal lidocaine, and adjuvant agents used to relieve neuropathic pain.[6] Although the acute pain due to VCF is generally tolerable or gone within 6 to 12 weeks, it is recommended that the pharmacological management be started with acetaminophen and/or NSAIDs. If pain does not decrease with the first-line medications, opioids can then be used (▶ Table 5.1). Finally, VCFs are more frequently found in elderly patients, and physicians should be aware of the pharmacological characteristics of these medications along with the possible adverse effects associated with the them in this particular patient population.

5.2 Nonsteroidal Anti-Inflammatory Drugs

NSAIDs are the most commonly prescribed medications for the treatment of pain. They have antipyretic, anti-inflammatory, and analgesic effects; the latter two explain their use in patients needing treatment for pain. The mechanism of action of NSAIDs is the inhibition of the prostaglandin synthesis through the inhibition of the cyclooxygenase (COX) enzymes (COX-1 and COX-2), which cause anti-inflammatory and analgesic effects. The COX-2 enzyme can be induced in some stressful conditions, such as nerve injury. Several organs such as the central nervous system and the kidney express COX-1 constitutively.[7] NSAIDs that inhibit both COX-1 and COX-2 include aspirin, indomethacin, sulindac, diclofenac, ibuprofen, naproxen, and piroxicam. Those that selectively inhibit COX-2 include celecoxib, etoricoxib, and nimesulide.[7] Although few studies have been published on the use of NSAIDs in patients with VCFs, there is some low-quality evidence that demonstrates immediate- and short-term effects of NSAID on reducing the pain of VCFs.[3] Additionally, in a systematic review of 65 randomized controlled trials of NSAIDs in different types of back pain, NSAIDs were more effective than placebo and acetaminophen. However, there was strong evidence that there were no differences between the effects of various types of NSAIDs including COX-2 NSAIDs.[8] Additionally, in a systematic review of 13 randomized controlled trials of NSAIDs in chronic low back pain, authors identified no difference in efficacy between different NSAID types.[9]

NSAIDs have a variety of side effects on various organ systems including the cardiovascular system (cardiovascular thrombosis, myocardial infarction, and stroke), the gastrointestinal tract (hemorrhagic gastric erosion and gastric ulcer), and the kidney (renal insufficiency, sodium and water retention, hypertension, and edema). The risk factors for NSAID-induced gastrointestinal complications include advanced age, history of ulcer, concomitant use of corticosteroids, high doses of NSAIDs, concomitant anticoagulants, serious systemic disorder, smoking, alcohol consumption, and concomitant infection with *Helicobacter pylori*.[10] The risk of renal toxicity increases with chronic NSAID use, multiple NSAID use, dehydration, volume depletion, congestive heart failure, vascular disease, hyperreninemia, shock, sepsis, systemic lupus erythematosus, hepatic disease, sodium depletion, nephrotic syndrome, diuresis, concomitant drug therapy, and an age of 60 years or older.[11]

Pharmacologically, COX-1 is involved in the formation of cytoprotective prostanoids and constitutively expressed in platelets and gastrointestinal tracts. Therefore, inhibition of COX-1 increases the risk of gastrointestinal bleeding. Gastric bleeding from preexisting gastric ulcers may also occur due to NSAID suppression of platelet aggregation.[12] Although the exact mechanism is not fully understood, video capsule endoscopy has found that NSAID-induced enteropathy occurs in the small intestine as well as the large intestine.[13] Moreover, the discovery of COX enzyme, COX-1, and COX-2 led to the production of selective COX-2 inhibitors. Compared with nonselective COX inhibitors, the incidence and complications associated with gastrointestinal tract ulcers are reduced. In a comparative study, the risk of gastrointestinal adverse events was lower in patients treated with a COX-2 selective NSAID (celecoxib) than in those receiving a nonselective NSAID (diclofenac) with omeprazole.[14] Celecoxib was also associated with significantly fewer small bowel mucosal breaks than ibuprofen plus omeprazole.[15,16] The preference for COX-2 selective agents to reduce gastrointestinal

tract complications, however, has likely given rise to increased cardiovascular side effects. The worrisome complications discovered by various studies resulted in the withdrawal of two of three COX-2 selective agents (rofecoxib and valdecoxib). Only celecoxib remains in the market with warnings regarding its cardiovascular profile.

The mechanism for the increase in cardiovascular risks is believed to result from an imbalance between pro- and antithrombotic prostaglandin. Thromboxane A2 is a platelet activator and vasoconstrictor, whereas prostacyclin (PGI2) is a platelet inhibitor and vasodilator. Platelet activity is maintained by the balance between thromboxane A2 effects on platelets and PGI2 effects on endothelium. Aspirin and nonselective NSAIDs inhibit both COX-1 and COX-2 and decrease both thromboxane A2 and PGI2. Conversely, COX-2 selective NSAIDs reduce PGI2 synthesis without affecting thromboxane A2 synthesis.[17,18] The antithrombotic unbalance may thereby cause the increased cardiovascular risk. Nonetheless, the Food and Drug Administration (FDA) announced labeled changes for all NSAIDs, both COX-2 selective and nonselective, that may have a similar cardiovascular risk. Consequently, patients without cardiovascular risk factors and low gastrointestinal tract risk can receive a monotherapy of an NSAID. However, patients with low cardiovascular risk without prophylactic aspirin but who are at high gastrointestinal tract risk should receive COX-2 selective NSAID or a traditional NSAID plus a proton-pump inhibitor.[19]

NSAIDs may also result in deterioration of renal function and renal failure. The mechanism of renal dysfunction is a decreased renal prostaglandin production, which leads to a reduction in renal blood flow and medullary ischemia.[20] The renal profile of NSAIDs is related to sodium retention and glomerular filtration rate changes. All NSAIDs have been associated with hypertension and edema, but most of these side effects improve with discontinuation of therapy.[11]

5.3 Acetaminophen

No studies have reported the efficacy of acetaminophen (paracetamol) for the management of VCFs. Its usage is based on tradition, low economic burden, optimal gastrointestinal safety profile, and uncommon side effects. Acetaminophen, known as paracetamol, is a *p*-aminophenol derivative with analgesic and antipyretic properties. The mechanism of action is not fully understood, but it is thought to act via central and peripheral mechanisms. Its ability to inhibit the central prostaglandin synthesis is similar to aspirin, but its peripheral inhibition of prostaglandin synthesis is not significant. Therefore, it lacks effectiveness for peripheral anti-inflammatory inhibition compared to aspirin for painful, inflammatory conditions.[21] Doses of 600 to 650 mg are more effective than doses of 300 to 350 mg, but better effects are not reported above 1,000 mg, indicating an analgesic ceiling effect.[22] A dose of 2,600 to 3,200 mg per day is adequate as a chronic daily dose, but the overall dose of acetaminophen should not exceed 4 g/d.[23] Nephrotoxicity may occur in relation to acetaminophen but less so than with NSAIDs. Acetaminophen is almost completely metabolized in the liver, and the minor metabolites in overdose are associated with hepatotoxicity.[7]

5.4 Opioid Analgesics

Opioids are the most potent analgesics available and play an important role in the management of acute and chronic pain. Nociceptive pain is more responsive to opioid analgesics than neuropathic pain. In general, there is sufficient evidence to suggest that opioid analgesia is safe and effective in treating patients with chronic low back pain for at least a short duration but should not be used chronically.[24–27] Although there is a lack of data and studies on nonsurgical management of VCFs, in a meta-analysis of study associated with nonsurgical management of osteoporotic compression fractures, the use of opioids (tramadol, oxycodone, and tapentadol) showed a significant improvement in pain compared with the use of placebo or Chinese medicine.[3] Opioids may be used in patients with inadequately treated pain that does not respond to the first-line medications. Opioid analgesia is usually continued until the acute pain is reduced, proper mobilization is possible, and no progressive deformity is confirmed.

Opioids function by binding to μ-, κ-, and δ-receptors in the central and peripheral nervous system. They are G protein-coupled receptors that modulate ionic channels and intracellular pathways.[28] Opioids are available in combination with NSAIDs, which have significant opioid dose-sparing effects.[29] Among the available opioids, meperidine is not appropriate due to its low oral bioavailability, potential metabolite accumulation, and toxicity with prolonged administration. Although opioid has no ceiling effect, high doses increase the occurrence of adverse effects and increase the risk of overdose; thus, a practical ceiling effect should be accounted in the clinical practice. The side effects of opioids include constipation, urinary retention, nausea and vomiting, itching, sedation, decreased libido, cognitive blunting, and respiratory depression. Among those, constipation is the most common side effect. Therefore, a high-fiber diet with a good bowel regimen should be advised, and often a laxative should be prescribed when using opioid therapy. The patients develop tolerance to some side effects of opioids, such as sedation, nausea, and respiratory depression, but not to other side effects including constipation, sweating, and urinary retention.

5.5 Muscle Relaxants

Muscle relaxants are a heterogeneous group of agents that mainly act on the central nervous system. Many patients with VCFs often present with muscle spasms, and muscle relaxants may be helpful in managing painful paravertebral muscle spasms. It is recommended that muscle relaxants be used only during the acute phase, and there is no information on the long-term outcomes in chronic low back pain.[30] The side effects of muscle relaxants include drowsiness, dizziness, dependence, and abuse in the long-term period.[31]

5.6 Calcitonin

A systematic review and meta-analysis on the use of calcitonin for the management of patients with recent osteoporotic vertebral fractures identified five randomized double-blind placebo-controlled trials involving a total of 246 patients and suggested that calcitonin appears to provide a significant improvement in pain control.[32] Calcitonin may be helpful in facilitating earlier mobilization during the time of hospitalization.[33] A number of mechanisms have been suggested to account for the analgesic action of calcitonin, including increased plasma β-endorphin release in the pituitary gland, decreased synthesis of prostaglandins or other humoral factors, modulation of pain perception through a central mechanism involving calcitonin-binding receptors in the central nervous system, and perhaps an effect on local pain mediators through calcitonin-binding sites in the periphery.[32,34]

5.7 Transdermal Lidocaine

Although no randomized trial has reported that transdermal lidocaine is beneficial for the management of patients with osteoporotic vertebral fractures, it is commonly used in the clinical practice.[6] The recommended maximum daily dose is three patches applied simultaneously every 12 hours. Transdermal lidocaine is not associated with side effects except for mild skin reactions. However, attention is required in patients who receive oral Class I antiarrhythmic agents (e.g., mexiletine) and in patients with severe hepatic dysfunction to avoid antagonistic cardiac effects or toxicity.[35]

5.8 Bisphosphonate

Bisphosphonates have been used for reducing back pain related to acute vertebral fracture. In a randomized, double-blind controlled trial comparing intravenous pamidronate (30-mg intravenous pamidronate daily for three consecutive days) and placebo, pamidronate provided rapid and sustained pain relief in patients with acute painful osteoporotic VCFs.[36] In a comparison study of the analgesic efficacy of intravenous pamidronate and calcitonin in osteoporotic VCFs, however, calcitonin was recommended because of no difference in analgesic effect between groups and the low cost of calcitonin.[37]

5.9 Anticonvulsants

Anticonvulsants, including gabapentin, carbamazepine, and pregabalin, have been traditionally used to treat chronic neuropathic pain. Although gabapentin was originally made as a structural analog of the inhibitory neurotransmitter gamma-aminobutyric acid (GABA), it does not bind to GABA receptors and its mechanism is not fully elucidated. Its analgesic effect is likely to act on the α2δ subunit of voltage-dependent calcium channels for which it has a substantial affinity and which are upregulated in the dorsal root ganglia and spinal cord after peripheral nerve injury.[38,39] Analgesic effects of gabapentin result from binding to and presynaptically inhibiting voltage-dependent calcium channels, preventing calcium influx, then inhibiting the release of excitatory amino acids such as glutamate from the presynaptic terminals.[40] Gabapentin has been shown to be effective in the treatment of a variety of chronic neuropathic pain. However, there is controversy regarding its therapeutic effect on acute pain and there has been no randomized controlled trial on the effect of gabapentin in acute painful VCFs. The use of gabapentin may be appropriate for the patients who have coexistence of both nociceptive and neuropathic pain, such as foraminal stenosis or tumor invasion. A meta-analysis showed that gabapentin significantly reduced pain and decreased the opioid usage in patients who perioperatively received gabapentin,[41] but there is little evidence in the literature regarding the use of anticonvulsants in painful vertebral compressed fractures, and more research in this matter is needed to formulate evidence-based recommendations.

5.10 Conclusion

VCFs may result in serious pain and deteriorate patients' health-related quality of life. Although the acute pain due to VCF is often alleviated within 6 to 12 weeks, it may persist and medical management of pain is recommended in both the acute and subacute phases. Pharmacological therapy should be started with acetaminophen and/or NSAIDs. Patients who do not respond to the first-line medications may be prescribed with opioids. Adjuvant medications can be added in patients who show signs of neuropathic pain. Physicians should be aware of the useful role and side effects associated with these medications to achieve the goals of optimal nonsurgical management, such as adequate pain control, early mobilization, prevention of deformity, and functional restoration.

References

[1] Esses SI, McGuire R, Jenkins J, et al. The treatment of symptomatic osteoporotic spinal compression fractures. J Am Acad Orthop Surg 2011;19(3):176–182

[2] McConnell CT Jr, Wippold FJ II, Ray CE Jr, et al. ACR appropriateness criteria management of vertebral compression fractures. J Am Coll Radiol 2014;11(8):757–763

[3] Rzewuska M, Ferreira M, McLachlan AJ, Machado GC, Maher CG. The efficacy of conservative treatment of osteoporotic compression fractures on acute pain relief: a systematic review with meta-analysis. Eur Spine J 2015;24(4):702–714

[4] Hazzard MA, Huang KT, Toche UN, et al. Comparison of vertebroplasty, kyphoplasty, and nonsurgical management of vertebral compression fractures and impact on US healthcare resource utilization. Asian Spine J 2014;8(5):605–614

[5] Eisenberg E, Peterson D. Neuropathic pain pharmacotherapy. In: Fishman S, Ballantyne J, Rathmell JP, eds. Bonica's Management of Pain. Philadelphia, PA: LWW; 2010:1194–11207

[6] Ensrud KE, Schousboe JT. Clinical practice. Vertebral fractures. N Engl J Med 2011;364(17):1634–1642

[7] Lipman A, Buvanendran A. Nonsteroidal anti-inflammatory drugs and acetaminophen. In: Fishman SJ, Ballantyne JC, Rathmell JP, eds. Bonica's Management of pain. Philadelphia, PA: LWW; 2010:1157–1171

[8] Roelofs PD, Deyo RA, Koes BW, Scholten RJ, van Tulder MW. Non-steroidal anti-inflammatory drugs for low back pain. Cochrane Database Syst Rev 2008(1):CD000396

[9] Enthoven WT, Roelofs PD, Deyo RA, van Tulder MW, Koes BW. Non-steroidal anti-inflammatory drugs for chronic low back pain. Cochrane Database Syst Rev 2016;2:CD012087

[10] Brune K, Patrignani P. New insights into the use of currently available non-steroidal anti-inflammatory drugs. J Pain Res 2015;8:105–118

[11] Ković SV, Vujović KS, Srebro D, Medić B, Ilic-Mostic T. Prevention of renal complications induced by non- steroidal anti-inflammatory drugs. Curr Med Chem 2016;23(19):1953–1964

[12] Hawkey CJ, Hawthorne AB, Hudson N, Cole AT, Mahida YR, Daneshmend TK. Separation of the impairment of haemostasis by aspirin from mucosal injury in the human stomach. Clin Sci (Lond) 1991;81(4):565–573

[13] Lanas A, Sopeña F. Nonsteroidal anti-inflammatory drugs and lower gastrointestinal complications. Gastroenterol Clin North Am 2009;38(2):333–352

[14] Chan FK, Lanas A, Scheiman J, Berger MF, Nguyen H, Goldstein JL. Celecoxib versus omeprazole and diclofenac in patients with osteoarthritis and rheumatoid arthritis (CONDOR): a randomised trial. Lancet 2010;376(9736):173–179

[15] Goldstein JL, Eisen GM, Lewis B, Gralnek IM, Zlotnick S, Fort JG; Investigators. Video capsule endoscopy to prospectively assess small bowel injury with celecoxib, naproxen plus omeprazole, and placebo. Clin Gastroenterol Hepatol 2005;3(2):133–141

[16] Goldstein JL, Eisen GM, Lewis B, et al. Small bowel mucosal injury is reduced in healthy subjects treated with celecoxib compared with ibuprofen plus omeprazole, as assessed by video capsule endoscopy. Aliment Pharmacol Ther 2007;25(10):1211–1222

[17] McGettigan P, Henry D. Cardiovascular risk with non-steroidal anti-inflammatory drugs: systematic review of population-based controlled observational studies. PLoS Med 2011;8(9):e1001098

[18] Trelle S, Reichenbach S, Wandel S, et al. Cardiovascular safety of non-steroidal anti-inflammatory drugs: network meta-analysis. BMJ 2011;342:c7086

[19] Scarpignato C, Lanas A, Blandizzi C, Lems WF, Hermann M, Hunt RH; International NSAID Consensus Group. Safe prescribing of non-steroidal anti-inflammatory drugs in patients with osteoarthritis: an expert consensus addressing benefits as well as gastrointestinal and cardiovascular risks. BMC Med 2015;13:55

[20] Ungprasert P, Cheungpasitporn W, Crowson CS, Matteson EL. Individual non-steroidal anti-inflammatory drugs and risk of acute kidney injury: a systematic review and meta-analysis of observational studies. Eur J Intern Med 2015;26(4):285–291

[21] Anderson BJ. Paracetamol (Acetaminophen): mechanisms of action. Paediatr Anaesth 2008;18(10):915–921

[22] Skoglund LA, Skjelbred P, Fyllingen G. Analgesic efficacy of acetaminophen 1000 mg, acetaminophen 2000 mg, and the combination of acetaminophen 1000 mg and codeine phosphate 60 mg versus placebo in acute postoperative pain. Pharmacotherapy 1991;11(5):364–369

[23] Bertin P, Keddad K, Jolivet-Landreau I. Acetaminophen as symptomatic treatment of pain from osteoarthritis. Joint Bone Spine 2004;71(4):266–274

[24] Peloso PM, Fortin L, Beaulieu A, Kamin M, Rosenthal N; Protocol TRP-CAN-1 Study Group. Analgesic efficacy and safety of tramadol/ acetaminophen combination tablets (Ultracet) in treatment of chronic low back pain: a multicenter, outpatient, randomized, double blind, placebo controlled trial. J Rheumatol 2004;31(12):2454–2463

[25] Hale ME, Ahdieh H, Ma T, Rauck R; Oxymorphone ER Study Group 1. Efficacy and safety of OPANA ER (oxymorphone extended release) for relief of moderate to severe chronic low back pain in opioid-experienced patients: a 12-week,randomized,double-blind,placebo-controlledstudy.JPain2007;8(2): 175–184

[26] Katz N, Rauck R, Ahdieh H, et al. A 12-week, randomized, placebo-controlled trial assessing the safety and efficacy of oxymorphone extended release for opioid-naive patients with chronic low back pain. Curr Med Res Opin 2007;23(1):117–128

[27] Vorsanger GJ, Xiang J, Gana TJ, Pascual ML, Fleming RR. Extended-release tramadol (tramadol ER) in the treatment of chronic low back pain. J Opioid Manag 2008;4(2):87–97

[28] Inturrisi CE, Lipman AG. Opioid analgesics. In: Fishman SJ, Ballantyne JC, Rathmell JP, eds. Bonica's Management of Pain. Philadelphia, PA: LWW; 2010:1172–1187

[29] Zhang Z, Xu H, Zhang Y, et al. Nonsteroidal anti-inflammatory drugs for postoperative pain control after lumbar spine surgery: a meta-analysis of randomized controlled trials. J Clin Anesth 2017;43:84–89

[30] Abdel Shaheed C, Maher CG, Williams KA, McLachlan AJ. Efficacy and tolerability of muscle relaxants for low back pain: systematic review and meta-analysis. Eur J Pain 2017;21(2):228–237

[31] Browning R, Jackson JL, O'Malley PG. Cyclobenzaprine and back pain: a meta-analysis. Arch Intern Med 2001;161(13):1613–1620

[32] Knopp JA, Diner BM, Blitz M, Lyritis GP, Rowe BH. Calcitonin for treating acute pain of osteoporotic vertebral compression fractures: a systematic review of randomized, controlled trials. Osteoporos Int 2005;16(10):1281–1290

[33] Lyritis GP, Paspati I, Karachalios T, Ioakimidis D, Skarantavos G, Lyritis PG. Pain relief from nasal salmon calcitonin in osteoporotic vertebral crush fractures. A double blind, placebo-controlled clinical study. Acta Orthop Scand Suppl 1997;275:112–114

[34] Plosker GL, McTavish D. Intranasal salcatonin (salmon calcitonin). A review of its pharmacological properties and role in the management of postmenopausal osteoporosis. Drugs Aging 1996;8(5):378–400

[35] Dworkin RH, O'Connor AB, Backonja M, et al. Pharmacologic management of neuropathic pain: evidence-based recommendations. Pain 2007;132(3): 237–251

[36] Armingeat T, Brondino R, Pham T, Legré V, Lafforgue P. Intravenous pamidronate for pain relief in recent osteoporotic vertebral compression fracture: a randomized double-blind controlled study. Osteoporos Int 2006;17(11): 1659–1665

[37] Laroche M, Cantogrel S, Jamard B, et al. Comparison of the analgesic efficacy of pamidronate and synthetic human calcitonin in osteoporotic vertebral fractures: a double-blind controlled study. Clin Rheumatol 2006;25(5):683–686

[38] Gee NS, Brown JP, Dissanayake VU, Offord J, Thurlow R, Woodruff GN. The novel anticonvulsant drug, gabapentin (Neurontin), binds to the alpha2delta subunit of a calcium channel. J Biol Chem 1996;271(10):5768–5776

[39] Newton RA, Bingham S, Case PC, Sanger GJ, Lawson SN. Dorsal root ganglion neurons show increased expression of the calcium channel alpha2delta-1 subunit following partial sciatic nerve injury. Brain Res Mol Brain Res 2001;95 (1–2):1–8

[40] Shimoyama M, Shimoyama N, Hori Y. Gabapentin affects glutamatergic excitatory neurotransmission in the rat dorsal horn. Pain 2000;85(3):405–414

[41] Hurley RW, Cohen SP, Williams KA, Rowlingson AJ, Wu CL. The analgesic effects of perioperative gabapentin on postoperative pain: a meta-analysis. Reg Anesth Pain Med 2006;31(3):237–247

6 Approaches to the Vertebral Body

D. Mitchell Self, James Mooney, John W. Amburgy, and M.R. Chambers

Summary

Percutaneous vertebral augmentation procedures and vertebral body biopsy may be performed using a variety of unilateral or bilateral image guided approaches. The choice of approach will depend on many factors, including fracture level and vertebral morphology, as well as operator experience and preference. Herein, we describe the approaches along with the indications, risks and benefits offered by each. As with any image-guided procedure, preoperative positioning of the patient and the fluoroscope is paramount and a detailed understanding of relevant anatomy is essential.

Keywords: vertebral augmentation, percutaneous, minimally invasive, transpedicular, extrapedicular, parapedicular, anterolateral, transoral, vertebral body biopsy

6.1 Introduction

The first vertebroplasty was performed in 1984 and then introduced in the literature by Galibert et al in 1987.[1] Polymethyl methacrylate (PMMA) cement was injected percutaneously via a transoral approach into a C2 vertebra that had been partially disrupted by an aggressive vertebral hemangioma. This injection of cement was effective in decreasing the patient's pain and discomfort for an extended period of time. In spite of the fact that the first vertebroplasty was accomplished via a transoral approach, this is currently one of the least commonly utilized approaches to the vertebral bodies that exist.

A posterolateral extrapedicular approach was subsequently used in the thoracic spine, but after cement leakage along the track of the needle induced a case of intercostal radiculopathy, the transpedicular needle approach was developed. With the transpedicular approach, the needle passed through the pedicle into the vertebral body and was thought to result in a lower risk of cement discharging posteriorly along the needle track.[2]

Since the introduction of vertebral augmentation procedures, many approaches have been explored to provide the safest and most effective treatment of pain and deformity resulting from many types of vertebral body compression fractures. In addition to the anterolateral procedure first described, approaches now include transpedicular, extrapedicular, parapedicular (▶Fig. 6.1), and modified extrapedicular and parapedicular approaches. In the cervical spine, the anterolateral approach has been employed (▶Fig. 6.2). The transpedicular approach directs the needle through the longitudinal axis of the pedicle into the vertebral body. The parapedicular path enters the vertebral body at the vertebral body/pedicle junction near the mid to superior point and traverses into the vertebral body without breaching the medial pedicle wall. Finally, the extrapedicular approach enters the vertebral body directly either just lateral to the transverse process at the level of the pedicle progressing horizontally into the vertebral body or accessing the vertebral body just anterior to the pedicle and just above the inferior end plate entering the vertebral body at a 45-degree angle. Both of these extrapedicular approaches are performed without passing through the pedicle. The choice of approach will depend on many factors, including fracture level and vertebral morphology, as well as operator experience and preference.

6.2 Indications

The most common indication for percutaneous vertebral augmentation is stabilization of a painful osteoporotic vertebral body compression fracture. Other common indications include fracture nonunion, pain from a primary tumor, osteolysis following malignant infiltration of a vertebra, pain from vertebral body involvement of an aggressive hemangioma, and a painful fracture resulting from osteonecrosis.[3-9]

6.3 Anatomy

Each vertebra consists of a body and a vertebral arch with articular, transverse, and spinous processes. The vertebral body consists primarily of cancellous bone and marrow encased by cortical bone at the margins, including the superior and

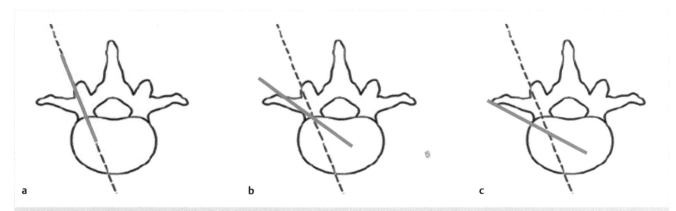

Fig. 6.1 Basic approaches: **(a)** transpedicular, **(b)** parapedicular, and **(c)** extrapedicular. Dashed line indicates the longitudinal axis of the pedicle.

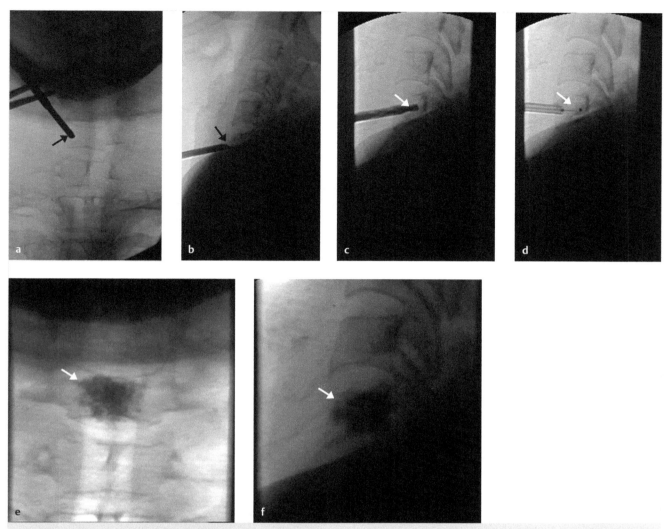

Fig. 6.2 Anteroposterior **(a)** and lateral **(b)** fluoroscopic views of the cervical spine shows an 11-gauge needle entering the anterolateral C6 vertebral body from the patient's right side (*black arrows* in **a** and **b**). Lateral fluoroscopic views of the cervical spine shows the needle in place in the anterior C6 vertebral body with the drill placed through the needle (*white arrow* in **c**) to create a channel for the inflatable bone tamp (*white arrow* in **d**). Anteroposterior **(e)** and lateral **(f)** fluoroscopic views shown after injection of polymethyl methacrylate (PMMA) into the C6 vertebral body shows the radiopaque cement present within the vertebral body (*white arrows* in **e** and **f**). The vertebral augmentation kyphoplasty at C6 was performed due to a painful aggressive hemangioma. (These images are provided courtesy of Dr. Douglas P. Beall.)

inferior end plates. The vertebral arch consists of right and left pedicles (which connect it to the body) and right and left laminae (▶ Fig. 6.3). The transverse processes project laterally at the junction of the pedicles and laminae, and the dorsal or posterior spinous process projects from the midline junction of the laminae. Postganglionic nerve roots exit bilaterally beneath the pedicle via foramina. Thoracic intercostal arteries and four pairs of lumbar arteries are located adjacent to the vertebrae.

6.3.1 Planning the Trajectory

The levels most commonly affected by vertebral compression fractures (VCFs) are at the mid-thoracic spine and thoracolumbar junction.[10] Bony landmarks are not reliably palpable; therefore, surgical planning and execution is dependent on imaging. Size of the pedicles can be important in determining needle gauge and trajectory. The pedicle angle of entry to the vertebra determines the trajectory. In the thoracic spine, the angles are steeper (more anteroposterior [AP]) than in the lumbar spine; therefore, the extrapedicular, modified extrapedicular, or parapedicular approaches may be indicated. In addition to the normal anatomy, changes caused by the fracture will also dictate the approach. For example, compression of the superior end plate may require a more caudal trajectory, while an inferior end plate deformity may require a more cranial entry point and horizontal direction. In the case of a biconcave fracture, the needle entry and trajectory should be equidistant from both end plates. A vertebra plana leaves little room for passage of a needle into the center of the vertebral body, but there is usually sparing of the more lateral portions of the vertebral body, which can be accessed despite prominent central compression. Breach of the vertebral posterior margin by a fracture risks cement escape into the spinal canal, but previous authors have shown that these fractures can be treated very safely.[11]

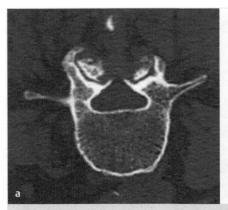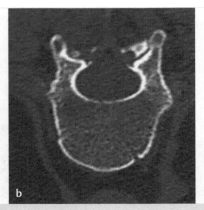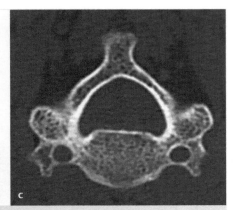

Fig. 6.3 Axial CT images of **(a)** lumbar, **(b)** thoracic, and **(c)** cervical vertebrae. (These images are provided courtesy of Dr. M. R. Chambers.)

6.4 Bilateral versus Unilateral Approach

There are substantial data supporting the bilateral approach for optimal outcomes in vertebral augmentation with balloon kyphoplasty; however, the unilateral approach may offer similar outcomes with reduced operative times and radiation exposure.

In a retrospective study of 296 patients with osteoporotic VCFs, Bozkurt et al identified significantly better height restoration following bilateral kyphoplasty compared to unilateral kyphoplasty and vertebroplasty.[12] The advantage of height restoration with a bilateral technique is also supported by a meta-analysis of five studies that reported a short-term follow-up.[13] Bilateral kyphoplasty had a significantly ($p = 0.03$) better degree of anterior vertebral height restoration than unilateral kyphoplasty.[13]

The unilateral approach was first introduced in an effort to overcome the challenge of visualizing superimposed cannulas and the second injection site in the lateral view. Depending on the fracture and vertebral morphology, pedicle size, pedicle angle of entry, bone quality, and experience of the operator, the unilateral approach has been used with equal success and favorable outcomes.

When multiple levels are being treated, they are typically all cannulated before the injection, allowing the bone fill material to be mixed once and injected in short order. If the levels to be treated are contiguous and the distance between levels is relatively small, the side of needle placement can be alternated for multiple unilateral approaches. This can significantly reduce operative time and radiation exposure to the operator as well as to give more working space for the needles than the same procedure with all of the levels done from the same side.

Several large systematic reviews of randomized control trials have examined the differences in height restoration, correction of kyphotic angulation, and patient ratings of pain associated with unilateral and bilateral approaches.

Favoring the unilateral approach, an analysis of 15 randomized controlled trials including 850 patients by Yang et al found no difference in quality of life or complications from surgery.[14] Chen et al found that the unilateral approach resulted in a shorter operative time, a smaller amount of cement injected, and a lower risk of cement leakage.[6] There was no statistically significant differences in Visual Analog Scale pain scores, height changes, or kyphotic angle changes between the groups.[15] Papanastassiou et al found no difference in clinical or radiological outcomes in multiple myeloma patients treated with the unilateral approach.[16] In a review of five studies including 253 patients, Huang et al found no clinically important differences but suggested that unilateral kyphoplasty is advantageous due to decreased operative time and cost.[17] Similarly, in a systematic review and meta-analysis including 563 patients, Sun et al noted that the unilateral approach led to decreased surgical time, cement consumption, and cement leakage; reduced radiation dose and hospitalization costs; and improved short-term general health.[9] In a comparison between unilateral transverse process-pedicle and bilateral puncture techniques in percutaneous kyphoplasty, Yan et al noted that both bilateral and unilateral approaches for kyphoplasty provide effective treatment for patients with painful osteoporotic VCFs.[18] However, patients treated with the unilateral procedure received significantly less radiation, had shorter operation time, fewer complications, and significantly less cement leakage. In this study, the unilateral approach offered a higher degree of deformity correction, local sagittal angle, and vertebral body height restoration (anterior and posterior). Although both techniques had the ability to restore vertebral height and to improve alignment, more postoperative height was restored in the unilateral group. This was attributed to the bone cement distribution, which was placed mainly in the anterior and middle vertebral bodies.[18]

In the bilateral group, 10.5% of patients had obvious pain in the puncture sites at 1 month postoperatively. With local block treatment, the pain disappeared in all patients at the last follow-up.[13] These complications were probably related to puncture technique as this issue has not been commonly reported. Compared with the bilateral technique, the puncture point of the unilateral technique was more lateral to the facet joint. Therefore, in the unilateral group, the violation of facet joint was rare and the bone cement was mainly distributed in the anterior and middle of the vertebral body.[13] There was no statistically significant difference in pain relief and functional improvement between the two groups during the 12-month follow-up. Similar clinical outcomes were achieved with either treatment procedure.[13]

In general, based on the above manuscripts and analyses, the unilateral approach provides the advantages of reduced procedure time, costs, radiation exposure, and cement leakage with improved short-term health. Kyphoplasty using a bilateral approach has been shown to provide significantly less vertebral height loss over 2 years than the same procedure performed via a unilateral approach.[19] There appears to be no significant difference in pain reduction or quality-of-life improvement when comparing the unilateral versus bilateral approaches.[18] Procedural complications, such as cement leakage, show varied results among studies and may be operator dependent and dependent on which imaging modality is used to detect this extravasation as computed tomography (CT) is more sensitive at detecting small amounts of extravasation as compared with plain film radiography or fluoroscopy.

6.5 Imaging and Equipment

The procedure is guided with single-plane or biplanar fluoroscopy or, in some cases, CT. In our experience, fluoroscopy is sufficient to identify the salient anatomy and affected vertebral bodies. If uncertainty remains about the fracture anatomy and extent of vertebral involvement, CT may be performed. Fracture age and anatomy can be assessed with magnetic resonance (MR)

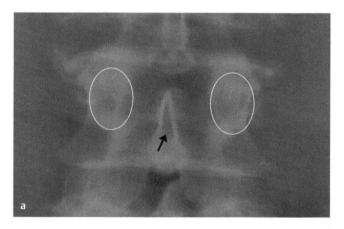

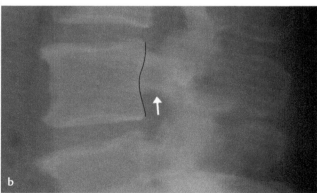

Fig. 6.4 (a) Anteroposterior and (b) lateral fluoroscopic images of a lumbar vertebra showing the spinous process in the center of the vertebral body on the anteroposterior (AP) view (*black arrow*) and the pedicles well seen and in the upper half of the vertebral body (*white ovals* in a). The posterior portion of the vertebral body is seen on the lateral view (*black line* in b) as is the pedicles, which are superimposed on one another (*white arrow* in b), indicating a direct lateral view.

imaging.[3,20] Nuclear bone scan imaging may also be helpful in characterizing a fracture, although the anatomic detail is limited and the spatial resolution poor.

6.6 Procedure

As with any image-guided procedure, preoperative positioning of the patient and fluoroscopes is paramount. Either conscious sedation or general anesthesia may be performed, but most patients with VCFs have multiple comorbidities and conscious sedation would be preferred over general anesthesia in this fragile patient population. The patient is positioned prone with shoulder and pelvis/hip bolsters. All pressure points are padded. The lateral image should be a "true lateral" that demonstrates the posterior margin of the vertebral body, spinal canal, and an optimized view of superimposed pedicles. The adjacent vertebrae can be used as guides if there is significant deformity of the fractured body. The AP view should be directed such that the spinous process is midline and both pedicles are visible and similar in size and shape and in the upper half of the incident vertebral body (►Fig. 6.4). In this way, two-dimensional imaging is used to guide a three-dimensional approach. Although we routinely use this fluoroscopic approach, some may prefer the en face approach, a view straight down the pedicle that demonstrates a circle or oval outline of the edges of the pedicle for guidance (►Fig. 6.5). This requires a 10- to 30-degree ipsilateral oblique angulation from the true AP. It is important to remember that the lateral imaging is used only for superior and inferior directional adjustments, while the AP image is only to be relied on for guidance with medial and lateral corrections.

All vertebral augmentation procedures require the establishment of a working channel for delivery of cement or an implant. Each of the following approaches begins with a small (~5 mm)

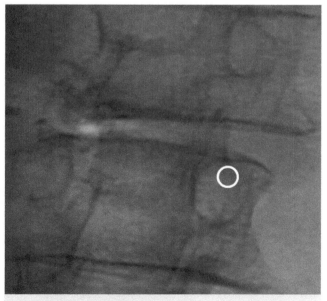

Fig. 6.5 Ipsilateral fluoroscopic view with a 25-degree ipsilateral angulation of the image intensifier shows the en face view of the pedicle with the target located in the upper outer portion of the pedicle (*white circle*).

skin incision and the introduction of a Jamshidi-style needle to establish the working channel extending into the vertebral body. An 11-gauge Jamshidi needle is generally used in the lumbar and lower thoracic spine. Smaller needles may be used in upper thoracic spine and as needed at other levels. Larger needles may be used in the lumbar spine or during the insertion of vertebral body implants. Needles are available in 10- to 15-mm lengths.

6.6.1 Potential Risks and Management of Complications

Each approach is associated with a unique set of indications and risks as described. Common to many of the approaches are the risks of rib or transverse process fractures, infection, hematoma,

pulmonary embolism, injury to surrounding organs, direct neural injury, and cement leakage with subsequent neural compression requiring immediate access to personnel and facilities for surgical decompression.

6.6.2 Transpedicular Approach

The basic bilateral transpedicular approach is considered standard for percutaneous access to the lumbar and lower thoracic vertebrae (▶Fig. 6.6). The transpedicular needle path offers protection for the surrounding tissues, including the postganglionic nerve roots, but is most likely to require bilateral needle insertion to accomplish proper balloon placement and adequate cement fill. In the upper thoracic spine, the transpedicular approach will not allow proper

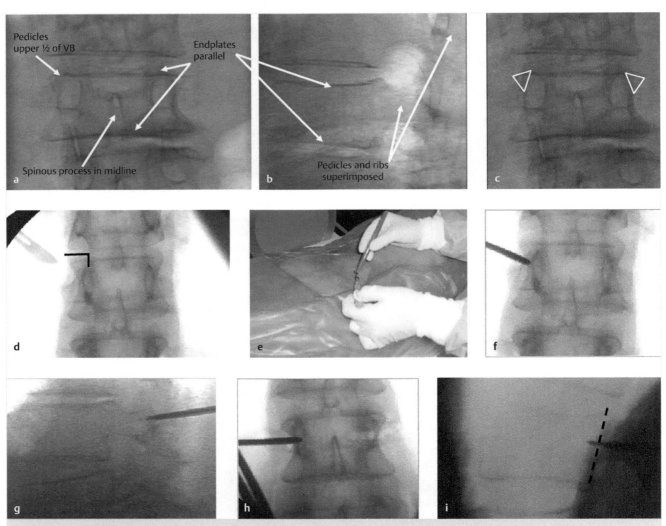

Fig. 6.6 Transpedicular approach for vertebral augmentation. (a) Anteroposterior (AP) and (b) lateral fluoroscopic images showing direct AP and lateral images with the appropriate bony landmarks labeled. These views will be common to any approach that uses AP and lateral views. The AP fluoroscopic view in (c) shows the pedicular targets at the 10 and 2 o'clock positions of the left and right pedicles, respectively, in the region of Kambin's safe triangle. A line is drawn 1 cm superior and 2 cm lateral (d) and an incision is placed at this point (e) after the appropriate needle starting point is fluoroscopically confirmed. The needle is then directed to the upper outer pedicle (f) and inserted a few millimeters into the bone with a mallet prior to confirming appropriate needle trajectory on the lateral view (g). The needle is advanced into the bone but before the medial wall of the pedicle is crossed (anteroposterior view in h), a lateral view is obtained to ensure the needle tip has entered into the posterior vertebral body wall (dashed line in i).

medial placement of the instruments and balloons placed too laterally will not achieve proper fracture reduction and may result in violation of the lateral cortex before fracture reduction is achieved.

Following sterile preparation and confirmation of appropriate imaging, the incision site just superior and lateral (1–2 cm) to the target pedicle is determined (►Fig. 6.6). The surgeon must visualize the passage of a working channel from that site through the length of the pedicle and two-thirds of the vertebral body, ending at or near the midline. The imagined course must not enter or traverse the spinal canal. Corresponding lateral and AP landmarks along the course (►Fig. 6.6) will ensure that instruments do not stray from the planned trajectory, risking injury.

Landmarks that must be identified include the pedicles, the spinous process, and the end plates (►Fig. 6.6). In a true AP view, the spinous process will be midline and the pedicles will be seen as symmetric ovals equidistant from the process and superimposed over the upper half of the vertebral body. End plates will be parallel (allowing for defects of the fracture). It is very important to locate these landmarks on true AP and lateral images before beginning (►Fig. 6.6). After injecting local anesthetic, a small approximately 5-mm stab incision is made (►Fig. 6.6). The Jamshidi needle is introduced and "docked" at the superolateral border of each pedicle ("10 and 2 o'clock positions"; ►Fig. 6.6). Just as the AP imaging demonstrates this starting point (►Fig. 6.6), lateral imaging should confirm that the needle tip is at the posterior margin of the pedicle (►Fig. 6.6). As the needle is advanced, it should reach mid-pedicle on both AP (►Fig. 6.6) and lateral imaging. As the needle reaches the medial aspect of the pedicle as seen on AP imaging (►Fig. 6.6), it should be seen in or near the posterior portion of the vertebral body on lateral imaging (►Fig. 6.6). The needle must not violate the medial pedicle wall, thereby entering the spinal canal and risking serious injury. After the Jamshidi needle is advanced via the pedicle into the vertebral body, a contralateral needle is placed if necessary. When performing a vertebroplasty, the needle(s) is/are advanced into the anterior one-third of the vertebral body and cement is then injected (►Fig. 6.7). During a balloon kyphoplasty procedure, the needles are place approximately 0.5 to 1.0 cm into the posterior portion of the vertebral body and then either a bone biopsy needle (if a biopsy is desired) or a drill is passed into the anterior

portion of the vertebral body up to within 0.3 to 0.5 cm of the anterior vertebral body wall cortex (►Fig. 6.8).

In the case of balloon kyphoplasty, the bone tamp (balloon) is inserted through the working channel and guided into the tract created by the drill (►Fig. 6.8). The radiopaque markers on the tamp are visualized distal to the cannula sheath on at least the lateral view (►Fig. 6.8) but preferably both the AP and lateral fluoroscopic images. This procedure is repeated on the contralateral side and each bone tamp is inflated (►Fig. 6.8) while being monitored with AP and lateral imaging. In the case of kyphoplasty, manometric controls are used to monitor the pressure of the balloons as they are inflated in small increments to the intended pressure. The inflation is done according to a combination of pressure, fracture characteristics, and balloon shape. The endpoint of balloon inflation is achieved when any of the following occurrences are seen: fracture reduction achieved, maximum inflation volume reached, maximum sustained balloon pressure achieved, cortical wall contact, or adequate cavity creation performed. The maximum balloon volume and balloon pressure will vary according to the balloon type and manufacturer.

After a void is created and height restoration is achieved as safely permitted, the bone tamps are removed and internal fixation is achieved through a low-pressure injection of bone void filler (►Fig. 6.8). After the cavity is filled and there is adequate interdigitation of cement into the interstices of the surrounding cancellous bone, the cannulas are removed.

6.6.3 Extrapedicular and Parapedicular Approaches

The transpedicular approach is effective in most cases, but it is difficult to achieve percutaneous access in certain situations. Reduced pedicle width and AP pedicular angle of the mid and upper thoracic vertebral pedicles compared to lumbar vertebrae often precludes a transpedicular approach in this area. Extrapedicular or parapedicular approaches are more appropriate for levels above T9. These approaches also accommodate placement of instruments too large for the transpedicular approach and can allow access to the vertebral body in a patient with existing hardware such as pedicle screws.[21] The extrapedicular approach is also more appropriate for a fracture that results in depression of the superior end plate to a location below the point of pedicle entry.[22]

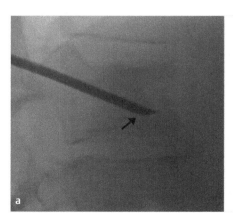
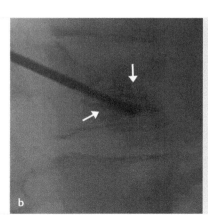

Fig. 6.7 Lateral fluoroscopic views showing the vertebral access needle placed into the anterior third of the vertebral body (*black arrow* in **a**) followed by injection of bone cement into the vertebral body (*white arrows* in **b**).

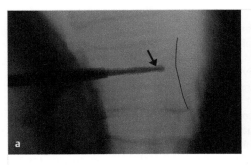
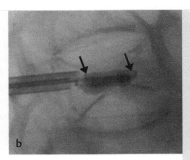
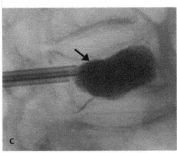
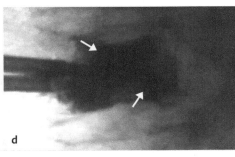

Fig. 6.8 Lateral fluoroscopic views showing the vertebral drill (*black arrow* in **a**) placed to within 0.5 cm of the anterior vertebral cortex (*black line* in **a**). Lateral fluoroscopic view showing the balloon being inserted with the anterior and posterior radiopaque marker bands completely through the needle and into the vertebral body (*black arrows* in **b**). The marker bands show the proximal and distal boundaries of the noninflated balloons. The balloon is then inflated with contrast (*black arrow* in **c**) with subsequent reduction of the vertebral body. After the balloons are deflated and removed, bone fillers are used to inject bone cement into the vertebral body (*white arrows* in **d**).

Downward-angled ribs sometimes limit extrapedicular access in the thoracic spine and the entry point may require the needle to pass under the rib, immediately adjacent to the intercostal neurovascular bundle. Further, wide pedicles at the L5 level as well as the obstructing presence of iliac crests make the extrapedicular approach particularly difficult at this level. However, the favorable needle trajectory allowed by the extrapedicular approach allows for a consistent and predictable approach to the vertebral body.

In the parapedicular approach, the entry site allows establishment of a working channel that effectively traverses the anterior portion of the pedicle at the pedicle–vertebral body junction rather than traveling within the pedicle throughout its course. The size of the cannula is therefore not limited by the diameter of the pedicle and the entry point anterior to the pedicle means there is decreased risk of pedicle fracture. Although this approach offers protection from medial canal breach at the pedicle–vertebral body junction, care must still be taken to avoid neural injury or injury to the pleura in the thoracic region given its more lateral entry point.[23]

6.6.4 Extrapedicular Modified Inferior End Plate Access

In 2016, Beall et al described a relatively avascular and aneural portion of the inferior vertebral body just anterior to the pedicle. They then treated a total of 96 thoracic and lumbar vertebral fractures using this extrapedicular modified inferior end plate access without any recognized clinical complications from the needle access or the instrumentation. This is an ideal approach when the vertebral body is very compressed superiorly or when a device larger than the size of the pedicle is to be inserted. The technique allows access around existing hardware and the authors noted that it could accommodate the placement of large instruments.[21]

For this approach, the AP fluoroscope is angled 45 degrees off midline for procedures involving the lumbar spine or 30 degrees off midline for procedures involving the thoracic spine for an oblique view (▶Fig. 6.9). The incision is made at a point just anterior to the pedicle, slightly above the inferior end plate (▶Fig. 6.9). The needle is advanced to the bone and subsequently just into the vertebral body. At this point, the AP view should be checked to confirm medial and lateral position (▶Fig. 6.9). The lateral view will confirm the needle tip to be in the middle to anterior third of the vertebral body. The needle should never go posterior to the pedicle on the oblique view, to avoid damage to the descending ventral ramus, and should never go into the paraspinal soft tissue adjacent to the thoracic spine without having the needle at a shallow angle to avoid damage to the pleura or entrance into the lung. An entry pint too far superior risks injury to the vertebral segmental artery. The operator should always line up the vertebral body in direct AP view (▶Fig. 6.6a) before arcing 45 degrees off midline in the lumbar spine and 30 degrees in the thoracic spine to ensure the angle of entry is appropriate.[21]

6.6.5 Parapedicular Approach

The parapedicular approach is also known as the transcostovertebral approach due to its course along the rib margin in the thoracic spine.[24] The needle passes lateral to the pedicle rather than through it and angles more toward the center of the vertebral body than with the transpedicular approach. The costotransverse and costovertebral junctions in the upper thoracic spine typically direct the trajectory of the needle more ipsilateral, thereby making the access to the center of the vertebral body with a unilateral approach more difficult. It is a useful approach if the pedicle is very thin, difficult to see, or affected by tumor. The size of the needle is not limited by the diameter of the pedicle and the risk of pedicle fracture is decreased. There is an increased risk of paraspinal hematoma and a decreased ability to control postprocedural bleeding by local tamponade. In a retrospective evaluation,

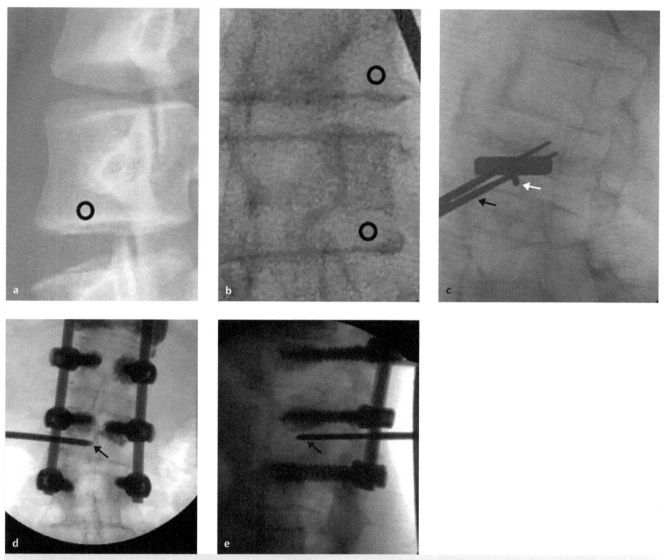

Fig. 6.9 The modified inferior end plate extrapedicular approach. The image intensifier is angled 45 degrees ipsilateral for the lumbar spine (a) and 30 degrees ipsilateral in the thoracic spine (b). The entry point is identified just anterior to the pedicle and just above the inferior end plate (*black circles* in a and b). At that point, a small skin incision is made and the needle (*white arrow* in c) is inserted and held by a Kelly or Kocher clamp (*black arrow* in c). The needle is advanced into the center of the vertebral body and the final needle tip position is confirmed on the anteroposterior and lateral views (*black arrows* in d and e, respectively).

Chiras and Deramond[25] and Chiras et al[26] reported parapedicular approach complication rates of 1% in patients with osteoporotic vertebral fracture and between 2.5 and 10% in patients with benign and malignant spinal tumors, respectively. Despite this relatively high complication rate reported in the 1990s, more recent data were reported in 2007 with 102 VCFs treated via a parapedicular access in patients between the ages of 17 and 96 with no nerve root injuries, hematomas, injury to spinal canal contents, or any other complications.[22] To avoid needle injury, the surgeon must be aware of nearby intercostal arteries in the thoracic spine and four pairs of lumbar arteries. In the thoracic region, there is also risk of injury to the pleura and a subsequent pneumothorax. As with the extrapedicular approach, wide pedicles of L5 level and occasionally the iliac crests make the parapedicular approach difficult at this level.[22]

6.6.6 Parapedicular Approach to the Vertebral Body

In 2007, to investigate and illustrate a variation on the traditional percutaneous access to the vertebral body via a parapedicular approach, Beall et al identified an effective parapedicular access technique that could safely and reliably guide the needle tip into the center of the vertebral body.[22] Developed from cadaver dissection observations for the purpose of clinical use, a total of 102 VCFs from T4 to L5 were treated via this parapedicular access between July 2005 and March 2006. There were 72 patients between the ages of 17 and 96 years (mean age: 68.2 years) who underwent treatment. The cadaver dissection revealed a relatively avascular and aneural portion of the vertebral body along the superior margin of the vertebral body–pedicle junction. A total

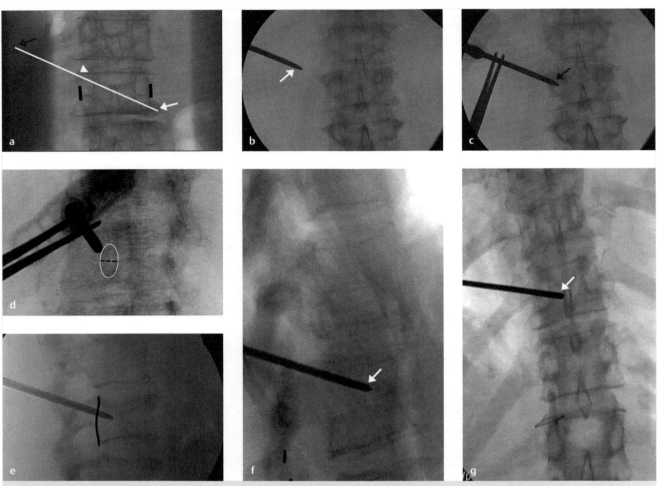

Fig. 6.10 (a) Parapedicular approach to the vertebral body. Anteroposterior (AP) view of the upper lumbar spine demonstrates a white line drawn from the contralateral inferior vertebral body corner (*white arrow*) to the ipsilateral superior vertebral body wall corner (*white arrowhead*). The line extends one vertebral body width (the distance between the *black vertical hash marks*) ipsilateral and superior to a point that serves as the skin entry point for parapedicular modified superior end plate access (*black arrow*). **(b–g)** The needle (*white arrow* in **b**) is advanced at a 45-degree angle to the upper outer portion of the pedicle (*black arrow* in **c**) at the pedicle–body junction. An ipsilateral oblique view is then obtained and the ideal needle tip position is just anterior to the pedicle (pedicle outlined by *white circle* in **d**) and just superior to the superoinferior midpoint of the pedicle (indicated by *black dashed line* in **d**). An AP view is then obtained (**c**) and the needle advanced. Prior to crossing the medial wall of the pedicle on the AP view, a lateral view is obtained to ensure that the needle tip has crossed the posterior vertebral body wall (*black line* in **e**). After advancing the needle into the vertebral body, the proper location is when the needle tip is halfway across the vertebral body in both the AP and lateral views (*white arrows* in **f** and **g**).

102 vertebral fractures were treated using this parapedicular access technique without any recognized clinical complications from the needle access or the instrumentation. This study showed that the thoracic and lumbar vertebral bodies may be safely, reliably, and reproducibly accessed using a percutaneous parapedicular access technique.[22]

Using a line extending from the contralateral inferior corner of the VB through the ipsilateral superior corner, a point along this line that is approximately one vertebral body width beyond the lateral aspect of the VB is identified (▶Fig. 6.10).[22] An incision is made at this point and the needle is the advanced inferiorly toward the vertebral body at a 45-degree angle (▶Fig. 6.10). If the approach is used for a thoracic vertebral body, the needle should be aligned with the medial rib insertion, as this allows passage adjacent to the costotransverse–costovertebral junction, which is the

path of least resistance to the center of the vertebral body. The operator should then look enface to ensure both proper needle trajectory and parapedicular location of the needle (▶Fig. 6.10). The operator can then return to the AP view and advance the needle along the selected trajectory. The needle tip should never cross the medial wall of the pedicle in this view prior to penetration of the posterior cortical wall of the vertebral body (▶Fig. 6.10). An AP view should be obtained to verify needle trajectory and position and ensure the medial aspect of the pedicle has not been violated. After confirming the needle tip is positioned within the posterior portion of the vertebral body, the needle can then be further advanced to the desired location within the vertebral body. The proper location is verified when the needle tip is halfway across the vertebral body in both the AP and lateral views (▶Fig. 6.10).[22]

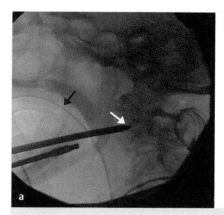 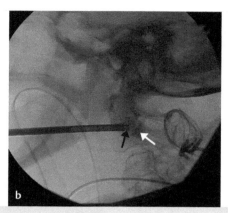 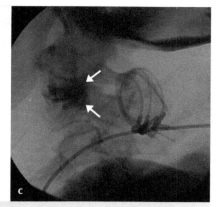

Fig. 6.11 Lateral fluoroscopic images showing the patient lying supine under general anesthesia and an endotracheal tube in place (*black arrow* in **a**). The needle was placed transorally into the anterior portion of the C2 vertebral body (*white arrow* in **a**) and cement (*white arrow* in **b**) was injected into the vertebral body via a bone filler (*black arrow* in **b**). Final lateral fluoroscopic images show cement filling the C2 vertebral body and dens (*white arrows* in **c**).

6.6.7 Approaches to the Cervical Spine

Of note, more on the approaches to the cervical spine can be seen in Chapter 10 (Cervical and Posterior Arch Augmentation).

Vertebroplasty has been shown to be beneficial for pain control and stabilization of multiple conditions affecting the cervical spine, including osteoporotic fracture, metastasis, aggressive hemangioma, and multiple myeloma.[27–30] In the upper cervical spine, the cervical pedicles are small and the vertebral arteries are near, so transpedicular access is difficult. Several variations of approach to the cervical spine have been described since the procedure was introduced by Galibert et al. These include the anterolateral, transoral, posteroanterior, posterolateral, and anterior retropharyngeal approaches.

The anterolateral approach (▶ Fig. 6.2), unlike the transoral approach, can be performed without general anesthesia or endotracheal intubation, and the risk of infection is also lower with the anterolateral approach. With manual retraction of the carotid artery and jugular vein laterally, the needle may be safely placed medial to the vessels.

The percutaneous inferior anterolateral approach involves placing a needle under the mandible (Chapter 10, ▶ Fig. 10.2). The needle is then directed cephalad and anteromedially into the vertebral body with manual traction of the adjacent vascular and nervous structures. This approach is technically challenging and risks injury to the vagal, spinal accessory, lingual, hypoglossal, marginal mandibular, and laryngeal nerves. The internal jugular vein and the vertebral and carotid arteries are also at risk.[27,31–33]

Lykomitros et al described the minimally invasive open approach whereby a small incision is made along the medial border of the sternocleidomastoid muscle. The platysma muscle is divided and the carotid sheath and sternocleidomastoid muscle retracted laterally. With fluoroscopic guidance and palpation of the airway, a guide pin is passed medial to the common carotid artery and advanced through the longus colli muscle and into the vertebral body. Positioning is guided by and confirmed with AP and lateral fluoroscopic imaging.[34]

In 2017, Bao et al retrospectively analyzed data from nine patients treated with percutaneous vertebroplasty via the anterolateral approach to treat late-stage metastatic

cancer to 22 cervical vertebrae (mean Tokuhashi score: 6.89 ± 2.14).[35] In each case, a small incision was made before a wire was passed medial to the sternocleidomastoid and carotid sheath and lateral to the esophagus and trachea. A working channel was established using the Seldinger technique. The mean volume of cement injected was 1.32 ± 0.49 mL). The cement leakage rate was 63.6% (14 of 22 vertebrae treated). No serious complications were observed, while significant pain relief was noted. VAS decreased from 8.11 ± 1.45 preoperatively to 2.22 ± 0.67) at 3 days after the procedure ($p < 0.001$).

High cervical vertebrae may be reached by using the anterolateral approach, but it is relatively difficult at the C2 level. Tong et al described the transoral approach to C2 in a patient with multiple myeloma resulting in complete pain relief and stabilization of the involved vertebra. According to the authors, the benefits of transoral vertebroplasty include precise needle placement and decreased risk to adjacent neurovascular structures.[33] Clarençon et al have also reported their early experience with the transoral approach, used to access C1.[36]

Although the transoral approach reduces the risk of neurovascular complications with a more direct route through the posterior oropharyngeal wall under fluoroscopic guidance into the VB of C2 (▶ Fig. 6.11), the route carries an increased risk of infection and should not be used in patients receiving or expected to receive radiation therapy that might interfere with wound healing. It requires general anesthesia and may require manual cervical stabilization and/or fiberoptic intubation.[31,33,37–39] Both anterolateral and transoral approaches have been successfully used in the upper cervical spine and while effective, both have potentially life-threatening complications.[32,40–43]

Wetzel et al described a technique for posteroanterior access to the lateral portion of C1 to treat osteolytic metastatic disease with precautions to protect the vertebrobasilar arterial supply.[44] Cianfoni et al have described a posterolateral approach to C1, also sparing the vertebral artery (VA), suggesting that it may be a therapeutic option in selected patients to avoid occipitocervical fusion but requiring good understanding of the anatomy and rigorous technique to avoid potential complications.[45]

In 2015, a novel anterior retropharyngeal approach was described by Yang et al as an effective alternative when the transoral approach is unsuitable or contraindicated. The approach involved passing the needle through the vertebral body of C2 into the C1 lateral mass to treat metastatic osteolytic vertebral lesions at each level.[46]

6.7 Vertebral Body Biopsy

A percutaneous approach with intraoperative imaging is an excellent minimally invasive method of vertebral body biopsy, offering high accuracy and low complication rates for both thoracic and lumbar vertebral body lesions.[47,48] In our practice, we routinely collect biopsies during vertebral augmentation, believing that it is in the best interest of each patient to identify any cause of pathologic fractures for timely and appropriate subsequent treatment. The majority of fractures are attributed to osteoporosis, but other etiologies include multiple myeloma, primary and metastatic disease, and osteomyelitis.[49] If infection is a concern, specimen should be submitted for culture and sensitivity.

With the transpedicular approach, an 11-gauge vertebral biopsy introducer needle is advanced and inserted into the posterior portion of the pedicle. It is important to appreciate the feel of the bone as bone affected by neoplasm, infection, or even osteoporosis may be softened, preventing reliable purchase and resistance. The introducer needle is carefully advanced through the pedicle by small, controlled, repetitive impacts with a mallet. The needle is advanced to the proximal edge of the lesion. The inner cannula is removed and biopsy needle advanced into the lesion. With gentle continuous aspiration from a 10- to 20-mL syringe, the biopsy needle is removed. If more tissue is required, the inner cannula is replaced and the introducer needle may be moved to a new location for repeat biopsy. If adequate specimen is obtained, the inner cannula is replaced and the introducer needle is removed under fluoroscopic guidance.

Different needle combinations may be used if it is difficult to obtain tissue. A soft-tissue core biopsy needle may be used through the outer bone needle. Some more resilient tissues may require the use of a high-speed drill. Coaxial technique will facilitate the use of different needles with different characteristics through the outer bone needle in whatever combination that is necessary to obtain an adequate biopsy specimen.

Any of the approaches described in this chapter may be used to access the vertebra of interest and obtain tissue for biopsy.

6.8 Conclusion

Percutaneous access to the vertebral body may be used for vertebral augmentation procedures to safely and effectively treat traumatic, neoplastic, or osteoporotic fractures. This minimally invasive access also allows vertebral body biopsy when infection or tumor is suspected. The approach employed will be specific to the patient and determined by many factors including fracture level, vertebral morphology, bone quality, and operator experience and preference. Each approach has specific indications and contraindications.

Planning and preparation are essential. Transpedicular approach is standard and straightforward. Both extrapedicular and parapedicular approaches are easily planned using landmarks that are fluoroscopically identifiable and a trajectory that places the entry point through relatively avascular and aneural tissues. Cervical anterolateral and transoral approaches have inherent risk of injury and, as with all approaches, require good understanding of the anatomy and rigorous technique. These approaches—in the hands of knowledgeable and skilled operators—are invaluable for safe and effective minimally invasive access to vertebrae for augmentation and diagnostic procedures.

References

[1] Galibert P, Deramond H, Rosat P, Le Gars D. Preliminary note on the treatment of vertebral angioma by percutaneous acrylic vertebroplasty Neurochirurgie 1987;33(2):166–168

[2] Mathis J, Belkoff S, Deramond H. Introduction: history and early development. In: Mathis J, Deramond H, Belkoff S, eds. Percutaneous Vertebroplasty and Kyphoplasty. New York, NY: Springer; 2006:1–5

[3] Röllinghoff M, Zarghooni K, Schlüter-Brust K, et al. Indications and contraindications for vertebroplasty and kyphoplasty. Arch Orthop Trauma Surg 2010;130(6):765–774

[4] Robinson Y, Heyde CE, Försth P, Olerud C. Kyphoplasty in osteoporotic vertebral compression fractures: guidelines and technical considerations. J Orthop Surg Res 2011;6:43

[5] Garfin SR, Yuan HA, Reiley MA. New technologies in spine: kyphoplasty and vertebroplasty for the treatment of painful osteoporotic compression fractures. Spine 2001;26(14):1511–1515

[6] Yu CW, Hsieh MK, Chen LH, et al. Percutaneous balloon kyphoplasty for the treatment of vertebral compression fractures. BMC Surg 2014;14:3

[7] Markmiller M. Percutaneous balloon kyphoplasty of malignant lesions of the spine: a prospective consecutive study in 115 patients. Eur Spine J 2015;24(10):2165–2172

[8] de Falco R, Bocchetti A. Balloon kyphoplasty for pure traumatic thoracolumbar fractures: retrospective analysis of 61 cases focusing on restoration of vertebral height. Eur Spine J 2014;23(23, Suppl 6):664–670

[9] Sun H, Lu PP, Liu YJ, et al. Can unilateral kyphoplasty replace bilateral kyphoplasty in treatment of osteoporotic vertebral compression fractures? a systematic review and meta-analysis. Pain Physician 2016;19(8):551–563

[10] Youmans JR, Winn HR. Youmans Neurological Surgery. Philadelphia, PA: Saunders; 2011

[11] Krüger A, Zettl R, Ziring E, Mann D, Schnabel M, Ruchholtz S. Kyphoplasty for the treatment of incomplete osteoporotic burst fractures. Eur Spine J 2010;19(6):893–900

[12] Bozkurt M, Kahilogullari G, Ozdemir M, et al. Comparative analysis of vertebroplasty and kyphoplasty for osteoporotic vertebral compression fractures. Asian Spine J 2014;8(1):27–34

[13] Feng H, Huang P, Zhang X, Zheng G, Wang Y. Unilateral versus bilateral percutaneous kyphoplasty for osteoporotic vertebral compression fractures: a systematic review and meta-analysis of RCTs. J Orthop Res 2015;33(11):1713–1723

[14] Yang S, Chen C, Wang H, Wu Z, Liu L. A systematic review of unilateral versus bilateral percutaneous vertebroplasty/percutaneous kyphoplasty for osteoporotic vertebral compression fractures. Acta Orthop Traumatol Turc 2017;51(4):290–297

[15] Chen H, Tang P, Zhao Y, Gao Y, Wang Y. Unilateral versus bilateral balloon kyphoplasty in the treatment of osteoporotic vertebral compression fractures. Orthopedics 2014;37(9):e828–e835

[16] Papanastassiou ID, Eleraky M, Murtagh R, Kokkalis ZT, Gerochristou M, Vrionis FD. Comparison of unilateral versus bilateral kyphoplasty in multiple myeloma patients and the importance of preoperative planning. Asian Spine J 2014;8(3):244–252

[17] Huang Z, Wan S, Ning L, Han S. Is unilateral kyphoplasty as effective and safe as bilateral kyphoplasties for osteoporotic vertebral compression fractures? A meta-analysis. Clin Orthop Relat Res 2014;472(9):2833–2842

[18] Yan L, Jiang R, He B, Liu T, Hao D. A comparison between unilateral transverse process-pedicle and bilateral puncture techniques in percutaneous kyphoplasty. Spine 2014;39(26, Spec No.):B19–B26

[19] Chung HJ, Chung KJ, Yoon HS, Kwon IH. Comparative study of balloon kyphoplasty with unilateral versus bilateral approach in osteoporotic vertebral compression fractures. Int Orthop 2008;32(6):817–820

[20] Schmidt R, Richter M, Puhl W, Cakir B. Vertebroplasty: basic science, indications and technique Zentralbl Chir 2005;130(5):476–484

[21] Beall DP, Parsons B, Burner S. Technical strategies and anatomic considerations for an extrapedicular modified inferior endplate access to thoracic and lumbar vertebral bodies. Pain Physician 2016;19(8):593–601

[22] Beall DP, Braswell JJ, Martin HD, Stapp AM, Puckett TA, Stechison MT. Technical strategies and anatomic considerations for parapedicular access to thoracic and lumbar vertebral bodies. Skeletal Radiol 2007;36(1):47–52

[23] Kim HS, Kim SW, Ju CI. Balloon kyphoplasty through extrapedicular approach in the treatment of middle thoracic osteoporotic compression fracture : T5-T8 level. J Korean Neurosurg Soc 2007;42(5):363–366

[24] Predey TA, Sewall LE, Smith SJ. Percutaneous vertebroplasty: new treatment for vertebral compression fractures. Am Fam Physician 2002;66(4):611–615

[25] Chiras J, Deramond H. Complications des vertebroplasties. In: Saillant G, Laville C, eds. Echecs et complication de la chirurgie du rachis. Montpillier, France: Saurmps Medical; 1995:149–153

[26] Chiras J, Depriester C, Weill A, Sola-Martinez MT, Deramond H. Percutaneous vertebral surgery. Technics and indications J Neuroradiol 1997;24(1):45–59

[27] Mont'Alverne F, Vallée JN, Cormier E, et al. Percutaneous vertebroplasty for metastatic involvement of the axis. AJNR Am J Neuroradiol 2005;26(7):1641–1645

[28] Murphy KJ, Deramond H. Percutaneous vertebroplasty in benign and malignant disease. Neuroimaging Clin N Am 2000;10(3):535–545

[29] Pilitsis JG, Rengachary SS. The role of vertebroplasty in metastatic spinal disease. Neurosurg Focus 2001;11(6):e9

[30] Weill A, Chiras J, Simon JM, Rose M, Sola-Martinez T, Enkaoua E. Spinal metastases: indications for and results of percutaneous injection of acrylic surgical cement. Radiology 1996;199(1):241–247

[31] Reddy AS, Hochman M, Loh S, Rachlin J, Li J, Hirsch JA. CT guided direct transoral approach to C2 for percutaneous vertebroplasty. Pain Physician 2005;8(2):235–238

[32] Dufresne AC, Brunet E, Sola-Martinez MT, Rose M, Chiras J. Percutaneous vertebroplasty of the cervico-thoracic junction using an anterior route. Technique and results. Report of nine cases J Neuroradiol 1998;25(2):123–128

[33] Tong FC, Cloft HJ, Joseph GJ, Rodts GR, Dion JE. Transoral approach to cervical vertebroplasty for multiple myeloma. AJR Am J Roentgenol 2000;175(5):1322–1324

[34] Lykomitros V, Anagnostidis KS, Alzeer Z, Kapetanos GA. Percutaneous anterolateral balloon kyphoplasty for metastatic lytic lesions of the cervical spine. Eur Spine J 2010;19(11):1948–1952

[35] Bao L, Jia P, Li J, et al. Percutaneous vertebroplasty relieves pain in cervical spine metastases. Pain Res Manag 2017;2017:3926318

[36] Clarençon F, Cormier E, Pascal-Moussellard H, et al. Transoral approach for percutaneous vertebroplasty in the treatment of osteolytic tumor lesions of the lateral mass of the atlas: feasibility and initial experience in 2 patients. Spine 2013;38(3):E193–E197

[37] Anselmetti GC, Regge D, Sardo E, et al. Minimally invasive treatment of C2 odontoid traumatic fracture with transoral percutaneous vertebroplasty. Eur Radiol 2007;17(3):850–851

[38] Martin JB, Gailloud P, Dietrich PY, et al. Direct transoral approach to C2 for percutaneous vertebroplasty. Cardiovasc Intervent Radiol 2002;25(6):517–519

[39] Sachs DC, Inamasu J, Mendel EE, Guiot BH. Transoral vertebroplasty for renal cell metastasis involving the axis: case report. Spine 2006;31(24):E925–E928

[40] Jensen ME, Evans AJ, Mathis JM, Kallmes DF, Cloft HJ, Dion JE. Percutaneous polymethylmethacrylate vertebroplasty in the treatment of osteoporotic vertebral body compression fractures: technical aspects. AJNR Am J Neuroradiol 1997;18(10):1897–1904

[41] Levine SA, Perin LA, Hayes D, Hayes WS. An evidence-based evaluation of percutaneous vertebroplasty. Manag Care 2000;9(3):56–60, 63

[42] Vender JR, McDonnel DE. Management of lesions involving the craniocervical junction. Neurosurg Q 2001;11:151–171

[43] Vieweg U, Meyer B, Schramm J. Tumour surgery of the upper cervical spine--a retrospective study of 13 cases. Acta Neurochir (Wien) 2001;143(3):217–225

[44] Wetzel SG, Martin JB, Somon T, Wilhelm K, Rufenacht DA. Painful osteolytic metastasis of the atlas: treatment with percutaneous vertebroplasty. Spine 2002;27(22):E493–E495

[45] Cianfoni A, Distefano D, Chin SH, Varma AK, Rumboldt Z, Bonaldi G. Percutaneous cement augmentation of a lytic lesion of C1 via posterolateral approach under CT guidance. Spine J 2012;12(6):500–506

[46] Yang JS, Chu L, Xiao FT, et al. Anterior retropharyngeal approach to C1 for percutaneous vertebroplasty under C-arm fluoroscopy. Spine J 2015;15(3):539–545

[47] Shrestha D, Shrestha R, Dhoju D. Fluoroscopy guided percutaneous transpedicular biopsy for thoracic and lumbar vertebral body lesion: technique and safety in 23 consecutive cases. Kathmandu Univ Med J (KUMJ) 2015;13(51):256–260 (KUMJ)

[48] Dave BR, Nanda A, Anandjiwala JV. Transpedicular percutaneous biopsy of vertebral body lesions: a series of 71 cases. Spinal Cord 2009;47(5):384–389

[49] Wang Y, Liu H, Pi B, Yang H, Qian Z, Zhu X. Clinical evaluation of percutaneous kyphoplasty in the treatment of osteolytic and osteoblastic metastatic vertebral lesions. Int J Surg 2016;30(30):161–165

7 Properties of Bone Cements and Vertebral Fill Materials: Implications for Clinical Use in Image-Guided Therapy and Vertebral Augmentation

David Nussbaum, Adam Thakore, and Kieran Murphy

Summary

Bone cement or polymethyl methacrylate (PMMA) is the primary stabilizing material used for treating painful vertebral compression fractures (VCFs). The PMMAs available are acrylic polymers comprised of different components that can be manipulated to maximize its utility in minimally invasive spine interventions. In addition to PMMA, there is also another cement type comprised of self-hardening calcium phosphate cements (CPCs) that have been used to treat VCFs. Unlike PMMA that hardens by a polymerization process converting methylmethacrylate (MMA) monomers to PMMA, CPCs dissolve with water into a paste that hardens at body temperature into hydroxyapatite (HA). The advantage of CPCs are that they are biocompatible and are resorbed over time but the disadvantages compared to PMMA is that they are difficult to inject, are weaker than PMMA, and are often too brittle to be used in high stress areas. Fill materials also include a glass ceramic tri-resin polymer that is hydrophilic, has lower exothermic temperatures, and mimics the mechanical properties of bone. While the hydrophilic properties result in a greater amount of interdigitation into the bone and less material injected, it tends to extravasate more easily than the hydrophobic cements. Cement properties can be tailored to the appropriate use by varying the cement ingredients and can have other added components such as antibiotics and other radiopacifying agents. The future of bone cements is likely with the addition of bioactive materials such as bioactive glass, bone morphogenic protein, platelet rich plasma, stem cells, and various growth factors to promote the osteogenic activity of the native bone and to improve the strength of the cement and its degree of bony incorporation.

Keywords: bone cement, polymethyl methacrylate, vertebral augmentation, osteogenic, calcium phosphate cement, vertebroplasty, kyphoplasty

7.1 Introduction

Advances in image-guided therapy for vertebral fractures and other bone-related disorders have made acrylic bone cement an integral part of the interventional tool kit. This chapter focuses on the chemistry of bone cement polymerization and the properties of components in PMMA based polymers, the most commonly used bone cements in interventional procedures such as percutaneous vertebroplasty (PVP) or vertebral augmentation. The effects of altering the concentration of the components such as MMA monomers, PMMA beads, benzoyl peroxide (BPO) activator, N,N-dimethyl-p-toluidine (DMPT) initiator, and radiopacifiers on the setting time, viscosity, polymerization temperature, and compressive strength of the cement are also considered. This information allows us to manipulate bone cement characteristics for specific applications and maximize the clinical potential of image-guided interventions. Most commercial cement kits used by radiologists were originally designed for joint replacement surgery, not vertebral fracture therapy. Novel applications such as VP require modifications of standard bone–cement mixtures—adjustments that can be made only by understanding the underlying chemical and material properties of these compounds. Our discussion will focus on the theoretical and practical aspects of polymerization chemistry, the basis for most bone cement solidification.

7.2 Bone Cement Types

There are two main types of bone cements: polymers and self-hardening CPCs. Both types are fillers that stabilize joint implants or fractures, but neither is adhesive. Polymers are most commonly used because of their proven track record of safety and efficacy. They are based on the polymerization of MMA monomers to polymethyl methacrylate (PMMA), a compound better known by the name Plexiglas. Unlike polymers, the first CPCs were developed in the late 1980s to remineralize early dental carries and were approved by the Food and Drug Administration for repairing cranial defects in 1996 as cavity void fillers.

The CPCs are potentially an ideal filling material for VP and balloon kyphoplasty (BKP) applications. CPCs function by a completely different chemical mechanism based on the solubility of reactants and products. Despite the large number of calcium phosphate (CaP) combinations in different CPC systems, the setting chemistry is similar and involves dissolution and reprecipitation. Based on the nature of the end hydration product, which depends on the pH of the cement paste, $Ca PO_4$ cements can be divided into two categories: apatite (HA) or calcium-deficient hydroxyapatite [CDHA], formed at pH > 4.2) and brushite (dicalcium phosphate dehydrate [DCPD]). Due to the short setting time, low mechanical strength, and inferior injection characteristics, brushite cements only have limited clinical applications. When tetracalcium phosphate and dicalcium phosphate are mixed with water into a paste, HA (the major mineral found in normal teeth) is rapidly formed and precipitates out of the solution, forming a hard mass at body temperature.[1,2] HA is a biocompatible material believed to be gradually replaced in vivo by new bone with no loss of volume.[3,4] On the downside, the cement is difficult to inject against high backpressure, and the bone resorption properties may actually cause long-term weakening in patients with osteoporosis. Additionally, it may be weaker than polymer cement[5] and too brittle to be used for load-bearing applications. Because there are no long-term data for CPC technology, this review will focus on PMMA bone cements.

The use of HA and CaP bone cements in an osteoporotic patient without the addition of anabolic parathyroid (PTH) analog medication is probably not a sound concept. The addition of systemic PTH allows bone activation and anabolic bone stimulation to integrate these cements in a way that the inert elderly osteoporotic cannot achieve otherwise.

Cortoss is a glass ceramic combeite tri-resin polymer, an injectable, synthetic, nonresorbable biomaterial that mimics the mechanical properties of cortical bone.[1] Cortoss has been clinically proven to match the safety and effectiveness of PMMA for VP and clinical trials with Cortoss report a low incidence of adjacent fractures,[2] lower exothermic temperatures, and less monomer release than PMMA. The safety and efficacy of Cortoss has been demonstrated in three U.S. clinical investigations and multiple European studies.[6,7] In patients with a first-time fracture at one level, there was a 43% reduction in adjacent-level fractures in the patient population that used Cortoss.[6] Compared to PMMA, Cortoss is more hydrophilic, which enables it to coat and augment the internal structure of the vertebral body. This interdigitating characteristic resulted in a 30% reduction in material injected when compared to PMMA in a controlled study. Despite the optimal characteristics allowing the interdigitation of Cortoss within the cancellous vertebral body bone, the hydrophilic properties of the fill material make it prone to extravasation outside the vertebral body.

7.2.1 Polymer Chemistry

Before the specifics of bone cement are discussed, we will briefly review polymer chemistry. Polymers are large molecules composed of individual repeating units (monomers). Proteins are classic examples of biologic polymers composed of smaller amino acid units.

Polymerization can occur by two different mechanisms: (1) in condensation reactions, a functional group on the monomer reacts with a functional group on the growing end of the polymer, lengthening the chain and releasing an extraneous molecule (▶ Fig. 7.1)[8] and (2) in addition reactions, the polymer chain grows by reacting directly with the double bond of a monomer and no extraneous molecules are created (▶ Fig. 7.2).

Polymerization begins by the addition mechanism in which a monomer becomes unstable by reacting with an initiator, a volatile molecule that is most commonly a radical (molecules that contain a single unpaired electron). Radicals bond with monomers, forming monomer radicals that can attack the double bond of the next monomer by the mechanism shown in ▶ Fig. 7.2, propagating the polymer chain.

Because radicals are so transient, initiators are often added in the form of an unreactive peroxide form that is stable in solution. Radicals are formed when heat or light cleaves the

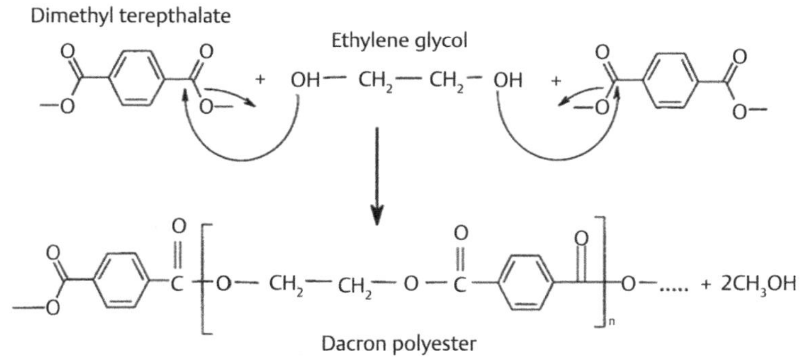

Fig. 7.1 Polymerization of Dacron polyester via a condensation reaction of dimethyl terephthalate and ethylene glycol. Note that methanol is released as a byproduct of the reaction.[9]

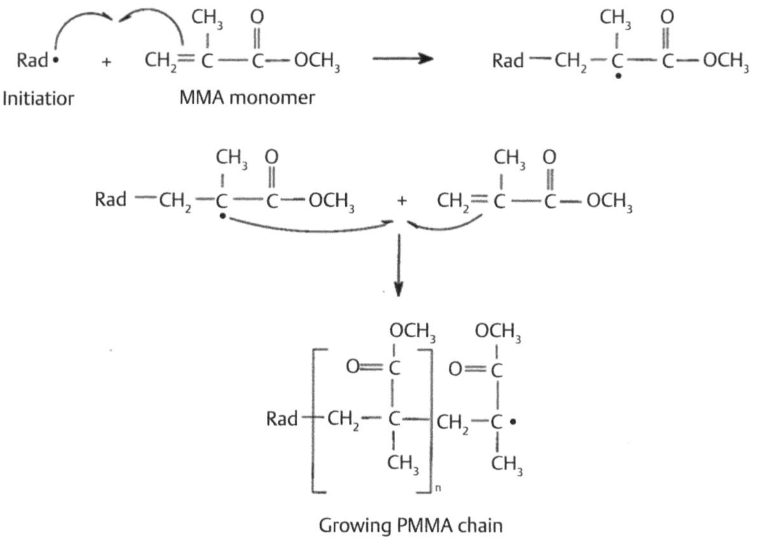

Fig. 7.2 Polymerization of polymethyl methacrylate (PMMA) by an addition reaction. Note that the methylmethacrylate (MMA) monomer reacts with a radical to form a secondary radical that can attack the double bond of another MMA monomer.

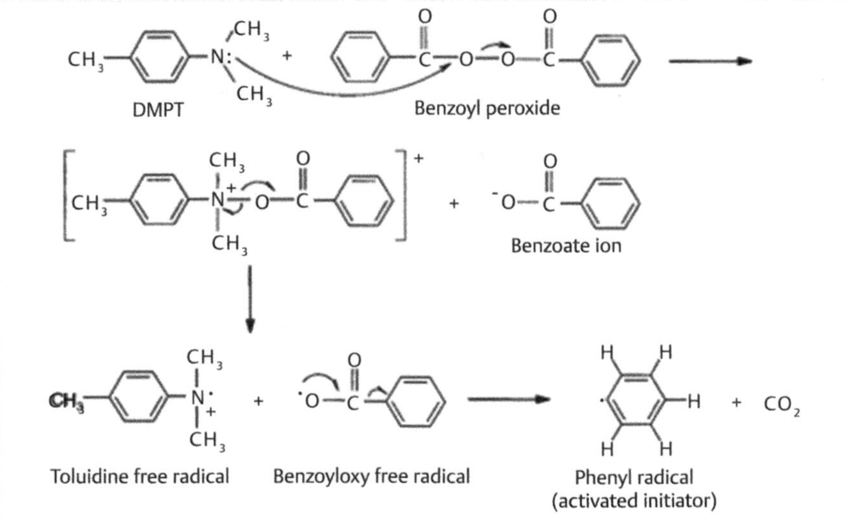

Fig. 7.3 Formation of phenyl radical by reaction of N,N-dimethyl-p-toluidine (DMPT) with the benzoyl peroxide (BPO) initiator. The phenyl radical goes on to react with methylmethacrylate (MMA) by the mechanism shown in ▶ Fig. 7.2.

Table 7.1 Components of commercially available cement mixtures[1]

Powder
• PMMA beads
• Benzoyl peroxide (BPO)
• Radiopacifier

Liquid
• MMA monomers
• Activator (DMPT)
• Hydroquinone 15–75 ppm

Abbreviations: DMPT, N,N-dimethyl-p-toluidine; MMA, methylmethacrylate; PMMA, polymethyl methacrylate.

peroxide molecule. For applications in which high temperatures are not practical (such as the use of bone cement in vivo), peroxide is cleaved by adding a chemical activator such as N, N-dimethyl-p-toluidine (DMPT; ▶ Fig. 7.3).[9]

7.2.2 PMMA-Based Bone Cements

Bone cements polymerize by radical-initiated addition reactions. Most commercially available cements have two separate components (▶ Table 7.1): a powder containing prepolymerized beads of PMMA (or PMMA/styrene copolymer) and a liquid containing MMA monomer. The BPO initiator is incorporated into the powder and the chemical activator (i.e., DMPT) is incorporated into the liquid, so peroxide cleavage and polymerization begin only when the two are mixed. To prevent spontaneous polymerization during storage, the easily oxidized molecule hydroquinone is also added to the liquid. The DMPT cleaves BPO initiator at room temperature, forming a phenyl radical (▶ Fig. 7.3) that attacks the double bond of the MMA monomer by the mechanism shown in ▶ Fig. 7.2. The growing polymer chains encapsulate the PMMA beads within a solid matrix.

Cement is made radiopaque by adding barium sulfate or zirconium dioxide compounds to the powder (▶ Table 7.2).

7.3 Cement Properties

To design cements with predictable intraoperative and postoperative behavior, we must understand how cement formulation affects the polymerization and material properties of the solid. Like any heterogeneous mixture, the characteristics of the whole differ markedly from those of its components. For example, one cannot calculate a priori the porosity and strength of building mortar based solely on the properties of its various pebbles and finely ground minerals. These individual particles form a complex intermolecular network whose characteristics can be identified only empirically. The effect of each component on the setting time, polymerization temperature, and material properties of bone cement is detailed in the following sections.

7.3.1 Liquid-to-Powder Ratio

Polymerization temperature and setting time can be studied by altering liquid-to-powder (L/P) ratios. Clinically, these are key properties to control. Predictable setting time is critical intraoperatively to prevent solidification before completion of the procedure. High polymerization temperatures are known to cause tissue necrosis and hinder the efficacy of joint prostheses.[1] In spite of adverse effects of cement heat in some situations, highly exothermic cements can be preferentially used in a patient with malignant disease and pathologic compression fractures to achieve local tumor kill. Exofix is a cement that polymerizes to 88°C and was designed specifically for this purpose. Early research showed that greater L/P ratios produce higher peak temperatures but increase setting time. One hypothesis was that, at high L/P ratios, an abundance of monomers react exothermically, increasing the peak polymerization temperature. However, the high L/P ratio also decreases the relative concentration of the initiator (a component of the powder), so the monomers are activated slowly,

Table 7.2 Different types of commercially available cements and their properties

Cement name/maker	Opacifier	Working time (min)	Viscosity
SpinePlex/Stryker	30% barium	10–12	Low
Osteopal/Heraeus	45% zirconium	8	Low
KyphX HV-R/Medtronic	30% barium	8	High
StabiliT Bone Cement/Merit	35% barium	30	High
Confidence/Depuy/J and J	30% barium	8–10	High
Vertifix plus/IZI Medical	25% barium 10% HA	12	Low-medium
Osteofix/IZI Medical	45 zirconium dioxide	18	Medium, high density
Thermalfix Oncology cement/IZI Medical	45% zirconium, 5% HA	10	Low-medium, highly exothermic
Cortoss/Stryker		Mix on demand	

Table 7.3 Cement component variations and how the changes affect the polymerization process and mechanical characteristics

Concentration characteristics	Setting time	Polymerization temperature	Compressive strength
High liquid-to-powder ratio	Increased	Increased	Decreased
High BPO concentration	Decreased	Slightly increased	Increased
High DMPT concentration	Decreased	Slightly increased	Increased
Large PMMA bead size	Decreased	Decreased	Increased
Increased Radiopacifier conc.	No impact	No impact	Decreased

Abbreviations: BPO, benzoyl peroxide; DMPT, N,N-dimethyl-p-toluidine; PMMA, polymethyl methacrylate.

increasing setting time.[10,11] Clearly, studies that vary monomer-to-polymer ratios independently of other cement components are needed (▶ Table 7.3).

7.3.2 Initiator-to-Activator Ratio

Altering the BPO-to-DMPT ratio has a significant effect on setting time, polymerization temperature, and strength (▶ Table 7.3). Unfortunately, strength and setting time are inversely related. Adjusting BPO and DMPT concentrations to maximize setting time reduces overall strength.[9,12]

The rate of radical formation is dependent on the concentrations of the activator (i.e., DMPT) and peroxide. Faster radical formation activates more monomers that act as nucleation sites for polymer chain growth. This has a number of downstream effects. First, this will speed up the overall polymerization process, decreasing setting time. Second, more nucleation sites imply that more individual polymer chains will form simultaneously. This will reduce the average molecular weight of each polymer chain and affect overall strength and tensile properties of the cement.

To determine the proper initiator/activator (i.e., BPO-to-DMPT) ratio, a system that uses two liquid solutions was developed. Use of two-part liquid solutions rather than conventional liquid/powder cements allows for better mixing and consistency among experimental samples and reduces porosity caused by the trapping of air while mixing liquid/powder cements. These air pockets act as fracture initiation sites that compromise the strength of the cement. Both parts contained dissolved PMMA powder and MMA monomers in a 4:5 ratio. BPO was added to the first solution and DMPT to the second. Samples with varying concentrations of BPO and DMPT were prepared for comparative testing.

Although BPO and DMPT concentrations had profound effects on setting time, the impact on polymerization temperature is unclear. Increasing the concentration of BPO from 0.5 g per 100-mL MMA to 2.75 g per 100-mL MMA (at a constant DMPT concentration of 0.2 mL per 100-mL MMA) decreased setting time from 28.30 ($\pm$ 3.34) to 9.26 minutes ($\pm$ 0.97). Similarly, increasing DMPT concentration from 0.2 mL per 100-mL MMA to 4.9 mL per 100-mL MMA (at a constant BPO concentration of 0.5 g per 100-mL MMA) decreased setting time from 28.20 ($\pm$ 3.34) to 5.50 minutes ($\pm$ 0.17). No statistically significant changes in polymerization temperature were observed in these experiments.

Pascual et al[13] reported conflicting results with use of the more conventional liquid/powder cement mix. Although boosting BPO concentration from 0.75 to 2.0% decreased setting time by 20%, polymerization temperature increased an average of 3 to 6°C. When DMPT was doubled from 1.0 to 2.0% and BPO increased from 0.75 to 2.0%, temperatures increased an average of 10°C.

Mechanical properties were also strongly related to BPO and DMPT concentrations. As the concentrations of BPO and DMPT increased, the mechanical strength of the cement cores also increased. Cements with the lowest concentrations of BPO (0.5 g per 100-mL MMA) and DMPT (0.2 mL per 100-mL MMA) were significantly weaker than other cements. At every BPO concentration, peak strength occurred at a DMPT concentration of 1.4 mL per 100-mL MMA. The maximum value (105–110 MPa) was achieved at a BPO-to-DMPT ratio of approximately 1:1. In a measure of durability, compounds containing 2.0 g BPO and 1.4 mL DMPT withstood more cycles of stress loading before structural failure than samples containing 2.0 g BPO and 4.9 mL DMPT.[12] Optimizing the BPO-to-DMPT ratio for cement strength decreases setting time and may increase polymerization temperature.

7.3.3 Radiopacifiers

Radiopacifiers such as barium sulfate and zirconium dioxide are present in standard bone cement mixes at low concentrations. Additional opacifiers are often added for interventional procedures such as VP, in which visibility is key. These heavy metals interrupt the polymerizing matrix and produce pores that can act as fracture initiation sites, diminishing overall cement strength with an unclear effect on polymerization temperature and setting time.[14,15] Adding 10% barium sulfate to Simplex P cement decreased tensile strength and fracture toughness by 10%. As the percentage of barium in samples of Cranioplastic cement increased from 0 to 12.5%, tensile strength decreased 10%, strain to failure (ability to compress before being destroyed) decreased by one-third, and the Young modulus (stress/strain, a measure of stiffness) increased 20%.[15]

The effect of metal radiopacifiers on cement fatigue is less clear. Dynamic fatigue refers to the behavior of materials under repeated loads over time and is measured by applying a cyclic load with constant amplitude and measuring the number of cycles until failure.[16] This is an important property for cement used in procedures such as VP in which vertebral bodies will be subjected to repeated loading and unloading of forces over a period of years. Although a number of studies have shown that barium decreases fatigue strength[17] and increases crack growth rate,[18] others report lower rates of fatigue crack growth with radiopaque cement.[19] This discrepancy may be caused by the fact that the latter study was performed in water to simulate an in vivo environment, whereas the other studies tested cement samples in air.

Clinicians can enhance the structural integrity of radiopacified cement in a number of ways. First, there are indications that zirconium is superior to barium structurally and may be the agent of choice.[15,20] Second, homogeneity of mixed cement is key; failure to disperse barium particles evenly leads to fracture formation.[21] Third, new cross-linking agents and preparation methods that enhance cement strength have been reported.[15,22] Incorporating these concepts into cement formulations will minimize any loss of strength or durability from radiopacifiers.

7.3.4 Polymethyl Methacrylate Bead Size

The average diameter and size distribution of PMMA beads play an important role in the cure properties of bone cement. Aside from its structural role as a component of the cement matrix, PMMA beads serve as a heat sink—dissipating energy released by the exothermic polymerization of MMA monomers. Samples containing PMMA particles with larger mean diameters and widespread distributions of particle size had lower peak polymerization temperatures and longer setting times.[13,23]

As particle diameter increased from 33 to 65 m and size range spread from 10 to 60 m to 10 to 140 m, peak polymerization temperature decreased from approximately 88 to 62°C and setting time doubled to 10 minutes.[13]

Structurally, bead size and distribution has less impact. Although an increase from 33 to 55 m did cause compressive strength to increase from 128 to 149 MPa with 1% DMPT and from 103 to 152 MPa with 2% DMPT, other parameters including elastic modulus and tensile strength were unaffected.[16] Creep resistance, a measure of the ability to withstand a load, increased when larger PMMA particles were used and when larger MMA/styrene copolymer beads were substituted for PMMA beads.[24] For this reason, many brands of commercial cement contain a large percentage of MMA/styrene copolymer in cement powder.

Therefore, use of PMMA beads with a larger mean diameter and wider size distribution has a number of beneficial effects. Unlike the BPO-to-DMPT ratio, proper bead size allows maximization of setting time and decrease of polymerization temperature without diminished cement strength.

7.4 Mixing Method

Aside from intrinsic factors related to composition, extrinsic factors such as mixing method have a large impact on cement properties. Depending on mixing technique, air may become trapped in the cement mixture, increasing porosity. Air weakens the cement and provides an interface for fractures and cracks to develop. Although the two-solution cement discussed earlier is effective at decreasing porosity, almost all commercially available cement requires mixing powder and liquid. For these situations, vacuum mixing devices have been shown to reduce porosity by more than 44% compared with mixing with a bowl and spatula. Centrifugation may also be an effective method for limiting porosity. Cement cores manufactured by centrifuging the powder/monomer mixture had increased fatigue life with greater consistency among different samples than cores created with use of the bowl and spatula mixing technique.[25] Consistent preparation methods will ensure uniform results and prevent uneven mixtures with variable mechanical properties.

7.5 Antibiotics

Antibiotics are sometimes added to the cement powder before injection to minimize infection.[26,27] These additives, like barium sulfate and zirconium dioxide, can affect the mechanical properties of the bone cement. Research has shown that adding various types of antibiotics to bone cement, in quantities less than 2 g per standard packet of bone cement, does not adversely affect some of the cement's mechanical properties (compressive or diametrical tensile strengths), although quantities exceeding 2 g did weaken them.[28,29] These findings were substantiated by another report that showed the addition of 0.5 g of erythromycin and 0.24 g of colistin to Simplex P was not detrimental to the cement's fatigue properties.[30]

As with other additives, the addition of antibiotics to the cement has produced conflicting results. In one study, the addition of 2 g of powdered gentamicin, oxacillin, or cefazolin to 60 g of Simplex P or Palacos produced no statistically significant difference in terms of short-term (<40 days) compressive and tensile strengths compared with the cement without powdered antibiotics.[31] However, another study found a significant decrease in mechanical strength between cements mixed with 250 or 500 mg of gentamicin in 6.25 or 12.5 mL of water and cements without aqueous antibiotics.[29] Although these reports showed no deleterious mechanical effects from the addition of powdered antibiotics, provided the quantity was less than 2 g, other investigators have reported that compression strength was compromised by the addition of 2 g of antibiotics (gentamicin or Keflin) per 60 g of Simplex P.[32]

One alternative, already used by some physicians performing VP or kyphoplasty, is the intravenous administration of antibiotics before vertebral augmentation,[33] which avoids the risk of potential changes to the cement's properties.

7.6 Pain Relief

Thermal necrosis of surrounding nerves was previously postulated as a mechanism of pain relief in VP. Research in laboratory animals indicates that thermal necrosis of bone tissue occurs when temperatures surpass 50°C for more than 1 minute.[34]

Deramond et al[35] measured temperatures at the anterior cortices, centers, and spinal canals of cadaveric vertebral bodies after bipedicular injections of Simplex P or Orthocomp (bisphenol glycidyl dimethacrylate/bisphenol ethoxy dimethacrylate/triethylene glycol dimethacrylate, a matrix composite cement reinforced with glass-ceramic), both of which were prepared according to the manufacturer's specifications. They found that, at the central location, Simplex P injection was associated with significantly higher temperatures and with temperatures exceeding 50°C for significantly longer times (61.8°C) than Orthocomp injection (51.2°C).[35] However, measurements at the anterior cortex and spinal canal locations showed no significant difference between the two cements. In fact, at the latter location, the temperature of cement did not exceed 41°C in either cement. The authors hypothesized that, given their results, it was unlikely the pain relief from VP was caused by intraosseous neural tissue damage.[35]

There is also additional evidence that pain relief from vertebral augmentation is provided by the reestablishment of the mechanical stability of the vertebral body rather than by any neurolysis of intravertebral nerves. In a kyphoplasty study with information from the Swiss registry, cement volume was a significant predictor for pain relief and the only operator modifiable variable.[36] This study showed a clear dose–outcome relationship between cement filling volumes and pain relief and the authors recommended a minimum of 4.5 mL of PMMA to achieve durable pain relief.

The Investigational Device Exemption trial comparing Cortoss versus PMMA had nearly superimposable graphs showing the mean Visual Analog Scale (VAS) pain reduction for Cortoss and PMMA.[6,7] Given that Cortoss has little to no exothermic reaction, it is very likely that all or most of the pain relief is caused by reestablished mechanical stability of the vertebral body.

In unpublished data from a patient cohort treated by vertebral augmentation with corticocancellous allograft bone, the mean VAS pain reduction scores decreased from 43 to 22 after osseous augmentation with allograft bone only. The amount of allograft bone injected per patient averaged 8.6 mL. This resulted in not only a pain decrease presumed to be from the increased mechanical stability but also a functional increase with the Oswestry Disability Index decreasing from 40 to 21.[37]

7.7 Bone Adherence

Conventional PMMA cements cannot adhere to existing bone,[38] but this disadvantage may not be as pertinent for VP as for arthroplasty. Because the cement is injected directly into the bone, and not used as an adhesive agent as in arthroplasty, cement loosening may not cause any noticeable problems. Results of one study indicated that, at long-term follow-up (average, 1.3 years) after VP with PMMA cements, the vertebrae were stable with respect to compression and the degree of kyphosis.[39] Only 1 of 20 vertebral levels showed signs of cement compression; the remaining 19 showed no change in cement morphology.[40] Another follow-up study (48 months after the procedure) showed no progression of vertebral deformity after VP.[38] However, if the cement loosens to such a degree that it compromises the structural integrity of the vertebral body, refracture of the vertebral body can occur around the injected cement.[40]

7.8 Bone Formation and Other New Developments

Although research has shown that PMMA cements cannot induce new bone formation,[38] some new bone cements show promise not only in terms of bone growth but also in terms of improved physical and mechanical properties, which could be beneficial for PVP. One recently developed cement consists of bioactive glass beads and a novel organic matrix of PMMA, which resulted in new bone formation around the beads and a significant increase in bending strength compared with PMMA cement without the beads.[40] Curing time and polymerization temperatures were not reported. Adding a glass-ceramic powder and bisphenol-a-glycidyl methacrylate (bis-GMA) resin to a PMMA-based cement has produced a bioactive acrylic bone cement that bonds directly to the bone after 4 to 8 weeks in vivo and has faster hardening times, lower curing temperatures, and significantly better physical properties.[41] In one study, investigators measured the stiffness and strength of fresh cadaveric thoracic and lumbar vertebrae injected with BoneSource (an HA bioactive bone cement) or Cranioplastic (a PMMA-based product) and then mechanically compressed.[42] The vertebrae injected with Cranioplastic had significantly greater strength compared with strength in the prefractured state, whereas those injected with BoneSource regained initial strength. However, both Cranioplastic and BoneSource resulted in a lower stiffness in all vertebrae compared with initial measurements.[42] A similar comparison of Simplex P and BoneSource showed that both cements resulted in significantly less stiffness than in the precompressed states.[5] However, Simplex P injections resulted in significantly greater strength compared with prefracture measurements, whereas BoneSource restored the vertebrae to their initial strength.[41] Despite these findings, in vitro studies comparing HA cements and PMMA products should be conducted to determine which is more suitable for use in VP as the HA cement can show osteoconversion in the porous portions of the cement at the bone or bone–cartilaginous junction without inflammatory activity and absence of a fibrous capsule surrounding the cement.[43] This may lead to a stronger bond to the native bone and increased durability over time.

Simplex P and Orthocomp were studied with respect to their ability to restore strength and stiffness of the vertebral body.[44] After initial measurements of strength and stiffness were made, mechanical compression was applied to osteoporotic cadaveric vertebral bodies posterior to the anterior wall.[45] Vertebrae were then injected with Simplex P or Orthocomp and retested to determine their augmented strength and stiffness. Injection with Simplex P or Orthocomp significantly increased vertebral body strength compared with the initial measurements. Initial vertebral body stiffness was restored by using Orthocomp, but vertebral bodies augmented with Simplex P were significantly less stiff than in their precrush condition.[46]

Similar studies have compared a PMMA cement (Palacos E-Flow) to a CaP experimental brushite cement (EBC) with respect to strength and stiffness.[44] Osteoporotic vertebral bodies harvested from cadavers were measured, axially compressed, injected with either Palacos E-Flow or EBC, and then retested for strength and stiffness. Injections of PMMA and EBC increased the average stiffness (in osteoporotic vertebrae only) by 174% (range, 10–159%) and 120% (range, 108–131%), respectively, and the average strength by 195% (range, 26–254%) and 113% (range, 104–126%), respectively. The study also showed that the cements' augmenting effects were proportional to the degree of filling, although the correlation was weak.[47]

Novel work is underway with cements containing bone morphogenic protein (BMP), a protein that belongs to the transforming growth factor (TGF) superfamily and found in bone matrix.[48] It is believed that BMP serves as a growth factor for adult articular cartilage matrix repair and synthesis. Although no work specific to PVP has been conducted, studies using BMP-impregnated cement implanted into bone have shown new bone or callus formation in a dose-dependent manner.[48–50] Additional research is required to determine what effect, if any, BMP has on the physical properties of the bone cement and its application in PVP.

7.9 The Future

PMMA bone cements usually lack sufficient osteoinductivity. Therefore, various bioactive osteogenic agents can be added in order to promote new bone formation. The incorporation of bioactive materials has been shown to improve the biological performance of CPCs by promoting bone metabolism. Because they are porous, CPCs can be used as carrier agents for stem cells and growth factors. These growth factors can include bone morphogenetic proteins (BMPs), basic fibroblast growth factor (bFGF), and vascular endothelial growth factor (VEGF). The growth factors may be mixed with CPC components alone, or can be encapsulated within microspheres of chitosan, gelatin, or hyaluronic acid before incorporation into the CPC for best preservation of their bioactivity. Plasmids or small interfering RNAs (siRNAs) may also be incorporated

into CPCs to achieve gene delivery to cells at the injection area. Recently, platelet-rich plasma (PRP), mesenchymal stem cells of umbilical origin, and autologous bone marrow concentrate have been used together with CPCs as autologous bone substitutes. Systemic subcutaneous or inhaled PTH in pulsed delivery mode has been shown in animals to augment CPC integration.

7.10 Conclusion

The percutaneous treatment of bone-related disorders is a fast-growing field within interventional radiology. We are beginning to expand beyond VP, performing cementoplasty of fractures and metastatic lesions in sites ranging from the acetabulum to the scapula.[51]

Many of these indications could take advantage of bone cements with specific attributes. Whereas cement mixtures with very high polymerization temperatures are useful for painful pelvic metastases to maximize necrosis of the tumor, treatment of vertebral or other weight-bearing fractures may, conversely, require cements that can withstand greater stress and fatigue. For procedures that have limited access or require a specific needle size, the cement viscosity and setting time are key characteristics. The theoretical principles and practical data discussed earlier identify numerous ways to perfect PMMA bone cement for different indications.

Modifying cement characteristics is only the first step toward improving patient health. Research is needed to determine which material properties are clinically relevant for each procedure. Bone cement strength may not be critical for most procedures, compared to other characteristics such as setting time and polymerization temperature. In fact, arguments could be made that weaker cements may be more beneficial for procedures such as VP. These questions would best be answered by studies and nationwide registries correlating cement formulation with long-term clinical outcomes. This would lead to the establishment of guidelines describing the safest and most effective formulations of bone cement for specific types of procedures.

Like any procedure, percutaneous treatments of bone disease such as VP are not immune to complications. Most problems are caused by the extravasation of bone cement into the spinal canal and venous system. Bone cement preparation may be one source of the problem. Cement that is too fluid or has a long setting time, for example, is more likely to escape its site of injection. By understanding the principles described in this review, these pitfalls can be avoided. Just as practitioners must understand the mechanism of action before prescribing a drug, interventional radiologists must have intimate knowledge of bone cement before injecting a compound that can be potentially fatal when used incorrectly.

7.11 Pearls

- When it comes to cement injection into a vertebral body, see it like an embolization of a venous space with a liquid polymer.
- You can always do more; you can never do less.
- This is civil engineering; think of the load distribution.
- If your little voice tells you to stop the injection, stop.
- Optimistic happy patients do better.

References

[1] Fukase Y, Eanes ED, Takagi S, Chow LC, Brown WE. Setting reactions and compressive strengths of calcium phosphate cements. J Dent Res 1990; 69(12):1852–1856

[2] Liu C, Shen W, Gu Y, Hu L. Mechanism of the hardening process for a hydroxyapatite cement. J Biomed Mater Res 1997;35(1):75–80

[3] Ishikawa K, Takagi S, Chow LC, Suzuki K. Reaction of calcium phosphate cements with different amounts of tetracalcium phosphate and dicalcium phosphate anhydrous. J Biomed Mater Res 1999;46(4):504–510

[4] Lim THL, Brebach GT, Renner SM, et al. Biomechanical evaluation of an injectable calcium phosphate cement for vertebroplasty. Spine 2002;27(12): 1297–1302

[5] Belkoff SM, Mathis JM, Jasper LE. Ex vivo biomechanical comparison of hydroxyapatite and polymethylmethacrylate cements for use with vertebroplasty. AJNR Am J Neuroradiol 2002;23(10):1647–1651

[6] Bae H, Hatten HP Jr, Linovitz R, et al. A prospective randomized FDA-IDE trial comparing Cortoss with PMMA for vertebroplasty: a comparative effectiveness research study with 24-month follow-up. Spine 2012;37(7):544–550

[7] Palussière J, Berge J, Gangi A, et al. Clinical results of an open prospective study of a bis-GMA composite in percutaneous vertebral augmentation. Eur Spine J 2005;14(10):982–991, 18, 2016

[8] Wade LG. Synthetic polymers. In: Wade LG, ed. Organic Chemistry. 3rd ed. Princeton, NJ: Prentice Hall; 1995:1231–1246

[9] Hasenwinkel JM, Lautenschlager EP, Wixson RL, Gilbert JL. A novel high-viscosity, two-solution acrylic bone cement: effect of chemical composition on properties. J Biomed Mater Res 1999;47(1):36–45

[10] Turner RC, Atkins PE, Ackley MA, Park JB. Molecular and macroscopic properties of PMMA bone cement: free-radical generation and temperature change versus mixing ratio. J Biomed Mater Res 1981;15(3):425–432

[11] Pascual B, Gurruchaga M, Ginebra MP, Gil FJ, Planell JA, Goñi I. Influence of the modification of P/L ratio on a new formulation of acrylic bone cement. Biomaterials 1999;20(5):465–474

[12] Hasenwinkel JM, Lautenschlager EP, Wixson RL, Gilbert JL. Effect of initiation chemistry on the fracture toughness, fatigue strength, and residual monomer content of a novel high-viscosity, two-solution acrylic bone cement. J Biomed Mater Res 2002;59(3):411–421

[13] Pascual B, Vázquez B, Gurruchaga M, et al. New aspects of the effect of size and size distribution on the setting parameters and mechanical properties of acrylic bone cements. Biomaterials 1996;17(5):509–516

[14] Topoleski LD, Ducheyne P, Cuckler JM. A fractographic analysis of in vivo poly(methyl methacrylate) bone cement failure mechanisms. J Biomed Mater Res 1990;24(2):135–154

[15] De S, Vazquez B. The effect of cross-linking agents on acrylic bone cements containing radiopacifiers. Biomaterials 2001;22(15):2177–2181

[16] Soltesz U, Richter H. Mechanical behavior of selected ceramics. In: Ducheyne PD, Hastings GH, eds. Metal and Ceramic Biomaterials. Vol. II: Strength and Surface. Boca Raton, FL: CRC Press; 1984

[17] Baleani M, Cristofolini L, Minari C, Toni A. Fatigue strength of PMMA bone cement mixed with gentamicin and barium sulphate vs pure PMMA. Proc Inst Mech Eng H 2003;217(1):9–12

[18] Owen AB, Beaumont PW. Fracture behaviour of commercial surgical acrylic bone cements. J Biomed Eng 1979;1(4):277–280

[19] Molino LN, Topoleski LDT. Effect of BaSO4 on the fatigue crack propagation rate of PMMA bone cement. J Biomed Mater Res 1996;31(1):131–137

[20] Rudigier J, Draenert K, Gruenert A, Ritter G. Effects of adding x-ray contrast materials to bone cements. Akt Traumatol 1977;7:35–48

[21] Bhambri SK, Gilbertson LN. Micromechanisms of fatigue crack initiation and propagation in bone cements. J Biomed Mater Res 1995;29(2):233–237

[22] Kim HY, Yasuda HK. Improvement of fatigue properties of poly (methyl methacrylate) bone cement by means of plasma surface treatment of fillers. J Biomed Mater Res 1999;48(2):135–142

[23] Lewis G, Carroll M. Rheological properties of acrylic bone cement during curing and the role of the size of the powder particles. J Biomed Mater Res 2002;63(2):191–199

[24] Treharne RW, Brown N. Factors influencing the creep behavior of poly(methyl methacrylate) cements. J Biomed Mater Res 1975;9(4):81–88

[25] James SP, Jasty M, Davies J, Piehler H, Harris WH. A fractographic investigation of PMMA bone cement focusing on the relationship between porosity reduction and increased fatigue life. J Biomed Mater Res 1992;26(5):651–662

[26] Jensen ME, Evans AJ, Mathis JM, Kallmes DF, Cloft HJ, Dion JE. Percutaneous polymethylmethacrylate vertebroplasty in the treatment of osteoporotic vertebral body compression fractures: technical aspects. AJNR Am J Neuroradiol 1997;18(10):1897–1904

[27] Murphy KJ, Deramond H. Percutaneous vertebroplasty in benign and malignant disease. Neuroimaging Clin N Am 2000;10(3):535–545

[28] Lautenschlager EP, Jacobs JJ, Marshall GW, Meyer PR Jr. Mechanical properties of bone cements containing large doses of antibiotic powders. J Biomed Mater Res 1976;10(6):929–938

[29] Lautenschlager EP, Marshall GW, Marks KE, Schwartz J, Nelson CL. Mechanical strength of acrylic bone cements impregnated with antibiotics. J Biomed Mater Res 1976;10(6):837–845

[30] Davies JP, O'Connor DO, Burke DW, Harris WH. Influence of antibiotic impregnation on the fatigue life of Simplex P and Palacos R acrylic bone cements, with and without centrifugation. J Biomed Mater Res 1989;23(4):379–397

[31] Marks KE, Nelson CL, Lautenschlager EP. Antibiotic-impregnated acrylic bone cement. J Bone Joint Surg Am 1976;58(3):358–364

[32] Nelson RC, Hoffman RO, Burton TA. The effect of antibiotic additions on the mechanical properties of acrylic cement. J Biomed Mater Res 1978;12(4): 473–490

[33] Amar AP, Larsen DW, Esnaashari N, Albuquerque FC, Lavine SD, Teitelbaum GP. Percutaneous transpedicular polymethylmethacrylate vertebroplasty for the treatment of spinal compression fractures. Neurosurgery 2001;49(5):1105–1114, discussion 1114–1115

[34] Eriksson RA, Albrektsson T, Magnusson B. Assessment of bone viability after heat trauma. A histological, histochemical and vital microscopic study in the rabbit. Scand J Plast Reconstr Surg 1984;18(3):261–268

[35] Deramond H, Wright NT, Belkoff SM. Temperature elevation caused by bone cement polymerization during vertebroplasty. [Suppl] Bone 1999;25(2, Suppl): 17S–21S

[36] Röder C, Boszczyk B, Perler G, Aghayev E, Külling F, Maestretti G. Cement volume is the most important modifiable predictor for pain relief in BKP: results from SWISSspine, a nationwide registry. Eur Spine J 2013;22(10):2241–2248

[37] Vertebral augmentation with Allograft bone: a clinical trial to assess treatment efficacy and patient response to therapy. 2007. Unpublished manuscript

[38] Freeman MAR, Bradley GW, Revell PA. Observations upon the interface between bone and polymethylmethacrylate cement. J Bone Joint Surg Br 1982;64(4):489–493

[39] Kallmes DF, Jensen ME. Percutaneous vertebroplasty. Radiology 2003; 229(1):27–36

[40] Molloy S, Mathis JM, Belkoff SM. The effect of vertebral body percentage fill on mechanical behavior during percutaneous vertebroplasty. Spine 2003;28(14):1549–1554

[41] Shinzato S, Nakamura T, Kokubo T, Kitamura Y. Bioactive bone cement: effect of silane treatment on mechanical properties and osteoconductivity. J Biomed Mater Res 2001;55(3):277–284

[42] Yamamuro T, Nakamura T, Iida H, et al. Development of bioactive bone cement and its clinical applications. Biomaterials 1998;19(16):1479–1482

[43] Kokoska MS, Friedman CD, Castellano RD, Costantino PD. Experimental facial augmentation with hydroxyapatite cement. Arch Facial Plast Surg 2004;6(5):290–294

[44] Belkoff SM, Mathis JM, Jasper LE, Deramond H. An ex vivo biomechanical evaluation of a hydroxyapatite cement for use with vertebroplasty. Spine 2001;26(14):1542–1546

[45] Grados F, Depriester C, Cayrolle G, Hardy N, Deramond H, Fardellone P. Long-term observations of vertebral osteoporotic fractures treated by percutaneous vertebroplasty. Rheumatology (Oxford) 2000;39(12):1410–1414

[46] Heini PF, Berlemann U, Kaufmann M, Lippuner K, Fankhauser C, van Landuyt P. Augmentation of mechanical properties in osteoporotic vertebral bones: a biomechanical investigation of vertebroplasty efficacy with different bone cements. Eur Spine J 2001;10(2):164–171

[47] Belkoff SM, Mathis JM, Erbe EM, Fenton DC. Biomechanical evaluation of a new bone cement for use in vertebroplasty. Spine 2000;25(9):1061–1064

[48] Alam I, Asahina I, Ohmamiuda K, Enomoto S. Comparative study of biphasic calcium phosphate ceramics impregnated with rhBMP-2 as bone substitutes. J Biomed Mater Res 2001;54(1):129–138

[49] Chubinskaya S, Kuettner KE. Regulation of osteogenic proteins by chondrocytes. Int J Biochem Cell Biol 2003;35(9):1323–1340

[50] Niedhart C, Maus U, Redmann E, Schmidt-Rohlfing B, Niethard FU, Siebert CH. Stimulation of bone formation with an in situ setting tricalcium phosphate/rhBMP-2 composite in rats. J Biomed Mater Res A 2003;65(1):17–23

[51] Dehdashti AR, Martin JB, Jean B, Rüfenacht DA. PMMA cementoplasty in symptomatic metastatic lesions of the S1 vertebral body. Cardiovasc Intervent Radiol 2000;23(3):235–237

8 Vertebroplasty

Nicole S. Carter, Hong Kuan Kok, Julian Maingard, Hamed Asadi, Lee-Anne Slater, Thabele Leslie-Mazwi, Joshua A. Hirsch, and Ronil V. Chandra

Summary

Vertebroplasty is a minimally invasive procedure that involves the injection of bone cement or other injectable fill material into vertebral compression fractures, with the aim of providing pain relief and improving functional status. Vertebroplasty is generally performed in the thoracic, lumbar, and sacral spine. Cervical vertebroplasty may also be performed but is less common. Most procedures are performed for osteoporotic vertebral compression fractures that are refractory to nonsurgical management, or for neoplasm-related fractures from metastatic disease, or multiple myeloma. Failure of nonsurgical management may be considered to have occurred when severe back pain or significantly compromised mobility persists following medical therapies, or when unacceptable adverse effects such as confusion or sedation occur with the analgesic doses required to alleviate pain. The essential equipment required for vertebroplasty includes the vertebroplasty needle system and bone cement. While multiple types of cement and osseous fill materials are commercially available, polymethyl methacrylate (PMMA) remains the most widely used. Analgesia and antibiotic prophylaxis are typically utilized for the procedure. Image guidance is vital for all vertebroplasty procedures, with fluoroscopy and/or computed tomography recommended as the imaging modalities of choice. This chapter outlines a practical guide to the procedural and the technical aspects of vertebroplasty. A description of the equipment required, fill materials utilized, considerations for performing cervical vertebroplasty, and optimal postprocedure care are discussed.

Keywords: vertebroplasty, vertebral compression fractures, bone cement, percutaneous, osteoporosis, metastasis, fluoroscopy

8.1 Introduction

Vertebroplasty is a percutaneous minimally invasive, image-guided procedure that involves the injection of bone cement into a fractured vertebral body (▶Fig. 8.1). Most vertebroplasty procedures are performed for osteoporotic vertebral compression fractures (VCFs) that remain symptomatic following failure of nonsurgical management (NSM). Procedures are also performed for pathologic fractures, in particular for osteolytic metastases, multiple myeloma, or vascular tumors. Failure of NSM can be defined as persistent pain to the extent that mobility or activities of daily living are substantially compromised, or when unacceptable adverse effects, such as confusion or sedation occur due to high analgesic doses required for pain control. The goals of vertebroplasty are pain relief, improved mobility and functional status, and restoration of vertebral height and stability. Image guidance is essential for all vertebroplasty procedures, with fluoroscopy being the primary recommended method of imaging guidance due to its capacity to provide rapid image acquisition and ability to produce continuous real-time monitoring during cement injection. Vertebroplasty may also be performed using computed tomography (CT) guidance either with or without fluoroscopy or CT fluoroscopy.

This chapter will review the technical aspects of percutaneous vertebroplasty, the materials required, and suggested postprocedure care.

8.2 Anatomic Features

Vertebroplasty requires a robust understanding of spinal anatomy as viewed on fluoroscopy. In the anteroposterior (AP) projection, the vertebral body is visualized as a rectangular-shaped bone with the superior and inferior borders located adjacent to the adjacent intervertebral disks. The ovoid pedicular margins are viewed medial to the lateral margins of the vertebral body. The medial and inferior cortices of the pedicle should be noted, as these are critical landmarks for planning and maintaining a safe needle trajectory. A true AP position is obtained by aligning the spinous processes midway between the pedicles. In the true lateral projection, the end plates and posterior margin of the vertebral body are sharply defined with the ribs superimposed.[1]

Cement leakage outside the vertebral body can occur, although the vast majority of leaks are limited and are

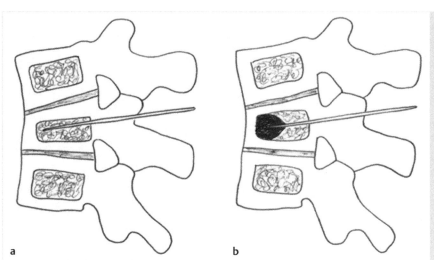

Fig. 8.1 (a, b) Vertebroplasty involves the percutaneous insertion of a needle into the vertebral body, followed by the injection of cement.

a

b

asymptomatic.[2-4] It is important to appreciate the posterior margin of the vertebral body on the lateral view and carefully observe for posterior leakage during cement injection. Maintaining a safe margin of 3 to 5 mm from the anterior border of the vertebral body also avoids damage to key structures anterior to the vertebral body, such as the aorta, inferior vena cava, and other retroperitoneal structures. Intradiskal leakage can be visualized as the cement extends through the superior or inferior end plates of the vertebral body.

8.3 The Procedure

8.3.1 Procedure Materials

Many forms of vertebroplasty needles are commercially available. Typically, needles are hollow, straight, and range from 10 to 15 gauge in caliber. Smaller systems may be necessary in small pedicles or in the upper thoracic or cervical spine. Needle tips are available in diamond-shaped, single-beveled, or multibeveled designs. The diamond-tip needle configuration provides optimal ease of needle penetration into cortical bone. Beveled needles have superior control and maneuverability, and are useful for changing the needle direction according to which direction the bevel is oriented. Curved needle systems have been recently developed that possess the ability to arc up to 90 degrees, allowing access to sites that are difficult to reach with straight needles. Polymethyl methacrylate (PMMA) remains the most common bone cement utilized.[5] The majority of vertebroplasty procedures are performed using fluoroscopic guidance. The procedure room should include equipment for patient monitoring, including electrocardiography, blood pressure and pulse oximetry, and cardiopulmonary resuscitation equipment. Patients commonly receive local anesthesia and moderate conscious sedation, as well as prophylactic antibiotics prior to the procedure. Preprocedural imaging should be available to ensure treatment of the correct vertebral levels. In the rare event of symptomatic complications during the procedure, it is important to have rapid availability of CT and magnetic resonance imaging (MRI) facilities. Modern fluoroscopic units may also have on-table cone beam CT functionality that can be useful in large or obese patients where fluoroscopic landmarks may be difficult to identify or where intraprocedural complications are suspected.

8.3.2 Sedation and Anesthetic Preparation

Analgesia is necessary for all vertebroplasty procedures. For the majority of patients, this is achieved by using a combination of local anesthetics (e.g., lidocaine and bupivacaine) and moderate conscious sedation (e.g., intravenous fentanyl and midazolam). The skin, subcutaneous tissues, and periosteum along the needle tract and at the bone entry point should be thoroughly infiltrated with local anesthetic to minimize pain. Some mild discomfort may be expected as the needle traverses periosteum during the initial cortical penetration. Additional discomfort may occur when the PMMA is injected; in these cases, additional intravenous analgesics may be required. The advantage of conscious sedation is it allows feedback from the patient, such as worsening pain or neurologic dysfunction, which may alert the operator to potential complications. However, general anesthesia may be required in some cases, such as in those with severe pain, high doses of opioid analgesia, or those at risk of cardiopulmonary complications from prone positioning. All cases require continuous monitoring of blood pressure, heart rate, and oxygen saturations. Patient monitoring and sedation are performed by the proceduralists, anesthesiologists, anesthetic nurses, or other certified nursing personnel. For patients with significant preprocedure cardiac or respiratory disease, evaluation by an anesthesiologist may be required to determine the requirements for additional monitored anesthesia care. In all patients, fasting from food and drink is required for at least 4 to 6 hours prior to the procedure.

8.3.3 Positioning

Thoracic and lumbar vertebroplasty is typically performed with the patient in the prone position. However, it is acceptable to allow the patient freedom to place themself in a prone oblique position to improve their comfort during the procedure. This may introduce approximately 10 to 15 degrees of obliquity. Cushion support should be applied under the upper chest and pelvis (▶ Fig. 8.2). This promotes patient comfort, allows clear access to the spine, reduces kyphosis, and maximizes extension of the fractured vertebral segments, which may widen and allow cement penetration.[6] The patient's arms should be placed toward the head to keep them out of the path of the fluoroscope beam. Analgesia should be considered prior to positioning the patient, as transfer from the bed to operating table may be painful. Particular care should be taken when positioning those who are elderly or have advanced osteoporosis or myelomatous infiltration, as transfer may result in new vertebral or rib fractures.

8.3.4 Antibiotic Prophylaxis and Skin Preparation

While no clear data currently support or opposes prevertebroplasty administration of antibiotics in nonimmunocompromised patients,[7] there are reports of postprocedure spinal infections that are rendered difficult to treat due to the use of PMMA cement.[8,9] Prophylactic antibiotics are thus commonly used. Typical regimens include intravenous doses of cefazolin (1–2 g),

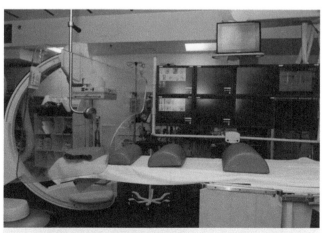

Fig. 8.2 Setup of the procedure room for a vertebral augmentation procedure. Note the cushion supports prepared on the procedural table for prone positioning.

or clindamycin (600 mg) in patients with penicillin allergy and gentamycin (80–160 mg). Infection risk is further minimized by following standard operating room guidelines for sterile skin preparation, draping, and operator scrubbing.

8.3.5 Needle Placement

The vertebroplasty needle is advanced via a small incision, through the skin and subcutaneous tissues and into the target vertebra. It is critical to maintain a needle trajectory that is lateral to the medial cortex and superior to the inferior cortex of the pedicle prior to entry of the needle into the posterior portion of the vertebral body. This prevents passage of the needle into the spinal canal or neural foramen, lowering the risk of spinal cord, cauda equina, or nerve root injury. Ideally, the final needle position should be at the midline of the vertebral body or tumoral target.

In thoracic and lumbar vertebroplasty, the needle may be placed via a transpedicular or parapedicular approach (▶Fig. 8.3). A transpedicular approach involves advancing the needle from the posterior surface of the pedicle, through the entire length of the pedicle, and into the vertebral body. This long intraosseous pathway protects the postganglionic nerve roots and surrounding soft tissues. This approach also provides a clear anatomic landmark for the operator that allows access from the skin into the vertebral body. However, the pedicle configuration can limit the ability to achieve an optimal final needle tip position. The parapedicular approach may permit a more medial placement of the needle tip, and is particularly useful when treating anatomically smaller pedicles, such as in the thoracic spine. The needle is directed along the lateral surface of the pedicle, penetrating the vertebral body at its junction with the pedicle.

Vertebroplasty can be performed with placement of bilateral needles or a single unilateral needle.[10] The aim in either approach is the midline spread of cement across the vertebral body from the superior to the inferior end plate. A single needle is often sufficient to achieve this. If the midline position is difficult to achieve due to anatomic constraints, a second needle may be placed on the contralateral side. When performing vertebroplasty, there is little difference in the clinical outcomes achieved with unipedicular versus bipedicular approaches and there are advantages to each approach.[11] The primary benefits of a unipedicular approach include reduced procedure time,

elimination of the risks associated with placement of a second needle, and lower rates of cement leakage.[12] The main advantage of a bipedicular approach is the capacity to inject a greater cement volume.[13,14]

8.3.6 Image Guidance

Vertebroplasty is typically performed using fluoroscopy. Advantages of fluoroscopic guidance include real-time needle positioning and adjustment, and the capacity for continuous monitoring during cement injection. The use of biplane fluoroscopy (two perpendicular image detectors used simultaneously) permits swift alternation between imaging planes without the necessity to move equipment or realign the projection. Alternatively, a single C-arm may be used with views obtained in both the AP and lateral views by simply rotating the C-arm. The goal with both types of fluoroscopic units is to keep the procedure time to a minimum, to adequately visualize the progress and results of the procedure, and to keep the radiation dose as low as possible. For either transpedicular or parapedicular approach, there are multiple image guidance strategies, typically an AP view, or a "down-the-barrel" (end-on) view. The latter technique uses ipsilateral oblique rotation of the image intensifier to place the fluoroscopy beam, pedicle, and needle tract parallel to each other. CT may be used as an adjunctive tool. This cross-sectional imaging modality has superior contrast resolution, and is thus useful for the detection of small cement leaks and, with CT fluoroscopy, allows for continuous real-time monitoring of needle and cement placement.[15,16]

8.3.7 Needle Insertion

The following description assumes the use of fluoroscopy for image guidance:
- Rotate the image detector to a true AP position by aligning the spinous process in the midline between the pedicles.
- Center the pedicles within the superior one half of the vertebral body or overlying a compressed vertebral body by adjusting the craniocaudal angulation. Use the lateral fluoroscopic view to assist in determining the correct craniocaudal adjustment required.
- For the end-on view, rotate the image detector approximately 20 to 30 degrees ipsilateral to the target pedicle, so that the medial cortex of the pedicle is at the middle third

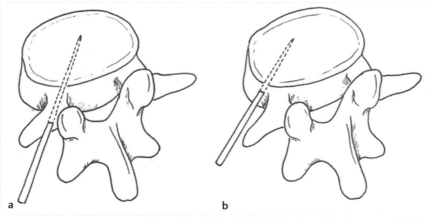

Fig. 8.3 Transpedicular and parapedicular approaches to the vertebral body. **(a)** The transpedicular approach takes the needle from the posterior surface of the pedicle, through the pedicle's length, and into the vertebral body. **(b)** The parapedicular advances the needle along the lateral surface of the pedicle, and penetrates the vertebral body at its junction with the pedicle. This approach may achieve a more medial position of the needle.

of the vertebral body. The vertebra adopts the "scottie dog" formation. Place the needle "end on" to the image detector, matching its angulation such that it appears as a dot.

- Plan the trocar trajectory. For the transpedicular approach, target the lateral margin of the pedicle, with an entry position at the 2 to 3 o'clock position of the right pedicle or at the 9 to 10 o'clock position of the left pedicle. For the parapedicular approach, the optimal entry position is just lateral to the transpedicular approach position. Preliminary planning of the needle trajectory and prediction of the ultimate route (▶ Fig. 8.4) allow operators to make alterations as the needle is advanced.
- Anesthetize the skin, subcutaneous tissues, and periosteum along the expected needle tract and bone entry point with subcutaneous lidocaine or bupivacaine via a 22-gauge needle.
- Make a small cutaneous incision, with the skin entry point decided based on preprocedural imaging and the approach being utilized. Advance the chosen needle to the periosteum.
- During the advancement of the needle to the bone surface, small corrections in the craniocaudal angulation can be made using a lateral view. In the parapedicular approach, the point at which bone is encountered (the junction of the pedicle with the vertebral body) will be more anterior on the lateral view.
- In the bone, advance the needle by gently tapping the handle of the needle with a mallet. The posterior wall of the vertebral body may be detected with a slight change to the "tapping" sound that occurs when advancing the needle with the mallet.[17] In soft osteoporotic bone, the needle may pass through with relative ease, with only light mallet strikes.
- If the end-on view was used initially, the needle should be kept as a dot during the initial placement through the pedicle. The needle should remain lateral to the medial cortex of the pedicle until it has navigated through the whole pedicle on the lateral view.
- After traversing the pedicle, if a diamond-tipped needle has been used, it may be replaced with a straight bevel-tipped needle or a curved needle, for improved maneuverability. Using the lateral projection, the needle is advanced further, to the anterior one-third of the vertebral body, and as close to midline

as possible or in the anterior portion of the lateral one-third of the vertebral body if a bilateral approach is planned. Confirm final positioning of the needle in both lateral and AP views prior to cement injection. The spinal canal has been cleared if the needle is anterior to the posterior margin of the verte-bral body.

8.3.8 Fill Materials

Several types of injectable bone cements are commercially available, including PMMA, composite glass ceramics, and calcium phosphate cements. These differ in terms of cost, polymerization times, biocompatibility, and radio-opacity. PMMA remains the most widely used cement for the treatment of osteoporotic and neoplastic VCFs. Key advantages of PMMA include good radio-opacity and low cost.[18] The PMMA cement is prepared by mixing a polymer powder and liquid monomer, resulting in liquid paste.[19] The polymerization of PMMA is an exothermic reaction, resulting in increasing thickness of the cement and increased cement temperature of up to 70 to 120°C. This may produce a local thermal cytotoxic effect on neoplastic cells.[18] Newer cement materials include composite and calcium phosphate cements. Composite cements do not cause the exothermic reaction of PMMA, and hence avoid potential risks of high cement temperatures and cytotoxic effects. As such, they may be less useful for the treatment of osseous metastases.[18] Composite cements have improved biocompatibility, yet have low viscosity that can lead to increased risk of leaks, and a rapid setting time that may lead to the needle staying cemented in the vertebra.[20] Calcium phosphate cements have superior biocompatibility, and stimulate new bone formation due to precipitation of crystals from the cement's injectable form. These cements, however, have longer setting times, higher cost, and lower radio-opacity, and are often less resistant to compression.[18,20]

Preparation of the cement takes place after needle(s) placement. When ready for injection, the consistency of PMMA cement should be similar to toothpaste with a matte appearance. A "shiny" or glossy appearance of the cement mixture indicates that it is too liquid for use. A "drip" test may be performed,

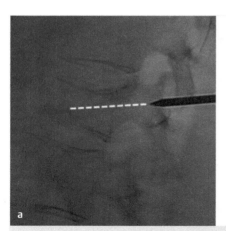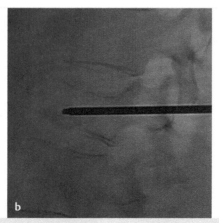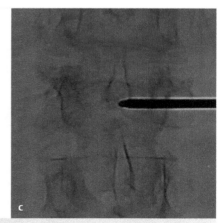

Fig. 8.4 Needle trajectory for a unilateral transpedicular approach in the lumbar spine. **(a)** Lateral fluoroscopic image of the vertebral body prior to vertebroplasty. The entire needle trajectory is extrapolated during initial transpedicular access to achieve optimal final needle position (*dotted line*). **(b)** The needle is advanced into the vertebral body. **(c)** Anteroposterior fluoroscopic image showing final needle position at midline.

whereby the cement should ball up at the end of the needle and not drip downward.[21] Automated mixing systems improve mixing consistency and can be used if available. Depending on the ambient temperature and specific PMMA formulation, working time varies from 10 to 20 minutes. Numerous delivery systems for the cement are available. These vary from 1-mL syringes with a spatula and mixing bowl to self-contained delivery devices. Injectors with long flexible delivery tubing have an advantage of minimizing operator exposure to radiation.[22]

8.3.9 Cement Injection

- The needle stylet is removed, and delivery system is connected and the cement is injected at a slow pace to avoid overpressurizing the delivery device with subsequent extravasation.
- Continuous monitoring with lateral and AP fluoroscopy is vital during cement injection, to ensure that the cement remains inside the vertebra and to rapidly identify leaks (▶Fig. 8.5). The risk of cement leakage is greater at the beginning of injection, when the cement is least viscous. New pain reported by the patient should prompt a pause in the procedure and the acquisition of additional imaging views. If cement is observed to pass into a vein, injection should be ceased for 1 to 2 minutes to allow the cement to solidify. The needle position can be adjusted slightly, then the cement may be reinjected to see if it is redirected safely within the vertebral body.[23] Larger leaks may necessitate placing additional needles or rarely even abandoning the procedure.
- Suggested endpoints for cement injection include passage of cement beyond the marrow space, and/or cement reaching the posterior wall of the vertebral body on the lateral view.

At the end of injection, cement should ideally form a column extending across midline to the contralateral pedicle and from end plate to end plate (▶Fig. 8.6).

- Care should be taken to avoid leaving a "tail" of cement upon concluding cement injection. This can be avoided by reinserting the needle stylet to deliver the residual portion of cement within the hollow cannula and leaving the needle in place for 1 to 2 minutes before removing it. The stylet may also be removed and reinserted to ensure that the cement is not backing up into the cannula. Finally, when withdrawing the needle, a gentle rocking and rotating motion may be employed to ensure the cement within the cannula separates at the cannula tip.

8.3.10 Volume of Cement Injected

The optimal volume of cement to inject remains is enough to alleviate pain as well as to restore the strength of the vertebral body and its stiffness. Based on the results of an in vitro biomechanical study, Mathis and Wong recommend aiming for 50 to 70% filling of the residual vertebral body volume.[24] Recent positive results from the VAPOUR (vertebroplasty for acute painful osteoporotic fractures) randomized controlled trial achieved with large volumes of cement (average 7.5 mL) have also supported larger-volume injections.[3] Much smaller volumes of cement have been shown to reduce pain similar to larger volumes and have inherently lower risk of cement extravasation, but more recent recommendations are to fill the vertebral body up to 15 to 25% of the native uncompressed amount.[25,26,38] In general, the goal should be maximum cement delivery with careful visual inspection to ensure injection is ceased well prior to complications occurring.

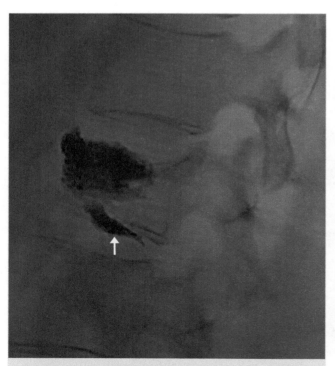

Fig. 8.5 Lateral fluoroscopic image showing minor diskal cement leakage (*white arrow*) following a vertebral augmentation procedure. Note that no posterior cement leakage has occurred.

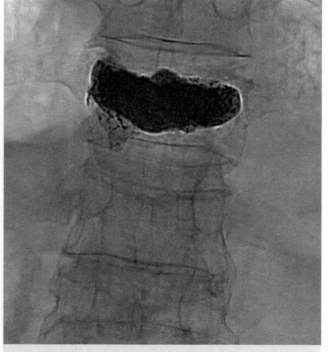

Fig. 8.6 Anteroposterior fluoroscopic image of the thoracic spine following vertebroplasty. Note that the injected cement forms a column extending across the midline.

8.4 Considerations in Cervical Vertebroplasty

Most vertebroplasty procedures are performed in the thoracic and lumbar spine. Cervical vertebroplasty is technically different due to the small size of target pedicles and vertebral bodies, and the anterior approach to the vertebral body. It is recommended that these procedures be undertaken by somewhat more experienced practitioners and, similar to thoracic or lumbar vertebroplasty, imaging guidance for cervical vertebroplasty may be with either fluoroscopy or CT.[27]

The precise approach for needle insertion in the cervical spine varies depending on the vertebral level. Procedures performed for C1 and C2 may use a direct transoral approach although a posterolateral approach to the C2 vertebral body has been reported.[27,28,39] As only a thin layer of tissue (pharyngeal constrictor muscles, pharyngobasilar fascia, and anterior longitudinal ligament) separates the posterior oropharynx from the upper cervical spine, this approach provides a direct route that avoids adjacent neurovascular structures.[27–29] After general anesthesia is provided, the patient is positioned supine on the fluoroscopy table and an oropharyngeal retractor is placed to expose the oropharynx. A large gauge (i.e., smaller diameter) needle is inserted through the posterior pharyngeal wall to gain access to the vertebral body.[28]

Below the level of C2, either anterolateral or posterior transpedicular approach may be used.[27] In the anterolateral approach, the needle trajectory must avoid the carotid sheath complex. The carotid artery should be located by palpation and manually retracted laterally by the operator's fingers. CT may also be used to visualize the carotid sheath and contents. The needle path ascends from below the angle of the mandible, and advances between the carotid complex, thyroid gland, and esophagus on the patient's right side. A small guide needle may be useful for confirming safe placement that avoids the carotid complex.[30] When the posterior transpedicular approach is used for the cervical spine, the operator should confirm that pedicles are large enough for access. Care is taken to avoid the vertebral artery, located lateral to the pedicle.

8.5 Postprocedure Care

8.5.1 Initial Postprocedure Care

The needles are removed once sufficient filling of the vertebral body has occurred. Manual pressure is immediately applied to the needle entry sites for enough time to promote hemostasis and prevent hematoma formation in the soft tissues. A sterile dressing is then applied. Transfer to the stretcher using log roll maneuvers or manual-assisted transfer can occur directly after the procedure, except in the case of vertebral cleft. In these cases, the patient should remain prone on the procedure table for 5 to 10 minutes to allow the cement to further polymerize in the expanded vertebral body.

Vital signs should be performed at regular intervals over the first few hours postprocedure, along with neurologic examinations. In recovery, the patient should remain flat and supine for the first hour, followed by a further 30 minutes to 1 hour with the head of the bed inclined approximately 30 degrees. Following this, patients can begin supervised mobilization

when their symptoms become tolerable and the effects of the anesthesia have waned. Initial postprocedure pain at the procedure site may occur and can be relieved with administration of acetaminophen or ketorolac, depending on renal function or ice. The patient is usually able to discriminate any new procedure-related pain, which typically relieves with simple analgesia over the next 24 to 72 hours. Assessment of the patient shortly after vertebroplasty commonly reveals improvement in fracture-related back pain. Persistent severe pain, new severe pain of a different character, or signs of spinal canal stenosis should prompt imaging with CT to exclude complications such as hematoma or cement leakage into neural foramina or spinal canal.

8.5.2 Discharge and Follow-Up

Most vertebroplasty procedures are performed on an outpatient basis, with the patient discharged later the same day following a satisfactory period of observation. More infirm patients may require overnight observation in the hospital. It is recommended to maintain bed rest and minimal activity for the first 24 hours. Regular diet and medications may be resumed on the same day. The patient is counseled to notify the appropriate medical professionals in the case of worsening pain or new pain, swelling, difficulty in walking, sensory changes in the hips and legs, or altered bowel or bladder function. Cross-sectional imaging should be performed in the event of these symptoms occurring, and surgical consult may be considered.

Tenderness may occur at the procedural site for 24 to 48 hours. Pain in the hours following vertebroplasty is typically procedure related. Delayed pain, either at the procedure or in a different location, should raise suspicion of new fracture. Up to one-third of patients will suffer a repeat fracture within 1 to 3 years, most occurring at adjacent vertebral levels.[31,32] However, a small percentage (0.6–2.4%) may suffer refracture at a vertebral level previously treated with vertebroplasty.[33,34] It should be noted that for up to one-third of patients, bone marrow edema is a normal MRI finding for up to 6 months postvertebroplasty.[35] Thus, caution should be taken when interpreting marrow edema at a previously treated level, as it may not indicate a new acute fracture.

Outpatient clinic follow-up should occur typically 2 to 4 weeks postprocedure. At this time, durability of the initial pain improvement, degree of patient mobility, and analgesic requirements are reviewed. The patient is assessed for signs of procedural complications. Subsequent follow-up appointments may take place as is indicated on a case-by-case basis. Management of the underlying cause of fracture is important to prevent future fractures. Optimal osteoporosis treatment should involve vitamin D and calcium supplementation, and medical management with an anabolic bone agent or other targeted therapy as indicated.[36,37]

8.6 Conclusion

Vertebroplasty is a safe and effective treatment for painful VCFs that are refractory to medical management or in patients who are severely debilitated by their vertebral fracture. Meticulous technique and accurate image visualization with fluoroscopy are important to achieve optimal outcomes. With attention to postoperative care and follow-up, the risks of complications are very low. Cervical vertebroplasty presents additional challenges, but may achieve similar success in the hands of experienced operators.

8.7 Key Points

- Vertebroplasty is a minimally invasive procedure that involves the percutaneous injection of cement into a fractured vertebral body.
- Vertebroplasty procedures are performed with image guidance. Fluoroscopy is recommended as it allows continuous monitoring during needle placement and cement injection.
- The trajectory taken to direct the needle into the vertebral body may be either transpedicular or parapedicular. There are advantages to each approach.
- Numerous types of bone cement are available, but PMMA remains the most widely used.
- Most procedures are performed in the thoracic and lumbar spine. Cervical vertebroplasty is less commonly performed and requires some additional considerations such as the type of approach and the size of the needles used.
- A repeat fracture at the treated level or adjacent level can occur and can be prevented with optimal osteoporosis control.
- Most patients report improvement in back pain shortly following vertebroplasty. Delayed pain following initial improvement, or new pain of a different character, should raise suspicion of new fracture.

References

[1] Syed MI, Shaikh A. Vertebroplasty: a systematic approach. Pain Physician 2007;10(2):367–380

[2] Klazen CAH, Lohle PNM, de Vries J, et al. Vertebroplasty versus conservative treatment in acute osteoporotic vertebral compression fractures (Vertos II): an open-label randomised trial. Lancet 2010;376(9746):1085–1092

[3] Clark W, Bird P, Gonski P, et al. Safety and efficacy of vertebroplasty for acute painful osteoporotic fractures (VAPOUR): a multicentre, randomised, double-blind, placebo-controlled trial. Lancet 2016;388(10052):1408–1416

[4] Lee IJ, Choi AL, Yie MY, et al. CT evaluation of local leakage of bone cement after percutaneous kyphoplasty and vertebroplasty. Acta Radiol 2010;51(6):649–654

[5] Ploeg WT, Veldhuizen AG, The B, Sietsma MS. Percutaneous vertebroplasty as a treatment for osteoporotic vertebral compression fractures: a systematic review. Eur Spine J 2006;15(12):1749–1758

[6] Teng MM, Wei CJ, Wei LC, et al. Kyphosis correction and height restoration effects of percutaneous vertebroplasty. AJNR Am J Neuroradiol 2003;24(9):1893–1900

[7] Moon E, Tam MDBS, Kikano RN, Karuppasamy K. Prophylactic antibiotic guidelines in modern interventional radiology practice. Semin Intervent Radiol 2010;27(4):327–337

[8] Kallmes DF, Jensen ME. Percutaneous vertebroplasty. Radiology 2003; 229(1):27–36

[9] Yu SW, Chen WJ, Lin WC, Chen YJ, Tu YK. Serious pyogenic spondylitis following vertebroplasty: a case report. Spine 2004;29(10):E209–E211

[10] Ortiz AO, Zoarski GH, Beckerman M. Kyphoplasty. Tech Vasc Interv Radiol 2002;5(4):239–249

[11] Kim AK, Jensen ME, Dion JE, Schweickert PA, Kaufmann TJ, Kallmes DF. Unilateral transpedicular percutaneous vertebroplasty: initial experience. Radiology 2002;222(3):737–741

[12] Kaufmann TJ, Trout AT, Kallmes DF. The effects of cement volume on clinical outcomes of percutaneous vertebroplasty. AJNR Am J Neuroradiol 2006;27(9):1933–1937

[13] Zhu SY, Zhong ZM, Wu Q, Chen JT. Risk factors for bone cement leakage in percutaneous vertebroplasty: a retrospective study of four hundred and eighty five patients. Int Orthop 2016;40(6):1205–1210

[14] Zhang L, Liu Z, Wang J, et al. Unipedicular versus bipedicular percutaneous vertebroplasty for osteoporotic vertebral compression fractures: a prospective randomized study. BMC Musculoskelet Disord 2015;16:145

[15] Caudana R, Renzi Brivio L, Ventura L, Aitini E, Rozzanigo U, Barai G. CT-guided percutaneous vertebroplasty: personal experience in the treatment of osteoporotic fractures and dorsolumbar metastases. Radiol Med (Torino) 2008;113(1):114–133

[16] Vogl TJ, Proschek D, Schwarz W, Mack M, Hochmuth K. CT-guided percutaneous vertebroplasty in the therapy of vertebral compression fractures. Eur Radiol 2006;16(4):797–803

[17] Jay B, Ahn SH. Vertebroplasty. Semin Intervent Radiol 2013;30(3):297–306

[18] Katsanos K, Sabharwal T, Adam A. Percutaneous cementoplasty. Semin Intervent Radiol 2010;27(2):137–147

[19] Lieberman IH, Togawa D, Kayanja MM. Vertebroplasty and kyphoplasty: filler materials. Spine J 2005;5(6, Suppl):305S–316S

[20] Pomrink GJ, DiCicco MP, Clineff TD, Erbe EM. Evaluation of the reaction kinetics of CORTOSS, a thermoset cortical bone void filler. Biomaterials 2003;24(6):1023–1031

[21] Wong W, Mathis J. Is intraosseous venography a significant safety measure in performance of vertebroplasty? J Vasc Interv Radiol 2002;13(2 Pt 1):137–138

[22] Komemushi A, Tanigawa N, Kariya S, Kojima H, Shomura Y, Sawada S. Radiation exposure to operators during vertebroplasty. J Vasc Interv Radiol 2005;16(10):1327–1332

[23] Mathis JM, Ortiz AO, Zoarski GH. Vertebroplasty versus kyphoplasty: a comparison and contrast. AJNR Am J Neuroradiol 2004;25(5):840–845

[24] Mathis JM, Wong W. Percutaneous vertebroplasty: technical considerations. J Vasc Interv Radiol 2003;14(8):953–960

[25] Kaufmann TJ, Trout AT, Kallmes DF. The effects of cement volume on clinical outcomes of percutaneous vertebroplasty. AJNR Am J Neuroradiol 2006;27(9):1933–1937

[26] Molloy S, Riley LH III, Belkoff SM. Effect of cement volume and placement on mechanical-property restoration resulting from vertebroplasty. AJNR Am J Neuroradiol 2005;26(2):401–404

[27] Tsoumakidou G, Too CW, Koch G, et al. CIRSE guidelines on percutaneous vertebral augmentation. Cardiovasc Intervent Radiol 2017;40(3):331–342

[28] Anselmetti GC, Manca A, Montemurro F, et al. Vertebroplasty using transoral approach in painful malignant involvement of the second cervical vertebra (C2): a single-institution series of 25 patients. Pain Physician 2012;15(1):35–42

[29] Kaminsky IA, Härtl R, Sigounas D, Mlot S, Patsalides A. Transoral C2 biopsy and vertebroplasty. Interv Med Appl Sci 2013;5(2):76–80

[30] Mathis JM, Golovac S, eds. Image-Guided Spine Interventions. New York, NY: Springer; 2010

[31] Tanigawa N, Kariya S, Komemushi A, et al. Percutaneous vertebroplasty for osteoporotic compression fractures: long-term evaluation of the technical and clinical outcomes. AJR Am J Roentgenol 2011;196(6):1415–1418

[32] Chandra RV, Maingard J, Asadi H, et al. Vertebroplasty and kyphoplasty for osteoporotic vertebral fractures: what are the latest data? AJNR Am J Neuroradiol 2018;39(5):798–806

[33] Chen LH, Hsieh MK, Liao JC, et al. Repeated percutaneous vertebroplasty for refracture of cemented vertebrae. Arch Orthop Trauma Surg 2011;131(7): 927–933

[34] Gaughen JR Jr, Jensen ME, Schweickert PA, Marx WF, Kallmes DF. The therapeutic benefit of repeat percutaneous vertebroplasty at previously treated vertebral levels. AJNR Am J Neuroradiol 2002;23(10):1657–1661

[35] Dansie DM, Luetmer PH, Lane JI, Thielen KR, Wald JT, Kallmes DF. MRI findings after successful vertebroplasty. AJNR Am J Neuroradiol 2005;26(6): 1595–1600

[36] Chandra RV, Meyers PM, Hirsch JA, et al; Society of NeuroInterventional Surgery. Vertebral augmentation: report of the Standards and Guidelines Committee of the Society of NeuroInterventional Surgery. J Neurointerv Surg 2014;6(1):7–15

[37] Chandra RV, Yoo AJ, Hirsch JA. Vertebral augmentation: update on safety, efficacy, cost effectiveness and increased survival? Pain Physician 2013;16 (4):309–320

[38] Martinčič D, Brojan M, Kosel F, et al. Minimum cement volume for vertebroplasty. Int Orthop 2015;39(4):727–733

[39] Sun HY, Lee JW, Kim KJ, Yeom JS, Kang HS. Percutaneous intervention of the C2 vertebral body using a CT-guided posterolateral approach. AJR Am J Roentgenol 2009;193(6):1703–1705

9 Sacroplasty: Management of Sacral Insufficiency Fractures

Kieran Murphy

Summary

Sacral insufficiency fractures are relatively common but are often underdiagnosed and undertreated. These fractures are a frequent cause of low back pain in the elderly patient population but are frequently missed on X-ray and cross sectional evaluation of the lumbosacral spine. The typical sacral insufficiency fractures (SIFs) characteristically involve the sacral ala and the S2 vertebral body. When SIFs are suspected, MR imaging is the single best imaging modality for diagnosing these fractures but a combination of nuclear medicine bone scan and CT can be used in patients who cannot have an magnetic resonance imaging (MRI). The management of SIFs should consist of treatments that allow for early and sustained mobilization of the patient including sacroplasty if necessary. There are various techniques and different ways of performing sacroplasty including the short-axis technique, long-axis technique, lateral approach technique, and the three needle technique. All of these techniques have been shown to be safe and effective and studies of sacroplasty have confirmed its safety and efficacy out to as long as ten years. Providing the option of sacroplasty to those patients who do not or cannot undergo non-surgical management can lead to better mobility, improved function, dramatically decreased pain, and less mortality.

Keywords: sacroplasty, sacrum, osteoporosis, sacral insufficiency fractures, osseous augmentation

9.1 Introduction

First described by Lourie et al in 1982,[1] SIFs are a common but often underdiagnosed source of low back pain in the elderly and/or the osteoporotic patient. Insufficiency fractures of the pelvis are a consequence of undue stress onto a weakened bone or of increased stress on a bone with marginally adequate bone mineral density. Risks of SIFs are very similar to that of vertebral compression fractures and include risk factors of osteoporosis, osteopenia, osteomalacia, renal osteodystrophy, prior radiation therapy, Paget's disease, previous lumbosacral fusion, total hip arthroplasty, and bone metabolic diseases known to weaken the skeletal system.[1,2] Osteoporosis is the most common cause of fractures of the pelvis and over 25 million people are affected in the United States. There is a strong female predominance for SIFs (10:1), and they can occur without an identifiable injury in someone with low bone mineral density and compromised bone strength.[3] The incidence of SIFs comprises approximately 1 to 2% of the pathologic fractures involving the spine and pelvis. This incidence, however, may be an underestimate as the diagnosis is often delayed or does not happen due to the relatively poor sensitivity of plain radiographs and the lack of adequate recognition of SIFs on cross-sectional imaging including both MR and CT imaging.

9.2 Fractures of the Sacrum: Anatomy

Anatomically, the sacrum is comprised of five fused segments. Weight transfers can occur through the lumbar spine into the sacrum and then through the ilium into the proximal femora with regions of stress in the second sacral segment and in the pubic rami. This stress pattern can produce insufficiency fractures that can have a unique but often characteristic appearance of SIFs.[4] In 1988, Denis et al classified the location of sacral fractures into three sacral zones (▶Fig. 9.1).[5] Zone 1 fractures are laterally located fractures that involve the sacral ala but do not traverse the foramina or the central sacral canal. Zone 2 fractures involve the sacral foramina but do not involve the central spinal canal. Zone 3 fractures extend into and involve the central spinal canal. A fracture to the central portion of the sacrum is typically associated with a higher energy type injury and patients with zone 3 fractures can present with saddle anesthesia and loss of sphincter tone as a result of cauda equina injury or can present with varying degrees of injuries including neuropraxia or injury to a single nerve root.[5] The most common location of SIFs are within zone 1, but a minority of the fractures can involve the sacral foramina. The SIFs typically run parallel to the sacroiliac joint along the entire sacral ala and can have a horizontal component that is usually located at the S2 level of the sacrum when present (▶Fig. 9.2). The most common fracture pattern is that of bilateral sacral alar fractures that primarily involve the S1 and S2 vertebrae. Unilateral fractures can also occur and can be present without a contralateral fracture or can progress to bilateral fractures. The appearance and

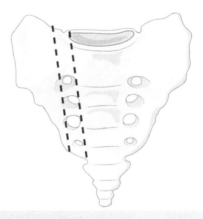

Fig. 9.1 Denis Fracture Classification. Zone 1 fractures are laterally located fractures that involve the sacral ala but do not traverse the foramina or central sacral canal. Zone 2 fractures involve the sacral foramina but do not involve the central spinal canal. Zone 3 fractures extend into and involve the central spinal canal. (Image created with BioRender.)

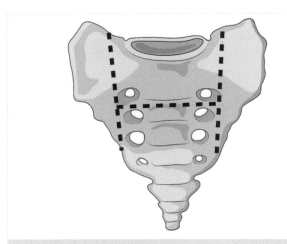

Fig. 9.2 The sacral insufficiency fractures typically run parallel to the sacroiliac joint along the entire sacral ala and can have a horizontal component that is usually located at the S2 level of the sacrum when present.

location of the fractures must be noted as well as the anatomic regions affected, as these factors can have significant implications in the repair of these fractures.

9.3 Sacral Insufficiency Fractures: Causes and Natural History

There are some studies that have examined the morbidity and mortality associated with SIFs. Park et al recently published their experience, looking at 325 patients with a mean follow-up of 51.5 months.[6] The mean age at time of diagnosis was 69.4 years. There was a history of malignancy in 43.1% of patients and 21.8% had undergone pelvic irradiation prior to the fracture. The 6-month mortality rate was 9.8% and the 1-year mortality rate was 17.5%, while mortality increased to 25.5% at 3 years. The sex- and age-adjusted mortality ratio increased after these fractures, and the overall 3-month standardized mortality ratio (SMR) was 8.9.

The major cause of SIFs is normal stress on an osteoporotic or otherwise weakened bone. Traumas, both minor and severe, are also causes of sacral fractures, but SIFs are a low-velocity, low-energy type of fractures that develop due to normal or slightly increased stress on a weak bone. When sacral fractures are associated with some type of inciting event, it is typically a low-velocity injury such as a fall on the sacrum and coccyx from a standing height or a minimal axial load impact like stepping off a curb. Patients will often notice a severe and immediate pain in their back or buttock.[7] The pain is often not severe and can be described as a dull ache that increases in severity over time. Other patients will feel pain primarily when sitting and will shift in their seats because their back and buttock hurts. Patients often develop an antalgic gait pattern due to the forces transmitted across the sacral ala that increase when the patient is walking. This pain may be quite debilitating and the patient may require a cane or walker to ambulate or may even be confined to a stretcher. Other patients with SIFs have severe localized pain in the low back or sacrum with a sciatica-type pain, usually in an S1 distribution.

9.4 History and Examination

Determining the cause and contributing factors to the SIFs is important and appropriate history taking is an essential element in identifying the risk factors as well as the inciting event. Important factors are whether the patient is on medications for osteoporosis,[8] whether they have had a recent dual energy X-ray absorptiometry (DEXA) scan or quantitative CT (QCT) to determine bone density, and if they have had previous fractures of the wrist, hip, or spine. Appropriate imaging studies are also necessary to evaluate the fracture pattern and surrounding anatomy.[4] A thorough laboratory evaluation should include a complete blood count and an extended blood chemistry along with measurements of ionized calcium, parathyroid hormone (PTH), and 1, 25-hydroxyvitamin D levels, alkaline phosphatase, albumin, free testosterone, thyroid-stimulating hormone, and serum protein electrophoresis. Other laboratory work for an osteoporosis should include urinary measurements of calcium and cortisol and a urinary protein electrophoresis. Obtaining a history of malignancy is also important and consideration should be given to whether the SIF may be related to a neoplastic process. If this is a concern, performing a biopsy during the process to treat the sacral fracture is warranted.

Physical examination techniques are also important in the diagnostic process and include the standing leg test and the presence of tenderness of the sacrum with compression of the pelvis. Typically, there is no muscle weakness or reflex changes and normal sphincter tone is most often present, but abnormalities of any of these must be documented. Patients with SIFs may be able to walk into the physician's clinic independently or with the aid of a walker or wheelchair and on a stretcher in some cases. If they are walking without assist devices, they most often have a slow antalgic gait. It is not unusual for older patients or patients with more severe SIFs to be unable to walk.

9.5 Imaging

If an SIF is suspected by history and/or physical examination, then the next step is to obtain the appropriate imaging. Spinal and/or pelvic radiographs have poor sensitivity and are of questionable value in the diagnosis of SIFs. The best imaging modality that yields the highest sensitivity and specificity is MR imaging.[9] Fractures of the sacrum are best shown on dedicated studies of the sacrum and on the axial and coronal images. Traditionally, MR imaging examinations of the lumbar spine may miss a fracture of the sacrum as the axial images may not extend far enough inferiorly to see the fractures in this plane and the sagittal images may not optimally show the fractures or the fractures may be confused with the sacroiliac joint. They can be seen on lumbar imaging, however, if close attention is paid to the symptoms and the findings.[9] Short tau inversion recovery (STIR) and non-fat saturated T1-weighted MR imaging sequences are the best imaging to diagnose these fractures as edema from the fractures are well seen on the STIR images and the fracture lines are most optimally demonstrated on the T1-weighted images (▶Fig. 9.3).

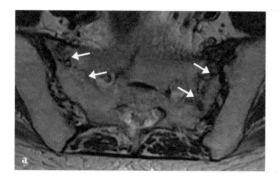

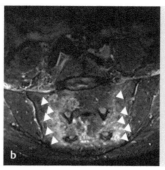

Fig. 9.3 Axial T1-weighted (**a**) and short tau inversion recovery (STIR; **b**) MR images show bilateral fracture lines (*white arrows* in a) that are well demonstrated on this T1-weighted image. The bilateral sacral insufficiency fractures are seen to be associated with considerable edema (*white arrowheads* in b) on the coronal STIR MR image.

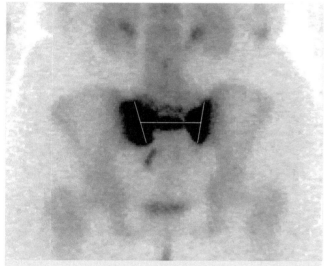

Fig. 9.4 Nuclear medicine bone scan showing increase uptake of radiotracer in an H pattern (*white lines*) that resembles the shape of the H on the front of Honda automobiles.

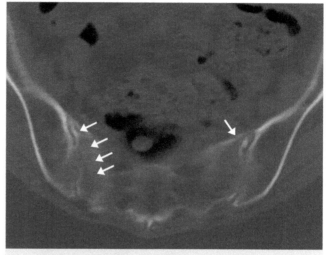

Fig. 9.5 Axial CT image shows bilateral sacral fractures with fracture lines (*white arrows*) causing cortical and cancellous bone disruption. This disruption is seen without much surrounding sclerosis, thereby making these fractures more subtle than those with a large amount of sclerosis surrounding the fractures.

Traditionally, the most sensitive but not specific imaging modality is a nuclear medicine bone scan[10]. A bone scan has increased activity of the radiotracer within the fracture and the pattern has classically been described as Honda's sign, a typical H-shaped pattern on bone scan that is pathognomonic for SIFs (▶Fig. 9.4). The pattern of increased uptake on the bone scan represents increased activity that is vertically oriented in the sacral ala and is joined by horizontal activity in the mid to upper portion of the sacrum usually located at the S2 level of the sacrum.[10] The H shape with the vertical components narrower at the inferior portion and wider at the superior portion resembles the shape of the H on the front of Honda automobiles (▶Fig. 9.4). A cross-sectional evaluation of a bone scan or a single-photon emission computed tomography (SPECT) scan may also be helpful in identifying and localizing SIFs. Despite the sensitivity of bone scans in detecting SIFs, MRI has replaced this modality in many departments, due largely to better availability of MR imaging.

If a patient has a pacemaker, cochlear implant, or something else that precludes from them getting an MRI, a CT scan is the necessary examination to compliment the bone scan. Any cross-sectional imaging examination may not highlight sacral fractures optimally and although CT scans can be more sensitive in detecting cortical breaks associated with SIFs, nondisplaced fractures without obvious reactive sclerosis may be missed[11] (▶Fig. 9.5).

9.6 Treatment

9.6.1 Conservative Treatment

The treatment of SIFs either can be interventional with a percutaneous approach, surgical, or can consist of nonsurgical management (NSM). Unstable fractures, especially high-velocity injuries with associated cauda equina syndrome, may require open reduction and internal fixation. As opposed to closed or percutaneous procedures, open procedures are associated with an increased risk of surgical and postsurgical complications including wound problems and infection.[12]

Historically, treatment has been limited to bed rest, oral narcotic medications, lumbosacral or pelvic corsets, and protected weight bearing with the patient using a walker in order to accomplish early mobilization.[4,13] If early mobilization is not possible, prolonged bed rest can lead to additional morbidities including deep venous thromboses, pulmonary emboli, reduced muscle strength, postural hypotension, impaired cardiac function, atelectasis, pneumonia, pressure ulcers, constipation, fecal impaction, depression, and side effects from opioids including altered sensorium, additional constipation, memory loss, and putting the patient at an increased risk for falling.[14] These morbidities are profoundly impactful and are known complications of periods of inactivity. In addition to the substantial impact of the morbidities associated with SIFs, the associated mortality is also significant, with studies estimating the 1- to 3-year mortality at 20 to 25%.[6,15] When patients respond promptly to NSM, the initial clinical improvement may occur quickly, but it is important to know that compete resolution of symptoms may not occur for up to 9 to 12 months. All these factors contribute to a clinical scenario that can be arduous for the patient to tolerate with the goal being to prevent or limit the spiral of immobility, followed by bed rest, deconditioning, secondary events (e.g., infections, venous thromboembolism), and other sequelae of the initial event.[16] In patients for whom the symptoms are sufficiently severe or debilitating, invasive treatments may benefit them and prevent the incapacitation that is often seen in patients with SIFs.

9.6.2 Osseous Augmentation

Chronic symptoms and disability related to osteoporotic insufficiency fractures are believed to be due to fracture nonunion, micro-motion, resultant deformity related to the original fracture deformity, or progressive deformity due to the inability of the weakened bone to promptly heal.[17,18] The percutaneous injection of polymethyl methacrylate (PMMA) into fractured vertebral bodies (osteoplasty or sacral vertebroplasty) has been safely performed to successfully treat painful osteoporotic vertebral fractures. A natural extension of the application of vertebroplasty is the percutaneous injection of PMMA into the fractured sacrum (sacroplasty) to treat persistent symptoms and disability associated with SIFs. Sacroplasty was first reported in the early 2000s as treatment for symptomatic sacral metastatic lesions,[19,20] and subsequent reports have documented its safe and effective performance. The initial short follow-up intervals and small study cohorts led to more definitive studies evaluating the safety and efficacy of the procedure and the durability of initial results.[21] More recently, studies with a greater number of patients and longer follow-up have clarified the treatment outcomes of sacroplasty regarding safety and long term efficacy.[22,23]

9.7 Techniques

Various techniques have been described for performing percutaneous sacroplasty, and these include both short- and long-axis approaches. Routinely, sacroplasty is performed with fluoroscopy, but CT guidance or a combination of both may be used. Many interventional radiologists who are well trained in CT-guided procedures advocate for performing sacroplasty with CT guidance. While CT is a viable method of performing imaging guidance, it is slower and more expensive as compared with fluoroscopy, which is cheaper, faster, and technically straightforward (▶Table 9.1). Fluoroscopic guidance, however, typically requires more experience to identify untoward cement extravasation. More recently, the routine use of cone-beam CT has allowed a combination of both approaches to be used.

Whitlow et al looked at technical considerations and analyzed PMMA injection under fluoroscopic guidance.[24] Sacroplasty was performed on cadaveric specimens using biplane fluoroscopy. The cadaveric specimens were evaluated with CT that was performed both before and after sacroplasty to examine needle placement and to assess for PMMA extravasation. The CT imaging demonstrated that needle placement and PMMA delivery may be done safely and is facilitated by orienting the needle parallel to the L5–S1 interspace and ipsilateral sacroiliac joint and targeting the superolateral sacral ala within an area whose borders are formed by a line just lateral to the posterior sacral foramina and a line along the medial edge of the sacroiliac joint (▶Fig. 9.6). In another assessment of this technique, Betts published an article on fluoroscopic anatomy landmarks and associated these landmarks with their gross anatomic structures as seen with open dissection.[25]

Table 9.1 Comparing the pros and cons of CT versus fluoroscopy when performing sacroplasty

	Fluoroscopic guidance	CT guided
Pros	Faster Cheaper Easier	Less steep learning curve Debatable reduction rate of complication
Cons	Require experience	Slower More expensive

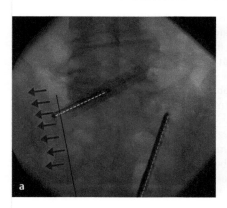
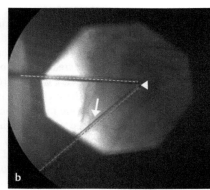

Fig. 9.6 (a, b) Short-axis target is shown on fluoroscopy with the left-sided needle (highlighted by *yellow dashed line* in **a** and **b**) targeting the superolateral left sacral ala between the outer border of the sacral foramina (*thin black line* in **a**) and the sacroiliac joint (*black arrows* in **a**). The short-axis technique involves placing the needle nearly parallel to the end plates of S1. The long-axis technique involves placing the needle (highlighted by *red dashed line* in **a** and **b**) between the outer border of the sacral foramina and the sacroiliac joint starting at the posteroinferior portion of S2 (*white arrow* in **b**) and advancing the needle anterosuperiorly to the midportion of the S1 vertebral body(*white arrowhead* in **b**).

9.7.1 Short-Axis Technique

In a 2007 manuscript reporting the results of sacroplasty in 37 patients, Frey et al described a variation of the short-axis technique for performing percutaneous sacroplasty.[26] All procedures were performed under fluoroscopic guidance using moderate sedation and every patient received preoperative antibiotics. The procedure time from the initial set up to the completion and patient recovery takes about an hour. At the start of the procedure, the patient is placed in a prone position and the image intensifier is placed in an oblique view along the axis of the ipsilateral sacroiliac joint (see ▶Fig. 9.6 and ▶Table 9.2 for details). This obliquity varies from patient to patient but is typically 5 to 20 degrees in mediolateral angulation. Next, two 13-gauge bone trocars were placed between the sacral foramina and the sacroiliac joint on the side of the fracture with an angle paralleling the sacroiliac joint (▶Fig. 9.7a,b). The needles were then inserted to approximately the midpoint of the sacrum on the lateral view, maintaining the initial angle. After mixing the cement, 3 to 5 mL of PMMA were injected through each trocars while monitoring the spread of the bone cement on the oblique anteroposterior fluoroscopic view. Care was taken when injecting the bone cement to avoid medial spreading of the cement toward the sacral nerve roots. Each patient was maintained in the prone position for 30 minutes after the procedure and prior to ambulation. The patients were then asked to stand on the affected leg to assess their pain improvement. If they had bilateral pain, they were asked to stand on each leg, one at a time to assess the level of pain they were having.

This study was a prospective, multicenter, observational cohort study of patients with a mean age of 76.6 years who had undergone and failed a trial of NSM for a mean of 34.4 days (range between 13 and 82 days). All patients were available at all follow-up intervals. The mean Visual Analog Scale (VAS) score at baseline was 7.7 and was 3.2 within 30 minutes after the procedure and 2.1 at 2 weeks, 1.7 at 4 weeks, 1.3 at 12 weeks, 1.0 at 24 weeks, and 0.7 at 52 weeks after the procedure [16]. Thirty minutes after the procedure, 5 patients reported

Table 9.2 Short-axis technique

Sacroplasty using the short-axis technique: step by step	
1	In the frontal plane, rotate the II cephalad to parallel the L5–S1 disk space. (This will usually require significant caudal angulation of the II)
2	Rotate the II so that the spinous processes are in the center of the vertebral body—a direct AP view
3	Rotate the II to the side opposite the treatment location, by about 25–30 degrees OR to an angle along the longitudinal axis of the SI joint that aligns the inferior portion of the joint
4	The starting position is chosen: halfway between the SIJ and a vertical line that joins the medial borders of the sacral neural foramina
5	Anesthetize the skin at the desired starting point and make a small incision
6	Insert the sacroplasty needle at the incision, advancing the needle parallel to the II
7	Using a mallet, slowly advance the needle tip just past the posterior sacral cortex and into the center one-third of the sacrum. It is important to keep the mediolateral angulation of the needle "as is," to avoid deviating from the trajectory chosen
8	Rotate the II to get a lateral view of the sacrum, and the needle within the S1 vertebral body. (If using biplane equipment, the lateral II can be used for this purpose)
9	When the PMMA has been mixed and a toothpaste consistency achieved, inject it into the sacrum using both lateral and oblique AP views to monitor PMMA distribution. On the lateral view, watch for anterior extravasation (i.e., anterior to the anterior body of the sacrum), while on the oblique AP view there should be little or no extravasation into the neural exit foramina
10	Deposit the PMMA in the sacrum trying to fill the center portion of the sacral ala (i.e., between the SIJ and the neural foramina), intermittently retracting the needle and depositing PMMA along the needle tract, i.e., along the longitudinal axis of the sacrum
11	If necessary, insert a second needle into the inferior half of the sacrum using the same technique (and mediolateral positioning) as the first needle
12	When the PMMA has been deposited adequately, remove all needles and place appropriate bandages over the puncture sites

Abbreviations: AP, anteroposterior; II, image intensifier; PMMA, polymethylmethacrylate; SIJ, sacroiliac joint.

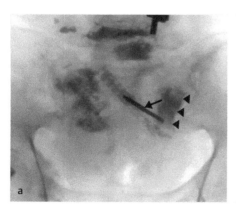
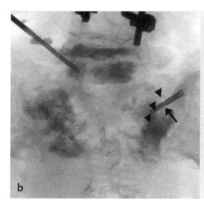

Fig. 9.7 (a, b) Anteroposterior fluoroscopic images show two needles place in sequence into the patient's right sacral ala (*black arrows*) using the short-axis technique to inject bone cement (*black arrowheads*) into the sacral ala.

complete pain relief, 10 patients reported no pain at 2 weeks, and 25 patients were pain free by 52 weeks after the procedure. Twenty patients were using narcotic analgesics at baseline and only 6 patients were using narcotics at 2 to 8 weeks following the procedure. One significant adverse event (SAE) was encountered during the procedure but none at any of the follow-up intervals. The single SAE involved a patient who developed S1 radicular pain during the procedure, necessitating termination of injection of the PMMA. Although the primary sacral pain was alleviated, the patient experienced persistent inferior buttock and posterior thigh pain that was completely relieved 7 days later by a selective nerve root injection consisting of 2.0 mL of preservative-free betamethasone (6 mg/mL) and 1.0 mL of 1.0% lidocaine injected in the epidural space around the S1 nerve root. Potential risks for sacroplasty include cement emboli, cement extravasation, sacral nerve root injury, and injury to the lumbosacral plexus. In February 2008, Frey et al published a subsequent study of 52 patients.[21] In this study, using the short-axis technique, more than 75% of the patients had their pain reduced by half or more 30 minutes after the procedure. This study provided strong additional support for the safety and efficacy of sacroplasty.

9.7.2 Long-Axis Technique

The long-axis technique can be used to access both the S1 and the S2 segments with one needle per side. The needle is placed between the sacroiliac joint and the lateral border of the neural foramen and directed superiorly at an oblique angle along the long axis of the sacrum (▶Fig. 9.6 and ▶Table 9.3). The long-axis technique can produce optimal cement distribution along the longitudinal axis of the fractures and can decrease the risk of violating the anterior border of the sacrum with the access needle. The starting point is at the posteroinferior portion of the S2 vertebral body between the lateral border of the sacral foramina and the sacroiliac joint. The needle is then advanced from the posteroinferior portion of S2 to the mid to superior portion of S1 (▶Fig. 9.6). The normal anatomy with the lordosis of the lumbosacral junction and the patient's prone position makes this approach technically straightforward and can be accomplished without extreme angulation of the needle. As with the short-axis approach, care should be taken not to violate the anterior cortex of the sacrum as the lumbosacral plexus traverses the sacral ala from superior to inferior just anterior to the anterior sacral cortex. Anterior extravasation of the cement can also cause damage to the lumbosacral plexus and should also be avoided. The cement is best injected from distal to proximal using cement with a thick viscous consistency. The steps of the long-axis approach are listed in sequence in ▶Table 9.3.

A variation of the long-axis technique is to add a third needle placed in the center of the osseous sacrum directed in a similar orientation to the needles in the sacral ala with the starting point of the needle inferior to the thecal sac (▶Fig. 9.8). This technique can be used in fractures that have a prominent horizontal component that the treating physician believes needs additional dedicated stabilization in addition to stabilizing the fractures of the sacral ala. The three-needle long-axis technique will allow the injection of a substantial amount of bone cement into the center of the sacrum as well as the sacral ala (▶Fig. 9.9).

9.7.3 Lateral Approach Technique

An alternative approach involves placing the needles perpendicular to the sacrum and approaching it from lateral to medial (i.e., in a horizontal plane, extending from one side to the other; see ▶Fig. 9.10). The patient is positioned prone and

Table 9.3 Long-axis technique	
Sacroplasty using the long-axis technique: step by step	
1	In the frontal plane, rotate the image intensifier cephalad to the AP plane
2	Rotate the II so that the spinous processes are in the center of the vertebral body—a direct AP view
3	Rotate the II to the side opposite the treatment location, by about 25–30 degrees OR to an angle along the longitudinal axis of the SIJ that aligns the inferior portion of the joint
4	The starting position is chosen: halfway between the SIJ and a vertical line that joins the medial borders of the sacral neural foramina
5	Anesthetize the skin at the desired starting point and make a small incision
6	Insert the sacroplasty needle at the incision, advancing the needle parallel to the II and angling the tip 20–40 degrees cranially
7	Using a mallet, slowly advance the needle tip just past the posterior sacral cortex. It is important to keep the mediolateral angulation of the needle "as is," to avoid deviating from the trajectory chosen
8	Rotate the II to get a lateral view of the sacrum, adjusting the superoinferior angulation of the needle so that it advances to the level of the mid to superior portion of the S1 vertebral body. (If using biplane equipment, the lateral II can be used for this purpose. If so, the next two steps can be skipped as the biplane equipment allows you to adjust both angles as you go)
9	Return to the angled AP view and ensure that the mediolateral angulation of the needle is appropriate
10	Return to the lateral view, and advance the needle tip to the level of the superior portion of the S1 vertebral body
11	When the PMMA has been mixed and a toothpaste consistency achieved, inject it into the sacrum using both lateral and oblique AP views to monitor PMMA distribution. On the lateral view, watch for anterior extravasation (i.e., anterior to the anterior body of the sacrum), while on the oblique AP view, there should be little or no extravasation into the neural exit foramina
12	Deposit the PMMA in the sacrum trying to fill the center portion of the sacral ala (i.e., between the SIJ and the neural foramina), intermittently retracting the needle and depositing PMMA along the needle tract, i.e., along the longitudinal axis of the sacrum
13	When the PMMA has been deposited adequately, remove all needles and place appropriate bandages over the puncture sites

Abbreviations: AP, anteroposterior; II, image intensifier; PMMA, polymethyl methacrylate; SIJ, sacroiliac joint.

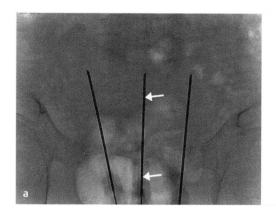
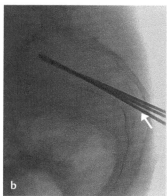

Fig. 9.8 Anteroposterior (a) and lateral (b) fluoroscopic views show the long-axis approach with a third needle (*white arrows* in **a** and **b**) placed in the center of the osseous sacrum directed in a similar orientation to the needles in the sacral ala with the starting point of the needle inferior to the thecal sac.

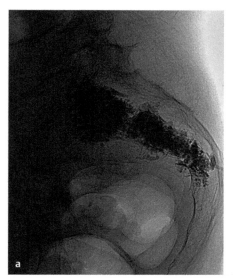
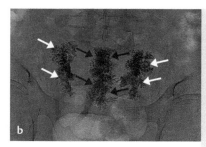
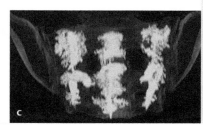

Fig. 9.9 Lateral (a) and anteroposterior (b) fluoroscopic images showing cement in the sacral ala (*white arrows* in **b**) and in the center portion of the sacrum (*black arrows* in **b**). Coronal CT reconstructed image (c) shows bone cement in the center of the sacrum as well as in the sacral ala.

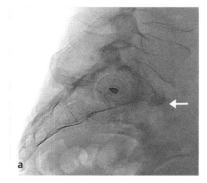
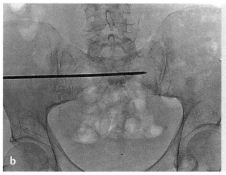

Fig. 9.10 Lateral (a) and anteroposterior (b) fluoroscopic images showing the needle positioning and trajectory for the long-axis approach. The *white arrow* denotes an anterior osteophyte (not to be mistaken for cement extravasation on the postsacroplasty images). A longer needle is used in this case (e.g., an 18-cm Murphy needle) in order to reach the contralateral sacral ala.

sterilely prepped and draped taking into consideration the direct lateral-to-medial approach. In addition to fluoroscopic guidance, a cone-beam CT can be performed for planning purposes and to adequately visualize the sacral neural foramina. The most common skin-entry site is overlying the midportion of S1 as seen on a direct lateral view. The midportion of S2 may also be accessed in an identical manner to S1. Following local analgesia, a 15- to 18-cm-long Murphy needle is then inserted horizontally perpendicular to the long axis of the sacrum, targeting the fracture lines. One or more needles can be used.[27] Once the needle(s) has crossed the target fracture lines, cement is deposited first in the contralateral ala and then the needle is progressively withdrawn while injecting aliquots of cement in continuity under real-time fluoroscopic guidance (▶ Fig. 9.11). Attention is paid to avoiding cement passing anterior to the cortex of the sacrum, and posteriorly to the inferior spinal canal.

9.8 Outcomes

Since initial publication of the technique, several more long-term studies have proven the safety, efficacy, and durability of the technique. For example, in 2012, Kortman et al[28] published their experience. They looked at 243 patients who were experiencing severe pain unresponsive to NSM. Patients were

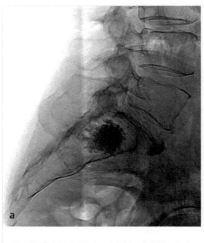 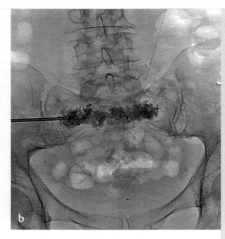

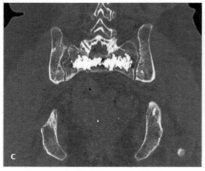 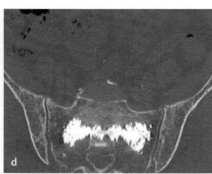

Fig. 9.11 Lateral **(a)** and anteroposterior (AP; **b**) fluoroscopic images showing polymethyl methacrylate (PMMA) deposition along the mediolateral axis of the S1 vertebrae. The AP view shows the sequential PMMA injection with injection of cement as the needle is being withdrawn. Coronal reformat **(c)** and axial **(d)** CT images showing PMMA distribution following the sacroplasty.

followed for at least 1 year after their procedure. The average pretreatment VAS was 9.2 ± 1.1. Following sacroplasty, this improved to 1.9 ± 1.7 in those patients with SIFs. There were no major complications (such as hemorrhage, significant extravasation, pulmonary emboli, or procedure-related deaths). Similarly, in the Gupta et al publication in 2014,[2,3] 53 patients were followed for a mean of 27 (±3.7) days. The patients were 83% females and the mean VAS pretreatment pain score was 9.0. This decreased to 3.0 following the sacroplasty. This group also highlighted the safety of the technique as there were no procedural complications or procedure-related mortalities.

Most recently, Frey et al[1] published a 10-year follow-up of the patients presenting for percutaneous sacroplasty beginning in 2004. Two hundred and forty-four patients with SIFs were evaluated. Two hundred and ten patients underwent sacroplasty and the 34 patients that were treated with NSM functioned as the control group. The patients' gender, age, preprocedure pain duration, analgesic use, pain level, and patient satisfaction were recorded at the following post-op intervals: immediately post procedure, 2, 4, 12, 24, and 52 weeks, and 2 years. Ten years later, the patients in the experimental group were contacted. The experimental group was found to have a statistically significant drop in VAS score between follow-ups up to 1 year and opioid use was significantly less than in the control group. There was a progressive decrease in pain from year 1 to 10 and pain level remained low with a pain level of 0.5 on the VAS. In conclusion, these studies all have established that sacroplasty allows for a decrease in the use of opioid pain medications and produces significant pain relief, greater mobility,

and improved patient satisfaction as compared with NSM. The long-term follow-up supports sacroplasty as being durable as well as safe and effective for patients suffering from SIFs. Other groups, such as Kamel et al, have documented significant increases in patient mobility. For example, in their group, 58% of patients returned to full mobility following the procedure.[29] This increase in postsacroplasty mobility has been confirmed by other authors such as Talmadge et al.[30]

Where they occur, the main complications have been extravasation of cement into the neural foramina, primarily the S1 neural foramen. The extravasations occurred in only a few scattered cases (1–2% in most series), and most of the symptoms from the cement extravasation resolved with conservative management.[31,32] A minority of these patients needed either a therapeutic nerve root injection or surgical decompression of the neural foramen to adequately address their symptoms.

Overall, sacral and pelvic insufficiency fractures are a relatively common problem that can be very debilitating to patients, causing them a host of morbidities and even mortality as a result of their deconditioning and immobility. In the last decade, more aggressive and definitive treatments such as sacroplasty have been advocated for these patients.

The literature evaluating sacroplasty has evolved over time with several reports containing patient cohorts ranging up to more than 200 patients. The existing literature shows good efficacy and minimal complications and good durability of the procedure even in long-term follow-up. Importantly, improvements in patient condition are many and the treatment definitive in the appropriate patient. Providing sacroplasty to debilitated patients or patients who are not optimally responsive to NSM can thus lead to decreased pain, improved functionality, decreased morbidities, and most importantly a lower risk of mortality.

References

[1] Lourie H. Spontaneous osteoporotic fracture of the sacrum. An unrecognized syndrome of the elderly. JAMA 1982;248(6):715–717

[2] Lin JT, Lane JM. Sacral stress fractures. J Womens Health (Larchmt) 2003;12(9):879–888

[3] Boufous S, Finch C, Lord S, Close J. The increasing burden of pelvic fractures in older people, New South Wales, Australia. Injury 2005;36(11):1323–1329

[4] Lyders EM, Whitlow CT, Baker MD, Morris PP. Imaging and treatment of sacral insufficiency fractures. AJNR Am J Neuroradiol 2010;31(2):201–210

[5] Denis F, Davis S, Comfort T. Sacral fractures: an important problem. Retrospective analysis of 236 cases. Clin Orthop Relat Res 1988;227(227):67–81

[6] Park JW, Park SM, Lee HJ, Lee CK, Chang BS, Kim H. Mortality following benign sacral insufficiency fracture and associated risk factors. Arch Osteoporos 2017;12(1):100

[7] Finiels H, Finiels P, Jacquot J, et al. Fractures of the sacrum caused by bone insufficiency. Meta-analysis of 508 cases. 1997;2;6(33):1568–1573

[8] Sambrook PN, Flahive J, Hooven FH, et al. Predicting fractures in an international cohort using risk factor algorithms without BMD. J Bone Miner Res 2011;26(11):2770–2777

[9] Kim YY, Chung BM, Kim WT. Lumbar spine MRI versus non-lumbar imaging modalities in the diagnosis of sacral insufficiency fracture: a retrospective observational study. BMC Musculoskelet Disord 2018;19(1):257

[10] Brahme SK, Cervilla V, Vint V, Cooper K, Kortman K, Resnick D. Magnetic resonance appearance of sacral insufficiency fractures. Skeletal Radiol 1990;19(7):489–493

[11] Matcuk GR Jr, Mahanty SR, Skalski MR, Patel DB, White EA, Gottsegen CJ. Stress fractures: pathophysiology, clinical presentation, imaging features, and treatment options. Emerg Radiol 2016;23(4):365–375

[12] Routt ML Jr, Simonian PT. Closed reduction and percutaneous skeletal fixation of sacral fractures. Clin Orthop Relat Res 1996(329):121–128

[13] Longhino V, Bonora C, Sansone V. The management of sacral stress fractures: current concepts. Clin Cases Miner Bone Metab 2011;8(3):19–23

[14] Mears SC, Berry DJ. Outcomes of displaced and nondisplaced pelvic and sacral fractures in elderly adults. J Am Geriatr Soc 2011;59(7):1309–1312

[15] Maier GS, Kolbow K, Lazovic D, et al. Risk factors for pelvic insufficiency fractures and outcome after conservative therapy. Arch Gerontol Geriatr 2016;67:80–85

[16] Taillandier J, Langue F, Alemanni M, Taillandier-Heriche E. Mortality and functional outcomes of pelvic insufficiency fractures in older patients. Joint Bone Spine 2003;70(4):287–289

[17] Butler CL, Given CA II, Michel SJ, Tibbs PA. Percutaneous sacroplasty for the treatment of sacral insufficiency fractures. AJR Am J Roentgenol 2005;184 (6):1956–1959

[18] De Smet AA, Neff JR. Pubic and sacral insufficiency fractures: clinical course and radiologic findings. AJR Am J Roentgenol 1985;145(3):601–606

[19] Garant M. Sacroplasty: a new treatment for sacral insufficiency fracture. J Vasc Interv Radiol 2002;13(12):1265–1267

[20] Pommersheim W, Huang-Hellinger F, Baker M, Morris P. Sacroplasty: a treatment for sacral insufficiency fractures. AJNR Am J Neuroradiol 2003; 24(5):1003–1007

[21] Frey ME, Depalma MJ, Cifu DX, Bhagia SM, Carne W, Daitch JS. Percutaneous sacroplasty for osteoporotic sacral insufficiency fractures: a prospective, multicenter, observational pilot study. Spine J 2008;8(2):367–373

[22] Frey ME, Warner C, Thomas SM, et al. Sacroplasty: a ten-year analysis of prospective patients treated with percutaneous sacroplasty: literature review and technical considerations. Pain Physician 2017;20(7):E1063–E1072

[23] Gupta AC, Chandra RV, Yoo AJ, et al. Safety and effectiveness of sacroplasty: a large single-center experience. AJNR Am J Neuroradiol 2014;35(11):2202–2206

[24] Whitlow CT, Yazdani SK, Reedy ML, Kaminsky SE, Berry JL, Morris PP. Investigating sacroplasty: technical considerations and finite element analysis of polymethylmethacrylate infusion into cadaveric sacrum. AJNR Am J Neuroradiol 2007;28(6):1036–1041

[25] Betts A. Sacral vertebral augmentation: confirmation of fluoroscopic landmarks by open dissection. Pain Physician 2008;11(1):57–65

[26] Frey M, ed. Atlas of Image-Guided Spinal Procedures. 1st ed. Philadelphia, PA: Elsevier; 2012

[27] Nicholson P, Hilditch C, Brinjikji W, et al. Single-needle lateral sacroplasty technique. AJNR Am J Neuroradiol 2019;40(2):382–385

[28] Kortman K, Ortiz O, Miller T, et al. Multicenter study to assess the efficacy and safety of sacroplasty in patients with osteoporotic sacral insufficiency fractures or pathologic sacral lesions. J Neurointerv Surg 2013;5(5):461–466

[29] Kamel EM, Binaghi S, Guntern D, Mouhsine E, Schnyder P, Theumann N. Outcome of long-axis percutaneous sacroplasty for the treatment of sacral insufficiency fractures. Eur Radiol 2009;19(12):3002–3007

[30] Talmadge J, Smith K, Dykes T, Mittleider D. Clinical impact of sacroplasty on patient mobility. J Vasc Interv Radiol 2014;25(6):911–915

[31] Bayley E, Srinivas S, Boszczyk BM. Clinical outcomes of sacroplasty in sacral insufficiency fractures: a review of the literature. Eur Spine J 2009;18(9): 1266–1271

[32] Pereira LP, Clarençon F, Cormier E, et al. Safety and effectiveness of percutaneous sacroplasty: a single-centre experience in 58 consecutive patients with tumours or osteoporotic insufficient fractures treated under fluoroscopic guidance. Eur Radiol 2013;23(10):2764–2772

10 Cervical and Posterior Arch Augmentation

Luigi Manfre, Nicole S. Carter, Joshua A. Hirsch, and Ronil V. Chandra

Summary

Cervical vertebroplasty is performed far less often than thoracic and lumbar vertebroplasty but is an important treatment for patients with fractures and neoplastic involvement of the cervical spine. Osseous augmentation of the cervical spine has greater technical challenges due to the surrounding neurovascular structures and the small size of the vertebral bodies and should be performed by experienced practitioners. Cervical vertebroplasty is typically performed under fluoroscopic or CT guidance with various approaches utilized such as the transoral, translateral, and transpedicular approaches. Posterior arch osseous augmentation can be performed for neoplastic and non-neoplastic pathologies located in the pedicles, laminae, and in the spinous process. Injection of cement into the pedicles or laminae must be done with care as important nerves and vessels are located directly adjacent to these osseous structures and CT guidance can be very useful when augmenting the posterior arch. Spinoplasty can be very useful prior to placement of interspinous spacers to augment the strength of the spinous process in patients at high risk of fracture or osseous erosion around the spacer.

Keywords: osseous augmentation, cervical, posterior arch, transoral, translateral, pediculoplasty, laminoplasty, spinoplasty

10.1 Cervical Augmentation

10.1.1 Introduction

Percutaneous vertebroplasty is widely considered an effective procedure in the treatment of selected patients with vertebral compression fractures (VCFs) related to osteoporotic disease, primary and secondary osteolytic tumors, and some cases of trauma.[1] The majority of vertebroplasty procedures are performed in the thoracic and lumbar spine by fluoroscopic or computed tomography (CT) guidance, where established radiological landmarks and approaches to the body allow safe and rapid augmentation. VCFs also occur in the cervical spine, in around 1% of patients affected by primary or secondary spinal neoplasms.[2,3] For these cases, cervical vertebroplasty presents an alternative or an adjunct treatment to radiotherapy (RT) or cervical spinal surgery in reducing pain and improving stability of the VCF. However, compared with thoracolumbar vertebroplasty, augmentation in the cervical spine presents technical challenges due to the small size of target vertebral bodies, the difficulty in visualizing bony landmarks, and the surrounding neurovascular and airway structures. Cervical vertebroplasty thus requires special considerations in regard to the procedural approach, sedation, and radiological guidance, and should be performed by experienced operators.[4]

Operative surgery of the cervical spine remains essential when the spinal canal is compromised and/or when there is spinal instability.[5,6] Even when cervical lesions generate instability, anterior fixation of the spine may not be well tolerated, particularly in patients with short life expectancy, immune compromise, or significant debilitation. Moreover, even in patients with longer life expectancy and greater baseline functional status, surgical treatment carries risk of restricted cervical movement, which may not be desirable for younger patients.

Palliative RT has demonstrated powerful effects in the treatment of secondary cervical lesions that require pain relief and vertebral bone remineralization.[7] It does not require general anesthesia, and can be performed in patients who are in extremely poor clinical condition. However, post radiation remineralization generally occurs in 3 to 6 months after treatment, with interval risk of vertebral collapse or radiation-specific complications such as radiation-induced myelitis or soft-tissue radionecrosis.[8]

10.1.2 Historical Perspective

The first vertebral augmentation procedure reported in the literature was performed in the cervical spine by Galibert et al, who performed vertebroplasty to treat an aggressive C2 hemangioma.[9] The procedure provided rapid, almost complete pain relief for the patient, leading to an increased uptake of the procedure and application to treat thoracolumbar fractures. It is currently considered highly effective for cervical lesions and can be considered the best treatment option after stringent patient selection, even in extremely aggressive osteolytic lesions (▶Fig. 10.1a, b).

10.1.3 Image Guidance

Conventional vertebroplasty can be safely performed under either fluoroscopic or CT guidance; the choice of either method is at the discretion of the practitioner. In cervical

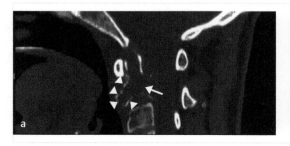
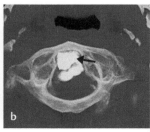

Fig. 10.1 Multiple myeloma with subtotal C2 osteolysis (*white arrow*). Only a faint cortical bone can be appreciated (*white arrowheads*), with dramatic cervical pain and need for immediate stabilization **(a)**. After the procedure, complete C2 augmentation, reproducing the dens (*black arrow*), is obtained, regaining the conventional C1–C2 joint function, avoiding more severe posterior occipital bone–C3 surgical fixation **(b)**.

vertebroplasty, both fluoroscopy and CT can be used if necessary along with multiplanar reconstructions. Prior to the procedure, comprehensive radiological analysis is advisable, including both CT and magnetic resonance imaging (MRI), with cervical vessel imaging with CT or MR angiography. Careful pre-procedural planning reduces the likelihood of complications.

10.1.4 Procedural Approaches

Transoral

The transoral approach (utilized by Galibert et al in the first cervical vertebroplasty procedures) is considered the preferred approach in the case of a lesion involving the upper cervical spine (C1–C4).[10–12] In this approach, the patient is positioned supine, with mild hyperextension of the neck and an oropharyngeal retractor utilized to achieve sufficient mouth opening. The needle is introduced directly through the oral cavity along the midline, traversing the oropharynx to reach the vertebral body directly (▶Fig. 10.2a). In certain cases, even the clivus can be reached through this method, allowing the treatment of large osteolytic lesions of the skull base.[13]

Benefits

In contrast to alternative approaches, the transoral method avoids almost all the main neurovascular cervical structures, as thin pharyngeal muscles, fascia, and anterior ligaments are the only structures that will be perforated by a correctly placed transoral needle.[14] This approach is a known neurosurgical route for treating intradural and extradural diseases and, despite not being a percutaneous approach, it remains one of the safest ways to reach the upper cervical vertebrae.

Limitations

General anesthesia and intubation are mandatory for the transoral approach. Oral intubation is possible but generally not recommended, as oral cavity should not be occupied by tools other than the vertebroplasty equipment; this allows more freedom when mediolateral or craniocaudal inclination of the needle is preferred, depending on the location of the disease. Nasotracheal intubation is thus accomplished, and may be performed with fiberoptic assistance. Infection is a key source of

potential complication in the transoral approach, with wound infections occurring in less than 2% and meningitis in less than 5%.[15,16] For this reason, perioperative and postoperative antibiotic prophylaxis is recommended for preventing infection, as preparation of the posterior oropharynx with iodine is not always sufficient to obtain 100% oral cavity sterility.

Translateral

Translateral approaches (TLAs; ▶Fig. 10.2c) have been described for cervical lesions at C1 to C5, and allow direct percutaneous treatment of the vertebral body. Three translateral methods are differentiated: the anterolateral approach (ALA), the TLA, and the posterolateral approach (PLA). In the ALA,[17,18] with moderate hyperextension of the head, the carotid is manually compressed and pushed laterally by the operator's fingers. The needle is carefully introduced under the mandibular angle, between the trachea and the carotid–jugular axis.[17,18] The TLA for vertebral augmentation has usually been described in the literature as a combined fluoroscopy-CT guided treatment. In some cases, this approach may be somewhat difficult to perform due to the risk of damaging nearby neurovascular structures.[17] The PLA[19,20] may be performed in certain cases: the needle is placed posterolaterally through the posterior cervical space, bypassing the main lateral neurovascular structures.[19,20] However, in the case of anatomical variations or tumoral mass displacement (▶Fig. 10.3), the vertebral artery may prevent the PLA from being utilized.[21]

Benefits

In some cases, translateral procedures can be performed under simple local anesthesia. Nevertheless, considering the difficult anatomical area to be accessed, sedation of the patient is strongly advised. Moreover, since these procedures utilize a fully percutaneous approach, there is no significant risk of infection, and a simple skin disinfection is considered sufficient for infection prevention. A TLA is typically the optimal choice in case of obese or short-necked patients.[22]

Limitations

TLAs require the needle has to be advanced slowly and carefully in the soft local neck tissues. In contrast to posterior thoracic or lumbar procedures, where the main paravertebral muscles offer

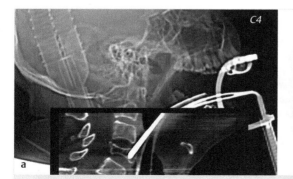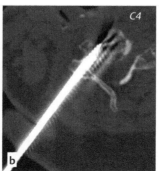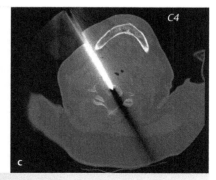

Fig. 10.2 Cervical vertebroplasty of C4: different technical approach. The same vertebra (C4 in this case) can be reached on different routes: transoral (a), transpedicular (b), or anterolateral (c).

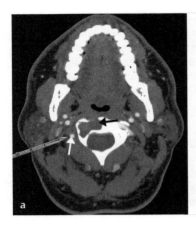
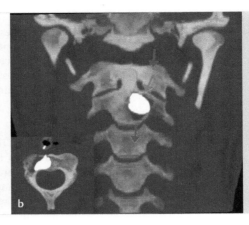

Fig. 10.3 Right-sided C2 osteolysis related to multiple myeloma. **(a)** A posterolateral approach, despite ostensibly easier than the transoral approach, can be extremely dangerous in the case of displacement of the vertebral artery (*white arrow*) by a tumor (*black arrow*). **(b)** In this patient, a transoral approach was selected and complete augmentation was obtained (*red arrow*) to sustain the axial load (*blue arrows*).

moderate resistance and support to maintain the needle position, in TLAs the needle almost immediately reaches deep structures under only mild pressure. Moreover, potential damage to the main vascular and neural structures of the neck presents a life-threating potential risk. These structures may even be located in nonstandard areas in the case of anatomical variation or displacement.

Transpedicular

A transpedicular approach can be utilized in some cases when the target lesion is located from C4 to C7. The fundamental requirement for this approach is a sufficiently large posterior vertebral pedicle, allowing transpedicular needle access (▶Fig. 10.2b). This approach is almost identical to the more familiar approach adopted for conventional thoracic and lumbar vertebroplasty.

Benefits

As in the TLA, there is minimal risk of infection for transpedicular procedures. The procedure may be performed under local anesthesia.

Limitations

Transpedicular approaches are not suitable when the cervical pedicles are very small or require a needle smaller than 15 gauge. As precision is required in needle placement, CT guidance may be utilized to protect against accidental damage to the vertebral artery or the spinal cord.

10.1.5 Prevention of Infection

In transoral approaches, a key potential risk is infection, generally related to disruption of the protective mucosal barrier, allowing pathogens to enter the deep neck tissues. The most common pathogens are *Staphylococcus aureus*, *Streptococcus*, *Candida*, as well as gram-negative bacteria including *Escherichia coli*, *Proteus*, and *Klebsiella*. Furthermore, even resident oral flora such as *Corynebacterium* and *Bacteroides* may cause infection, considering that many patients that undergo treatment are immunocompromised patients due to underlying neoplastic disease and/or chemoradiotherapy treatments.[23] It is important to recognize that the oral cavity cannot be sterilized completely and that systemic antibiotic treatment is important for infection prevention.

After the retracting forceps have been applied, the oral cavity is sterilized, generally using chlorhexidine or Betadine. For antibiotic prophylaxis, we generally use cefazolin (1–2 g, IV in adults, or 3 g in patients weighing in excess of 120 kg) immediately administered 30 to 60 minutes before the beginning of the surgical procedure. Alternatively, other protocols include a combination of 600-mg clindamycin and 500-mg levofloxacin 30 minutes preprocedure or a combination of 1,200-mg clindamycin and gentamycin (2 mg/kg). Regardless, antibiotics should be continued for at least 48 hours postprocedure after transoral needle access. For translateral and transpedicular approaches, the initial preprocedure antibiotic prophylaxis is usually sufficient.

10.1.6 Complications

There is little existing literature on the complications of cervical vertebroplasty. Chiras described a 16.7% complication rate (2 out of 12 patients in his series): 1 patient had a C1–C2 perivertebral leakage and occipital neuralgia, and the other patient had cerebellar symptoms related to polymethyl methacrylate (PMMA) embolization seen after treatment of their hypervascular pheochromocytoma metastasis. In both cases, symptoms regressed after a few weeks.[24] One fatal complication has been described in a 4-year-old patient affected by a C2 aneurysmal bone cyst, with leakage into the venous compartment and embolization of the vertebrobasilar system.[25] For this reason, an injection of contrast media directly into the vertebra body is useful prior to the injection of PMMA, to detect possible retrograde filling of the vertebrobasilar system.[26]

10.1.7 Conclusion

Cervical vertebroplasty plays an important role in the management of VCFs due to disease of the cervical spine. Successful implementation of the procedure requires a specific approach to preoperative planning, procedural techniques, and postoperative care. When patients are carefully selected, and meticulous care is taken in procedural technique, vertebroplasty can be considered a safe procedure for the treatment of osteoporotic, traumatic, and neoplastic fractures in the cervical spine. It may be utilized not only for simple pain relief but also for mechanical stabilization and prevention of life-threatening vertebral collapse.[27]

10.2 Posterior Arch Augmentation

10.2.1 Introduction

Lesions located in the posterior arch have previously been considered a contraindication to vertebral augmentation. However, posterior arch procedures have been described by several authors as a safe and effective option for pain relief in both neoplastic and non-neoplastic lesions.[28–30]

10.2.2 Pediculoplasty

The pedicle can be involved both in traumatic (stress fracture with or without osteoporosis) and metastatic or neoplastic disease. The risk of vertebral body collapse is related not only to the volume of disease within the vertebral body but also to the direct involvement of the pedicle. This is particularly significant in the case of disease in the thoracic spine where, according to several biomechanical studies, fracture risk increases with pedicle or costovertebral involvement. Posterior arch augmentation of the pedicle thus should be considered not only an adjunct procedure to vertebral body augmentation but as a key treatment option to stabilize the vertebral body in thoracic-level fractures.[31]

Pediculoplasty in Vertebral Tumors

The pediculoplasty procedure requires additional technical considerations. When the pedicle is involved by an osteolytic lesion, conventional radiological landmarks can no longer be reliably detected on fluoroscopy. Moreover, injecting PMMA cement inside the pedicle by fluoroscopic guidance could potentially be considered unsafe, as it is not possible to detect potential leakage inside the spinal canal or neural foramina. Thus, the CT-guided technique can be used to optimize patient safety in performing augmentation of the pedicle. The needle (generally 13–15 gauge in size) is introduced into the pedicle deep to the vertebral body, followed by the slow injection of a small volume of PMMA (approximately 1 mL) while the needle is gently retrieved from the vertebral body (▶ Fig. 10.4). As the delivery of the PMMA can be directed from the tip of the needle, the use of a beveled needle is advised.[32]

Pediculoplasty in Spondylolysis

Pedicle discontinuity is found with lysis of a portion of the pedicle. This is sometimes associated with listhesis. Unilateral involvement is possible, which reduces the stability of the local spinal unit and acts as an important trigger point for pain. Stress fractures of the pedicle related to intense sport activity have also been described.[33] Fractures of the pedicles have also been reported to result from abnormal stresses resulting from posterior screw and rod instrumentation.[34,35] In these patients, pediculoplasty is a potential treatment option to provide pain relief and improved stability. The combination of percutaneous posterior intrapedicular screw fixation and PMMA injection, a treatment originally named "Buck's technique,"[36] has been described as a highly successful solution for restoring vertebral stability.[37]

Pediculoplasty in Osteoporotic Disease

Pedicular involvement is not typically reported on routine radiological studies for osteoporotic disease, as attention is generally focused on the vertebral body. However, the association between more typical osteoporotic VCFs and unsuspected pedicular fractures has been reported in the literature.[38] Jung et al reported involvement of the pedicle in 51% of patients affected by vertebral body fracture (▶ Fig. 10.5), with typical bone discontinuity on CT scan as well as signal abnormalities of the bone marrow on MR imaging.[39] Osteoporotic fractures of the pedicle may also be detected as double symmetrical uptake spots on bone scanning.[40] In patients with this type of fracture, pedicle strength can be significantly improved by cement injection in which the PMMA-filled needle is pulled out while the stylet remains unreplaced, thereby creating a long continuous tube of cement within the pedicle.[38]

10.2.3 Laminoplasty and Spinoplasty

New-generation interspinous spacers generally cause minimal stress to the spinous process and laminae. However, particularly in the case of full PEEK systems, larger interspinous implants or in elderly patients with advanced osteoporosis, bone remodeling or fracture of the spinous process can occur. Younger patients treated with interspinous spacers for spinal canal stenosis or spinal foramina stenosis may suffer a posterior element fracture due to the effects of stress upon the bone

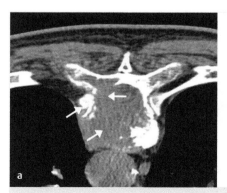
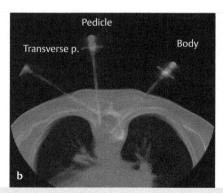
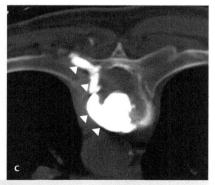

Fig. 10.4 Metastasis at the level of T9, with extensive osteolysis of the left vertebral body, pedicle, and costovertebral process (*white arrows*; a): three needles were introduced into the vertebral body, the left pedicle, and the left costovertebral process **(b)**. **(c)** PMMA injection was performed, with total bone remodeling of the osteolytic area (*white arrowheads*).

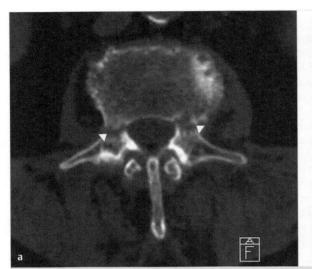
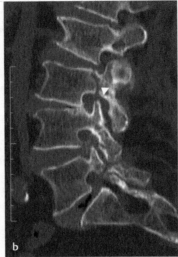
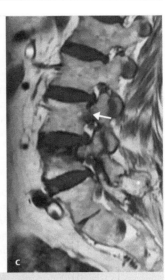

Fig. 10.5 Bilateral L3 pedicle fractures in a patient with severe osteoporotic disease (*white arrowheads*). On axial (**a**) and 2D recon sagittal (**b**) CT scans, interruption of the cortical bone can be appreciated on both the pedicles of the third lumbar vertebra (*white arrowheads*). Signal abnormality is easily depicted on sagittal T1-weighted scan (**c**; *white arrow*).

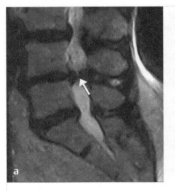
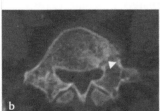
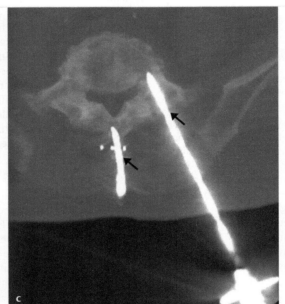
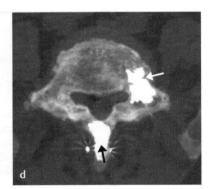
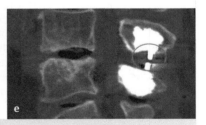

Fig. 10.6 Prophylactic spinoplasty and pediculoplasty in a patient affected by severe L4–L5 spinal canal stenosis (SCS) associated with left pedicle stress fracture. On sagittal T2-weighted scan (**a**), grade D spinal canal stenosis (according to Schizas' classification) was detected (*white arrow*). Pre-op axial CT scan of L4 revealed left pedicle stress fracture (*white arrowhead*) as an incidental finding (**b**). Two needles were introduced on a sagittal route inside the spinous processes of L4 and L5 (*black arrow*), and a third needle was introduced into the left L4 pedicle (*black arrow*; **c**). After injection of PMMA, spinoplasty of L4 and L5 (*black arrow*) as well as left-side pediculoplasty of L4 (*white arrow*) was obtained (**d**), making possible the subsequent safe introduction of the interspinous spacer (*blue circle*; **e**).

surrounding the device. Bone remodeling of the posterior laminae has been described in approximately 13% of patients undergoing interspinous spacer insertion.[41]

To perform spinoplasty, PMMA can be prophylactically introduced directly into the spinous processes via CT or fluoroscopic guidance with a small needle (13–15 gauge). In the case of a very thin spinous processes, an oblique posterolateral route may be utilized to reach the laminae crus for retrograde filling of the spinous process (▶Fig. 10.6). As this area is far from the main neural structures, and the bone cortex of the laminae crus is particularly compact (which protects the spinal canal and foramina), no significant contraindication or complication generally

occurs.[42] By performing prophylactic spinoplasty, bone remodeling and fracture related to interspinous spacers can be decreased or avoided, increasing the efficacy of the spacer itself.[42]

10.2.4 Key Points

- Vertebroplasty (cervical).
- Vertebroplasty (pedicle).
- Spinoplasty.
- Prophylaxis.
- Transoral.
- Spondylolisthesis.

References

[1] Jensen ME, Evans AJ, Mathis JM, Kallmes DF, Cloft HJ, Dion JE. Percutaneous polymethylmethacrylate vertebroplasty in the treatment of osteoporotic vertebral body compression fractures: technical aspects. AJNR Am J Neuroradiol 1997;18(10):1897–1904

[2] Sherk HH. Lesions of the atlas and axis. Clin Orthop Relat Res 1975(109):33–41

[3] Moulding HD, Bilsky MH. Metastases to the craniovertebral junction. Neurosurgery 2010;66(3, Suppl):113–118

[4] Cotten A, Boutry N, Cortet B, et al. Percutaneous vertebroplasty: state of the art. Radiographics 1998;18(2):311–320, discussion 320–323

[5] Delank KS, Wendtner C, Eich HT, Eysel P. The treatment of spinal metastases. Dtsch Arztebl Int 2011;108(5):71–79, quiz 80

[6] Boschi V, Pogorelić Z, Gulan G, Perko Z, Grandić L, Radonić V. Management of cement vertebroplasty in the treatment of vertebral hemangioma. Scand J Surg 2011;100(2):120–124

[7] Rades D, Schild SE, Abrahm JL. Treatment of painful bone metastases. Nat Rev Clin Oncol 2010;7(4):220–229

[8] Guedea F, Majó J, Guardia E, Canals E, Craven-Bartle J. The role of radiation therapy in vertebral hemangiomas without neurological signs. Int Orthop 1994;18(2):77–79

[9] Galibert P, Deramond H, Rosat P, Le Gars D. Preliminary note on the treatment of vertebral angioma by percutaneous acrylic vertebroplasty Neurochirurgie 1987;33(2):166–168

[10] Gailloud P, Martin JB, Olivi A, Rüfenacht DA, Murphy KJ. Transoral vertebroplasty for a fractured C2 aneurysmal bone cyst. J Vasc Interv Radiol 2002;13(3):340–341

[11] Tong FC, Cloft HJ, Joseph GJ, Rodts GR, Dion JE. Transoral approach to cervical vertebroplasty for multiple myeloma. AJR Am J Roentgenol 2000;175(5):1322–1324

[12] Reddy AS, Hochman M, Loh S, Rachlin J, Li J, Hirsch JA. CT guided direct transoral approach to C2 for percutaneous vertebroplasty. Pain Physician 2005;8(2):235–238

[13] Wright CH, Kusyk D, Rosenberg WS, Sweet JA. Percutaneous transoral clivoplasty and upper cervical vertebroplasties for multifocal skeletal lymphangiomatosis resulting in complete resolution of pain: case report. J Neurosurg Spine 2017;26(2):171–176

[14] Menezes AH, VanGilder JC. Transoral-transpharyngeal approach to the anterior craniocervical junction. Ten-year experience with 72 patients. J Neurosurg 1988;69(6):895–903

[15] Kingdom TT, Nockels RP, Kaplan MJ. Transoral-transpharyngeal approach to the craniocervical junction. Otolaryngol Head Neck Surg 1995;113(4):393–400

[16] Hadley MN, Spetzler RF, Sonntag VK. The transoral approach to the superior cervical spine. A review of 53 cases of extradural cervicomedullary compression. J Neurosurg 1989;71(1):16–23

[17] Anselmetti GC, Manca A, Chiara G, Regge D. Painful osteolytic metastasis involving the anterior and posterior arches of C1: percutaneous vertebroplasty with local anesthesia. J Vasc Interv Radiol 2009;20(12):1645–1647

[18] Wetzel SG, Martin JB, Somon T, Wilhelm K, Rufenacht DA. Painful osteolytic metastasis of the atlas: treatment with percutaneous vertebroplasty. Spine 2002;27(22):E493–E495

[19] Huegli RW, Schaeren S, Jacob AL, Martin JB, Wetzel SG. Percutaneous cervical vertebroplasty in a multifunctional image-guided therapy suite: hybrid lateral approach to C1 and C4 under CT and fluoroscopic guidance. Cardiovasc Intervent Radiol 2005;28(5):649–652

[20] Sun G, Jin P, Li M, et al. Percutaneous vertebroplasty for treatment of osteolytic metastases of the C2 vertebral body using anterolateral and posterolateral approach. Technol Cancer Res Treat 2010;9(4):417–422

[21] Sun HY, Lee JW, Kim KJ, Yeom JS, Kang HS. Percutaneous intervention of the C2 vertebral body using a CT-guided posterolateral approach. AJR Am J Roentgenol 2009;193(6):1703–1705

[22] Guo WH, Meng MB, You X, et al. CT-guided percutaneous vertebroplasty of the upper cervical spine via a translateral approach. Pain Physician 2012;15(5):E733–E741

[23] Todar K. The normal bacterial flora of humans. In: Todar K, ed. Todar's Online Textbook of Bacteriology (online book). Madison, WI: Keith Todar; 2008–2012

[24] Mont'Alverne F, Vallée JN, Cormier E, et al. Percutaneous vertebroplasty for metastatic involvement of the axis. AJNR Am J Neuroradiol 2005;26(7):1641–1645

[25] Peraud A, Drake JM, Armstrong D, Hedden D, Babyn P, Wilson G. Fatal ethibloc embolization of vertebrobasilar system following percutaneous injection into aneurysmal bone cyst of the second cervical vertebra. AJNR Am J Neuroradiol 2004;25(6):1116–1120

[26] Turowski B, Schellhammer F, Herdmann J, Rommel F. Fatal Ethibloc embolization of vertebrobasilar system following percutaneous injection into aneurysmal bone cyst of the second cervical vertebra. AJNR Am J Neuroradiol 2005;26(7):1883–1884

[27] De la Garza-Ramos R, Benvenutti-Regato M, Caro-Osorio E. Vertebroplasty and kyphoplasty for cervical spine metastases: a systematic review and meta-analysis. Int J Spine Surg 2016;10:7

[28] Anselmetti GC, Bonaldi G, Carpeggiani P, Manfrè L, Masala S, Muto M. Vertebral augmentation: 7 years' experience. In: Alexandre A, Masini M, Menchetti P, eds. Advances in Minimal Invasive Therapy of the Spine and Nerves. Vienna: Springer; 2011:147–161

[29] Reyes M, Georgy M, Brook L, et al. Multicenter clinical and imaging evaluation of targeted radiofrequency ablation (t-RFA) and cement augmentation of neoplastic vertebral lesions. J Neurointerv Surg 2018;10(2):176–182

[30] Manfrè L. Posterior arch and extravertebral augmentation. Neuroradiology 2014;56(1):109–110

[31] Taneichi H, Kaneda K, Takeda N, Abumi K, Satoh S. Risk factors and probability of vertebral body collapse in metastases of the thoracic and lumbar spine. Spine 1997;22(3):239–245

[32] Martin JB, Wetzel SG, Seium Y, et al. Percutaneous vertebroplasty in metastatic disease: transpedicular access and treatment of lysed pedicles—initial experience. Radiology 2003;229(2):593–597

[33] Guillodo Y, Botton E, Saraux A, et al. Contralateral spondylolysis and fracture of the lumbar pedicle in an elite female gymnast. Spine 2000;25(19):2541–2543

[34] Maurer SG, Wright KE, Bendo JA. Iatrogenic spondylolysis leading to contralateral pedicular stress fracture and unstable spondylolisthesis. Spine 2000;25(7):895–898

[35] Macdessi SJ, Leong AK, Bentivoglio JEC. Pedicle fracture after instrumented posterolateral lumbar fusion: a case report. Spine 2001;26(5):580–582

[36] Buck JE. Direct repair of the defect in spondylolisthesis. Preliminary report. J Bone Joint Surg Br 1970;52(3):432–437

[37] Rajasekaran S, Subbiah M, Shetty AP. Direct repair of lumbar spondylolysis by Buck's technique. Indian J Orthop 2011;45(2):136–140

[38] Eyheremendy EP, De Luca SE, Sanabria E. Percutaneous pediculoplasty in osteoporotic compression fractures. J Vasc Interv Radiol 2004;15(8):869–874

[39] Jung HS, Jee WH, McCauley TR, Ha KY, Choi KH. Discrimination of metastatic from acute osteoporotic compression spinal fractures with MR imaging. Radiographics 2003;23(1):179–187

[40] Traughber PD, Havlina JM Jr. Bilateral pedicle stress fractures: SPECT and CT features. J Comput Assist Tomogr 1991;15(2):338–340

[41] Miller JD, Miller MC, Lucas MG. Erosion of the spinous process: a potential cause of interspinous process spacer failure. J Neurosurg Spine 2010;12(2):210–213

[42] Manfrè L. Posterior arch augmentation (spinoplasty) before and after single and double interspinous spacer introduction at the same level: preventing and treating the failure? Interv Neuroradiol 2014;20(5):626–631

11 Balloon Kyphoplasty

James Mooney, John W. Amburgy, D. Mitchell Self, Leah J. Schoel, and M.R. Chambers

Summary

Balloon kyphoplasty is a minimally invasive vertebral augmentation procedure used to treat painful vertebral compression fractures. The goal of any vertebral augmentation procedure is pain reduction, stabilization of the fracture, and improvement in patient function. Unique to balloon kyphoplasty is restoration of vertebral body height and reduction of kyphotic angulation through the use of inflatable bone tamps. In addition, the balloon tamps reduce the risk of cement leakage by facilitating an injection that follows the path of least resistance into and around the cavity created by the balloon. In this chapter, the diagnostic criteria, techniques, indications, and contraindications are discussed. Materials, equipment, imaging, and the procedure itself are described in detail. In addition, the importance of sagittal balance restoration and realignment is addressed as it relates to the risk of adjacent fractures. The risks and benefits of balloon kyphoplasty are summarized.

Keywords: balloon kyphoplasty, vertebral augmentation, vertebral compression fracture, bone cement, vertebral height, kyphotic angulation, sagittal balance, minimally invasive

11.1 Introduction

Vertebral augmentation is a category of surgical procedures used to treat vertebral fractures and includes vertebroplasty, kyphoplasty, and implants. The goal of any vertebral augmentation procedure is the minimally invasive reduction and stabilization of a painful vertebral compression fracture (VCF). Unique to balloon kyphoplasty is restoration of vertebral body height and reduction of kyphotic angulation through the use of inflatable bone tamps. The balloon tamps reduce the risk of cement leakage by facilitating an injection that follows the path of least resistance into and around the cavity created by the balloon.

11.2 Materials

The surgical equipment is available through numerous sources. A comprehensive list of manufacturers, materials, and equipment for kyphoplasty can be found in ▶ Table 11.1. Components available from Medtronic Kyphon are listed in the following sections and shown in ▶ Fig. 11.1.

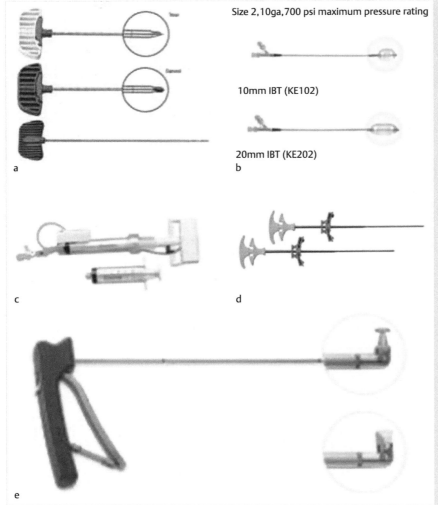

Size 2,10ga,700 psi maximum pressure rating

10mm IBT (KE102)

20mm IBT (KE202)

Fig. 11.1 Kyphon Balloon Kyphoplasty devices. **(a)** Kyphon Osteo Introducers (Diamond introducer, Bevel introducer, and drill shown). **(b)** Kyphon inflatable bone tamps. **(c)** Kyphon inflation syringe. **(d)** Kyphon cement delivery system. **(e)** Kyphon Latitude II Curette.

Table 11.1 Providers of materials and equipment for balloon kyphoplasty

Balloon kyphoplasty
Ackermann
Alphatec Spine
BM Korea
BPB Medico
Biopsybell
Depuy Synthes
G-21
iMedicom
KMC-Maxxspine
Medtronic (Kyphon)
Osseon
Panmed US
Rontis
Taeyeon
Synimed

11.2.1 Bone Access Tools

- **Jamshidi-style needle:** Typically, an 11- or 13-gauge cannulated needle used to gain access to the vertebral body via the pedicle or a peripedicular approach. The internal stylet may have a variety of bevel tips for increased penetration capability or for directional control. Once in position, the inner trocar is removed.
- **Kirschner's wire (K-wire):** It is placed in the cannula, which is then removed for a Seldinger-technique establishment of the working channel.
- **Osteointroducer:** An 8- or 10-gauge cannulated introducer or working channel is placed over the K-wire, which is then removed. The osteointroducer may be beveled for directional control.
- **Drill:** It is used to cut and channel through cancellous bone for placement of the balloon.
- **Curette:** It is used to expand the cavity created by the drill to accommodate the expansion of the balloon.

11.2.2 Balloons Tamps and Inflation Devices

- **Inflatable bone tamps:** These are available for use with 8- and 10-gauge introducers in three lengths (10, 15, and 20 mm) with volumes ranging from 3 to 6 mL and pressure ratings ranging from 300 to 700 psi.
- **Inflation device:** It has a manometer with a digital pressure gauge for controlled inflation.
- **Cement delivery cannulas:** It is an 8- or 10-gauge coaxial delivery system with an outer cannula and an inner rod or "pusher" for expelling cement.

11.2.3 Bone Cement

Acrylic bone cement (ABC) is the most commonly used cement for vertebral augmentation. The main components of ABC are solid and liquid acrylic compounds that cure rapidly when mixed at room temperature and even faster when exposed to body temperature. A number of brands are commercially available. Disadvantages of using ABC include non-biodegradability and significant mechanical mismatch with the osseous components of the vertebral body.[1] Efforts have been made to improve the mechanical characteristics, porosity, and biodegradability of the products. Polymethyl methacrylate (PMMA) is the most popular bone cement. A modern version of PMMA was first used in the United Kingdom by Dr. John Charnley in total hip replacement surgery[2] and was Food and Drug Administration (FDA) approved for treating VCFs in 2004.

In 2017, calcium phosphate cement (CPC) was redesigned by incorporating starch and $BaSO_4$ to create a new cement. Biomechanical strengths measured by in vitro and in vivo models were not less than that of PMMA, while its biodegradability and osseointegrative capacities were significantly enhanced compared to PMMA.

Other less commonly used bone cements include CPC, calcium sulfate cement (CSC), and magnesium phosphate cement (MPC). Chapter 7 provides a detailed discussion of the various cements and fill materials.

11.3 Diagnosis and Preoperative Preparation

A patient with an acute or subacute vertebral body compression fracture will almost always complain of severe back pain. Physical examination will reveal tenderness to palpation and percussion over the corresponding spinous process. Subsequent radiographs, CT, MR, and/or nuclear bone scan imaging are used to confirm and characterize a fracture. Short tau inversion recovery (STIR) and T1-weighted sequences on MR imaging are considered the gold standard for evaluating VCFs. There is a high degree of correlation between increased STIR signal and a pain-generating fracture and the T1-weighted images well demonstrate fracture lines and marrow signal changes (▶Fig. 11.2). If MR imaging is not possible, nuclear bone scan imaging may be used to demonstrate radionuclide uptake in an acute or subacute fracture and can be used in combination with CT scanning for accurate anatomic characterization of the fracture.

Patients undergoing kyphoplasty are often elderly, are deconditioned, and have inherent vulnerability to perioperative stress. For example, inhalation agents are affected by the minimum alveolar anesthetic concentration, which decreases approximately 6% for every decade. Clearance and the volume of the central compartment decrease with age. Metabolism of medications and their durations of action depend on renal or hepatic excretion. It is important to titrate doses and prudent to use short-acting drugs. Preoperative assessment of organ function and reserve is essential to know how the patient might react with anesthesia.[3] Although preoperative laboratory studies and testing will vary from patient to patient, we routinely include CBC with differential, chemistries, coagulation studies, anteroposterior (AP) chest radiograph, and an ECG.

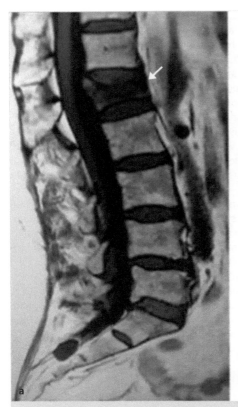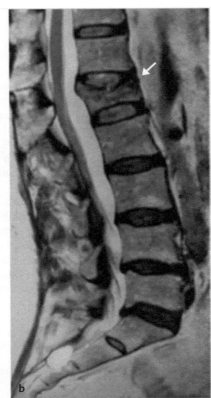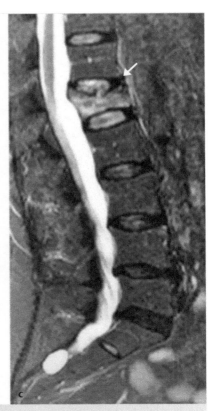

Fig. 11.2 Sagittal **(a)** T1 turbo spin echo (TSE), **(b)** T2 TSE, and **(c)** T2 short tau inversion recovery (STIR) images of an acute L1 vertebral compression fracture (*white arrows*). Bone marrow edema is hypointense on T1-weighted and hyperintense on T2 STIR images. (These images are provided courtesy of Dr. M. R. Chambers).

11.4 Indications and Contraindications

Indications for kyphoplasty include intractable severe pain or moderate to severe persistent pain associated and correlating with a VCF. In 2017, a multidisciplinary expert panel of orthopaedic and neurosurgeons, interventional radiologists, and pain specialists, using the RAND/UCLA Appropriateness Method (RUAM), developed the Clinical Care Pathway (CCP), defining patient-specific recommendations for vertebral fragility fractures (VFF). The panel assessed the relative importance of signs and symptoms for the suspicion of VFF, the relevance of diagnostic procedures, and the appropriateness of vertebral augmentation versus nonsurgical management for a variety of clinical scenarios (▶Fig. 11.3). Their report included the following guidelines for relative and absolute contraindications (▶Table 11.2).

Absolute contraindications include active infection at the surgical site and untreated blood-borne infections. Strong contraindications include osteomyelitis, pregnancy, allergy to fill material, coagulopathy, spinal instability, myelopathy from the fracture, neurologic deficit, and neural impingement. Although dependent on degree, fracture repulsion and canal compromise are not generally a contraindication. Relative contraindications include cardiorespiratory compromise such that safe sedation or anesthesia cannot be achieved and in such cases the procedure may need to be done under local anesthesia. Breach of posterior vertebral cortex by tumor and tumor extension into the spinal canal are also relative contraindications for percutaneous vertebral augmentation techniques due to the potential for leakage of cement and/or displacement of tumor posteriorly.

11.5 Procedure

Kyphoplasty may be performed under general anesthesia or monitored anesthesia care (MAC) with conscious sedation and local anesthetic. In our practice, with rare exceptions, we perform kyphoplasty under general endotracheal anesthesia. In patients who cannot tolerate general anesthesia due to severe cardiopulmonary disease, for example, sedation with MAC is used with caution to avoid oversedation and respiratory compromise.

The patient is positioned prone on the operating table with shoulder and hip bolsters to aid in spinal extension and vertebral height restoration. All pressure points are padded and checked. With fluoroscopic guidance for localization, the area of planned surgery is prepped and draped in the usual sterile fashion. Appropriate prophylactic antibiotics are administered. Fluoroscopy is used to identify the pedicles and fractured vertebral body. Fluoroscopic views include true AP and lateral views. Another technique includes the en face view, directed down the longitudinal axis of the pedicle (▶Fig. 11.4).

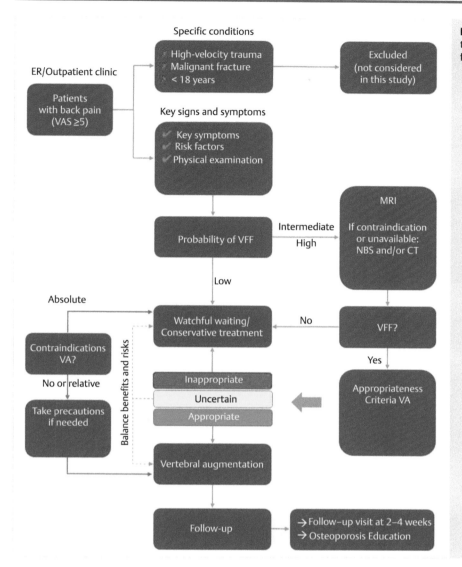

Fig. 11.3 The clinical care pathway (CCP) for the management of vertebral compression fractures.

Table 11.2 Absolute and relative contraindications for kyphoplasty

Condition	Panel recommendation
Active infection at surgical site	Absolute contraindication for curent vertebral augmentation (VA).
Untreated blood-borne infection	Absolute contraindication. Preoperative antibiotic (parenteral) therapy is required. Once cultures are negative, following an appropriate period of antibiotic therapy, one can proceed with caution.
Osteomyelitis	Usually a strong contraindication for VA. In rare situations, VA may be considered, for example, if the patient is not stable for an open procedure and the infection is chronic and caused by a less virulent organism. The infection may then be controlled locally with antibiotic-loaded cement and long-term antibiotic suppression.
Pregnancy	Although VA is usually contraindicated in pregnant patients, there may be exceptional situations in which benefits could prevail over risks. Radiation exposure to the fetus should be minimized.
Allergy to fill material	Relative contraindication, depending on the severity of the allergy. If prior reactions were not associated with severe anaphylaxis, the allergy can be pretreated with steroids, Tylenol, and Benadryl. Alternatively, another fill material can be chosen.
Coagulopathy	Relative contraindication. Try to normalize/correct clotting function if possible (international normalized ratio [INR] < 1.7). The risk of bleeding should be balanced against the complications from bed rest. Caution in patients with thrombocytopenia (platelets less than 30,000/µL).
Spinal instability	Relative contraindication, depending on the degree of instability and level of fracture. If needed, plan an additional intervention to address instability, possibly but not necessarily in the same session.
Myelopathy from the fracture	Relative contraindication. Decompression and stabilization is the preferred option, but VA may be considered if the patient is unable to undergo surgery. Coordination with spine surgeon and neurologist is mandatory.

(Continued)

Table 11.2 (*Continued*) Absolute and relative contraindications for kyphoplasty

Condition	Panel recommendation
Neurologic deficit	Relative contraindication. Additional decompression with or without stabilization may be required. Patients should be informed about the risk of cement in the spinal canal. Coordination with spine surgeon and neurologist is mandatory.
Neural impingement	Relative contraindication, depending on the degree. Take extra care to avoid delivery of cement into canal or neural foramen. May need an additional open procedure.
Fracture retropulsion/canal compromise	Generally not a contraindication. Avoid hyperextension or aggravating stenosis. A CT scan may be used to determine integrity of posterior wall.

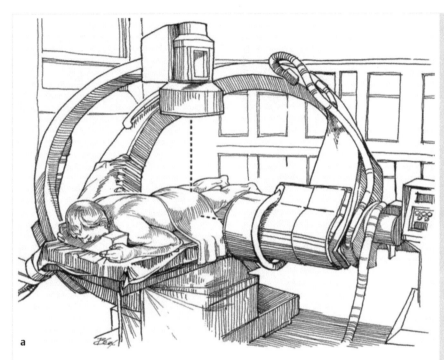

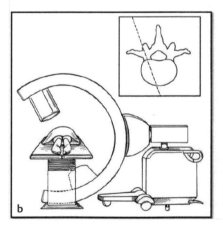

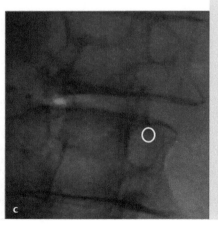

Fig. 11.4 **(a)** Proper positioning of patient and anteroposterior and lateral fluoroscopy for kyphoplasty procedure. (Source: Kim CW, Garfin SR. Percutaneous cement augmentation techniques [vertebroplasty, kyphoplasty]. In: Vaccaro AR, Albert TJ. Spine Surgery: Tricks of the Trade. New York, NY: Thieme; 2009:250–254.) **(b)** The en face view provides an angle directly down the axis of the pedicle. (Source: Resnick DK, Barr JD, and Garfin SR. Vertebroplasty and Kyphoplasty. 1st ed. New York, NY: Thieme Publishers; 2005.) **(c)** Fluoroscopic view: 20-degree ipsilateral right-sided oblique; starting position on the upper outer pedicle (*white circle*).

Local anesthetic is injected and a small stab incision is made with a no. 15 or a no. 11 blade approximately 1 cm superior and 2 cm lateral to the superior pedicle border. For a standard transpedicular approach, the Jamshidi needle is inserted and guided under direct fluoroscopy through the pedicle into the vertebral body. Other approaches and access techniques may also be used (see Chapter 6). The inner cannula is removed and replaced with a K-wire. Using the Seldinger technique, the Jamshidi cannula is removed and the cannulated osteointroducer is passed over the K-wire and advanced through two-thirds of the AP vertebral body diameter. The K-wire and inner cannula are removed when the outer cannula position is confirmed. The drill is passed manually with fluoroscopic guidance to create a void for the bone tamp and to obtain biopsy material for pathology. Core bone biopsies may be obtained through the introducer or a biopsy cannula (▶Fig. 11.1).

Next, a 10- or 15-mm bone tamp connected to a syringe prefilled with iodinated contrast is inserted through the cannula and, under direct fluoroscopic guidance, guided into the tract created by the drill. The radiopaque markers on the balloon tamp are visualized distal to the cannula sheath in both AP and lateral fluoroscopic images. When a bilateral approach is used, this procedure is repeated identically on the contralateral side.

The use of balloon tamps allows for safe and gentle end plate reduction, displacement of trabecular bone, and the creation of a void. The balloon tamps are incrementally inflated while being monitored with AP and lateral imaging. Digital manometers incorporated into the inflation devices demonstrate increases in pressure with each increase in volume. The pressure then gradually diminishes as the trabecular bone is displaced. This process is repeated as safely tolerated. Fracture reduction is guided by the degree of end plate distraction, height restoration, and reduction of kyphotic angulation. Pressure, volume, and fluoroscopic images will all dictate an endpoint. There should be no breach of lateral wall or anterior cortex of the vertebral body. The final balloon volume is recorded and one or both tamps are deflated and removed. The cement-delivery cannula is inserted through the working channel and advanced until the tip of the cannula reaches the anterior extent of the void created by the tamp, preferably just posterior to the anterior cortical wall of the vertebral body. The rod is used to expel cement from the cannula. As cement is delivered, the cannula and rod are retracted gently to allow room for the cement to fill the void. As the cement extends posteriorly, the injection should be slow to watch for extravasation. The cement should extend from superior to inferior end plate and be located between the pedicles. The cement can extend up to the posterior vertebral body wall, but it is important to watch for and recognize extension of cement beyond this margin. This process is repeated on each side until an adequate fill is achieved. As the cement begins to harden, the cannulas are removed. The internal fixation and stabilization of the vertebrae is achieved through the hardening of the cement injected into the vertebral body. Final fluoroscopic images are taken to document the final cement position. Wounds are dressed with Dermabond or Steri-Strips (▶Fig. 11.5).

11.5.1 Bilateral versus Unilateral Approach

Several large systematic reviews of randomized control trials have examined the difference between bilateral and unilateral approaches for kyphoplasty. Some differences were observed between the two approaches in terms of height restoration, correction of kyphotic angulation, and patient ratings of pain.[4,5]

In an analysis of 15 randomized control trials including 850 patients, Yang et al found no difference in quality-of-life or complications from surgery between bilateral and unilateral kyphoplasty.[4] Chen et al found that the unilateral approach resulted in a shorter operative time, smaller amount of cement injected, and lower risk of cement leakage.[5] There were no statistically significant differences in visual analog scale pain scores, height changes, or kyphotic angle changes between the groups.[5] Papanastassiou et al examined the differences between unilateral and bilateral kyphoplasty in multiple myeloma patients and found no difference in clinical or radiological outcomes.[6] Huang et al in a review of five studies including 253 patients found no clinically important differences but suggested that unilateral kyphoplasty is advantageous due to decreased operative time and cost.[7] Similarly, in a systematic review and meta-analysis including 563 patients, Sun et al noted that unilateral approach led to decreased surgical time, cement consumption, and cement leakage; reduced radiation dose and hospitalization costs; and improved short-term general health.[8]

There are also substantial data supporting the bilateral approach for optimal outcomes in vertebral augmentation with balloon kyphoplasty. In a retrospective study of 296 patients with osteoporotic VCFs, Bozkurt et al showed that although there was no statistically significant difference between unilateral kyphoplasty and vertebroplasty regarding height restoration of the fractured vertebral body, there was a further advantage of significant height restoration of bilateral kyphoplasty compared to the other two techniques.[9] The advantage of height restoration with a bilateral technique is also supported by a meta-analysis of five studies that reported a short-term follow-up that indicated bilateral balloon

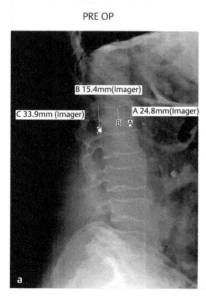

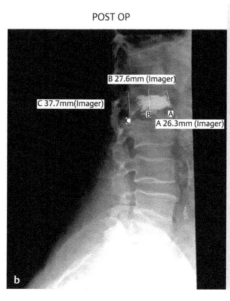

Fig. 11.5 Pre- and postoperative images demonstrating cement filling and height restoration after kyphoplasty of an L1 compression fracture. Measurements are made at three points from posterior (measurement on **a**) to anterior (measurement on **b**). The height of the three points of the vertebral body is listed in millimeters. (These images are provided courtesy of Dr. M. R. Chambers.)

kyphoplasty had a significantly (p = 0.03) better degree of anterior vertebral height restoration than unilateral balloon kyphoplasty.[10]

In general, based on the above studies and analyses, a unilateral approach provides an advantage regarding procedure time, procedure and hospital costs, radiation dose, and improved short-term health and cement extravasation. Additionally, there appears to be no significant difference in the unilateral versus bilateral approach with respect to pain reduction, quality-of-life improvement, or procedural complications. Finally, balloon kyphoplasty using a bilateral approach has been shown to provide significantly better short-term height restoration than the same procedure performed via a unilateral approach.

11.6 Risks and Benefits

As with any surgical procedure, possible adverse events include infection, hemorrhage, cardiac arrest, and stroke. Other risks specific to kyphoplasty include cement leakage and emboli, spinal cord compression, and nerve injury. Risks related to balloon failure are generally minimal. With failure or rupture of the balloon, pressure will rapidly drop to or near zero and a small amount of contrast medium and saline escape. The balloon may be gently removed after deflation. Fortunately, the complication rate for kyphoplasty is very low and this procedure has been shown to lead to significant and sustained reduction of pain, disability, and opioid analgesic usage, which results in a significantly improved quality of life.[11–16]

11.7 Importance of Sagittal Balance Restoration and Kyphosis Correction

The physical consequences of vertebral deformity, sagittal imbalance, and kyphosis include reduced pulmonary function, early satiety and gastric distress, difficulty with balance, postural compensation with altered gait and reduced velocity, chronic back pain, reduced activity and function, increased fracture risk independent of bone mineral density, and increased mortality.[9,10,17–28]

Sagittal balance is recognized as an important factor in determining outcomes following spine surgery and is included in the radiographic assessment of spinal deformity.[29–32] Many patients with VCFs present with sagittal imbalance due to the kyphosis caused by the compression fracture itself. Sagittal balance is determined with respect to a plumb line drawn from the middle of the C7 vertebral body. In normal sagittal balance, the line will pass through a point at the posterosuperior aspect of the S1 vertebral body. A patient is in positive balance if the line passes greater than 2 cm anterior to this point and in negative balance if the line passes greater than 2cm posterior to the same point (▸Fig. 11.6).

Few studies have directly examined the relationship between kyphoplasty and sagittal vertical axis (SVA) correction. Pradhan et al retrospectively reviewed 65 patients undergoing level 1 to 3 kyphoplasty procedures to examine the effects of single and multilevel kyphoplasty on local and overall sagittal alignment of the spine. The authors found that the majority of kyphosis correction by kyphoplasty was limited to the vertebral body treated

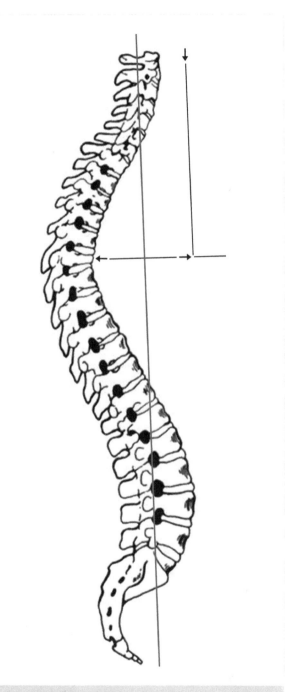

Fig. 11.6 Sagittal balance is determined by the C7 plumb line, which is a vertical line drawn from the center of the C7 vertebral body. Positive sagittal balance occurs when this line falls greater than 2 cm anterior to the posterosuperior corner of S1. Negative sagittal balance occurs when the line falls greater than 2 cm posterior to this point. (Source: Dickson R, Harms J, eds. Pathogenesis. In: Modern Management of Spinal Deformities: A Theoretical, Practical, and Evidence-Based Text. 1st ed. New York, NY: Thieme; 2018.)

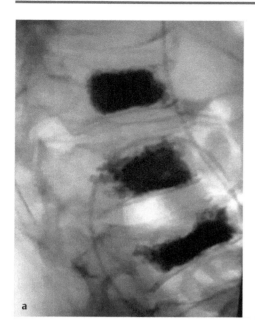
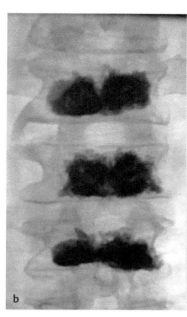

Fig. 11.7 (a, b) Postoperative images following a three-level kyphoplasty procedure. (Source: Resnick DK, Barr JD, and Garfin SR. Vertebroplasty and Kyphoplasty. 1st ed. New York, NY: Thieme Publishers; 2005.)

and that correction over longer spans with multilevel kyphoplasties could achieve improved sagittal balance.[33] In a study of 21 patients who underwent kyphoplasty, Yokoyama et al found that the preoperative SVA was 7 ± 3.9 cm, demonstrating a significant shift to anterior (positive) sagittal balance as compared to a healthy group that measured 1.45 ± 2.7 cm. After kyphoplasty, the SVA decreased to 5.02 ± 2.91 and this decrease correlated with the kyphotic reduction of the treated vertebrae.[34]

Reports examining the correlation between restoration of sagittal balance alignment and clinical outcome parameters have been mixed. Several studies have shown that improvements in sagittal balance after kyphoplasty are correlated with surgical outcomes involving pain and quality-of-life scores.[35-37] Particularly in patients with adult degenerative spinal deformity, correlations between sagittal balance correction and surgical outcomes have been strong. However, other studies have demonstrated no relationship between sagittal balance alignment restoration and clinical outcome parameters.[38-42] The FREE trial, a randomized, nonblinded trail comparing kyphoplasty with nonsurgical management of acute painful vertebral fractures, reported that patients with the greatest quality-of-life improvement, based on the SF-36 PCS (physical component summary) scores, had the better kyphosis correction (5.18 degrees) compared with the subgroup having the least quality-of-life improvement (1.98 degrees of angulation correction). Similarly, patients with the highest kyphotic angulation correction had higher SF-36 PCS quality-of-life improvement.[35]

11.8 Adjacent Fractures

Additional fractures have been reported following vertebral augmentation procedures, but the causal relationship between the procedures and subsequent adjacent vertebral fractures is doubtful as patients with osteoporosis who do not undergo surgery also develop additional fractures.[43-53] A fracture rate above that of the natural history of osteoporosis

has not been demonstrated. Additional fractures occur more quickly in patients who have undergone augmentation as compared to those who have not. This may explain the perception that augmented patients fracture more often (▶ Fig. 11.7).[20,54-56]

Regardless of bone mineral density, age, and other clinical risk factors, vertebral fractures confirmed radiographically—even if asymptomatic—signal-impaired bone quality and strongly predict new vertebral and other nonvertebral fractures. The presence of a single vertebral fracture increases the risk of subsequent vertebral fractures fivefold and the risk of hip and other fractures twofold to threefold.[57] Following an initial fracture, osteoporotic patients not treated with systemic anti-osteoporosis therapy develop an additional fracture at twice the rate (20%) of those on antiresorptive medication and even fewer vertebral fractures are seen in patients receiving anabolic bone agents with dramatic absolute and relative risk reductions of 3.6 and 86%, respectively.[52,55,58,59]

Vertebral augmentation may serve to decrease additional or adjacent-level fractures. Numerous studies have demonstrated a lower incidence of adjacent fractures in patients treated with kyphoplasty (4.2%), compared to published rates in untreated patients with osteoporotic fractures (20%).[15] In retrospectively analyzing 240 patients with painful VCFs, Baek et al found that risk for adjacent-level fractures after vertebral augmentation decreased significantly when the SVA was less than 6 cm and the segmental kyphotic angle was less than 11 degrees.[60] In a matched prospective study, Palombaro reported a 6-month adjacent fracture rate of 37% in patients treated with balloon kyphoplasty and 65% in nonsurgically treated patients.[61]

Kyphosis resulting from a wedge-shaped fracture shifts the center of gravity of the upper body forward. This increases the flexion bending moment and leads to a compensatory stance with hamstrings foreshortened (knees bent) and paraspinal muscle activity increased in the effort to maintain balance. In a finite element study, Rohlmann et al measured intradiskal pressure (IDP) in the disks adjacent to a fractured vertebra before and after augmentation. The elastic modulus of PMMA varied between 1,000 and 3,000 MPa and the volume between 4 and 10 mL. The effects of volume and elastic modulus of bone cement on IDP were negligible. Augmentation of the fractured vertebral body with bone cement had a much smaller effect on IDP than did the vertebral fracture itself (with or without compensatory upper-body shift). In cadaveric studies completed in 2005, Berlemann et al described a "stress riser" effect weakening a functional spinal unit (two vertebral bodies and the intervening disk), whereby increased stiffness of the treated vertebra altered the load transfer to the noncemented adjacent level.[55] Much more pronounced than any stiffness increase resulting from cement injection is the effect on spinal load resulting from the fracture and upper-body shift.[62] Restoration of anterior vertebral body height and correction of kyphosis reduces the compressive forces by reducing the bending moment.[63]

Luo et al analyzed "stress profiles" of 28 cadaveric spine specimen comprising three thoracolumbar vertebrae and intervening disks and ligaments before and after compression injury to one of the three vertebrae, and again after vertebroplasty. Induction of the injury reduced IDP to an average of 47% of prefracture value at the affected level and 73% of baseline values at adjacent levels. Injury also transferred compressive load bearing from the nucleus to the annulus and from the disk to the neural arch. Vertebroplasty partially reversed these changes, increasing mean IDP to 76 and 81% of baseline values at fractured and adjacent levels, respectively. Following injury, a 14-fold increase in creep deformation of the vertebral body under load was noted. Vertebroplasty also reversed these changes, reducing deformation of the anterior vertebral body by 62% at the fractured level and 52% at the adjacent level, compared to postfracture values.[64]

Balloon kyphoplasty has been shown to significantly ($p < 0.001$) restore more than 80% of the original vertebral height following a wedge fracture and to correct vertebral wedge fracture deformity in up to 92% of patients[65,66] with changes remaining stable for at least two years following surgery.[65] Local kyphosis reduction continues to be one of the advantages of balloon kyphoplasty over vertebroplasty. Reduction of kyphosis with kyphoplasty has been shown to be greater than that for vertebroplasty (3.7–8 degrees vs. 0.5–3 degrees) and this kyphotic correction allows for a more effortless upright posture leading to relaxation of the paraspinal muscles, reduced pain, and fewer additional VCFs.[12]

Although there is limited evidence that postural reduction (preoperative positioning) is the most important factor for kyphosis correction,[67] there is strong evidence that the balloon tamps used in kyphoplasty enhance reduction greater than 4.5-fold over positioning maneuvers alone and account for over 80% of the reduction.[35–37,40–42,68–79]

More information on additional or adjacent VCFs after vertebral augmentation can be found in Chapter 17.

11.9 Postoperative Care

Although it is customary to perform kyphoplasty as an outpatient procedure, many affected patients are elderly and have multiple medical comorbidities; thus, an overnight admission may be indicated. Elderly patients have an inherent progressive loss of functional reserve in all organ systems. Common causes of postoperative morbidity include atelectasis, bronchitis, pneumonia, delirium, heart failure, and myocardial infarction.[3]

Increased vulnerability to perioperative stress favors minimally invasive surgery with shorter operative times and a shorter hospital stay. Meticulous intraoperative management of coexisting disorders and postoperative pain control will help mitigate patient stress. When treating elderly patients, the clinician should always keep in mind that changes in pharmacokinetics and pharmacodynamics render some medications more potent in geriatric patients. Morphine clearance, for example, is decreased in the elderly, leading to a decreased narcotic requirement for pain relief. There is an increase in brain sensitivity to opioids with age.[3]

Patients are encouraged at discharge to resume all of their typical daily activities as soon as feasible with few restrictions. Patients are examined at 2 weeks postoperatively to evaluate their response to the procedure, their progress in healing, and to determine the need for additional care including physical therapy. Back-strengthening programs are often useful in these patients after kyphoplasty. All patients presenting with VFF should be referred for bone mineral density monitoring and osteoporosis education with treatment as indicated. The treatment of their underlying disorder of osteoporosis will be discussed in greater detail in Chapter 34. If their pain is not resolved or significantly diminished following kyphoplasty, re-evaluation with imaging is indicated. There are countless nonsurgical causes of back pain as well as frequent additional vertebral fractures after the initial vertebral augmentation procedure.

11.10 Conclusion

Kyphoplasty is a minimally invasive procedure designed to relieve pain and improve function in patients with pain and disability associated with VCFs. Results of numerous studies have demonstrated significant and durable pain relief, reduced disability, improved function, and enhanced quality of life after kyphoplasty in patients with VCFs resulting from a wide range of etiologies. In addition, restoration of vertebral height, correction of kyphotic angulation, and improved sagittal balance may decrease the risk of future vertebral fractures.

Performed under general anesthesia or MAC with sedation and local anesthetic, kyphoplasty has an extremely low complication rate in experienced hands and has been shown to significantly improve the rates of patient morbidity and mortality. Kyphoplasty remains a first-line treatment option for patients with painful VCFs unresponsive to medical therapy.

References

[1] He Z, Zhai Q, Hu M, et al. Bone cements for percutaneous vertebroplasty and balloon kyphoplasty: Current status and future developments. J Orthop Translat 2014;3(1):1–11

[2] Charnley J. Anchorage of the femoral head prosthesis to the shaft of the femur. J Bone Joint Surg Br 1960;42-B:28–30

[3] Kanonidou Z, Karystianou G. Anesthesia for the elderly. Hippokratia 2007;11(4):175–177

[4] Yang S, Chen C, Wang H, Wu Z, Liu L. A systematic review of unilateral versus bilateral percutaneous vertebroplasty/percutaneous kyphoplasty for osteoporotic vertebral compression fractures. Acta Orthop Traumatol Turc 2017;51(4):290–297

[5] Chen H, Tang P, Zhao Y, Gao Y, Wang Y. Unilateral versus bilateral balloon kyphoplasty in the treatment of osteoporotic vertebral compression fractures. Orthopedics 2014;37(9):e828–e835

[6] Papanastassiou ID, Eleraky M, Murtagh R, Kokkalis ZT, Gerochristou M, Vrionis FD. Comparison of unilateral versus bilateral kyphoplasty in multiple myeloma patients and the importance of preoperative planning. Asian Spine J 2014;8(3):244–252

[7] Huang Z, Wan S, Ning L, Han S. Is unilateral kyphoplasty as effective and safe as bilateral kyphoplasties for osteoporotic vertebral compression fractures? A meta-analysis. Clin Orthop Relat Res 2014;472(9):2833–2842

[8] Sun H, Lu PP, Liu YJ, et al. Can Unilateral Kyphoplasty Replace Bilateral Kyphoplasty in Treatment of Osteoporotic Vertebral Compression Fractures? A Systematic Review and Meta-analysis. Pain Physician 2016;19(8):551–563

[9] Bozkurt M, Kahilogullari G, Ozdemir M, et al. Comparative analysis of vertebroplasty and kyphoplasty for osteoporotic vertebral compression fractures. Asian Spine J 2014;8(1):27–34

[10] Feng H, Huang P, Zhang X, Zheng G, Wang Y. Unilateral versus bilateral percutaneous kyphoplasty for osteoporotic vertebral compression fractures: A systematic review and meta-analysis of RCTs. J Orthop Res 2015;33(11):1713–1723

[11] Eidt-Koch D, Greiner W. Quality of life results of balloon kyphoplasty versus non surgical management for osteoporotic vertebral fractures in Germany. Health Econ Rev 2011;1(1):7

[12] Papanastassiou ID, Phillips FM, Van Meirhaeghe J, et al. Comparing effects of kyphoplasty, vertebroplasty, and non-surgical management in a systematic review of randomized and non-randomized controlled studies. Eur Spine J 2012;21(9):1826–1843

[13] Wardlaw D, Cummings SR, Van Meirhaeghe J, et al. Efficacy and safety of balloon kyphoplasty compared with non-surgical care for vertebral compression fracture (FREE): a randomised controlled trial. Lancet 2009;373(9668):1016–1024

[14] Van Meirhaeghe J, Bastian L, Boonen S, Ranstam J, Tillman JB, Wardlaw D; FREE investigators. A randomized trial of balloon kyphoplasty and non-surgical management for treating acute vertebral compression fractures: vertebral body kyphosis correction and surgical parameters. Spine 2013;38(12):971–983

[15] Kicielinski KP, Pritchard Patrick R, Ruiz H, et al. Patient Experience Following Kyphoplasty: Safety, Efficacy and Patient Satisfaction. J Adv Med Med Res 2015;10(1):1–11

[16] Feltes C, Fountas KN, Machinis T, et al. Immediate and early postoperative pain relief after kyphoplasty without significant restoration of vertebral body height in acute osteoporotic vertebral fractures. Neurosurg Focus 2005;18(3):e5

[17] Kanis JA, Oden A, Johnell O, De Laet C, Jonsson B. Excess mortality after hospitalisation for vertebral fracture. Osteoporos Int 2004;15(2):108–112

[18] Johnell O, Kanis JA, Odén A, et al. Mortality after osteoporotic fractures. Osteoporos Int 2004;15(1):38–42

[19] Hillier TA, Lui LY, Kado DM, et al. Height loss in older women: risk of hip fracture and mortality independent of vertebral fractures. J Bone Miner Res 2012;27(1):153–159

[20] Lindsay R, Silverman SL, Cooper C, et al. Risk of new vertebral fracture in the year following a fracture. JAMA 2001;285(3):320–323

[21] Nevitt MC, Ettinger B, Black DM, et al. The association of radiographically detected vertebral fractures with back pain and function: a prospective study. Ann Intern Med 1998;128(10):793–800

[22] van Schoor NM, Smit JH, Twisk JW, Lips P. Impact of vertebral deformities, osteoarthritis, and other chronic diseases on quality of life: a population-based study. Osteoporos Int 2005;16(7):749–756

[23] Hallberg I, Rosenqvist AM, Kartous L, Löfman O, Wahlström O, Toss G. Health-related quality of life after osteoporotic fractures. Osteoporos Int 2004;15(10):834–841

[24] Silverman SL. The clinical consequences of vertebral compression fracture. Bone 1992;13(Suppl 2):S27–S31

[25] Sinaki M, Brey RH, Hughes CA, Larson DR, Kaufman KR. Balance disorder and increased risk of falls in osteoporosis and kyphosis: significance of kyphotic posture and muscle strength. Osteoporos Int 2005;16(8):1004–1010

[26] Schlaich C, Minne HW, Bruckner T, et al. Reduced pulmonary function in patients with spinal osteoporotic fractures. Osteoporos Int 1998;8(3):261–267

[27] Culham EG, Jimenez HA, King CE. Thoracic kyphosis, rib mobility, and lung volumes in normal women and women with osteoporosis. Spine 1994;19(11):1250–1255

[28] Leech JA, Dulberg C, Kellie S, Pattee L, Gay J. Relationship of lung function to severity of osteoporosis in women. Am Rev Respir Dis 1990;141(1):68–71

[29] Booth KC, Bridwell KH, Lenke LG, Baldus CR, Blanke KM. Complications and predictive factors for the successful treatment of flatback deformity (fixed sagittal imbalance). Spine 1999;24(16):1712–1720

[30] Berven SH, Deviren V, Smith JA, Hu SH, Bradford DS. Management of fixed sagittal plane deformity: outcome of combined anterior and posterior surgery. Spine 2003;28(15):1710–1715, discussion 1716

[31] Park SJ, Lee CS, Chung SS, Kang KC, Shin SK. Postoperative changes in pelvic parameters and sagittal balance in adult isthmic spondylolisthesis. Neurosurgery 2011;68(2, Suppl Operative):355–363, discussion 362–363

[32] Endo K, Suzuki H, Tanaka H, Kang Y, Yamamoto K. Sagittal spinal alignment in patients with lumbar disc herniation. Eur Spine J 2010;19(3):435–438

[33] Pradhan BB, Bae HW, Kropf MA, Patel VV, Delamarter RB. Kyphoplasty reduction of osteoporotic vertebral compression fractures: correction of local kyphosis versus overall sagittal alignment. Spine 2006;31(4):435–441

[34] Yokoyama K, Kawanishi M, Yamada M, et al. Postoperative change in sagittal balance after Kyphoplasty for the treatment of osteoporotic vertebral compression fracture. Eur Spine J 2015;24(4):744–749

[35] Ranstam J, Turkiewicz A, Boonen S, Van Meirhaeghe J, Bastian L, Wardlaw D. Alternative analyses for handling incomplete follow-up in the intention-to-treat analysis: the randomized controlled trial of balloon kyphoplasty versus non-surgical care for vertebral compression fracture (FREE). BMC Med Res Methodol 2012;12:35

[36] Grohs JG, Matzner M, Trieb K, Krepler P. Minimal invasive stabilization of osteoporotic vertebral fractures: a prospective nonrandomized comparison of vertebroplasty and balloon kyphoplasty. J Spinal Disord Tech 2005;18(3):238–242

[37] Dong R, Chen L, Gu Y, et al. Improvement in respiratory function after vertebroplasty and kyphoplasty. Int Orthop 2009;33(6):1689–1694

[38] Dong R, Chen L, Tang T, et al. Pain reduction following vertebroplasty and kyphoplasty. Int Orthop 2013;37(1):83–87

[39] Berlemann U, Franz T, Orler R, Heini PF. Kyphoplasty for treatment of osteoporotic vertebral fractures: a prospective non-randomized study. Eur Spine J 2004;13(6):496–501

[40] Rollinghoff M, Siewe J, Zarghooni K, et al. Effectiveness, security and height restoration on fresh compression fractures: a comparative prospective study of vertebroplasty and kyphoplasty Minim Invasive Neurosurg 2009;52(5–6):233–237

[41] Lovi A, Teli M, Ortolina A, Costa F, Fornari M, Brayda-Bruno M. Vertebroplasty and kyphoplasty: complementary techniques for the treatment of painful osteoporotic vertebral compression fractures. A prospective non-randomised study on 154 patients. Eur Spine J 2009;18(Suppl 1):95–101

[42] Kasperk C, Hillmeier J, Nöldge G, et al. Treatment of painful vertebral fractures by kyphoplasty in patients with primary osteoporosis: a prospective nonrandomized controlled study. J Bone Miner Res 2005;20(4):604–612

[43] Ettinger B, Black DM, Mitlak BH, et al; Multiple Outcomes of Raloxifene Evaluation (MORE) Investigators. Reduction of vertebral fracture risk in postmenopausal women with osteoporosis treated with raloxifene: results from a 3-year randomized clinical trial. JAMA 1999;282(7):637–645

[44] Zoarski GH, Snow P, Olan WJ, et al. Percutaneous vertebroplasty for osteoporotic compression fractures: quantitative prospective evaluation of long-term outcomes. J Vasc Interv Radiol 2002;13(2, Pt 1):139–148

[45] Uppin AA, Hirsch JA, Centenera LV, Pfiefer BA, Pazianos AG, Choi IS. Occurrence of new vertebral fracture after percutaneous vertebroplasty in patients with osteoporosis. Radiology 2003;226(1):119–124

[46] Syed MI, Patel NA, Jan S, Harron MS, Morar K, Shaikh A. New symptomatic vertebral compression fractures within a year following vertebroplasty in osteoporotic women. AJNR Am J Neuroradiol 2005;26(6):1601–1604

[47] Legroux-Gérot I, Lormeau C, Boutry N, Cotten A, Duquesnoy B, Cortet B. Long-term follow-up of vertebral osteoporotic fractures treated by percutaneous vertebroplasty. Clin Rheumatol 2004;23(4):310–317

[48] Kobayashi K, Shimoyama K, Nakamura K, Murata K. Percutaneous vertebroplasty immediately relieves pain of osteoporotic vertebral compression fractures and prevents prolonged immobilization of patients. Eur Radiol 2005;15(2):360–367

[49] Jensen ME, Dion JE. Percutaneous vertebroplasty in the treatment of osteoporotic compression fractures. Neuroimaging Clin N Am 2000;10(3):547–568

[50] Heini PF, Wälchli B, Berlemann U. Percutaneous transpedicular vertebroplasty with PMMA: operative technique and early results. A prospective study for the treatment of osteoporotic compression fractures. Eur Spine J 2000;9(5):445–450

[51] Diamond TH, Bryant C, Browne L, Clark WA. Clinical outcomes after acute osteoporotic vertebral fractures: a 2-year non-randomised trial comparing percutaneous vertebroplasty with conservative therapy. Med J Aust 2006;184(3):113–117

[52] Frankel BM, Monroe T, Wang C. Percutaneous vertebral augmentation: an elevation in adjacent-level fracture risk in kyphoplasty as compared with vertebroplasty. Spine J 2007;7(5):575–582

[53] Grados F, Depriester C, Cayrolle G, Hardy N, Deramond H, Fardellone P. Long-term observations of vertebral osteoporotic fractures treated by percutaneous vertebroplasty. Rheumatology (Oxford) 2000;39(12):1410–1414

[54] Lindsay R, Burge RT, Strauss DM. One year outcomes and costs following a vertebral fracture. Osteoporos Int 2005;16(1):78–85

[55] Berlemann U, Ferguson SJ, Nolte LP, Heini PF. Adjacent vertebral failure after vertebroplasty. A biomechanical investigation. J Bone Joint Surg Br 2002;84(5):748–752

[56] Yi X, Lu H, Tian F, et al. Recompression in new levels after percutaneous vertebroplasty and kyphoplasty compared with conservative treatment. Arch Orthop Trauma Surg 2014;134(1):21–30

[57] Gold DT. The nonskeletal consequences of osteoporotic fractures. Psychologic and social outcomes. Rheum Dis Clin North Am 2001;27(1):255–262

[58] Hoenig HM, Rubenstein LZ. Hospital-associated deconditioning and dysfunction. J Am Geriatr Soc 1991;39(2):220–222

[59] Miller PD, Hattersley G, Riis BJ, et al; ACTIVE Study Investigators. Effect of Abaloparatide vs Placebo on New Vertebral Fractures in Postmenopausal Women With Osteoporosis: A Randomized Clinical Trial. JAMA 2016;316(7):722–733

[60] Baek SW, Kim C, Chang H. The relationship between the spinopelvic balance and the incidence of adjacent vertebral fractures following percutaneous vertebroplasty. Osteoporos Int 2015;26(5):1507–1513

[61] Palombaro KM. Effects of walking-only interventions on bone mineral density at various skeletal sites: a meta-analysis. J Geriatr Phys Ther 2005;28(3):102–107

[62] Rohlmann A, Zander T Jony, Weber U, Bergmann G. [Effect of vertebral body stiffness before and after vertebroplasty on intradiscal pressure] Biomed Tech (Berl) 2005;50(5):148–152

[63] Disch AC, Schmoelz W. Cement augmentation in a thoracolumbar fracture model: reduction and stability after balloon kyphoplasty versus vertebral body stenting. Spine 2014;39(19):E1147–E1153

[64] Luo J, Annesley-Williams DJ, Adams MA, Dolan P. How are adjacent spinal levels affected by vertebral fracture and by vertebroplasty? A biomechanical study on cadaveric spines. Spine J 2017;17(6):863–874

[65] Ledlie JT, Renfro MB. Kyphoplasty treatment of vertebral fractures: 2-year outcomes show sustained benefits. Spine 2006;31(1):57–64

[66] Gaitanis IN, Hadjipavlou AG, Katonis PG, Tzermiadianos MN, Pasku DS, Patwardhan AG. Balloon kyphoplasty for the treatment of pathological vertebral compressive fractures. Eur Spine J 2005;14(3):250–260

[67] Pflugmacher R, Bornemann R, Koch EM, et al. [Comparison of clinical and radiological data in the treatment of patients with osteoporotic vertebral compression fractures using radiofrequency kyphoplasty or balloon kyphoplasty] Z Orthop Unfall 2012;150(1):56–61

[68] Movrin I. Adjacent level fracture after osteoporotic vertebral compression fracture: a nonrandomized prospective study comparing balloon kyphoplasty with conservative therapy. Wien Klin Wochenschr 2012;124(9–10):304–311

[69] Kasperk C, Grafe IA, Schmitt S, et al. Three-year outcomes after kyphoplasty in patients with osteoporosis with painful vertebral fractures. J Vasc Interv Radiol 2010;21(5):701–709

[70] Grafe IA, Da Fonseca K, Hillmeier J, et al. Reduction of pain and fracture incidence after kyphoplasty: 1-year outcomes of a prospective controlled trial of patients with primary osteoporosis. Osteoporos Int 2005;16(12):2005–2012

[71] Grafe IA, Baier M, Nöldge G, et al. Calcium-phosphate and polymethylmethacrylate cement in long-term outcome after kyphoplasty of painful osteoporotic vertebral fractures. Spine 2008;33(11):1284–1290

[72] Xing D, Ma JX, Ma XL, et al. A meta-analysis of balloon kyphoplasty compared to percutaneous vertebroplasty for treating osteoporotic vertebral compression fractures. J Clin Neurosci 2013;20(6):795–803

[73] Liu JT, Liao WJ, Tan WC, et al. Balloon kyphoplasty versus vertebroplasty for treatment of osteoporotic vertebral compression fracture: a prospective, comparative, and randomized clinical study. Osteoporos Int 2010;21(2):359–364

[74] Kumar K, Nguyen R, Bishop S. A comparative analysis of the results of vertebroplasty and kyphoplasty in osteoporotic vertebral compression fractures. Neurosurgery 2010;67(3, Suppl Operative):ons171–ons188, discussion ons188

[75] Li X, Yang H, Tang T, Qian Z, Chen L, Zhang Z. Comparison of kyphoplasty and vertebroplasty for treatment of painful osteoporotic vertebral compression fractures: twelve-month follow-up in a prospective nonrandomized comparative study. J Spinal Disord Tech 2012;25(3):142–149

[76] Schofer MD, Efe T, Timmesfeld N, Kortmann HR, Quante M. Comparison of kyphoplasty and vertebroplasty in the treatment of fresh vertebral compression fractures. Arch Orthop Trauma Surg 2009;129(10):1391–1399

[77] Pflugmacher R, Kandziora F, Schröder R, et al. [Vertebroplasty and kyphoplasty in osteoporotic fractures of vertebral bodies -- a prospective 1-year follow-up analysis] RoFo Fortschr Geb Rontgenstr Nuklearmed 2005;177(12):1670–1676

[78] Movrin I, Vengust R, Komadina R. Adjacent vertebral fractures after percutaneous vertebral augmentation of osteoporotic vertebral compression fracture: a comparison of balloon kyphoplasty and vertebroplasty. Arch Orthop Trauma Surg 2010;130(9):1157–1166

[79] Shindle MK, Gardner MJ, Koob J, Bukata S, Cabin JA, Lane JM. Vertebral height restoration in osteoporotic compression fractures: kyphoplasty balloon tamp is superior to postural correction alone. Osteoporos Int 2006;17(12):1815–1819

12 Vertebral Augmentation with Implants

Dimitrios K. Filippiadis, Stefano Marcia, and Alexios Kelekis

Summary

Implant augmentation was developed after vertebroplasty and balloon kyphoplasty and is indicated when improvement of the post-fracture kyphotic angle is a primary treatment goal. Correction of the kyphotic angle and having optimal stabilization of the vertebral body is associated with a decreased rate of additional fractures and greater improvement of pain. The indications and contraindications for vertebral body implants are similar to those for vertebroplasty and balloon kyphoplasty and implants are indicated for fractures associated with trauma, osteoporosis, and neoplasia. The currently used vertebral implants used to treat fractures include the vertebral body stent, the SpineJack, Osseofix, VerteLift, and the Kiva implant. Vertebral implants are typically placed through larger diameter systems so the size of the pedicle should be considered when placing the implant via a transpedicular approach or the physician may opt to use an extrapedicular approach. Implant augmentation is typically slightly more complex than the precursor forms of vertebral augmentation and all of the implants are placed bilaterally except for the Kiva implant which is placed through unilateral access. The main advantages of implant augmentation over vertebroplasty and balloon kyphoplasty include better reduction of the compressed vertebral body, better pain improvement, and less adjacent or additional vertebral compression fractures. Additional investigation into the cost-effectiveness of implant augmentation will need to be done as well as additional development of smaller implants for use in the upper thoracic and cervical spine.

Keywords: implant augmentation, vertebral body stenting, SpineJack, Kiva, Osseofix, VerteLift

12.1 Introduction

Apart from pain and mobility impairment, vertebral compression fractures (VCFs) result in deformities that in the long term can cause potential systemic complications as well as increased chance of future vertebral fractures of either the adjacent vertebral segments or other vertebral bodies.

One of the indications for use of intraosseous implants is the attempt to correct the kyphotic angle. Mechanical effects of kyphosis include decreased thoracic and abdominal space, anterior shift of the craniothoracic center of gravity, and a compensatory counterkyphotic stance with subsequent clinical consequences such as decreased appetite with resultant nutritional impact, frailty, increased future VCF risk, and secondary chronic back pain due to constant paraspinal muscular contraction.[1-4] With current evidence, it is clear that percutaneous vertebroplasty and balloon kyphoplasty (BKP) are more efficient than conservative therapy for the management of painful fractures, prolonging survival, and preventing morbidity in these patients.[1] Use of vertebral implants, combined with cement injection, is intended to provide analgesic and stabilizing effects along with kyphotic angle correction and vertebral height restoration. Correction of the kyphotic angle may be associated with optimal spinal alignment, paraspinal muscle relaxation, a more upright posture, and reduced pain along with a significantly higher improvement in function and quality of life.[4,5]

Another potential use of the intraosseous implants is to provide stabilization of the fracture along with the improved sagittal alignment to optimize and decrease the stress on the adjacent vertebral bodies. The prospect of stabilizing the vertebral body by using vertebroplasty or even kyphoplasty might be associated with a higher risk of refracture due to the less optimal restoration of the vertebral height.[1,6] In fractures where simple augmentation is contraindicated, the use of an alternative material with different mechanical properties than polymethyl methacrylate (PMMA) can have an additive effect to normalize the spinal compression forces.

The purpose of this chapter is to describe the most commonly used vertebral implants and the implantation procedures associated with placing these implants. The advantages and disadvantages of different products will be addressed.

12.2 The Implants

Vertebral implants for fracture treatment include stents, jacks, polyether ether ketone (PEEK) cages, and fracture reduction systems. Indications for implants include osteoporotic or traumatic fractures as well as primary or metastatic neoplastic spine disease.[6,7] The contraindications are similar to those for standard vertebral augmentation techniques, including asymptomatic fractures, pain relief with conservative therapy, local or systemic infection, severe coagulopathy, and severe cardiorespiratory disease.[6,7]

Vertebral body stenting (VBS): VBS is a minimally invasive percutaneous technique during which an expandable cobalt–chromium device is deployed inside the vertebral body (▶ Fig. 12.1). The stent access kit includes guidewires, trocars,

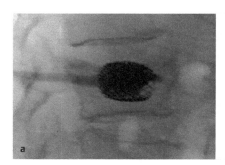
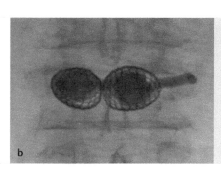

Fig. 12.1 (a) Lateral and (b) posteroanterior fluoroscopy views post implantation and cement injection of vertebral body stents.

and working sleeves, drill and blunt plungers, vertebral body balloons and inflation system, vertebral body catheters and stents, as well as cement and a cement delivery system. The balloons and stents are available in three sizes; size selection is based on the preoperative planning via computed tomography scan. Usually, the stents are nonretrievable once expanded.

SpineJack: The concept of SpineJack is to achieve a superoinferior restoration of the vertebral body including cortical rings and end plates. The expansion of the implant is progressive and can be maintained until the cement is injected (▶Fig. 12.2). Additionally, in order to best fit for each fracture's shape and patient's anatomy, it is possible to expand the implant under the most compressed portion of the VCF. The access kit for spine jack implant includes trocar, Kirschner's wire, reamer and template, the implant introduction system, and the cement delivery system. Once Spine Jack is expanded, there is no retrieval of the implant.

Osseofix: Osseofix (Alphatec Spine, Carlsbad, CA) is an intravertebral expandable titanium mesh cylinder (▶Fig. 12.3). During expansion, the surrounding trabecular bone is compacted and the vertebral height is partially restored and the kyphotic deformity decreased.[7] The implant acts as scaffold augmenting the vertebral fracture stabilization and creating channels for subsequent cement injection. Osseofix is indicated for compression fractures at the T6–L5 levels. Once Osseofix is expanded, there is no retrieval of the implant.

VerteLift: This is a nitinol implant of different sizes and configurations in order to fit each fracture and patient. The implant also has the feature of being able to be repositioned. This nitinol implant is composed of super-elastic struts designed for vertebral end plate support and fracture reduction, which is maintained until bone cement is injected (▶Fig. 12.4). During cement injection, the polymer flows around and through the struts interdigitating with the cancellous bone.

KIVA system: This is a spiraled coiled PEEK-OPTIMA implant loaded with 15% barium sulfate (▶Fig. 12.5). The implant has a distal marker and is indicated for treatment of thoracic and lumbar spinal fractures (T6–L5 levels). The access kit of the KIVA system includes needles, guide pins, a working cannula, a deployment system containing the nitinol coil, and the PEEK

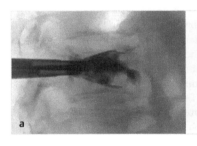 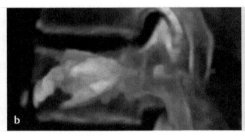

Fig. 12.2 Lateral fluoroscopy view (a) and cone beam 3D CT reconstruction (b) post implantation and cement injection of SpineJack.

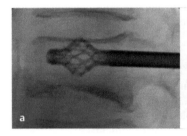 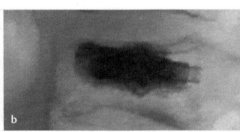

Fig. 12.3 Lateral fluoroscopy view during deployment (a) and post cement injection of Osseofix (b).

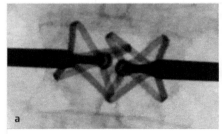 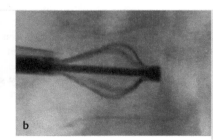

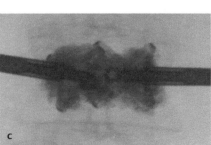 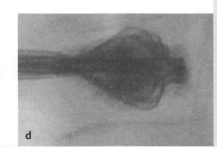

Fig. 12.4 (a, b) Posteroanterior and lateral fluoroscopy views during deployment of (c, d). Posteroanterior and lateral fluoroscopy views during cement injection in VerteLift.

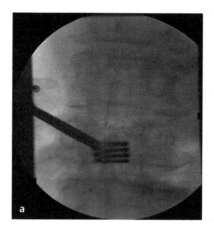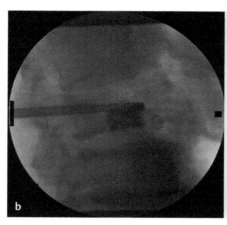

Fig. 12.5 (a) Posteroanterior fluoroscopy view during deployment of KIVA and (b) lateral fluoroscopy view during cement injection.

Table 12.1 Summary of most commonly used percutaneous vertebral implants

Implant	Type	Company	Approach
Vertebral body stenting	Expandable, intrasomatic, titanium stent	DePuy Synthes, Synthes GmbH, Switzerland	Bilateral
Osseofix	Deformable metallic component	ATEC Spine Inc., Carlsbad, CA, United States	Bilateral (1 study of unilateral approach)
SpineJack	Deformable metallic component with a direct lift mechanism with the ability to produce a large force of elevation	STRYKER, VEXIM Balma, France	Bilateral
KIVA system	PEEK polymer cage forming a continuous, spiral loop inside the vertebral body	Benvenue Medical Santa Clara, CA, United States	Unilateral
VerteLift	Nitinol (nickel/titanium alloy) cage	SpineAlign Medical Inc, San Jose, CA, United States	Bilateral

polymer cage as well as a cement delivery system. During the expansion of the nitinol coil, the system is retrievable and repositionable. Once the PEEK material is deployed, there is no possibility of withdrawal. The most commonly used percutaneous vertebral implants are listed in ▶Table. 12.1.

12.3 The Procedures

From a technical point of view, introduction of these devices is performed through working cannulas of larger diameters than the standard trocars used in vertebroplasty and therefore size of the pedicle is an important feasibility and success factor when the proceduralist chooses a transpedicular approach. In some cases, where there is a preference for the use of implants, an extrapedicular approach can be opted for. Additionally, deployment of each implant is a more complex procedure when compared to standard augmentation techniques often requiring a learning curve for optimal performance. In all cases and for all products, the patient is placed in a prone position and implantation is performed via fluoroscopic guidance.

VBS: Vertebral body stents are placed through an extra- or transpedicular approach. The trocars are inserted inside the vertebral body, thus creating a pathway for positioning of the instruments in a single step. The final position of the trocars should be such that it allows placement of the two stents symmetrically toward the midline. The trocar is exchanged for a working cannula over a wire. The drill and the blunt plunger are sequentially inserted through the working cannula in order to create space and an access channel for the stents (in the distal tip of the plunger, there are three grooves that correspond to the different stent lengths available). Following this, a vertebral body balloon catheter (selected on the basis of stent size) is inserted through the working sleeve and positioned to the anticipated stent location. After dilatation with the inflation system, the balloon catheters are retrieved and the vertebral body stent catheters are inserted and deployed.[8] After catheter removal, PMMA is injected under real-time fluoroscopic control in, and around, the implant (▶Fig. 12.1). The cement preferentially fills the cavity created by the balloons and supported by the stents.[8,9]

SpineJack: Needles are inserted into the vertebral body via a transpedicular approach. The needles are then exchanged over a guidewire for a drill and a working cannula. The drill is used to create a channel inside the vertebral body. The working cannula is left in place after removal of the drill and a template is then used for removing residual bone fragments in the implant's location. A cannula plug is inserted for any potential bleeding and a radiopaque marker in the cannula plug allows the operator to visualize the implant's depth. A SpineJack implant is then inserted and cement is injected using bone fillers through the expander (▶Fig. 12.2).[10]

Osseofix: Targeting needles are inserted into the posterior portion of the vertebral body. This is followed by sequential exchanges over guidewires, and drill sleeves are introduced. The drill creates an access channel. The diameter of the drill corresponds to the diameter of a nonexpanded implant. The drill is then removed and the sleeve is replaced by the working cannula through which the nonexpanded implant is inserted and then subsequently expanded (the system has a stop mechanism to prevent excessive expansion). Once the implant is dilated, it cannot be percutaneously removed. Finally, cement is injected into the implant though the working cannula (▶ Fig. 12.3).[11,12]

VerteLift: Access cannulas for the VerteLift system are inserted through the access needles and a manual drill is used to create the implant's delivery pathway. The implants are delivered, positioned, and deployed using a multifunctional handle attached to the delivery system. After correct positioning of the implant, the delivery system is detached and injection of cement follows (▶ Fig. 12.4).[13]

KIVA system: A standard needle is inserted into the vertebral body using a transpedicular approach. The needle is place ipsilaterally and horizontally aligned with the unfractured end plate aiming at the lateral portion of the vertebral body. A guide pin is used to exchange the needle cannula with a drilling dilator and that is then introduced into the vertebral body. The drilling dilatory is placed up to 3 to 5 mm from the anterior vertebral body all which leaves the shorter working cannula positioned just anterior to the posterior vertebral body wall. The appropriate implant deployment device is then chosen for either a right-sided or a left-sided insertion and the nitinol wire is then inserted into the vertebral body by twisting the blue knob on the side of the deployment device. After the nitinol wire is placed, the PEEK implant is inserted into the vertebral body over the coiled wire by twisting the white knob on the other side of the deployment device. After the PEEK implant is delivered over the guidewire in a continuous, spiral loop, the wire is removed and the PEEK cage is filled with cement (▶ Fig. 12.5).[4]

12.4 Bilateral versus Unilateral Approach

According to the manufacturer's guidelines, the vast majority of vertebral implants should be placed in pairs inside the vertebral body through a bilateral access. The KIVA system is the only implant, according to the manufacturer's guidelines, that is designed to be placed via a unilateral transpedicular approach. Pua et al have proposed the "central stentoplasty" approach inserting the Osseofix titanium mesh cage system into vertebral bodies using cone-beam CT guidance.[15] Unilateral approaches receive less radiation dose and operation time, being similarly effective in alleviating the back pain, but a unilateral approach may be less effective at reducing the vertebral fracture and reestablishing the prefracture vertebral height. There is a paucity of data; however, comparing unilateral and bilateral approaches for implant placement and additional randomized controlled trials would be needed to assess for safety, efficacy, biomechanical stability, and adverse events related to unilateral and bilateral approaches.

12.5 Advantages and Disadvantages of Vertebral Implants

Implants aim to provide long-term vertebral height restoration and correction of kyphosis, as well as additional support compared to standard augmentation. In selected cases of extreme fractures, implants can work as anchors, thus providing extra support against shearing forces, where the risk of cement failure is higher. Thus far, there are no completed and published clinical studies proving the concept of structural support superiority to standard cement or evidence of superiority of one device over the other. Despite this, preliminary data available at the time of this writing from the 151-patient randomized placebo-controlled SAKOS trial comparing the SpineJack to the KyphX Xpander Inflatable Bone Tamp suggest that both SpineJack and BKP had comparable effects on function improvement and QOL, but SpineJack appears to be significantly better than BKP for pain relief, VB height restoration, and in decreasing the rate of adjacent fractures.[20]

Most biomechanical and other clinical comparative studies versus standard augmentation techniques thus far report noninferiority of spine implants with a reduced volume of injected cement.[14] In addition to optimal fracture repair, Noriega et al reported that restoration of the previous spinal alignment at the fractured segment seems to be a crucial factor for the maintenance of normal disk diffusion.[16] In another study comparing an early version of vertebral stents with BKP, Werner et al reported that vertebral body stents are associated with significantly higher pressures during balloon inflation and more material-related complications. This was a relatively small study with only 100 fractures assessed, but the results showed no clear beneficial effect of the stent over that of traditional BKP.[17]

The disadvantage of all implants is their higher initial cost when compared to that of standard vertebral augmentation techniques. The smaller proportion of VCF patients who are treated with implants can cost up to 70% of the total budget for vertebral augmentation.[6,7,18] At the moment, there is no study reporting cost-effectiveness of vertebral implants over standard techniques, so the final determination as to the relative cost-effectiveness is uncertain. Cost-effectiveness assessments are essential as it has been shown that despite an initially higher cost, BKP was found to be more cost-effective than vertebroplasty within 2 years in a U.S. study by Ong et al and within 4 years in a European study by Lange et al.[21,22]

Cost-effectiveness is determined by many factors including quality of treatment effect, so a greater benefit provided to the patient could give rise to greater cost-effectiveness over time relative to technologies with a lower initial cost. Other disadvantages of vertebral implant include the aspect that it is somewhat more invasive, the implants are irretrievable, and there is an absence of adapted material for implantation in the cervical and upper thoracic spine and in the sacrum.[18]

12.6 Postprocedure Care

Depending on the product used, the injection of the cement should be done according to the manufacturer's guidelines; in the first 2 hours, vital signs and neurological evaluations mainly of the extremities should be routinely monitored.[19] A CT scan can be used to evaluate the anatomic outcome of the fracture treatment including the vertebral reduction, kyphotic angle correction and any potential cement leakage, device migration/fracture, or any spinal canal compromise or bony retropulsion. If the patient has persistent significant pain after vertebral augmentation, MRI can be used for additional assessment.[19]

References

[1] Filippiadis DK, Marcia S, Masala S, Deschamps F, Kelekis A. Percutaneous vertebroplasty and kyphoplasty: current status, new developments and old controversies. Cardiovasc Intervent Radiol 2017;40(12):1815–1823

[2] Schlaich C, Minne HW, Bruckner T, et al. Reduced pulmonary function in patients with spinal osteoporotic fractures. Osteoporos Int 1998;8(3):261–267

[3] Sinaki M, Brey RH, Hughes CA, Larson DR, Kaufman KR. Balance disorder and increased risk of falls in osteoporosis and kyphosis: significance of kyphotic posture and muscle strength. Osteoporos Int 2005;16(8):1004–1010

[4] Silverman SL. The clinical consequences of vertebral compression fracture. Bone 1992;13(Suppl 2):S27–S31

[5] Kado DM, Lui LY, Ensrud KE, Fink HA, Karlamangla AS, Cummings SR; Study of Osteoporotic Fractures. Hyperkyphosis predicts mortality independent of vertebral osteoporosis in older women. Ann Intern Med 2009;150(10):681–687

[6] Guglielmi G, Andreula C, Muto M, Gilula LA. Percutaneous vertebroplasty: indications, contraindications, technique, and complications. Acta Radiol 2005;46(3):256–268

[7] Muto M, Perrotta V, Guarnieri G, et al. Vertebroplasty and kyphoplasty: friends or foes? Radiol Med (Torino) 2008;113(8):1171–1184

[8] Heini PF, Teuscher R. Vertebral body stenting / stentoplasty. Swiss Med Wkly 2012;142:w13658

[9] Aparisi F. Vertebroplasty and kyphoplasty in vertebral osteoporotic fractures. Semin Musculoskelet Radiol 2016;20(4):382–391

[10] Sietsma MS, Hosman AJ, Verdonschot NJ, Aalsma AM, Veldhuizen AG. Biomechanical evaluation of the vertebral jack tool and the inflatable bone tamp for reduction of osteoporotic spine fractures. Spine 2009;34(18):E640–E644

[11] Ender SA, Gradl G, Ender M, Langner S, Merk HR, Kayser R. Osseofix system for percutaneous stabilization of osteoporotic and tumorous vertebral compression fractures: clinical and radiological results after 12 months. RoFo Fortschr Geb Rontgenstr Nuklearmed 2014;186(4):380–387

[12] Ender SA, Wetterau E, Ender M, Kühn JP, Merk HR, Kayser R. Percutaneous stabilization system Osseofix for treatment of osteoporotic vertebral compression fractures: clinical and radiological results after 12 months. PLoS One 2013;8(6):e65119

[13] Anselmetti GC, Manca A, Marcia S, et al. Vertebral augmentation with nitinol endoprosthesis: clinical experience in 40 patients with 1-year follow-up. Cardiovasc Intervent Radiol 2014;37(1):193–202

[14] Tutton SM, Pflugmacher R, Davidian M, Beall DP, Facchini FR, Garfin SR. KAST study: the Kiva system as a vertebral augmentation treatment—a safety and effectiveness trial: a randomized, noninferiority trial comparing the kiva system with balloon kyphoplasty in treatment of osteoporotic vertebral compression fractures. Spine 2015;40(12):865–875

[15] Pua U, Quek LH, Ng LC. Central stentoplasty: technique for unipedicular single midline vertebral body stent implantation. Cardiovasc Intervent Radiol 2014;37(3):810–814

[16] Noriega DC, Marcia S, Ardura F, Lite IS, Marras M, Saba L. Diffusion-weighted mri assessment of adjacent disc degeneration after thoracolumbar vertebral fractures. Cardiovasc Intervent Radiol 2016;39(9):1306–1314

[17] Werner CM, Osterhoff G, Schlickeiser J, et al. Vertebral body stenting versus kyphoplasty for the treatment of osteoporotic vertebral compression fractures: a randomized trial. J Bone Joint Surg Am 2013;95(7):577–584

[18] Muto M, Marcia S, Guarnieri G, Pereira V. Assisted techniques for vertebral cementoplasty: why should we do it? Eur J Radiol 2015;84(5):783–788

[19] Tsoumakidou G, Too CW, Koch G, et al. CIRSE Guidelines on Percutaneous Vertebral Augmentation. Cardiovasc Intervent Radiol 2017;40(3):331–342

[20] U.S. National Library of Medicine; ClinicalTrials.gov. A prospective multicenter, randomized, comparative clinical study to compare the safety and effectiveness of two vertebral compression fracture (VCF) reduction techniques: the SpineJack and the KyphX Xpander Inflatable Bone Tamp. Interim clinical study report. Available at: https://clinicaltrials.gov/ct2/show/NCT02461810. Published May 1, 2018. Accessed June 17, 2018

[21] Ong KL, Lau E, Kemner JE, Kurtz SM. Two-year cost comparison of vertebroplasty and kyphoplasty for the treatment of vertebral compression fractures: are initial surgical costs misleading? Osteoporos Int 2013;24(4):1437–1445

[22] Lange A, Kasperk C, Alvares L, Sauermann S, Braun S. Survival and cost comparison of kyphoplasty and percutaneous vertebroplasty using German claims data. Spine 2014;39(4):318–326

13 Radiation Exposure and Protection: A Conversation Beyond the Inverse Square Law, Thermoluminescent Dosimeters, and Lead Aprons

Kieran Murphy, Susannah Ryan, Marie-Constance Lacasse, Adam Thakore, and Danyal Khan

Summary

Although patient protection from radiation is important, interventionalists have a daily and career long exposure to radiation and the protection from this radiation is critically important to limit its adverse effects. Some of the more common adverse effects include cataract formation and the development of both benign and malignant tumors. Radiation can cause damage to the deoxyribonucleic acid (DNA) contained within genes which can lead to genetic mutations that will give rise to various types of cancer. Recently occupational limits to radiation have been decreased by the International Commission on Radiological Protection (ICRP) but interventionalists and technologists are known to far exceed these limits. Protection from radiation-induced mutation can include screening for genetic mutations that impair the reparation of damaged DNA. It should be noted and understood that chronic low dose radiation exposure is not benign and the risk associated with working with radiation should be acknowledged by the institutions in which we work and mitigated by safety regulations developed by the medical professionals working in this environment. The radiation dose obtained by performing vertebral augmentation can be substantially reduced by using certain equipment such as cement injectors that allow the operator to stand back from the radiation field rather than by using syringes that places the operator directly in the radiation field when injecting. The knowledge of the damaging effects of ionizing radiation and how to effectively limit and control this exposure is key to the safe and effective continuation of vertebral augmentation and procedures like it.

Keywords: radiation safety, thermoluminescent dosimeter, gray Sievert, Oncogenes, DNA, radiation-induced mutation

13.1 Introduction

Most scholarly writing about radiation and procedures focuses on the dose to the patient. However, patients have episodic and rare exposure in the millisievert (mSv) range. We as a profession have daily, career-long, low-dose exposure and amass over years an accumulate dose that in a busy interventionalist practice can be in the therapeutic range and measured in gray (Gy). Familiarity with current guidelines and radiation protection devices is a vital prerequisite to working with radiation. However, these preventive measures are often less than rigorously adhered to, leading to continuous everyday exposure to low-rate doses of radiation. This results in a significant accumulated exposure over a lifetime. Certain procedures in particular, including aortic intervention, cardiac electrophysiology, and neurointervention can, result in large doses to the operators. Rationalization of the inherent risk by interventionalists is common, as are ready excuses such as not wearing their radiation protection badge because it was misplaced badges or not wearing the appropriate radiation protection because of an estimated short duration of the procedure, significant muscular strain and spasm caused by the heaviness of lead aprons, decreased dexterity with lead gloves, or discomfort in wearing lead protective glasses. Most of this dismissive and cavalier attitude, however, is most likely due to the innate inability to feel threatened by something they cannot see or feel, a duty to the patient at any cost, and a workplace culture that supports and encourages their actions.

In recent years, many notable interventionalists have broadcasted their own personal stories on the detrimental consequences of chronic radiation exposure to their long-term health. In a documentary produced by the Organization for Occupational Radiation Safety in Interventional Fluoroscopy (ORSIF), Dr. Ted Diethrich, world renowned cardiovascular surgeon, revealed he had previously felt invincible to the effects of radiation, before being diagnosed with radiation-induced cataracts, premature left carotid artery atherosclerosis, and a left brain oligodendroglioma.[1] Dr. Lindsay Machan, inventor of the drug-eluting coronary stent, has warned his colleagues for years that there is no safe level of radiation exposure and of the need to fully protect oneself against it, having himself suffered from bilateral radiation-induced cataracts.[2]

There is recent, substantial evidence on the increased risk of radiation-induced cataracts even at low doses of radiation. The ICRP modified its eye lens dose thresholds in 2011, to a lifetime limit of 0.5 Gy and a yearly limit of 20 mSv/y, with no single year to surpass 50 mSv.[3] This is a far stricter reduction of the previous annual average level, which allowed 150 mSv/y to the lens.[4]

Moreover, chronic radiation exposure and the advancement of radiation-induced tumors have been suggested by new peer-reviewed data to have a causal relationship. A recent case study recorded 31 individual cases of interventionists diagnosed with various brain and neck tumors, showing 17 professionals affected with glioblastoma multiforme, 5 with meningiomas, and 2 with astrocytomas.[5] These three types of primary tumors are well known for their potential to be radiation induced. Furthermore, a striking finding in this report was that there was 85% left-sided predominance of the lesions, hypothesized to be secondary to the X-ray beam being on the interventionalist's left during the procedures. Reeves et al also reported that radiation received to the left side of the head was 16 times higher than that to the right.[6]

13.2 Gene Mutation and Radiation Effects on DNA Leading to the Development of Cancer

The mutation of one or more genes within a cell is the origin of all cancers. This alteration in the sequence of DNA, if not corrected, can result in the production of proteins with different or lost amino acid sequences, drastically affecting protein function. In some cases, it can result in a complete lack of protein being produced at all. Genetic mutations fall under two categories: acquired and germ line. Acquired mutations are the most common cause of cancer and arise from direct or indirect damage to the DNA of somatic cells and are acquired over the course of a person's life. Acquired mutations are found in a group(s) of somatic cells all arising from the same progenitor, rather than in sex cells, and are thus not heritable mutations. Germ line mutations are less regular, heritable, and arise from mutations in reproductive cells. This can result in the possibly cancer-inducing mutations being present throughout every cell in the organism, including those reproductive cells of the ensuing progeny.

Our DNA is consistently being attacked by the products of cellular metabolism, viral infections, ultraviolet (UV) radiation, chemical exposure, and replication errors, all of which frequently cause genetic mutations. Of course, there exists a multitude of cellular repair mechanisms to rectify these DNA-induced mutations. It is the failure of these systems to recognize or repair DNA damage, or to trigger apoptosis where the damage may not be mended. This can result in the accumulation of mutations, which can lead to cancer and other genetic diseases. Cancer is therefore unlikely to be caused by a single mutation; rather, it will take numerous mutations acquired over a lifetime for a cancer to form. Ionizing radiation is a confirmed and long-standing mutagen, producing mutation through a variety of molecular mechanisms including single-stranded DNA breaks, double-stranded DNA breaks, nucleotide substitution, and sugar ribose alterations.[7,8]

Many of the genes central to the development of cancer can be grouped into three categories: tumor suppressor genes, oncogenes, and DNA repair genes. Tumor suppressor genes are responsible for restricting cell growth by modulating cell mitosis, repairing certain kinds of DNA mismatch, or inducing apoptosis if the damage cannot be fixed. Tumor suppressor mutations tend to be loss of function, which allows cells to grow and undergo mitosis at an unchecked rate, resulting in tumor formation. Oncogenes can be defined as any gene that when mutated or expressed at suitably high levels contributes to the transformation of a normal cell into a cancer cell. Oncogenic mutations are not heritable and are acquired over time. Finally, DNA repair genes fix any mistakes and replication errors before cell division takes place. Mutations in repair genes lead to repair failure and ensuing accumulation of potentially cancer-causing mutations.

A considerable amount of peer-reviewed literature exists that focuses on the effects of solar and cosmic radiation on the long-term health of airline crew members. The ICRP has set them an occupational limit of 20 mSv/y, and they routinely aggregate between 3 and 7 mSv/y.[9] However, in comparison to ground crew and the normal population, their risk of cancer has been increased by between 1 in 130 and 1 in 4,800 for specific tumor types, depending on the number of hours worked and the altitudes reached on the airline routes taken. The higher the altitude, the greater the radiation received. The relationship between flight distance and altitude is well associated with the risk of chromosomal translocations that could manifest into cancer.[10] Comparatively, Canadian radiation workers are exposed to a cumulative dose of 6.3 mSv/y,[11] and thus incur a

significant level of risk of developing mutations that contribute to cancer. A small proportion of Danish radiation workers even managed to exceed 50 mSv/y,[12] again increasing the risk of developing cancerous mutations. Interventionalists and technologists alike are known to routinely far surpass these radiation levels.

Propagation of radiation-induced mutation is prevented by efficient DNA damage repair mechanisms operating within the cell. Any form of inherited impairment of these repair mechanisms will potentially increase risk of cancer induction by radiation-induced mutation, especially in those health care professionals working with various forms of ionizing radiation. One approach that could feasibly minimize risk to interventionalists and technologists is to make available, when requested, and only with the appropriate ethical and genetic support, screening for genetic mutations that impair radiation-induced DNA damage repair. Screening for specific mutations or alleles of genes is already a well-established practice in breast cancer and colorectal cancer, and is a useful way to reveal someone's genetic predisposition to cancer development. In theory, the screening process would take place before a graduate enters their residency, or fellowship, with an intent to provide an objective assessment of the individual risk incurred by pursuing a medical career in interventional radiology, interventional cardiology, vascular surgery, interventional pain management, or neuroradiology. Germline mutations to be screened for would include mutation types in BRCA1, BRCA2, MLH1, MSH2, MSH6, PMS2, APC, MYH, TP53, PTEN, CDKN2A, and RET. However, this is by no means a comprehensive list, as there are a myriad of potential alleles and mutations that could be screened for. This would have to be done in the appropriate ethical context with a focus centered on the well-being of the trainee.

Chronic low-dose radiation exposure is not benign. As interventionalists and surgeons, it is our collective responsibility to establish radiation protection awareness and promote stricter adherence to guidelines created to ensure our safety. The vast increase in demand for interventional services has increased our professional exposure. Our institutions and health care systems need to acknowledge our inherent risk of working with radiation and we should act as our own regulators so that every professional can safely practice without compromising their health.

13.3 Radiation Dose to the Operator and Patient During Vertebroplasty/Kyphoplasty

During these procedures, both the patient and the operator are subjected to radiation exposure. The hands and body of the physician are the areas primarily targeted by this exposure.

Radiation received by physicians during such procedures differs with the use of different equipment.[13] Using an injection device instead of a 1-mL syringe to inject the bone cement into the fractured vertebral body can significantly reduce the dose of radiation to the operator's hands per unit time of injection.[14] A study by Kallmes et al. found that the mean radiation dose during injection is approximately 100 ± 145 mrem (range: 0–660 mrem) when using a 1-mL syringe and 55 ± 43 mrem (range: 0–130 mrem) when using an injection device. Per minute of lateral fluoroscopy, the average injection dose is 23.6 mrem with the use of the 1-mL syringe and 7.3 mrem for the injection device.[14] An additional study by Komemushi et al found that the mean radiation doses outside the lead apron were 320.8 µSv when using a 1-mL syringe and 116.2 µSv using a bone cement injector. This study also concluded that the use of bone cement injector was effective at reducing the dose of radiation the physician is exposed to.[13] However, as the procedural time is longer when using the injection device, the total dose per injection for the two methods is similar.[14]

Schils et al found that the use of a new cement delivery system (CDS) reduced the radiation dose to the finger, wrist, and leg of the operator by greater than 80% when performing balloon kyphoplasty procedures when compared to the classical bone filler injection mechanism. They claim that the use of the CDS would allow surgeons to operate far below the most severe annual radiation exposure limits.[15]

An additional study by Kruger et al stated that the average radiation dose per vertebroplasty procedure was 2.04 mSv/vertebrae to the hands and 1.44 mSv/vertebrae to the whole body before the implementation of radiation-reducing techniques. A significant reduction to the dose of radiation was seen after implementing these radiation-reduction techniques such as the use of shielding devices that provide maximum protection from scatter radiation to the physician's hands, upper extremities, and eyes. The dose of radiation to the operator's hands was reduced to 0.074 mSv/vertebrae per procedure and the dose to the whole body was reduced to 0.004 mSv/vertebrae.[16]

The dose of radiation decreases as the distance from the source increases. Von Wrangel et al discovered that moving the X-ray tube to the side of the patient opposite from the side of the operator reduced the radiation dose to the operator from lateral fluoroscopy at the thoracic and lumbar levels by a factor of 4 to 5. They also found a 30 to 40% reduction in radiation dose to the hands of the operator when wearing protective gloves.[17]

A 2004 study by Perisinakis et al found that the mean total fluoroscopy time for kyphoplasty was 10.1 ± 2.2 minutes and that the mean effective radiation dose to patients undergoing kyphoplasty was 8.5 to 12.7 mSv. They also determined that the mean gonadal dose ranged from 0.04 to 16.4 mGy, which was dependent on the level of the vertebra being treated. They also stated that skin injuries were more likely if the source of radiation was less than 35 cm from the skin or if there was an extended total fluoroscopy time per injection.[18]

Given that protective precautions and technique play a substantial role in minimizing radiation to the operator, knowledge of this equipment and these factors can help formulate a strategy to keep the radiation dose as low as reasonably allowable. The goal is to keep the quality of work as high as possible while keeping the radiation dose to the patient and operator as low as possible.

Acknowledgment

We would like to thank J. Beam, J. Coltrane, and E. Clapton for inspiration.

References

[1] ORSIF. Invisible Impact: The Risk of Ionizing Radiation on Cath Lab Staff [Video File]. United States, Trillium Studios. May 15, 2015.Available at: https://www.youtube.com/watch?v=rXgt0bF3GJM

[2] There is no safe dose of radiation. In: Interventional News. Issue 59. London, UK: Biba Publishing; 2015:6

[3] International Commission on Radiological Protection (ICRP). Statement on Tissue Reactions. ICRP ref. 4825-3093-1464. 2011. Available at: http://www.icrp.org/docs/icrp%20statement%20on%20tissue%20reactions.pdf

[4] International Commission on Radiological Protection (ICRP). The 2007 Recommendations of the International Commission on Radiological Protection. Publication 103 Ann ICRP 2007;37(2–4):1–332

[5] Roguin A, Goldstein J, Bar O, Goldstein JA. Brain and neck tumors among physicians performing interventional procedures. Am J Cardiol 2013;111(9):1368–1372

[6] Reeves RR, , Ang L, Bahadorani J, et al. Interventional cardiologists are exposed to greater left sided cranial radiation: the BRAIN study (brain radiation exposure and attenuation during invasive cardiology procedures). JACC Cardiovasc Interv 2015;8(9):1197–1206

[7] Bhogal N, Jalali F, Bristow RG. Microscopic imaging of DNA repair foci in irradiated normal tissues. Int J Radiat Biol 2009;85(9):732–746

[8] Gudkov AV, Komarova EA. The role of p53 in determining sensitivity to radiotherapy. Nat Rev Cancer 2003;3(2):117–129

[9] Friedberg W, Duke FE, Snyder L, et al. The cosmic radiation environment at air carrier flight altitudes and possible associated health risks. Radiat Prot Dosimetry 1993;48(1):21–25

[10] Yong LC, Sigurdson AJ, Ward EM, et al. Increased frequency of chromosome translocations in airline pilots with long-term flying experience. Occup Environ Med 2009;66(1):56–62

[11] Ashmore JP, Krewski D, Zielinski JM, Jiang H, Semenciw R, Band PR. First analysis of mortality and occupational radiation exposure based on the National Dose Registry of Canada. Am J Epidemiol 1998;148(6):564–574

[12] Andersson M, Engholm G, Ennow K, Jessen KA, Storm HH. Cancer risk among staff at two radiotherapy departments in Denmark. Br J Radiol 1991;64(761):455–460

[13] Komemushi A, Tanigawa N, Kariya S, Kojima H, Shomura Y, Sawada S. Radiation exposure to operators during vertebroplasty. J Vasc Interv Radiol 2005;16(10):1327–1332

[14] Kallmes DF, O E, Roy SS, et al. Radiation dose to the operator during vertebroplasty: prospective comparison of the use of 1-cc syringes versus an injection device. AJNR Am J Neuroradiol 2003;24(6):1257–1260

[15] Schils F, Schoojans W, Struelens L. The surgeon's real dose exposure during balloon kyphoplasty procedure and evaluation of the cement delivery system: a prospective study. Eur Spine J 2013;22(8):1758–1764

[16] Kruger R, Faciszewski T. Radiation dose reduction to medical staff during vertebroplasty: a review of techniques and methods to mitigate occupational dose. Spine 2003;28(14):1608–1613

[17] von Wrangel A, Cederblad A, Rodriguez-Catarino M. Fluoroscopically guided percutaneous vertebroplasty: assessment of radiation doses and implementation of procedural routines to reduce operator exposure. Acta Radiol 2009;50(5):490–496

[18] Perisinakis K, Damilakis J, Theocharopoulos N, Papadokostakis G, Hadjipavlou A, Gourtsoyiannis N. Patient exposure and associated radiation risks from fluoroscopically guided vertebroplasty or kyphoplasty. Radiology 2004;232(3):701–707

14 Appropriateness Criteria for Vertebral Augmentation

Alexios Kelekis and Dimitrios K. Filippiadis

Summary

Clinical practice decisions regarding how to treat certain fractures remain heterogeneous and traditionally there has been little consensus of what type of vertebral augmentation procedure should be used to treat specific fracture types. Various medical societies have produced their own recommendations for treating vertebral compression fractures but the most important document that has been developed to establish a clinical care pathway for the treatment of

Vertebral compression fractures (VCFs) has been the UCLA/RAND appropriateness criteria recommendations published in 2018 by a multispecialty group of physicians. These criteria included clinical signs and symptoms of VCFs that need vertebral augmentation as well as imaging criteria for choosing vertebral augmentation over nonsurgical management (NSM). There were seven key factors identified that determined the appropriateness of proceeding with vertebral augmentation as opposed to treating with NSM. The treatment choice was strongly influenced by the clinical variables and the difference in patient characteristics. The clinical factors that determined the overall choice of treatment included the clinical exam and imaging findings, the duration of pain, the impact of the VCF on daily functioning, the degree of height reduction, and kyphotic deformity, whether there was progressive vertebral body height loss and the overall evolution of symptoms. The contraindications for performing vertebral augmentation were also narrowed and refined and treatment recommendations were put forth for dealing with the underlying condition (i.e. osteoporosis) that gave rise to the fracture.

Keywords: appropriateness criteria, Magerl classification, UCLA/RAND methodology, clinical care pathway

14.1 Introduction

VCFs can be related to osteoporosis, trauma, or malignancy. The end result is pain and mobility impairment with a high impact on life quality as well as morbidities resulting in reduced life expectancy.[1] Therapeutic options include NSM (pain medication, bracing, bed rest, etc.) and vertebral augmentation by means of vertebroplasty (VP), balloon kyphoplasty (BKP), or spinal implants (stents, jacks, peek cages, etc.).[1,2] The wide variety in the causes and the characteristics of a VCF necessitate a tailored-based therapeutic approach taking into account both the advantages and limitations of each treatment. At the moment, clinical practice decisions are driven by operator's preference and/or international guidelines, which can be divergent and sometimes contradictory. There is no predictive tool available that will be able to identify the ideal therapeutic approach for a given VCF with specific characteristics. Furthermore, there is a clear lack of appropriateness criteria that will govern a therapy based on the expected benefits that should outweigh the potential complications by a sufficient margin in order to render the technique worth doing. A recent systematic review of evidence-based guidelines for the management of VCFs showed considerable inconsistencies in the treatment recommendations as well as in the recommendations for the diagnostic evaluation and the prevention of future fractures.[3]

14.2 Indications, Guidelines, and Recommendations

Standard indications for vertebral augmentation include symptomatic (painful) type A fractures according to the Magerl classification (most commonly type A1 fractures) with bone edema on MRI (►Fig. 14.1) and/or positive bone scan scintigraphy. The patient should be an adult reporting at least moderate pain (Visual Analog Scale >4 units) at the respective level, with absence of neurologic impairment and no absolute contraindications to therapy (e.g., active infection at the surgical site or the presence of an untreated blood borne infection).[1,2,4] Depending on the fracture's specific characteristics, different techniques of vertebral augmentation can be utilized.

Although many scientific organizations have published guidelines regarding the indications for vertebral augmentation, none provides a tailored approach based upon the unique characteristics of a specific vertebral fracture. Furthermore, almost all the documents mention standard

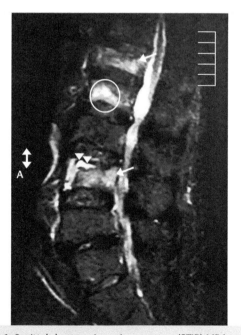

Fig. 14.1 Sagittal short tau inversion recovery (STIR) MR image showing acute or subacute vertebral compression fractures with bone marrow edema (areas of increased signal as shown by the *white arrows*). In L1 vertebral body there is suspected initial cavity formation with high signal intensity in the center (area within *white oval*). A fluid-filled cavity is seen under the upper end plate of L3 vertebral body (*white arrowheads*).

VP and balloon augmentation omitting spinal implants, which constitute a paradigm shift away from cement injection performed either with or without using bone tamps. According to the 2013 NICE guidelines and position paper 5, standard VP and balloon augmentation without stenting should be offered to patients with severe ongoing pain and in whom the pain has been confirmed to be at the level of the fracture by physical examination and imaging after a recent, unhealed vertebral fracture that continues to produce significant discomfort despite optimal pain management.[5] According to a position paper released by multiple scientific societies including the Society of Interventional Radiology (SIR), American Society of Neuroradiology (ASNR), American College of Radiology (ACR), American Association of Neurological Surgeons (AANS), Congress of Neurological Surgeons (CNS), American Society of Spine Radiology (ASSR), Canadian Interventional Radiology Association (CIRA), and the Society of NeuroInterventional Surgery (SNIS), vertebral augmentation remains a proven medically appropriate therapy for treatment of painful VCFs refractory to nonoperative medical therapy and for vertebrae weakened by neoplasia when performed for the medical indications outlined in the published standards.[6–10] The American Academy of Orthopaedic Surgeons (AAOS) guidelines are a distinct outlier with recommendations against VP and for BKP as a treatment option for painful VCFs.[11] According to ACR guidelines, both vertebral augmentation techniques are similar and should be offered as a second-line therapy after NSM with balloon augmentation resulting in better angular correction and fracture reduction.[12] The Standards and Guidelines Committee of the SNIS reports that both VP and kyphoplasty are indicated in symptomatic osteoporotic or cancer-related VCFs refractory to medical therapy.[13] The Cardiovascular and Interventional Radiological Society of Europe (CIRSE) in the recently published guidelines for vertebral augmentation include in the indications for VP painful osteoporotic fractures, painful vertebrae due to benign tumors or malignant

infiltration, Kummels' disease, symptomatic vertebrae plana, acute stable A1 and A3 fractures according to the Magerl classification, and chronic traumatic fractures (▶Fig. 14.2, ▶Fig. 14.3, ▶Fig. 14.4). In the same document, indications for balloon augmentation include all the aforementioned, but it is reported that the best indication for the technique is a traumatic acute (<7–10 days) fracture (particularly Magerl A1) with a local kyphotic angle less than 15 degrees.[4] The CIRSE guidelines include indications for the application of spinal implants that, according to the authors, can be used in all the indications valid for VP and balloon augmentation.[4] The spine metastatic disease working group suggests that vertebral augmentation can be proposed in the

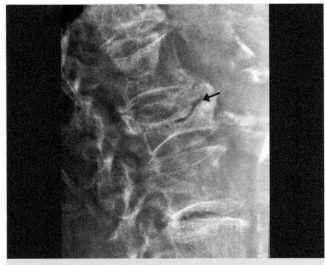

Fig. 14.2 Lateral X-ray view of the lumbar spine showing vacuum cleft phenomenon (*black arrow*) in an upper lumbar vertebral body indicative of a fracture nonunion and an unstable vertebral body.

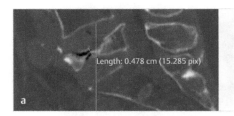
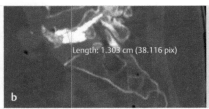

Fig. 14.3 Sagittal CT reconstructions of the lumbar spine showing a vertebra plana at L5 in a symptomatic patient **(a)** before and **(b)** after vertebral augmentation. The height of the midportion of the vertebral body was measured at 0.478 cm prior to vertebral augmentation and 1.303 cm afterward.

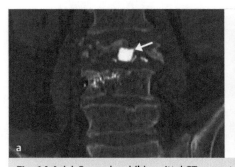
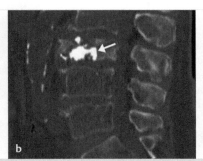
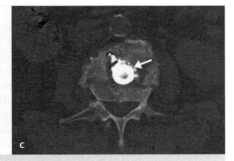

Fig. 14.4 **(a)** Coronal and **(b)** sagittal CT reconstructions and **(c)** an axial CT image of the lumbar spine showing a Magerl A3.3 vertebral fracture treated with a vertebral implant (Kiva device) and PMMA (polymethyl methacrylate; *white arrows*).

cases in which there is no metastatic epidural spinal cord compression and in the cases of fracture prophylaxis after radiation therapy or after percutaneous ablation for local tumor control.[14] These recommendations are especially important in patients with relatively good prognoses.[14] Additionally, according to the same authors, vertebral augmentation techniques are recommended for first-line pain palliation treatment, related to stable pathologic VCFs.[14] The American Society for Radiation Oncology (ASTRO) guidelines comment that there are no prospective data suggesting that either kyphoplasty or VP would obviate the need for EBRT (external beam radiotherapy) for painful bone metastases, but these two different therapies can certainly be complimentary.[15]

14.3 Appropriateness Criteria

In order to establish a clinical care pathway for VCFs, criteria to be considered include clinical signs and symptoms, imaging criteria for choosing vertebral augmentation techniques over NSM, contraindications for vertebral augmentation, and posttherapy follow-up.[16] Decisive variables for performing or not performing vertebral augmentation as well as for selecting one technique over the other include time passed since the fracture occurrence, MR imaging findings including number and type of fractured vertebrae, computed tomography (CT) findings of bone deformity, impact of the fracture on daily functioning, evolution of symptoms, spinal deformity (including kyphotic angle), proof of ongoing fracture process, and pulmonary dysfunction. An international, multispecialty utilization review showed excellent applicability of and good adherence to RAND/UCLA-based recommendations on treatment choice in osteoporotic VCFs. The treatment choice was strongly associated with the clinical variables used in the panel study. Differences in patient characteristics largely determined the different treatment decisions made by the clinicians and time since fracture was the most dominant clinical factor.[17] The UCLA/RAND recommendations published in 2018 by a multispecialty group of physicians from the United States found several key factors in determining the clinical appropriateness of vertebral augmentation, but in these recommendations (▶Fig. 14.5) duration of time since fracture occurrence was considered far less relevant for determining the appropriate treatment choice (▶Table. 14.1).[16] Overall some of the

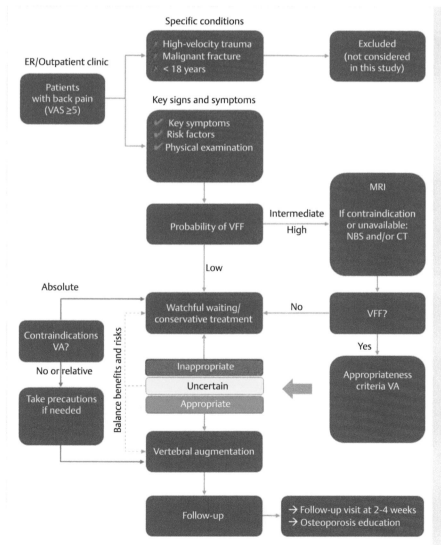

Fig. 14.5 Clinical care pathway for the treatment of osteoporotic vertebral compression fractures.[16]

important clinical factors that determine the treatment choice for the patient are as follows:

- The clinical exam should include pain, tenderness on palpation or closed fist percussion, vertebral height reduction and progression of height loss, as well as evolution of symptoms.[16]
- MR imaging should be the preferred imaging modality for the evaluation of VCFs, although scintigraphy can help indicate

Table 14.1 Key factors in determining the appropriateness of vertebral augmentation*[16]

Variable	Value	p-value
Duration of pain	<1 wk† 1–3 wk 3–6 wk >6 wk	<0.001
Advanced image findings	Negative† Positive	<0.001
Impact of vertebral fragility fracture on daily functioning	Moderate† Severe	<0.001
Degree of height reduction	Mild (<25%)† Moderate (25–40%)	<0.001
Kyphotic deformity	Severe (>40%)	<0.01
Progression of height loss	No† Yes	<0.001
Evolution of symptoms	No† Yes	<0.001

* Outcomes of logistic regression analysis for the panel outcome that VA = appropriate (vs. NSM = appropriate + equivocal/uncertain).
† Reference category.

the appropriate level. CT can be used for bone fragment identification.

- Timing of the fracture (acute or chronic) should not be confused with the presence of bone edema on the short tau inversion recovery (STIR) sequence of the MR imaging examination. Both acute and chronic fractures can show bone edema (illustrated as increased signal intensity in STIR sequence), which is a sign of bone marrow activity.
- According to the literature, vertebral body height restoration and kyphotic angle correction seem to be better achieved by BKP.[18–20] However, the number of vertebrae to be treated is significant for kyphotic angle correction with a proportionally greater improvement in sagittal alignment seen with the treatment of a greater number of vertebral bodies.[21]
- Standard techniques of vertebral augmentation are effective in treating low-velocity burst fractures but, at the same time, there is an increased risk of secondary in situ fracture.[22] Spinal implants along with cement could work as an additional intrinsic support structure providing the extra stability necessary in these cases.
- The impact of the fracture on daily functioning, evolution of symptoms, progression of vertebral body height loss, pulmonary dysfunction, and the degree of spinal and kyphotic deformity are important decision-making factors for performance of vertebral augmentation (▶Fig. 14.6).[16] The clinical consequences of kyphosis and vertebral fractures include decreased pulmonary function, decreased appetite with resultant nutritional impact, frailty, and increased future VCF risk, as well as central nervous system symptoms such as increased sensitivity and intolerance to pain and balance problems.[23,24]
- A cavity containing either vacuum phenomenon or fluid is an indication for vertebral augmentation.

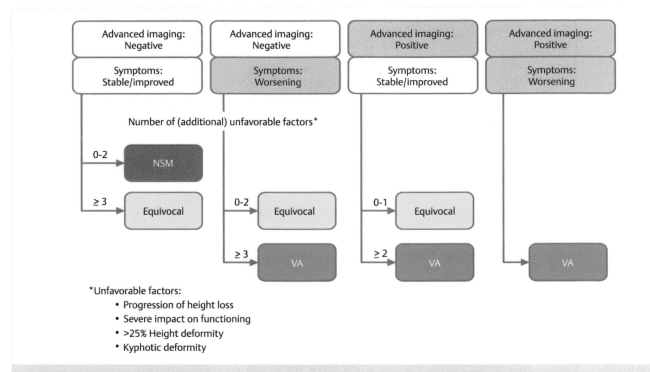

*Unfavorable factors:
- Progression of height loss
- Severe impact on functioning
- >25% Height deformity
- Kyphotic deformity

Fig. 14.6 Vertebral augmentation is appropriate in patients with positive imaging findings, with worsening symptoms and in patients with two to four unfavorable factors.

Table 14.2 Absolute and relative contraindications for vertebral augmentation (VA)[16]

Condition	Panel recommendation
Active infection at surgical site	**Absolute contraindication** for current VA.
Untreated blood-borne infection	**Absolute contraindication.** Preoperative antibiotic (parenteral) therapy is required. Once cultures are negative, following an appropriate period of antibiotic therapy, one can proceed with caution.
Osteomyelitis	Usually a **strong contraindication** for VA. In rare situations, VA may be considered, for example, if the patient is not stable for an open procedure and the infection is chronic and caused by a less virulent organism. The infection may then be controlled locally with antibiotic-loaded cement and long-term antibiotic suppression.
Pregnancy	Although VA is **usually contraindicated** in pregnant patients, there may be exceptional situations in which benefits could prevail over risks. Radiation exposure to the fetus should be minimized.
Allergy to fill material	**Relative contraindication**, depending on the severity of the allergy. If prior reactions were not associated with severe anaphylaxis, the allergy can be pretreated with steroids, Tylenol, and Benadryl. Alternatively, another fill material can be chosen.
Coagulopathy	**Relative contraindication.** Try to normalize/correct clotting function if possible (INR [international normalized ratio] < 1.7). The risk of bleeding should be balanced against the complications from bed rest. Caution in patients with thrombocytopenia (platelets < 30,000/µL).
Spinal instability	**Relative contraindication**, depending on the degree of instability and level of fracture. If needed, plan an additional intervention to address instability, possibly but not necessarily in the same session.
Myelopathy from the fracture	**Relative contraindication.** Decompression and stabilization is the preferred option, but VA may be considered if the patient is unable to undergo surgery. Coordination with spine surgeon and neurologist is mandatory.
Neurologic deficit	**Relative contraindication.** Additional decompression with or without stabilization may be required. Patients should be informed about the risk of cement in the spinal canal. Coordination with spine surgeon and neurologist is mandatory.
Neural impingement	**Relative contraindication**, depending on the degree. Take extra care to avoid delivery of cement into canal or neural foramen. An additional open procedure may be needed.
Fracture retropulsion/canal compromise	**Generally not a contraindication.** Avoid hyperextension or aggravating stenosis. A CT scan may be used to determine integrity of the posterior wall.

Table 14.3 Patient follow-up after vertebral augmentation (VA) for Vertebral compression fracture (VCF)

Follow-up after treatment for VCF

1. After either vertebral augmentation (VA) or conservative treatment, a follow-up visit should be planned at 2–4 wk.

2. In patients with a satisfactory result of VA at first follow-up (2–4 wk after the procedure), there is generally no need for further postoperative monitoring. Follow-up for management of the underlying pathology does not need to be managed by the proceduralist.

3. All patients presenting with VCF should be referred for evaluation of bone mineral density and osteoporosis education for subsequent treatment as indicated.

4. All patients with VCF should be instructed to take part in an osteoporosis prevention/treatment program.

5. If symptoms are not resolved at follow-up, repeat imaging (preferably MRI) is mandatory.

6. If the pain is not resolved after VA, repeat augmentation (at the same level) may be considered, but it does require a careful diagnostic evaluation to identify any other sources of pain (additional fractures, facet arthropathy, etc.).

- Absolute contraindications for vertebral augmentation include infection at the surgical site such as diskitis/osteomyelitis or an untreated blood-borne infection and relative contraindications are listed in ▶Table 14.2.[16]
- Follow-up evaluation should be performed at 2 to 4 weeks after treatment. Usually no further follow-up for fracture treatment is needed upon a satisfactory result, but the patient will almost always need further treatment for the underlying disorder (i.e., osteoporosis) that produced the fracture (▶Table 14.3).[16]

A literature meta-analysis comparing VP and kyphoplasty for single-level VCF treatment concludes that both techniques are similar in terms of long-term pain relief, function outcome, and new adjacent fracture rate, but there is superiority with kyphoplasty in terms of injected cement volume, short-term pain relief, improvement in short- and long-term kyphotic angle, and a lower cement leakage rate. This superiority comes at the cost of longer procedural times and higher material expenses.[18] Similar results have been reported by Evans et al and Liu et al in two prospective randomized trials.[19,20] At the moment, according to the literature, there is no clearly proven superiority of one technique over the other. An alternative approach may be that of modeling detailed treatment algorithms for patients with specific fracture types and clinical characteristics including the variables mentioned in this chapter.

References

[1] Filippiadis DK, Marcia S, Masala S, Deschamps F, Kelekis A. Percutaneous vertebroplasty and kyphoplasty: current status, new developments and old controversies. Cardiovasc Intervent Radiol 2017;40(12):1815–1823

[2] Filippiadis DK, Marcia S, Ryan A, et al. New implant-based technologies in the spine. Cardiovasc Intervent Radiol 2018;41(10):1463–1473

[3] Parreira PCS, Maher CG, Megale RZ, March L, Ferreira ML. An overview of clinical guidelines for the management of vertebral compression fracture: a systematic review. Spine J 2017;17(12):1932–1938

[4] Tsoumakidou G, Too CW, Koch G, et al. CIRSE guidelines on percutaneous vertebral augmentation. Cardiovasc Intervent Radiol 2017;40(3):331–342

[5] NICE guidance. Percutaneous vertebroplasty and percutaneous balloon kyphoplasty for treating osteoporotic vertebral compression fractures. Technology appraisal guidance. 2013. Available at: nice.org.uk/guidance/ta279

[6] Barr JD, Jensen ME, Hirsch JA, et al; Society of Interventional Radiology. American Association of Neurological Surgeons. Congress of Neurological

Surgeons. American College of Radiology. American Society of Neuroradiology. American Society of Spine Radiology. Canadian Interventional Radiology Association. Society of Neurointerventional Surgery. Position statement on percutaneous vertebral augmentation: a consensus statement developed by the Society of Interventional Radiology (SIR), American Association of Neurological Surgeons (AANS) and the Congress of Neurological Surgeons (CNS), American College of Radiology (ACR), American Society of Neuroradiology (ASNR), American Society of Spine Radiology (ASSR), Canadian Interventional Radiology Association (CIRA), and the Society of NeuroInterventional Surgery (SNIS). J Vasc Interv Radiol 2014;25(2):171–181

[7] Barr JD, Mathis JM, Barr MS, et al. Standard for the performance of percutaneous vertebroplasty. In: American College of Radiology Standards 2000–2001. Reston, VA: American College of Radiology; 2000:441–448

[8] McGraw JK, Cardella J, Barr JD, et al; SIR Standards of Practice Committee. Society of Interventional Radiology quality improvement guidelines for percutaneous vertebroplasty. J Vasc Interv Radiol 2003;14(7):827–831

[9] Lewis CA, Barr JD, Cardella JF, et al. Practice Guidelines for the Performance of Percutaneous Vertebroplasty. Reston, VA: American College of Radiology; 2005

[10] McGraw JK, Barr JD, Cardella JF, et al. Practice Guidelines for the Performance of Percutaneous Vertebroplasty. Reston, VA: American College of Radiology; 2009

[11] Esses SI, McGuire R, Jenkins J, et al. The treatment of symptomatic osteoporotic spinal compression fractures. J Am Acad Orthop Surg 2011;19(3):176–182

[12] ACR Appropriateness Criteria. Management of vertebral compression fractures. 2013. Available at: https://acsearch.acr.org/docs/70545/Narrative/

[13] Chandra RV, Meyers PM, Hirsch JA, et al. Society of NeuroInterventional Surgery. Vertebral augmentation: report of the Standards and Guidelines Committee of the Society of NeuroInterventional Surgery. J Neurointerv Surg 2014;6(1):7–15

[14] Wallace AN, Robinson CG, Meyer J, et al. The metastatic spine disease multidisciplinary working group algorithms. Oncologist 2015;20(10):1205–1215

[15] Lutz S, Balboni T, Jones J, et al. Palliative radiation therapy for bone metastases: update of an ASTRO evidence-based guideline. Pract Radiat Oncol 2017;7(1):4–12

[16] Hirsch JA, Beall DP, Chambers MR, et al. Management of vertebral fragility fractures: a clinical care pathway developed by a multispecialty panel using the RAND/UCLA appropriateness method. Spine J 2018;18(11):2152–2161

[17] Schupfner R, Stoevelaar HJ, Blattert T, et al. Treatment of Osteoporotic Vertebral Compression Fractures: Applicability of Appropriateness Criteria in Clinical Practice. Pain Physician 2016;19(1):E113–E120

[18] Wang H, Sribastav SS, Ye F, et al. Comparison of percutaneous vertebroplasty and balloon kyphoplasty for the treatment of single level vertebral compression fractures: a meta-analysis of the literature. Pain Physician 2015;18(3):209–222

[19] Evans AJ, Kip KE, Brinjikji W, et al. Randomized controlled trial of vertebroplasty versus kyphoplasty in the treatment of vertebral compression fractures. J Neurointerv Surg 2016;8(7):756–763

[20] Liu JT, Liao WJ, Tan WC, et al. Balloon kyphoplasty versus vertebroplasty for treatment of osteoporotic vertebral compression fracture: a prospective, comparative, and randomized clinical study. Osteoporos Int 2010;21(2):359–364

[21] Pradhan BB, Bae HW, Kropf MA, Patel VV, Delamarter RB. Kyphoplasty reduction of osteoporotic vertebral compression fractures: correction of local kyphosis versus overall sagittal alignment. Spine 2006;31(4):435–441

[22] Nieuwenhuijse MJ, Putter H, van Erkel AR, Dijkstra PD. New vertebral fractures after percutaneous vertebroplasty for painful osteoporotic vertebral compression fractures: a clustered analysis and the relevance of intradiskal cement leakage. Radiology 2013;266(3):862–870

[23] Silverman SL. The clinical consequences of vertebral compression fracture. Bone 1992;13(Suppl 2):S27–S31

[24] Kado DM, Lui LY, Ensrud KE, Fink HA, Karlamangla AS, Cummings SR; Study of Osteoporotic Fractures. Hyperkyphosis predicts mortality independent of vertebral osteoporosis in older women. Ann Intern Med 2009;150(10):681–687

15 Literature Analysis of Vertebral Augmentation

Nicole S. Carter, Hong Kuan Kok, Julian Maingard, Hamed Asadi, Lee-Anne Slater, Thabele Leslie-Mazwi, Joshua A. Hirsch, and Ronil V. Chandra

Summary

Vertebral augmentation procedures (vertebroplasty and kyphoplasty) provide benefit for debilitating vertebral compression fractures (VCFs) or fractures refractory to nonsurgical management (NSM). These procedures involve the image-guided reduction of the vertebral fracture and injection of cement into the vertebral body. The key goals are the relief of back pain, enhancement of functional status, and biomechanical stabilization of the vertebral body. Successful integration of vertebral augmentation into clinical practice is assisted by a good understanding of the current evidence in the medical literature. Although historically there has been occasional controversy over the efficacy of vertebroplasty for VCFs, there is now high-quality evidence from well-designed, large randomized controlled trials to support its use for acute osteoporotic VCFs with intractable pain despite medical therapy or for VCFs secondary to spinal neoplasm. Moderate-quality evidence supports vertebral augmentation to treat chronic and subacute osteoporotic VCFs. The current evidence suggests that vertebroplasty and kyphoplasty are both effective in providing pain relief although kyphoplasty has a small advantage in pain relief and is significantly better for improving patients' quality of life. The risk of major complications associated with vertebral augmentation is low with rare reports described across large trials. The risk of morbidity and mortality of patients treated with NSM has been reported in multiple analyses to be significantly higher than those patients treated with vertebroplasty or kyphoplasty. This chapter provides an analysis of the current literature on the safety and efficacy of vertebral augmentation procedures. The design, inclusion criteria, outcomes, and limitations of major randomized controlled trials on efficacy are presented along with data on procedural safety, complication rates, cement extravasation, and secondary fracture.

Keywords: vertebral augmentation, vertebral compression, fracture, vertebroplasty, kyphoplasty, osteoporosis, metastasis

15.1 Introduction

Vertebral augmentation procedures (vertebroplasty [VP] and kyphoplasty) involve the image-guided injection of polymethyl methacrylate (PMMA) cement into a fractured vertebral body. The majority of these minimally invasive procedures are performed for a subset of vertebral compression fractures (VCFs) that are refractory to nonsurgical management (NSM) or that are severely debilitating to the patient. The key goals are the relief of back pain, the enhancement of functional status, and biomechanical stabilization of the vertebral body. Vertebral augmentation was first described in 1987, and early enthusiasm was driven by positive results in observational studies. Since that time, over 3,000 articles have been published on vertebral augmentation procedures, and a number of randomized controlled trials (RCTs) have investigated the efficacy and safety of VP and kyphoplasty. The most recent literature provides high-quality evidence that vertebral augmentation procedures are safe and effective in the treatment of VCFs due to osteoporosis and malignancy.

The aim of this chapter is to analyze the current literature on vertebral augmentation procedures. A historical background is presented using early observational data. The design, key outcomes, and limitations of major RCTs are examined. High-quality data on procedural safety outcomes, including overall complication rates, cement leakage, and secondary fracture, are reviewed.

15.2 Early Data

VP was first performed in 1984 but not reported in literature until 1987 by Galibert et al, for the treatment of an aggressive vertebral hemangioma at C2.[1] The procedure provided complete pain relief for the patient, and was subsequently performed for six other patients. Shortly thereafter, the procedure was applied to treat the pain associated with osteoporotic and neoplastic compression fractures.[2] Following further success in small European series, Jensen et al introduced VP to the United States. In 1997, they published results from 29 patients with 47 painful osteoporotic compression fractures. Almost all (90%) patients reported pain relief and improved mobility within 24 hours of the procedure. The publication of several series followed.[3] In 2006, a pooled analysis of VP studies from 1989 to 2004 included 2,086 patients. In the 19 studies that reported pain outcomes from VP, there was significant postprocedure reduction of pain (mean visual analog scale [VAS] reduction of 8.1 to 2.6; $p < 0.001$) and serious complications occurred in less than 1%.[4]

Kyphoplasty was first described in 2001 by Lieberman et al as an alternative procedure with potentially lower risks of cement extravasation and a potential for greater height restoration of the vertebral body.[5] A pooled analysis of 26 kyphoplasty studies that included 1,710 patients found significant postprocedure improvements in pain intensity, mobility, and functional capacity. Vertebral alignment was also improved, with increased anterior vertebral height and reduction of kyphosis.[6]

These promising early data led medical societies to support vertebral augmentation as an effective treatment for osteoporotic VCF refractory to medical management.[7] However, there remained a lack of robust RCT data to support the efficacy of VP over NSM.

15.3 Evidence for Efficacy

15.3.1 Vertebroplasty

Early uptake of VP was rapid and driven by positive early data from observational studies and meta-analyses. However, two RCTs having a total of approximately 200 patients across both studies published in the New England Journal of Medicine (NEJM) found that VP offered no significant benefit over NSM. Since that time, these articles have been widely discredited and downgraded in their level of evidence category, but they have provided incentive for additional investigation of the efficacy of VP. Several large randomized trials have been released in recent years, focusing on rigorous inclusion criteria and minimizing methodological limitations. The key findings of the main prospective VP trials are summarized in ►Table 15.1.

The 2007 VERTOS trial was the first multicenter prospective RCT to compare VP to medical management for pain relief in osteoporotic VCFs.[8] Inclusion criteria included severe back pain persisting despite medical therapy for at least 6 weeks, fracture aged less than 6 months, focal tenderness on physical examination, and bone marrow edema on MRI. In total, 34 patients were randomized to receive VP (n = 18) or conservative management (n = 16). The primary outcome measures were back pain intensity (as measured by the VAS) and analgesic use at 1 day and 2 weeks. Analgesic requirement was quantified by assigning ordinal variables to different analgesic types: 0 (no analgesia required), 1 (paracetamol/acetaminophen), 2 (nonsteroidal anti-inflammatory medications) or 3 (opioids).

VP resulted in significant pain relief at 1 day postprocedure, with reduction in the baseline mean VAS from 7.1 to 4.7 (difference between groups –2.4 in favor of VP). While this effect was not maintained at the 2-week endpoint, 88% of patients from the conservative group had crossed over to the VP group. Analgesic

use was reduced in the VP group (–1.4; 95% confidence interval [CI] –2.1 to –0.8). Secondary outcomes of disability—defined by Roland–Morris Disability Questionnaire (RMDQ)—and quality of life (QOL; Quality of Life Questionnaire of the European Foundation for Osteoporosis [QUALEFFO]) were also significantly improved in the VP group.

The main limitations of the VERTOS trial were its small size and lack of blinding. No long-term follow-up was possible, as crossover was permitted after 2 weeks and 14 out of 16 patients in the conservative group requested crossover to VP.

In 2009, two RCTs comparing VP to a sham procedure for osteoporotic VCFs were published in the NEJM.[9,10] The results of both trials contrasted with earlier observational and meta-analysis data, and called into question the efficacy of VP. The Investigational Vertebroplasty Safety and Efficacy Trial (INVEST) screened 1,812 patients to randomize 131 to receive either VP (n = 68) or a sham procedure (n = 63).[9] Due to low initial recruitment, the proposed sample size was reduced from 250 to 130 patients, and the inclusion criteria were broadened. Inclusion criteria were as follows: age older than 50 years, pain intensity of ≥3/10 on numerical rating scale (NRS), and fracture age less than 1 year. Undetermined fracture ages were confirmed using MRI or radionuclide bone scan. The sham procedure involved the injection of local anesthetic onto the periosteum of the pedicle, combined with placing pressure

Table 15.1 Major prospective trials evaluating vertebroplasty for osteoporotic vertebral compression fractures

	INVEST	Buchbinder et al	VERTOS II	VAPOUR
Publication year	2009	2009	2010	2016
Total enrolment (n)	131	78	202	120
Comparator	Sham (periosteal anesthetic)	Sham (periosteal anesthetic)	Conservative management	Sham (subcutaneous anesthetic)
Mean (SD) age (y)	73.8 (9.4)	76.6 (12.1)	75.2 (9.8)	80.5 (7)
Pain score threshold	NRS ≥ 3/10	None	VAS ≥ 5/10	NRS ≥ 7/10
Mean (SD) baseline pain score (0–10 scale)	7.0 (1.9)	7.3 (2.2)	7.8 (1.5)	8.6
Number (%) with severe pain (0–10 scale)	61 (47%) ≥ 8	38 (49%) ≥ 8	NR	120 (100%) ≥ 7
Fracture age threshold (wk)	<52	<52	<6	<6
Mean (SD) fracture age (wk)	22.5 (16.3)	11.7 (11.1)	5.6	2.6
Number (%) with fractures <6 wk	26 (20%)	31 (40%)	202 (100%)	120 (100%)
Advanced imaging (MRI, SPECT) required?	No	Yes	Yes	Yes
Mean PMMA volume (mL)	NR	2.8	4.1	7.5
Primary endpoint	Pain relief and RMDQ at 1 month	Pain relief at 3 mo	Pain relief at 1 mo	Percent NRS <4/10 at 2 wk
Primary outcome	No difference	No difference	Vertebroplasty superior	Vertebroplasty superior
Notable secondary endpoints	Quality of life (EQ-5D)	Disability (RMDQ), quality of life (QUALEFFO, EQ-5D)	Disability (RMDQ), quality of life (QUALEFFO)	Disability (RMDQ), quality of life (QUALEFFO), analgesic use
Secondary outcomes	No difference	No difference	Vertebroplasty superior	Vertebroplasty superior

Abbreviations: MRI, magnetic resonance imaging; NR, not reported; NRS, numerical rating scale; PMMA polymethyl methacrylate; QUALEFFO, Quality of Life Questionnaire of the European Foundation for Osteoporosis; RMDQ, Roland–Morris Disability Questionnaire; SD, standard deviation; SPECT, single-photon emission computed tomography.

on the patient's back and opening a container of methacrylate monomer to replicate PMMA odor. At 1-month follow-up, there was no difference between groups in back pain NRS ($p = 0.19$) or disability (measured by RMDQ score; $p = 0.06$). No long-term follow-up was feasible due to crossover; by 3 months, 27 patients (43%) in the control group had crossed to the VP arm.

Key limitations of the INVEST were that the trial was underpowered and suffered from prominent selection bias (screened 1,812 patients to enroll 131), the crossover of patients in the INVEST trial was far greater for those patients crossing over from sham to VP (51%) as compared to the VP patients crossing over to sham (13%), the inclusion of fractures up to 12 months old, and the lack of inclusion requirements for physical examination or advanced imaging with MRI or radionuclide bone scan. The clinical and imaging diagnostic criteria for inclusion were very different from those of most RCTs, with patients having a pain score of 3 or more on the VAS being eligible for inclusion. There was no description of a clinical examination used to determine if the pain came from the VCF itself or from another issue. There was also criticism that the INVEST trial was not a true sham, with 63% of the sham patients correctly guessing their treatment, and with the injection performed using a paraspinal injection of local anesthetic that has been used to successfully palliate patients' pain from VCFs for up to 8 weeks.[11] Despite all of these limiting factors, if the same response rate for the 131 patients had been carried out to the originally intended 250 patients, VP would have been found to be significantly better than sham treatment at a p-value of less than 0.01. Additionally, if only one patient had reported a different response (i.e., a favorable response in the VP group or an unfavorable response in the sham group), VP would have been found to be significantly better than sham with a p-value of less than 0.04.

A second multicenter sham-controlled RCT on VP for osteoporotic VCFs was published in the NEJM in 2009, by Buchbinder et al.[10] This trial included patients with back pain of less than 12 months' duration and fracture confirmed on MRI with bone marrow edema or fracture line. A total of 78 patients were enrolled from four recruiting centers, and randomized to VP ($n = 38$) or sham procedure ($n = 40$) groups. The sham procedure did not involve the injection of anesthetic; a needle was inserted onto the lamina, with the sharp stylet replaced by a blunt stylet. To further simulate VP, the vertebral body was lightly tapped, and PMMA was mixed in the room but not injected. No significant difference between groups in pain scores was observed at 1 week, 3 months, or 6 months. There was also no difference in disability and quality-of-life (QOL) scores.

As with INVEST, Buchbinder and colleagues did not require a physical examination component and there was no description of a clinical examination used to ascertain VCF-related pain. The Buchbinder trial assessed "overall pain" rather than spine-related pain, undermining the validity of the measurement in this population replete with potentially comorbid painful conditions. Both subacute and chronic fractures (up to 12 months old) were included, with only 32% of patients having fractures less than 6 weeks old. Similar to the INVEST, the Buchbinder trial experienced difficulties with enrolment, taking 4.5 years to enroll only 78 patients, and making this trial subject to selection bias. Additionally, 68% of patients in the study were recruited at one of the four centers, with two of the remaining

centers recruiting only five patients. This may have caused outcomes to be weighted to the treatment effect at a single center. This single center tended to inject only small amounts of PMMA with the mean volume of cement being 2.8 mL. A later review by Boszczyk et al concluded that the data strongly indicate that the treatment arm included patients who were not treated in a reasonably effective manner.[12]

In 2012, a meta-analysis was published that included prospective randomized and nonrandomized trials comparing VP to NSM or sham therapy for osteoporotic VCFs.[13] Nine trials were analyzed, including INVEST, Buchbinder et al, and VERTOS II, with a total of 886 patients. No difference in pain relief was found between VP and sham procedure groups due to the reliance on the previously discussed VP versus sham trials as the only two trials of this type. When compared to the NSM used to treat patients with painful VCFs, however, VP was found to be superior to NSM at all time points studied, in both pain relief and QOL measures.

Several authors expressed dissatisfaction with the findings of the 2009 trials, raising concerns about the inclusion and exclusion criteria, the use of small volumes of PMMA cement, the selection bias, the precarious statistical calculations, the high rate of crossover, the low initial pain scores, the inclusion of worker compensation patients, the use of a sham that is a known active treatment, the absence of an appropriate physical examination component, and the lack of long-term follow-up.[14-16] In response, in 2013 Comstock et al published a study that followed up the INVEST cohort over 12 months to determine long-term outcomes.[17] At 1 year, there was a modest pain reduction in the VP arm, although no differences in disability measures were found. The potential for the INVEST sham group to have acted as an "active control," thus confounding results, was also raised.[18,19] The same year, a meta-analysis by Anderson et al was published that analyzed both NEJM sham studies and downgraded them to level II data based on flawed inclusion criteria (in both studies) and a subsequent high crossover rate (in the Comstock et al study). This downgrade was based on the Cochrane Risk of Bias table and Levels of Evidence for Primary Research as adopted by the North America Spine Society.[20]

There remained no large multicenter RCT comparing VP with medical management, until the 2010 publication of VERTOS II by Klazen and colleagues.[21] Addressing some previous concerns from the 2009 trials, it included fractures of less than 6 weeks' duration, with pain severity of ≥5/10, focal tenderness on examination, and bone marrow edema on MRI. The 202 enrolled patients were randomized equally into VP and conservative management groups. At 1 month, VP resulted in significantly reduced back pain. The mean reduction in VAS score was 2.6 greater (95% CI: 1.74–3.37; $p < 0.0001$) in the VP arm than in the conservative arm, and this effect was durable at 1 year. VP also resulted in improved QOL (as measured by several standardized questionnaires) and significant (VAS reduction >3 points) pain relief was achieved earlier in VP (30 vs. 116 days; $p < 0.0001$).

Farrokhi et al followed with a trial comparing VP and medical management for osteoporotic VCFs in 2011.[22] Inclusion criteria included severe pain despite NSM for 4 weeks, fractures aged 4 weeks to 1 year, focal tenderness on examination, and bone marrow edema or fracture cleft on MRI. Eighty-two patients were randomized to receive VP ($n = 40$) or NSM. At 1 week, there was reduction in VAS (difference of −3.1; $p < 0.001$)

and improvement in the QOL measures in the VP arm. Pain relief was durable to 6 months, while QOL outcomes sustained to 36 months. All VP patients were able to ambulate at 24 hours postprocedure, compared with 2% in the conservative group. VP also resulted in increased vertebral body height (mean 8 mm) and reduction in kyphosis (mean 8 degrees).

A further RCT comparing VP with medical management for osteoporotic VCFs followed in 2012, by Blasco and colleagues.[23] Inclusion criteria were moderate pain (VAS ≥ 4/10), fractures aged ≤12 months, and edema on MRI or increased uptake on radionuclide bone scan. A total of 125 patients were enrolled and randomized to VP ($n = 64$) or NSM ($n = 61$) arms. VP resulted in greater VAS and lower requirement for rescue analgesia (5% of patients requiring rescue analgesia compared with 25% of the medical arm).

In 2016, the VAPOUR (Vertebroplasty for Acute Painful Osteoporotic Fractures) trial aimed to compare VP with a sham procedure while addressing some of the limitations of earlier trials.[24,25] An appropriately higher pain threshold was utilized (>7/10 compared with >3 in INVEST and no pain threshold in Buchbinder et al), all fractures were less than 6 weeks old, and all fractures were imaged with MRI or single photon emission computed tomography (SPECT). In total, 120 patients were randomized to receive VP ($n = 61$) or a sham procedure involving subcutaneous injection of local anesthetic ($n = 59$). At 2 weeks, VP resulted in significant pain reduction, with NRS scores decreasing to less than 4/10 in 44% of VP patients. This effect was sustained at 1 and 6 months. VP also led to improved QOL questionnaire scores, reduced functional disability, reduced analgesic requirements, and increased height of the vertebral body.

In a 2016 prospective trial, Yang et al randomized 135 patients aged ≥70 years to receive VP or conservative therapy.[26] Early VP resulted in faster and greater pain relief and improved QOL, at 1 week, 1, 3, and 6 months, and 1 year ($p < 0.0001$). Surveys conducted at follow-up revealed that patients in the VP arm had greater overall satisfaction with their given treatment.

There are fewer high-quality studies available for VP in the treatment of neoplasm-related VCFs. A 2011 systematic review of 30 studies, with a total of 987 patients, found reductions in back pain ranging from 20.3 to 78.9% at 1 month following VP. At 6 months, pain reduction ranged between 47 and 87%.[27] A 2016 systematic review performed by Health Quality Ontario included 78 studies, with a total of 2,545 VP patients with fractures due to spinal metastases, multiple myeloma, or hemangioma.[28] They reported an overall rapid (within 48 hours) reduction in mean pain intensity scores following VP, along with parallel reduction in disability measures and opioid use.

15.3.2 Kyphoplasty

The Fracture Reduction Evaluation (FREE) trial, published in 2009, was a multicenter prospective randomized trial comparing kyphoplasty to NSM for VCFs.[29] Inclusion criteria were severe back pain (≥4/10) for ≤3 months, focal tenderness on examination, and MRI findings of bone marrow edema, vertebral body height loss, or pseudoarthrosis. A total of 300 patients were randomized to receive kyphoplasty ($n = 149$) or conservative management ($n = 151$). The primary outcome was QOL at 1 month, as measured by change in short-form 36 questionnaire (SF-36) physical component summary (PCS)

scale. These measures, along with back pain intensity scores and disability (RMDQ), were also evaluated at 1, 3, 6, and 12 months.

Kyphoplasty resulted in significant improvement in QOL when compared to NSM, with mean SF-36 scores improving 5.2 points more in the kyphoplasty group than the NSM arm (95% CI: 2.9–7.4; $p < 0.0001$). This outcome was durable at 3 and 6 months ($p < 0.0008$; $p < 0.0064$), but not at 12 months ($p = 0.208$). Kyphoplasty also led to significantly reduced back pain scores at 1 week ($p < 0.0001$) and 12 months ($p = 0.0034$). Analgesic use was reduced in the kyphoplasty group at 1 and 6 months. Two-year outcome data released by the FREE authors revealed that there remained a significant reduction in back pain scores for patients undergoing kyphoplasty ($p = 0.009$). However, there were no significant differences in SF-36 or RMDQ scores. The FREE trial also included both osteoporotic and neoplastic fractures, but only 4 of 300 patients had pathologic fractures.

The Cancer Patient Fracture Evaluation (CAFE) RCT compared kyphoplasty with NSM for malignant VCFs.[30] Inclusion criteria included pain intensity of ≥4/10, RMDQ disability score of ≤10, and vertebral fracture demonstrated on plain radiographs or MRI. Patients with index fractures due to primary or osteoblastic bone tumors were excluded. A total of 134 patients were enrolled and received either kyphoplasty ($n = 70$) or NSM ($n = 64$). At 1 month, there was a significant reduction in RMDQ scores in the kyphoplasty arm (difference between groups of 8.4 in favor of kyphoplasty), meeting the primary outcome. Kyphoplasty also resulted in greater pain relief, reduced analgesic use, and improved QOL (measured by SF-36), at all time points throughout the 12-month follow-up period.

A limitation of the CAFE trial was the lack of histological confirmation of fracture etiology. Although all participants were cancer patients, it was not known whether the fracture was caused by metastasis, osteoporosis, radionecrosis, or a combination thereof. The trial featured an opportunity for patients to crossover at 1 month with 38 of the 52 (73%) patients in the conservative group that completed the 1-month evaluation crossing over to kyphoplasty and 55% of these patients crossed over within 1 week after their 1-month visit.

The 2019 EVOLVE study, the largest trial of kyphoplasty efficacy conducted to date, compared 12-month disability and safety outcomes in a Medicare-eligible population.[31] A total of 350 patients enrolled at 24 U.S. sites received kyphoplasty for painful VCFs. Four primary endpoints were evaluated: NRS back pain scores, disability (represented by Owestry Disability Index [ODI] score), and QOL (EQ-5D and SF-36 scores). At 3 months, there were significant improvements in all primary outcomes. Mean NRS improved from 8.7 to 2.7, while ODI improved from 63.4 to 27.1. These effects were significant at all other time points measured (7 days and 1, 3, 6, and 12 months). Of all treated patients, only 5 procedure-related complications were reported; each event resolved with treatment.

Kyphoplasty may involve the adjunct use of a curet before or after inflation of the balloon tamp in an attempt to scrape away sclerotic bone that may impede the restoration of vertebral body height. The 2013 randomized trial comparing 2 techniques of balloon kyphoplasty and curette use for obtaining vertebral body height restoration and angular-deformity correction in vertebral compression fractures due to osteoporosis (SCORE) trial randomized patients with osteoporotic VCFs to receive kyphoplasty procedures in which the curet was used prior to balloon inflation (n = 57), or following inflation, followed by a second balloon tamp (n = 55).[32] Vertebral body height restoration and pain relief were significantly improved in both treatment approaches, with no significant difference between groups.

15.3.3 Vertebroplasty Compared with Kyphoplasty

The randomized trial comparing balloon kyphoplasty and vertebroplasty for vertebral compression fractures due to osteoporosis (KAVIAR) trial, published in 2014, directly compared VP and kyphoplasty in the treatment of osteoporotic VCFs.[33] A total of 381 patients with acute painful VCFs due to osteoporosis were randomly assigned to receive VP (n = 190) or kyphoplasty (n = 191), and were not blinded to the treatment received. All fractures were confirmed by imaging with MRI, radioisotope bone scan, or CT. The trial was terminated early, significantly short of the enrolment target of 1,234 with only 404 patients. Despite the lack of statistical power needed to demonstrate the difference between VP and kyphoplasty, both techniques resulted in statistically significant and sustained clinical improvement from baseline for pain, function, and QOL measurements.

Liu et al also compared VP and kyphoplasty for the treatment of painful VCFs in their 2010 prospective RCT.[34] One-hundred patients with osteoporotic VCFs were randomized to receive VP or kyphoplasty (comprising 50 in each group). Both procedures resulted in significantly reduced VAS pain scores, as well as improvements in vertebral height and kyphotic wedge angle. While there was no significant difference between groups in clinical outcomes, kyphoplasty resulted in higher periprocedural costs.

Röllinghoff et al found comparable results in their prospective study of 90 patients with VCFs treated with VP or kyphoplasty.[35] Both procedures provided significant benefits in QOL and pain relief (p < 0.001), with no statistically significant difference between the two in these clinical outcomes. However, kyphoplasty resulted in greater restoration of vertebral body height than VP, while the rate of cement leakage was lower in the VP group.

A 2015 meta-analysis (including eight studies with 845 total patients) found that VP and kyphoplasty were similar with regard to long-term pain relief, short- and long-term functional improvement, and risk of new adjacent VCF.[36] Kyphoplasty was superior to VP in short-term pain reduction, improvement of the kyphotic angle, and also resulted in lower rates of cement leakage.

The most complete meta-analysis published in 2012 examined the English-language articles and found that out of 1,587 vertebral augmentation manuscripts there were 27 level I and II articles including 8 randomized studies.[37] There were nine articles that compared VP to kyphoplasty. Pooled patient data were combined into one analyzable study group. Following this analysis of the highest quality data available, the authors concluded that kyphoplasty decreased pain to a greater degree than VP (5.07 vs. 4.55 points on the VAS) and resulted in significantly better improvement in QOL than both VP and NSM.

15.3.4 The Kiva System

The 2015 KAST study evaluated the Kiva system, a novel vertebral augmentation implantation device used to treat painful VCFs with minimal cement leakage.[38] A total of 300 patients with painful osteoporotic VCFs were randomized to receive Kiva (n = 153) or kyphoplasty (n = 147). At 12-month follow-up, Kiva was shown to be noninferior to kyphoplasty with regard to the primary outcomes of back pain (VAS) and disability (ODI) reduction. Secondary outcomes included cement volume usage, cement leakage, and adjacent vertebral fracture; analysis of these endpoints revealed superiority of the Kiva system over kyphoplasty.

15.4 Evidence for Safety

15.4.1 Overall Complications

The overall risk of serious complications from vertebral augmentation is very low.[39-42] Although uncommon, potential major complications that have been reported in the literature include neurologic damage from nerve or spinal cord injury, pulmonary embolism from cement or fat emboli, infection, hematoma, allergic or idiosyncratic reactions, hemothorax, pneumothorax, and fracture to vertebrae, ribs, or sternum.[43-47] Mortality from vertebral augmentation is exceedingly rare, with no procedural mortalities across all RCTs reviewed. Rare cases of death from cement anaphylaxis or cardiovascular collapse have been reported.[48]

Across major RCTs of vertebral augmentation for osteoporotic fractures, the rate of major complications was approximately 1%.[40-42] In the VERTOS II trial, the only complications occurring in the 101 patients referable to VP were 1 urinary tract infection (UTI) and 1 case of asymptomatic cement leakage into a segmental pulmonary artery. Buchbinder et al reported one thecal sac injury that did not require any specific treatment, while INVEST reported one case of osteomyelitis in a patient who did not receive prophylactic antibiotics. In the VAPOUR trial, there was one case of respiratory arrest following sedation prior to the procedure. This patient was treated with vertebral augmentation uneventfully 48 hours later. One patient in the VP group sustained a humeral fracture during transfer onto the procedure table. Conversely, two patients in the conservative arm had interval vertebral collapse with spinal cord compression. In the FREE trial, the only complications referable to kyphoplasty from the 149 patients were 1 soft-tissue hematoma and 1 UTI.

In the 2013 meta-analysis by Anderson et al, which examined prospective RCTs (including VERTOS, VERTOS II, INVEST, Buchbinder et al, and FREE) comparing VP or kyphoplasty to sham or conservative treatment for osteoporotic fractures,[20] there were no statistically significant differences in adverse events between vertebral augmentation and conservative arms. Minor adverse events reported from augmentation included asymptomatic cement leaks, soft-tissue hematoma, and vasovagal events.

15.4.2 Cement Leakage

Extraosseous leakage of PMMA cement is the major source of complications from vertebral augmentation. Asymptomatic leakage is common on postprocedural CT imaging; cement embolization may occur frequently, while symptomatic leakage is rare.[43-49] In VERTOS II, 72% of treated vertebral bodies had cement leakage on CT, with all patients remaining asymptomatic. Most leaks were diskal or into segmental veins, while none occurred in the spinal canal.[21] Reported rates of cement extravasation were lower in other RCTs, occurring in 36% of patients in the trial by Buchbinder et al and 34% in VAPOUR, likely related to the assessments with conventional radiography.[10,24]

While embolization to the pulmonary arteries has previously been characterized as an adverse event, it in fact can occur quite commonly, with reported rates of 5 to 23% of all patients.[50–52] It is important to note, however, that the vast majority of embolisms and extravasation are neither symptomatic nor produce adverse outcomes.[53]

Kyphoplasty has been shown to result in lower rates of cement extravasation, as inflation of the balloon tamp creates a path of least resistance into which cement is subsequently injected. In the FREE study, cement leakage occurred in 27% of treated vertebrae on imaging with intraoperative fluoroscopy and postoperative radiographs. All patients remained asymptomatic.[29] Cement extravasation occurred in only 2 of 70 patients in the CAFE trial; 1 case was asymptomatic, while the other, a diskal leakage, was associated with adjacent-level fracture on day 1 postprocedure.[30]

Malignant tumors frequently lead to regions of destroyed bone at the vertebral cortex, which may increase the risk of cement leakage into the surrounding tissues.[4] In a retrospective study of CT-guided VP for malignant vertebral fractures, local cement leak was evident in 59% of vertebrae (194 of 331).[54] Six percent of leaks occurred into the spinal canal through the posterior cortex, despite osteolysis of the posterior wall being apparent in 49%. Pulmonary cement emboli were demonstrated in 2% (1 of 53) of chest radiographs and 11% (10 of 88) of chest CT scans.[47] In a prospective study of 106 patients with multiple myeloma treated with VP, cement leakage was detected on CT in 23% of vertebrae.[55] Most leaks occurred into perivertebral veins (85%), and all events of leakage were asymptomatic. Pulmonary cement emboli were detected in 5% of patients.[48]

15.4.3 Subsequent Fractures

It is very unlikely that vertebral augmentation increases the risk of new or adjacent-level VCF compared to NSM.[49,56] An initial single-arm prospective study by Tanigawa et al followed up 194 patients with 500 osteoporotic VCFs treated by VP over the long term.[57] New VCFs were detected in 33.5% of patients using conventional radiographs. Of the new fractures, 63.1% were in adjacent vertebrae, and 36.9% in nonadjacent vertebrae. Of note, 12 patients with new VCFs diagnosed remained asymptomatic. No significant link was noted between the volume of cement injected and the rates of adjacent VCF. In a retrospective study of 88 postmenopausal women treated with VP, 14 patients suffered collapse of an adjacent vertebra within 1 month. Risk of collapse was significantly associated with advanced age and decreased lumbar and hip bone mineral density (BMD).[58]

However, in a 2017 meta-analysis of 12 comparative studies encompassing 1,328 patients, Zhang et al compared the incidence of new VCFs following vertebral augmentation and conservative management. No significant difference was seen between the two cohorts in either total new vertebral fractures or adjacent fractures.[59] Comparable results were displayed in the meta-analysis by Anderson et al, which found no significant differences between vertebral augmentation and conservative arms with regard to rates of subsequent fracture.[20] Shi et al, who performed a meta-analysis of prospective trials comparing VP with sham or conservative management for osteoporotic VCFs, also found no difference between arms in the risk of new VCF ($p = 0.82$).[13] In a larger meta-analysis, Papanastassiou et al analyzed all of the level I and II data on vertebral augmentation and determined that the additional fracture rate for those patients treated with vertebral augmentation was 12% compared with 23% for those patients treated with NSM.[37] A 2014 prospective study of 290 patients receiving vertebral augmentation or NSM found no significant difference between groups in additional VCFs.[60] However, additional VCFs occurred sooner in the vertebral augmentation group. This temporal difference in fracture appearance after vertebral augmentation could explain the perception that vertebral augmentation can predispose the patient to more subsequent fractures because the subsequent fractures after vertebral augmentation happen sooner than in patients treated with NSM. In a meta-analysis of 19 studies, Xiao et al compared postprocedure complication rates between VP and kyphoplasty. The authors of this study found no significant difference between procedures in subsequent adjacent-level fractures.[61]

A 2017 biomechanical study on cadaveric spines aimed to assess how fractures and VP affect vertebral deformation and loading.[62] Fracture of the vertebrae caused deformations to both the fractured and adjacent levels, and transferred compressive load onto the neural arch. These effects were significantly reduced by VP, which reduced anterior vertebral body deformation by 62% at fractured levels and 52% at adjacent levels.

The potential benefits of prophylactic VP to reduce postaugmentation adjacent-level fracture was investigated by Eichler et al in a retrospective study.[63] Thirty-seven patients treated with kyphoplasty for osteoporotic VCFs were included; 19 patients received kyphoplasty alone and 18 were treated with additional VP at the adjacent level. Prophylactic VP at adjacent levels did not reduce the rate of subsequent fractures after kyphoplasty. The authors concluded that adjacent-level fractures following vertebral augmentation are most likely related to underlying osteoporosis rather than the procedure itself.

15.5 Mortality Benefit

The excess mortality risk from osteoporotic VCF is considerable, ranging from 2 to 42% in the first year following fracture.[64] An analysis of the U.S. Medicare population (97,142 patients with VCF and 428,956 controls) revealed 3- and 5-year mortality rates of 46 and 69%, respectively, in VCF patients, compared with 22 and 36% in the control group.[65]

While none of the currently published large RCTs were powered to evaluate mortality reduction, there is some evidence that vertebral augmentation may confer a mortality benefit. A 2017 review of U.S. Medicare data, encompassing 261,756 kyphoplasty patients and 117,232 VP patients, evaluated vertebral augmentation utilization and VCF mortality risk.[6] In the years following the 2009 sham-controlled RCTs, there was a sharp decline in vertebral augmentation procedures. This time period was associated with elevated mortality risk in VCF patients when compared with the years preceding 2009, which saw higher uptake of vertebral augmentation procedures.

The first longitudinal, population-based comparison of mortality risk between interventional and NSM groups was performed in 2011 and included 858,978 patients treated with kyphoplasty, VP, or NSM.[67] Patients who received augmentation had a significantly higher survival rate than the NSM group (60.8% compared with 50%; $p < 0.001$). At 4-year follow-up, median life expectancy was 2.2 to 7.3 years greater across the vertebral augmentation groups than for NSM. However, due to its retrospective, observational design, this study was limited by the inability to evaluate causal relationships between surgical management, NSM, and patient survival.

In 2015, the same authors published a similar retrospective study of the U.S. Medicare population that identified 1,038,956 VCF patients, of which 141,343 underwent kyphoplasty and 75,365 underwent VP.[68] The nonoperated cohort had a 55% higher mortality risk than those treated with kyphoplasty, and a 25% higher risk than those treated with VP ($p < 0.001$). Of note, the nonoperated cohort had higher rates of pneumonia, UTI, deep vein thrombosis, and cardiac complications than the kyphoplasty cohort. In an analysis of Taiwanese health insurance data, 10,785 patients with painful VCF were identified. The mortality risk was 39% higher in those receiving medical management than in those treated with VP.[69] In a similar analysis of German claims data (including 3,607 VCF patients), those who received vertebral augmentation had a 43% lower mortality risk over the 5-year period.[70]

A comparative study of 5,766 VCF patients, of which 17% underwent kyphoplasty, revealed that kyphoplasty was associated with greater likelihood of discharge home (38.4 vs. 21% for NSM) and lower in-hospital mortality rate (26.1 vs. 34.8%).[71] In 2011, a retrospective study of a large hospital patient database compared mortality rates after vertebral augmentation with inpatient pain management and bracing.[72] Augmentation significantly improved survival for up to 2 years compared with NSM, regardless of patient age or gender, the number of VCFs, or comorbidity profile.

Contrasting results were found by McCullough et al, who selected 9,017 pairs from Medicare claims data treated with vertebral augmentation or NSM, matched by patient demographics and comorbidities.[73] While initial mortality and rates of medical complications were lower in the vertebral augmentation group, there were no significant differences between groups in mortality at 1 year, and the vertebral augmentation group had higher rates of health care utilization. However, this study is potentially subject to methodological limitations. The authors hypothesized that vertebral augmentation patients are healthier than patients given NSM, and hence attempted to control for selection bias by matching comorbidities between groups. Yet patient selection only considered a limited set of baseline comorbidities, and did not account for other conditions that may have led to VCFs. Furthermore, data showed that the control group, theorized to have poorer health compared

with augmentation patients, had significantly lower Quan comorbidity scores and lower rates of prior inpatient admissions; this is suggestive of improved health in the control group. To investigate preprocedure health status, the authors selected a subgroup of 3,023 patients who had not yet undergone augmentation by 30 days post-VCF. This excluded patients who may have needed emergent care, and thus may have led to a misleading estimation of preprocedure health status. Finally, the authors concluded that there was no mortality improvement for patients after vertebral augmentation despite three of their four analysis points showing statistically significant mortality improvement and the fourth point was close to statistical significance at $p = 0.18$. Their conclusion of no mortality benefit was at odds with their own data that suggest otherwise.

15.6 Conclusion

There is robust evidence to support vertebral augmentation as a safe and effective option to improve patients' pain, function, and QOL on those individuals presenting with moderate to severe pain and functional debilitation due to a VCF. Evidence for the efficacy of VP in osteoporotic VCFs has evolved over time. Early sham-controlled RCTs were designed to mitigate the possible placebo effects, but they had very problematic methodological limitations. More recent studies, including a large sham-controlled RCT that utilized rigorous inclusion criteria, have shown treatment benefits. Two large RCTs comparing kyphoplasty with conservative therapy have demonstrated benefits in both osteoporotic and neoplastic fractures, although a trial comparing kyphoplasty to a sham procedure has not yet been performed and may never be performed given the ethical concerns over the higher rates of morbidity and mortality in patients treated with NSM rather than vertebral augmentation. The risks of serious complications from vertebral augmentation are very low, and mortality directly related to the procedure is exceedingly rare. There is recent evidence to suggest that the complication rate, rate of morbidity, and rate of mortality are significantly less for patients undergoing vertebral augmentation than those patients undergoing NSM.

15.7 Key Points

- Vertebral augmentation procedures provide pain relief, functional improvement, and improved QOL in patients with painful VCFs refractory to medical management.
- There is high-quality evidence to support the use of VP for pain relief in acute osteoporotic VCFs. While two large sham-controlled randomized trials found no benefit from VP, these were flawed by serious methodological limitations, and more recent RCTs have demonstrated significant improvements in pain, disability, and QOL.
- There are data from large RCTs to support the use of kyphoplasty for VCFs.
- The risk of complications is exceedingly low. Complications generally result from unrecognized extravasation of bone cement and may include nerve or spinal cord injury,

pulmonary embolism, or infection. However, the vast majority of cement extravasations are asymptomatic. Mortality from vertebral augmentation is exceptionally rare.

- VCFs cause considerable excess mortality in patients with osteoporosis and vertebral neoplasm. There is recent evidence showing that vertebral augmentation confers a significant morbidity and mortality benefit in those patients treated with augmentation as opposed to those patients treated. with NSM.

References

[1] Galibert P, Deramond H, Rosat P, Le Gars D. Preliminary note on the treatment of vertebral angioma by percutaneous acrylic vertebroplasty Neurochirurgie 1987;33(2):166–168

[2] Bascoulergue Y, Duquesnel J, Leclercq R, et al. Percutaneous injection of methyl methacrylate in the vertebral body for the treatment of various diseases: percutaneous vertebroplasty. [abstract] Radiology 1988;169:372

[3] Jensen ME, Evans AJ, Mathis JM, Kallmes DF, Cloft HJ, Dion JE. Percutaneous polymethylmethacrylate vertebroplasty in the treatment of osteoporotic vertebral body compression fractures: technical aspects. AJNR Am J Neuroradiol 1997;18(10):1897–1904

[4] Hochmuth K, Proschek D, Schwarz W, Mack M, Kurth AA, Vogl TJ. Percutaneous vertebroplasty in the therapy of osteoporotic vertebral compression fractures: a critical review. Eur Radiol 2006;16(5):998–1004

[5] Lieberman IH, Dudeney S, Reinhardt MK, Bell G. Initial outcome and efficacy of "kyphoplasty" in the treatment of painful osteoporotic vertebral compression fractures. Spine 2001;26(14):1631–1638

[6] Bouza C, Lopez T, Magro A, et al. Efficacy and safety of balloon kyphoplasty in the therapy of osteoporotic vertebral compression fractures. Eur Radiol 2006;16:998–1004

[7] Jensen ME, McGraw JK, Cardella JF, Hirsch JA. Position statement on percutaneous vertebral augmentation. J Vasc Interv Radiol 2007;18(3):325–330

[8] Voormolen MH, Mali WP, Lohle PNM, et al. Percutaneous vertebroplasty compared with optimal pain medication treatment: short-term clinical outcome of patients with subacute or chronic painful osteoporotic vertebral compression fractures. The VERTOS study. AJNR Am J Neuroradiol 2007;28(3):555–560

[9] Kallmes DF, Comstock BA, Heagerty PJ, et al. A randomized trial of vertebroplasty for osteoporotic spinal fractures. N Engl J Med 2009;361(6):569–579

[10] Buchbinder R, Osborne RH, Ebeling PR, et al. A randomized trial of vertebroplasty for painful osteoporotic vertebral fractures. N Engl J Med 2009;361(6):557–568

[11] Wang B, Guo H, Yuan L, Huang D, Zhang H, Hao D. A prospective randomized controlled study comparing the pain relief in patients with osteoporotic vertebral compression fractures with the use of vertebroplasty or facet blocking. Eur Spine J 2016;25:3486–3494

[12] Boszczyk B. Volume matters: a review of procedural details of two randomised controlled vertebroplasty trials of 2009. Eur Spine J 2010;19(11):1837–1840

[13] Shi MM, Cai XZ, Lin T, Wang W, Yan SG. Is there really no benefit of vertebroplasty for osteoporotic vertebral fractures? A meta-analysis. Clin Orthop Relat Res 2012;470(10):2785–2799

[14] Aebi M. Vertebroplasty: about sense and nonsense of uncontrolled "controlled randomized prospective trials." Eur Spine J 2009;18(9):1247–1248

[15] Noonan P. Randomized vertebroplasty trials: bad news or sham news? AJNR Am J Neuroradiol 2009;30(10):1808–1809

[16] Bono CM, Heggeness M, Mick C, Resnick D, Watters WC III. North American Spine Society: newly released vertebroplasty randomized controlled trials: a tale of two trials. Spine J 2010;10(3):238–240

[17] Comstock BA, Sitlani CM, Jarvik JG, Heagerty PJ, Turner JA, Kallmes DF. Investigational vertebroplasty safety and efficacy trial (INVEST): patient-reported outcomes through 1 year. Radiology 2013;269(1):224–231

[18] Manchikanti L, Boswell MV, Kaye AD, Helm Ii S, Hirsch JA. Therapeutic role of placebo: evolution of a new paradigm in understanding research and clinical practice. Pain Physician 2017;20(5):363–386

[19] Manchikanti L, Knezevic NN, Boswell MV, Kaye AD, Hirsch JA. Epidural injections for lumbar radiculopathy and spinal stenosis: a comparative clinical review and meta-analysis. Pain Physician 2016;19(3):E365–E410

[20] Anderson PA, Froyshteter AB, Tontz WL Jr. Meta-analysis of vertebral augmentation compared with conservative treatment for osteoporotic spinal fractures. J Bone Miner Res 2013;28(2):372–382

[21] Klazen CA, Lohle PN, de Vries J, et al. Vertebroplasty versus conservative treatment in acute osteoporotic vertebral compression fractures (Vertos II): an open-label randomised trial. Lancet 2010;376(9746):1085–1092

[22] Farrokhi MR, Alibai E, Maghami Z. Randomized controlled trial of percutaneous vertebroplasty versus optimal medical management for the relief of pain and disability in acute osteoporotic vertebral compression fractures. J Neurosurg Spine 2011;14(5):561–569

[23] Blasco J, Martinez-Ferrer A, Macho J, et al. Effect of vertebroplasty on pain relief, quality of life, and the incidence of new vertebral fractures: a 12-month randomized follow-up, controlled trial. J Bone Miner Res 2012;27(5):1159–1166

[24] Clark W, Bird P, Gonski P, et al. Safety and efficacy of vertebroplasty for acute painful osteoporotic fractures (VAPOUR): a multicentre, randomised, double-blind, placebo-controlled trial. Lancet 2016;388(10052):1408–1416

[25] Hirsch JA, Chandra RV. Resurrection of evidence for vertebroplasty? Lancet 2016;388(10052):1356–1357

[26] Yang EZ, Xu JG, Huang GZ, et al. Percutaneous vertebroplasty versus conservative treatment in aged patients with acute osteoporotic vertebral compression fractures: a prospective randomized controlled clinical study. Spine (Phil Pa 1976) 2016;41(8):653–660

[27] Chew C, Craig L, Edwards R, Moss J, O'Dwyer PJ. Safety and efficacy of percutaneous vertebroplasty in malignancy: a systematic review. Clin Radiol 2011;66(1):63–72

[28] Pron G, Holubowich C, Kaulback K; Health Quality Ontario. Vertebral augmentation involving vertebroplasty or kyphoplasty for cancer-related vertebral compression fractures: a systematic review. Ont Health Technol Assess Ser 2016;16(11):1–202

[29] Wardlaw D, Cummings SR, Van Meirhaeghe J, et al. Efficacy and safety of balloon kyphoplasty compared with non-surgical care for vertebral compression fracture (FREE): a randomised controlled trial. Lancet 2009;373(9668):1016–1024

[30] Berenson J, Pflugmacher R, Jarzem P, et al; Cancer Patient Fracture Evaluation (CAFE) Investigators. Balloon kyphoplasty versus non-surgical fracture management for treatment of painful vertebral body compression fractures in patients with cancer: a multicentre, randomised controlled trial. Lancet Oncol 2011;12(3):225–235

[31] Beall DP, Chambers MR, Thomas S, Amburgy J, Webb JR, Goodman BS, et al. Prospective and multicenter evaluation of outcomes for quality of life and activities of daily living for balloon kyphoplasty in the treatment of vertebral compression fractures: the EVOLVE trial. Neurosurg 2019;84(1):169–178

[32] Bastian L, Schils F, Tillman JB, Fueredi G; SCORE Investigators. A randomized trial comparing 2 techniques of balloon kyphoplasty and curette use for obtaining vertebral body height restoration and angular-deformity correction in vertebral compression fractures due to osteoporosis. AJNR Am J Neuroradiol 2013;34(3):666–675

[33] Dohm M, Black CM, Dacre A, Tillman JB, Fueredi G; KAVIAR investigators. A randomized trial comparing balloon kyphoplasty and vertebroplasty for vertebral compression fractures due to osteoporosis. AJNR Am J Neuroradiol 2014;35(12):2227–2236

[34] Liu JT, Liao WJ, Tan WC, et al. Balloon kyphoplasty versus vertebroplasty for treatment of osteoporotic vertebral compression fracture: a prospective, comparative, and randomized clinical study. Osteoporos Int 2010;21(2):359–364

[35] Röllinghoff M, Siewe J, Zarghooni K, et al. Effectiveness, security and height restoration on fresh compression fractures: a comparative prospective study of vertebroplasty and kyphoplasty. Minim Invasive Neurosurg 2009;52(5–6):233–237

[36] Wang H, Sribastav SS, Ye F, et al. Comparison of percutaneous vertebroplasty and balloon kyphoplasty for the treatment of single level vertebral compression fractures: a meta-analysis of the literature. Pain Physician 2015;18(3):209–222

[37] Papanastassiou ID, Phillips FM, Van Meirhaeghe J, et al. Comparing effects of kyphoplasty, vertebroplasty, and non-surgical management in a systematic review of randomized and non-randomized controlled studies. Eur Spine J 2012;21(9):1826–1843

[38] Tutton SM, Pflugmacher R, Davidian M, Beall DP, Facchini FR, Garfin SR. KAST study: the Kiva system as a vertebral augmentation treatment—a safety and effectiveness trial: a randomized, noninferiority trial comparing the Kiva system with balloon kyphoplasty in treatment of osteoporotic vertebral compression fractures. Spine (Phila Pa 2976) 2015;40(12):865–875

[39] McGirt MJ, Parker SL, Wolinsky JP, Witham TF, Bydon A, Gokaslan ZL. Vertebroplasty and kyphoplasty for the treatment of vertebral compression fractures: an evidenced-based review of the literature. Spine J 2009;9(6):501–508

[40] McGraw JK, Cardella J, Barr JD, et al. Society of Interventional Radiology Standards of Practice Committee quality improvement guidelines for percutaneous vertebroplasty. J Vasc Interv Radiol 2003;14(1):311–315

[41] Chandra RV, Yoo AJ, Hirsch JA. Vertebral augmentation: update on safety, efficacy, cost effectiveness and increased survival? Pain Physician 2013;16(4):309–320

[42] Nussbaum DA, Gailloud P, Murphy K. A review of complications associated with vertebroplasty and kyphoplasty as reported to the Food and Drug Administration medical device related web site. J Vasc Interv Radiol 2004;15(11):1185–1192

[43] Yazbeck PG, Al Rouhban RB, Slaba SG, Kreichati GE, Kharrat KE. Anterior spinal artery syndrome after percutaneous vertebroplasty. Spine J 2011;11(8):e5–e8

[44] Ratliff J, Nguyen T, Heiss J. Root and spinal cord compression from methylmethacrylate vertebroplasty. Spine 2001;26(13):E300–E302

[45] Laredo JD, Hamze B. Complications of percutaneous vertebroplasty and their prevention. Skeletal Radiol 2004;33(9):493–505

[46] Barragán-Campos HM, Vallée JN, Lo D, et al. Percutaneous vertebroplasty for spinal metastases: complications. Radiology 2006;238(1):354–362

[47] Yu SW, Chen WJ, Lin WC, Chen YJ, Tu YK. Serious pyogenic spondylitis following vertebroplasty: a case report. Spine 2004;29(10):E209–E211

[48] Childers JC Jr. Cardiovascular collapse and death during vertebroplasty. Radiology 2003;228(3):902–903, author reply 902–903

[49] Chandra RV, Meyers PM, Hirsch JA, Abruzzo T, Eskey CK, Hussain MS. Vertebral augmentation: report of the Standards and Guidelines Committee of the Society of NeuroInterventional Surgery. J Neurointerv Surg 2013;0:1–9

[50] Bernhard J, Heini PF, Villiger PM. Asymptomatic diffuse pulmonary embolism caused by acrylic cement: an unusual complication of percutaneous vertebroplasty. Ann Rheum Dis 2003;62(1):85–86

[51] Choe DH, Marom EM, Ahrar K, Truong MT, Madewell JE. Pulmonary embolism of polymethyl methacrylate during percutaneous vertebroplasty and kyphoplasty. AJR Am J Roentgenol 2004;183(4):1097–1102

[52] Duran C, Sirvanci M, Aydoğan M, Ozturk E, Ozturk C, Akman C. Pulmonary cement embolism: a complication of percutaneous vertebroplasty. Acta Radiol 2007;48(8):854–859

[53] Hee HT. Percutaneous vertebroplasty: current concepts and local experience. Neurol India 2005;53(4):475–482

[54] Trumm CG, Pahl A, Helmberger TK, et al. CT fluoroscopy-guided percutaneous vertebroplasty in spinal malignancy: technical results, PMMA leakages, and complications in 202 patients. Skeletal Radiol 2012;41(11):1391–1400

[55] Anselmetti GC, Manca A, Montemurro F, et al. Percutaneous vertebroplasty in multiple myeloma: prospective long-term follow-up in 106 consecutive patients. Cardiovasc Intervent Radiol 2012;35(1):139–145

[56] Uppin AA, Hirsch JA, Centenera LV, Pfiefer BA, Pazianos AG, Choi IS. Occurrence of new vertebral body fracture after percutaneous vertebroplasty in patients with osteoporosis. Radiology 2003;226(1):119–124

[57] Tanigawa N, Kariya S, Komemushi A, et al. Percutaneous vertebroplasty for osteoporotic compression fractures: long-term evaluation of the technical and clinical outcomes. AJR Am J Roentgenol 2011;196(6):1415–1418

[58] Takahara K, Kamimura M, Moriya H, et al. Risk factors of adjacent vertebral collapse after percutaneous vertebroplasty for osteoporotic vertebral fracture in postmenopausal women. BMC Musculoskelet Disord 2016;17:12

[59] Zhang H, Xu C, Zhang T, Gao Z, Zhang T. Does percutaneous vertebroplasty or balloon kyphoplasty for osteoporotic vertebral compression fractures increase the incidence of new vertebral fractures? A meta-analysis. Pain Physician 2017;20(1):E13–E28

[60] Yi X, Lu H, Tian F, et al. Recompression in new levels after percutaneous vertebroplasty and kyphoplasty compared with conservative treatment. Arch Orthop Trauma Surg 2014;134(1):21–30

[61] Xiao H, Yang J, Feng X, et al. Comparing complications of vertebroplasty and kyphoplasty for treating osteoporotic vertebral compression fractures: a meta-analysis of the randomized and non-randomized controlled studies. Eur J Orthop Surg Traumatol 2015;25(Suppl 1):S77–S85

[62] Luo J, Annesley-Williams DJ, Adams MA, Dolan P. How are adjacent spinal levels affected by vertebral fracture and by vertebroplasty? A biomechanical study on cadaveric spines. Spine J 2017;17(6):863–874

[63] Eichler MC, Spross C, Ewers A, Mayer R, Külling FA. Prophylactic adjacent-segment vertebroplasty following kyphoplasty for a single osteoporotic vertebral fracture and the risk of adjacent fractures: a retrospective study and clinical experience. J Neurosurg Spine 2016;25(4):528–534

[64] Sattui SE, Saag KG. Fracture mortality: associations with epidemiology and osteoporosis treatment. Nat Rev Endocrinol 2014;10(10):592–602

[65] Lau E, Ong K, Kurtz S, Schmier J, Edidin A. Mortality following the diagnosis of a vertebral compression fracture in the Medicare population. J Bone Joint Surg Am 2008;90(7):1479–1486

[66] Ong KL, Beall DP, Frohbergh M, Lau E, Hirsch JA. Were VCF patients at higher risk of mortality following the 2009 publication of the vertebroplasty "sham" trials? Osteoporos Int 2018;29(2):375–383

[67] Edidin AA, Ong KL, Lau E, Kurtz SM. Mortality risk for operated and nonoperated vertebral fracture patients in the medicare population. J Bone Miner Res 2011;26(7):1617–1626

[68] Edidin AA, Ong KL, Lau E, Kurtz SM. Morbidity and mortality after vertebral fractures: comparison of vertebral augmentation and nonoperative management in the Medicare population. Spine 2015;40(15):1228–1241

[69] Lin JH, Chien LN, Tsai WL, Chen LY, Chiang YH, Hsieh YC. Early vertebroplasty associated with a lower risk of mortality and respiratory failure in aged patients with painful vertebral compression fractures: a population-based cohort study in Taiwan. Spine J 2017;17(9):1310–1318

[70] Lange A, Kasperk C, Alvares L, Sauermann S, Braun S. Survival and cost comparison of kyphoplasty and percutaneous vertebroplasty using German claims data. Spine 2014;39(4):318–326

[71] Zampini JM, White AP, McGuire KJ. Comparison of 5766 vertebral compression fractures treated with or without kyphoplasty. Clin Orthop Relat Res 2010;468(7):1773–1780

[72] Gerling MC, Eubanks JD, Patel R, Whang PG, Bohlman HH, Ahn NU. Cement augmentation of refractory osteoporotic vertebral compression fractures: survivorship analysis. Spine 2011;36(19):E1266–E1269

[73] McCullough BJ, Comstock BA, Deyo RA, Kreuter W, Jarvik JG. Major medical outcomes with spinal augmentation vs conservative therapy. JAMA Intern Med 2013;173(16):1514–1521

16 Cost-Effectiveness of Vertebral Augmentation

Andrew Brook, Gregory Parnes, David Kramer, Steven M. Henick, Allan L. Brook, and Derrick D. Wagoner

Summary

Vertebral compression fractures (VCFs) are common and are becoming even more common with the aging of the population. There is a substantial cost burden to treat these fractures and the treatment typically involves either non-surgical management (NSM), vertebroplasty, or kyphoplasty. Providing cost effective treatment is important to ensure that the treatment will be both effective and sustainable. It has been shown in a number of studies around the world that vertebroplasty is cost effective compared to NSM mainly due to an earlier hospital discharge and a decreased number of days spent in the hospital. In addition to less days spent in the hospital vertebral augmentation also has a positive effect in decreasing the mortality rate associated with VCFs. There are a number of studies of large patient populations showing the cost effectiveness of vertebral augmentation compared to NSM especially when the benefits of improved quality of life and decreased mortality are taken into account. When comparing the types of vertebral augmentation most of the data has shown that kyphoplasty is more cost effective compared to vertebroplasty primarily due to a better quality of treatment effect and less health care expenditures after the kyphoplasty procedure. Although there is less data regarding the cost effectiveness of vertebral augmentation in treating neoplastic fractures it appears that the same advantage exists for vertebral augmentation versus NSM in the treatment of fractures related to cancer in that treating these patients with vertebral augmentation is more cost effective than managing them with NSM.

Keywords: cost effectiveness, vertebral augmentation, quality adjusted life years, incremental cost-effectiveness ratio

16.1 Introduction

VCFs are the most commonly occurring fractures worldwide in osteoporotic patients.[1] The incidence of vertebral fractures is substantial and is often quoted as affecting one-third to one-half of patients over 50 years of age.[1] In cancer patients, the incidence of vertebral fractures is more specific to the type and site of the primary cancer, but metastatic disease is common especially with some types of cancer including breast cancer where 20 to 50% of patients develop bony metastases, and 65% of bony metastases in breast cancer involve the spine.[2] Vertebral fractures impose enormous societal costs, disrupt quality of life (QoL), and are associated with significant short-term mortality.[3,4]

The burden of vertebral fractures on health care cost, QoL, morbidity, and mortality has resulted in a variety of studies to evaluate the cost-effectiveness of treatment options. The treatments most commonly advocated for treating vertebral fractures are NSM, kyphoplasty, vertebroplasty, and instrumented fusion with or without surgical decompression. This review will focus solely on the first three treatments since cost-effectiveness of surgical decompression and instrumented fusion is beyond the focus of this chapter. Vertebral augmentation includes both kyphoplasty and vertebroplasty. For the purpose of this review, cost-effectiveness will be defined as the overall dollar expenditure as well as reduction in length of hospital stay, improvement in QoL, and decreased mortality per health care dollar spent. Because this review is inclusive of different disease states and both inpatient and outpatients, the review will summarize the best data available to make our conclusions as clear as possible.

Most patients admitted to the hospital with a painful VCF are managed with NSM. NSM has been shown to be not only ineffective in treating the symptoms of a painful VCF, but also more expensive due to the costs associated with prolonged bed rest, lengthier hospitalizations, and higher readmission rates.[5–8] For example, a systematic review of 622,675 hospitalized patients with VCFs reports an average length of stay of 10 days with approximately one-quarter of these patients hospitalized for greater than 2 weeks.[9] Additionally, 20% of patients hospitalized with VCF who were treated with NSM required readmission within 30 days.[10,11]

One of the only prospective evaluations of the cost of vertebral augmentation for osteoporotic compression fractures was done in Japan and published in 2017.[12] This prospective series assessed the cost-effectiveness and improvement in QoL. They prospectively followed 163 patients with acute compression fractures and measured the health-related QoL and pain during 52 weeks' observation using the European Quality of Life–5 Dimensions (EQ-5D), the Rolland–Morris Disability Questionnaire (RMD), the 8-item Short-Form health survey (SF-8), and visual analog scale (VAS).

They calculated the direct medical cost through the accounting system of the hospital and the Japanese health insurance system. The cost analysis did not take into account the lost time and money from work. They included the cost of the procedure (labor and material costs), hospitalization costs, examination and diagnosis (including imaging such as MR imaging, CT, biopsy, etc.), and other costs that could be counted such as meals were also included. The cost of the average vertebroplasty was listed as US$ 1,549, an amount that is similar to other Western countries.[12]

They reported rapid improvement in the EQ-5D, SF-8, RMD, and VAS scores.[12] Their findings suggest that vertebroplasty was cost-effective at improving QoL and pain in patients with acute osteoporotic compression fractures in Japan.

An analysis of several large cohort retrospective reviews from around the world presented data that supported reduced hospital stays and lower 30-day readmissions rates for patients with VCFs who were treated with vertebral augmentation. An analysis of 13,624 patients from *The French Hospital National Database* demonstrated that a greater number of patients who received vertebroplasty were discharged within a week in comparison to those who received NSM (68% for vertebral augmentation vs. 47% for NSM; $p < 0.0001$).[13] A nationwide cohort study from Taiwan involving 9,238 patients found a reduction in hospital length of stay by 2 days as well as a decrease in readmission rates at 7 and 30 days for patients who underwent vertebroplasty.[11] The National Medicare Database in the United

States has shown an average length of stay of 3 to 6 days for patients receiving augmentation, which is on average a 4- to 7-day reduction in length of stay when compared to traditional NSM data as presented above.[9,10] Intuitively, the length-of-stay decreases lead to less cost.

16.2 Cost-Effectiveness

We can clearly see that vertebral augmentation is associated with decreased short- and long-term mortality, but does it reduce cost? The most informative data on the cost-effectiveness of vertebral augmentation is derived from retrospective analyses of large patient populations (▶Table 16.1).[14–19] A review of this retrospective literature, while somewhat limited

in sample size and breadth of scope, does indicate that vertebral augmentation is more cost-effective when compared to NSM.[20–23] This is particularly apparent when the mortality benefit of vertebral augmentation is included in this cost analysis.

Cost-effectiveness models comparing vertebral augmentation to NSM have also been performed and calculated that the cost per life-year gained ranged from US$ 1,863 to 13,543 for vertebral augmentation.[20] A cohort study from the United Kingdom looked at patients hospitalized for VCFs and found that the cost per quality-adjusted life year of kyphoplasty versus vertebroplasty was €19,706 and concluded that kyphoplasty may be more cost-effective than both NSM and vertebroplasty (▶Table 16.2).[21] If one simply looks at health care dollars expended, NSM may *appear* more cost-effective, but when

Table 16.1 Review of literature

Study	Stevenson et al[24]	Svedbom et al[21]	Ström et al[25]	Klazen et al[26]	Fritzell et al[22]
Nation	United Kingdom	United Kingdom	United Kingdom	The Netherlands	Sweden
Year	2010–2011	2009	2008	2008	2008
Comparators	VP, BKP, NSM and operational local anesthesia	BKP, VP, NSM	BKP, NSM	VP, NSM	BKP, NSM
Base case target patient group	70-y-old women with a T-score of –3 SD	70-y-old-women with a T-score of –3.0 and a prevalent VCF	70-y-old UK men and women with a T-score of –2.5 and at least one VCF	75 y of age with prevalent VCF and back pain <6 wk)	72 y in BKP arm and 75 y in control arm
Time horizon	Lifetime	Lifetime	Lifetime	Within trial	Within trial
Study design	Markov's cohort model	Markov's cohort model	Markov's cohort model	Within trial	Within trial
Discounting	3.5%/y	3.5%/y	3.5%/y	None	None
Perspective	Health care	Health care	Health care	Health care	Societal
Outcomes	QALYs	QALYs	QALYs	QALYs	QALYs
Source for differential QoL	Combination	FREE, VERTOS II	FREE trial	VERTOS II	FREE (Swedish patients)
Underlying mechanism for determining QoL	Combination	EQ-5D (UK tariff)	EQ-5D (UK tariff)	EQ-5D (Dutch tariff)	EQ-5D (UK tariff)
Duration of differential effect	Different scenarios	2 y followed by 1-y decline to zero effect	1 y followed by 2-y decline to zero effect	1 y	2 y
Other differential effects	Differing hospital stay, mortality, refracture rate	Yes, reduced hospitalization days and mortality with BKP and VP vs. NSM	Yes, reduced hospitalization days with BKP	No	No
Adverse events considered	Yes	No	No	Unknown	Yes

Abbreviations: BKP, balloon kyphoplasty; EQ-5D: EQ-5D Health Questionnaire; NSM, nonsurgical management; QALYs, quality-adjusted life years; QoL, quality of life; SD, standard deviation; VCF, vertebral compression fracture; VP, vertebroplasty.

Table 16.2 Base case results in Svedbom et al[21]

	Total costs in euros	Total quality-adjusted life years	Incremental costs in € (ICER)	Quality-adjusted life-year gained	ICER vs. NSM (€)	ICER BKP vs. NSM (€)
BKP	11,483	5.473	26,58	0.14	3,337	19,706
VP	8,825	5.338	–1,001	0.36	Cost-saving	
NSM	9,826	4.976				

Abbreviations: BKP, balloon kyphoplasty; NSM, nonsurgical management; VP, vertebroplasty.

factoring the cost-effectiveness benefits of improved QoL and reduced mortality gained from vertebral augmentation, vertebral augmentation is clearly shown to be more cost-effective than NSM.[21] A prospective multicenter study from Sweden that lacked some of these adjustments and included only 63 patients failed to show the cost-effectiveness of kyphoplasty and computed an outrageously high cost per quality-adjusted life year of US$ 134,000.[22]

Borgström et al conducted a systematic analysis of peer-reviewed investigations of the cost-effectiveness of vertebral augmentation in patients with VCFs and osteoporosis.[23] When compared to NSM, vertebral augmentation was found to be cost-effective in three of the five studies reviewed. Incremental cost-effectiveness ratios ranged from €3,337 to 92,154 (US$ 3,799–104,914) in four out of the five studies analyzed.[23] Variations in cost-effectiveness were most affected by the time horizon of the study, time to realization of treatment effect, effect of treatment on QoL, reduction in length of stay, and mortality after vertebral augmentation.[23]

A cost analysis using Medicare claims from January 2005 to December 2008 in the United States found that the vertebral augmentation for the treatment of VCFs proves once again to be cost-effective.[27] In this analysis, while all forms of vertebral augmentation proved cost-effective, kyphoplasty could impart more cost savings when compared with vertebroplasty. The differences in cumulative median costs for vertebroplasty and kyphoplasty compared with nonoperative management were US$ 8,300 to 28,820 for vertebroplasty and US$ 12,580 to 18,500 for kyphoplasty.[27] These results were dependent on age and gender. The cost per life-year gained for kyphoplasty compared with NSM was US$ 1,863 to 6,687, and the cost per life-year gained for vertebroplasty compared with NSM was US$ 2,452 to 13,543.[27] The cost-per-life-year-gained when comparing kyphoplasty versus vertebroplasty was US$ 284 to 2,399 for females and US$ 2,763 to 4,878 for males.[27] These findings clearly indicate a lower cost-per-life-year-gained for kyphoplasty. Some variables including the cost of equipment and cost of the hospital vary greatly depending on the manufacturer, the location of the hospital, and the comorbidities of each patient. In addition, the lost work hours and the family cost of care to each patient are not represented and represent additional cost saving when appropriately taken into account.

A retrospective study by Masala et al showed that percutaneous vertebroplasty (PVP) in patients with osteoporotic vertebral fractures was more cost-effective than NSM.[28] In the European Union, vertebral fractures are responsible for 8% of the hospital costs of all osteoporotic fractures, and the hospital cost of a vertebral fracture treated by NSM is approximately 63% of the mean hospital cost of a femoral fracture.[28] In a patient population of 153 patients, 58 of which underwent PVP and 95 underwent NSM, Masala et al found PVP to be superior in outcome effectiveness, cumulative costs, and overall cost-effectiveness at 1 week and 3 and 12 months postprocedure.[28] Cost-effectiveness was measured as the average cost per patient per reduction of 1 point on a reduction of pain (VAS) or improvement in the activities of daily living (ADL) scale. Costs were evaluated for each group by adding hospital care costs to all outpatient costs. PVP was more cost-effective at all three time points, statistically significant in all three categories at 1 week,

and statistically significant for improved ADL scale at 3 months. It was also associated with earlier pain reduction, improvement of ambulation, and improvement of ability to perform ADL in the short and long term. The factors that most influenced cost were days of hospitalization, physical therapy, and the back brace for the NSM group. In the PVP group, costs were mainly affected by the hospital expenses of the procedure.[28] Masala et al concluded that the improved clinical outcomes, along with the lower cost-effectiveness ratio of PVP in the short term and its comparable cost-effectiveness ratio with that of NSM in the long term make PVP a preferable procedure to NSM.[28]

When dealing with metastatic disease and vertebral pathologic compression fractures, there is even less long-term prospective data than with osteoporotic VCFs. The best literature review is by the Health Quality Ontario assessment done in May 2016.[29] The objective of the Health Quality Ontario analysis was to determine the cost-effectiveness and budgetary impact of kyphoplasty or vertebroplasty compared with NSM for the treatment of VCFs in patients with cancer.

Upon completing a systemic review of health economic studies, they performed a primary cost-effectiveness analysis to assess the clinical benefits and costs of kyphoplasty or vertebroplasty compared with NSM in the same population from published sources. They also performed a 1-year budget impact analysis using data from the Health Quality Ontario administrative sources. They found that kyphoplasty and vertebroplasty used in patients with cancer may be a cost-effective strategy at commonly accepted willingness-to-pay thresholds.[29]

In conclusion, vertebral fractures are extremely common in patients older than 50 years, especially in patients with osteoporosis and metastatic cancer. The overall review of the literature supports vertebral augmentation as a cost-effective method that is superior and more cost-effective than NSM in patients with VCFs. Some of the major influences are the decreased length of stay and the overall lower rate of narcotic usage over time.

References

[1] Ballane G, Cauley JA, Luckey MM, El-Hajj Fuleihan G. Worldwide prevalence and incidence of osteoporotic vertebral fractures. Osteoporos Int 2017;28(5):1531–1542

[2] Fontanella C, Fanotto V, Rihawi K, Aprile G, Puglisi F. Skeletal metastases from breast cancer: pathogenesis of bone tropism and treatment strategy. Clin Exp Metastasis 2015;32(8):819–833

[3] Lau E, Ong K, Kurtz S, Schmier J, Edidin A. Mortality following the diagnosis of a vertebral compression fracture in the Medicare population. J Bone Joint Surg Am 2008;90(7):1479–1486

[4] Sattui SE, Saag KG. Fracture mortality: associations with epidemiology and osteoporosis treatment. Nat Rev Endocrinol 2014;10(10):592–602

[5] Rzewuska M, Ferreira M, McLachlan AJ, Machado GC, Maher CG. The efficacy of conservative treatment of osteoporotic compression fractures on acute pain relief: a systematic review with meta-analysis. Eur Spine J 2015;24(4):702–714

[6] Kim HJ, Yi JM, Cho HG, et al. Comparative study of the treatment outcomes of osteoporotic compression fractures without neurologic injury using a rigid brace, a soft brace, and no brace: a prospective randomized controlled non-inferiority trial. J Bone Joint Surg Am 2014;96(23):1959–1966

[7] Bailey CS, Dvorak MF, Thomas KC, et al. Comparison of thoracolumbosacral orthosis and no orthosis for the treatment of thoracolumbar burst fractures: interim analysis of a multicenter randomized clinical equivalence trial. J Neurosurg Spine 2009;11(3):295–303

[8] Phillips S, Fox N, Jacobs J, Wright WE. The direct medical costs of osteoporosis for American women aged 45 and older, 1986. Bone 1988;9(5):271–279

[9] Papaioannou A, Adachi JD, Parkinson W, Stephenson G, Bédard M. Lengthy hospitalization associated with vertebral fractures despite control for comorbid conditions. Osteoporos Int 2001;12(10):870–874

[10] Ong T, Kantachuvesiri P, Sahota O, et al. Characteristics and outcomes of hospitalised patients with vertebral fragility fractures: a systematic review. Age and Aging 20 18;47(1):17–25

[11] Tsai YW, Hsiao FY, Wen YW, et al. Clinical outcomes of vertebroplasty or kyphoplasty for patients with vertebral compression fractures: a nationwide cohort study. J Am Med Dir Assoc 2013;14(1):41–47

[12] Takura T, Yoshimatsu M, Sugimori H, et al. Cost-effectiveness analysis of percutaneous vertebroplasty for osteoporotic compression fractures. Clin Spine Surg 2017;30(3):E205–E210

[13] Maravic M, Taupin P, Roux C. Hospital burden of vertebral fractures in France: influence of vertebroplasty. Osteoporos Int 2013;24(7):2001–2006

[14] Ong KL, Lau E, Kemner JE, Kurtz SM. Two-year cost comparison of vertebroplasty and kyphoplasty for the treatment of vertebral compression fractures: are initial surgical costs misleading? Osteoporos Int 2013;24(4):1437–1445

[15] Lange A, Kasperk C, Alvares L, Sauermann S, Braun S. Survival and cost comparison of kyphoplasty and percutaneous vertebroplasty using German claims data. Spine 2014;39(4):318–326

[16] Lin JH, Chien LN, Tsai WL, Chen LY, Chiang YH, Hsieh YC. Early vertebroplasty associated with a lower risk of mortality and respiratory failure in aged patients with painful vertebral compression fractures: a population-based cohort study in Taiwan. Spine J 2017;17(9):1310–1318

[17] Zampini JM, White AP, McGuire KJ. Comparison of 5766 vertebral compression fractures treated with or without kyphoplasty. Clin Orthop Relat Res 2010;468(7):1773–1780

[18] Edidin AA, Ong KL, Lau E, Kurtz SM. Mortality risk for operated and nonoperated vertebral fracture patients in the Medicare population. J Bone Miner Res 2011;26(7):1617–1626

[19] Edidin AA, Ong KL, Lau E, Kurtz SM. Life expectancy following diagnosis of a vertebral compression fracture. Osteoporos Int 2013;24(2):451–458

[20] Owens DK. Interpretation of cost-effectiveness analyses. J Gen Intern Med 1998;13(10):716–717

[21] Svedbom A, Alvares L, Cooper C, Marsh D, Ström O. Balloon kyphoplasty compared to vertebroplasty and nonsurgical management in patients hospitalised with acute osteoporotic vertebral compression fracture: a UK cost-effectiveness analysis. Osteoporos Int 2013;24(1):355–367

[22] Fritzell P, Ohlin A, Borgström F. Cost-effectiveness of balloon kyphoplasty versus standard medical treatment in patients with osteoporotic vertebral compression fracture: a Swedish multicenter randomized controlled trial with 2-year follow-up. Spine 2011;36(26):2243–2251

[23] Borgström F, Beall DP, Berven S, et al. Health economic aspects of vertebral augmentation procedures. Osteoporos Int 2015;26(4):1239–1249

[24] Stevenson M, Gomersall T, Lloyd Jones M, et al. Percutaneous vertebroplasty and percutaneous balloon kyphoplasty for the treatment of osteoporotic vertebral fractures: a systematic review and cost-effectiveness analysis. Health Technol Assess 2014;18(17):1–290

[25] Ström O, Leonard C, Marsh D, Cooper C. Cost-effectiveness of balloon kyphoplasty in patients with symptomatic vertebral compression fractures in a UK setting. Osteoporos Int 2010;21(9):1599–1608

[26] Klazen CA, Lohle PN, de Vries J, et al. Vertebroplasty versus conservative treatment in acute osteoporotic vertebral compression fractures (Vertos II): an open-label randomised trial. Lancet 2010;376(9746):1085–1092

[27] Edidin AA, Ong KL, Lau E, Schmier JK, Kemner JE, Kurtz SM. Cost-effectiveness analysis of treatments for vertebral compression fractures. Appl Health Econ Health Policy 2012;10(4):273–284

[28] Masala S, Ciarrapico AM, Konda D, Vinicola V, Mammucari M, Simonetti G. Cost-effectiveness of percutaneous vertebroplasty in osteoporotic vertebral fractures. Eur Spine J 2008;17(9):1242–1250

[29] Health Quality Ontario. Vertebral augmentation involving vertebroplasty or kyphoplasty for cancer-related vertebral compression fractures: an economic analysis. ont health technol assess ser 2016;16(12):1–34

17 Additional and Adjacent Level Fractures after Vertebral Augmentation

Scott Kreiner

Summary

Vertebral compression fractures (VCFs) are common as are the occurrence of additional vertebral fractures that happen after the incident level fracture. There are several reasons that predispose patients to additional vertebral fractures including the anatomy of the fracture and the use of corticosteroids but the primary determinate factors are low bone mineral density and spinopelvic imbalance. Prior vertebral compression fractures also increase the risk of an additional fracture substantially with an increased risk up to 75 times higher for patients with three or more fractures. There is ample data showing no increased risk of additional fractures after vertebral augmentation but certain procedural features may predispose to adjacent level fractures such as cement extravasation into the disk.

Keywords: vertebral augmentation, adjacent level fractures, bone mineral density, spinopelvic balance, kyphotic deformity

17.1 Introduction

Compression fractures of the spine are a large problem, affecting between 700,000 and a million persons in the United States annually, and 25% of women in their lifetime.[1,2] Treatment of these compression fractures should not only focus on the index fracture but also on preventing further fractures in the future. To better understand how to prevent future fractures, it is imperative that we know what puts patients at risk for developing new fractures.

17.2 Risk Factors for Additional or Adjacent-Level Fractures

There are several risk factors associated with the development of additional or adjacent-level fractures. These risk factors are similar to the risk of initial fractures discussed in Chapter 4. Decreased bone mineral density (BMD) is the primary determinant in the development of additional or adjacent fractures whether they are treated or untreated.[3–15] In fact a prominent decline in BMD of 2 SD is associated with a fourfold to sixfold increase in risk of additional fracture.[15,16] In addition, the use of chronic corticosteroids has been associated with a propensity for developing VCFs and recurrent compression fractures[11,17] via their effects promoting osteoclastic activity, inhibiting osteoblastic activity, and the interference on the small intestine's ability to absorb calcium. The presence of prior fracture is also predictive of future fractures. A single compression fracture increases the risk of another fracture by 3.2 to 5 times, the presence of two or more fractures increases the risk of another fracture by a multiple of 10 to 12, and the presence of three or more fractures increases the risk of another fracture by a very substantial 23 to 75 times.[15,18,19] A combination of low BMD and more than two prior fractures increases the risk of a new vertebral fracture to at least a factor of 75-fold, relative to women with a BMD in the top 67th percentile and no prior fracture.[15]

However, it is not just the presence of a prior fracture that increases the risk of future fracture; there are biomechanical effects directly related to the index fracture that are associated with the increased risk of future fracture. End plate fracture itself affects the biomechanics of the spine by disrupting the ability of the intervertebral disk to pressurize, which increases the compressive loading on the anterior wall of the adjacent vertebrae, predisposing it to fracture.[20] The correction of end plate deformity by reducing the end plate and stabilizing it with polymethyl methacrylate (PMMA) decreases this force and is an important factor in decreasing adjacent-level fractures.[20] An even more important factor in causing additional and adjacent-level fractures is the kyphotic angle formed by the index fracture. This kyphotic deformity causes the body mass from above the fracture to deviate anterior to the typical center of balance, thereby increasing the effective pressure on adjacent vertebrae.[21] Additionally, to maintain equilibrium, the paraspinal muscles must supply a force equal and opposite to this anterior mass movement in direct proportion to the lever arm. So, as the kyphotic deformity increases, so do the downward forces on the spine especially on the anterior portion of the vertebral body.

Clinically, these biomechanical factors have been shown to be directly related to the occurrence of additional and adjacent-level fractures. Lunt et al[19] showed that the shape of the fracture (►Table 17.1) strongly influences the risk of future fracture, with more kyphotic deformity increasing the risk of fracture by a factor of 5.9 as compared with a compression fracture without kyphotic deformity that increases the risk of future fracture by a factor of only 1.6. In addition to the focal anatomic changes caused by a VCF, Baek et al[22] further defined the relationship between postfracture spinopelvic balance and the development of new fractures. The presence of a segmental kyphotic angle (SKA; ►Fig. 17.1) of over 11 degrees is associated with increased risk of fracture regardless of whether the vertebral body has undergone augmentation. Other spinopelvic parameters associated with increased fracture risk include a sagittal vertical axis (SVA; ►Fig. 17.2) of greater than 6 cm, sacral slope (SS; ►Fig. 17.3) less than 25 degrees, and a lumbar lordosis (LL) of less than 25 degrees.

17.3 Possible Influences of Vertebral Augmentation Technique

There has been some concern that the placement of PMMA in the spine, adjacent to osteoporotic vertebrae, increases the risk of adjacent-level fracture.[23] This perception is likely because, as

Table 17.1 Risk of future fracture based on shape of incident fracture

Shape of deformity		Relative risk of future fracture
Central fracture with global/posterior flattening	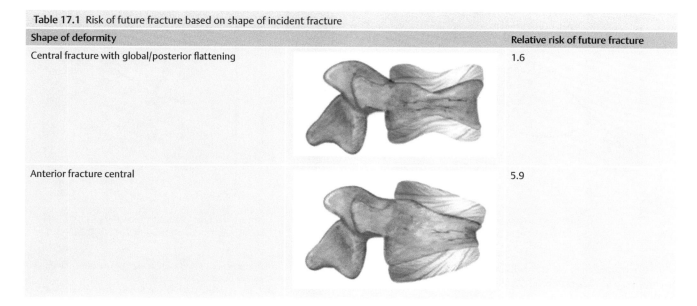	1.6
Anterior fracture central		5.9

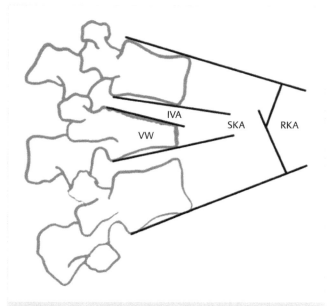

Fig. 17.1 Measurement techniques for assessment of regional deformity (RKA/SKA). (IVA, intervertebral angle; VW, vertebral wedging; SKA, segmental kyphosis angle; RKA, regional kyphosis angle.) IVA + VW = SKA. (Reproduced with permission of Koller H, Acosta F, Hempfing A, et al. Long-term investigation of nonsurgical treatment for thoracolumbar and lumbar burst fractures: an outcome analysis in sight of spinopelvic balance. Eur Spine J 2008;17:1073.)

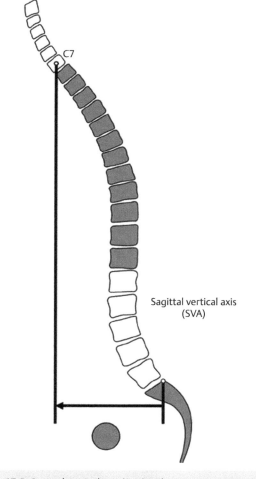

Fig. 17.2 Sagittal vertical axis (SVA) is the most common measurement of global alignment. (Reproduced with permission of Diebo BG, Varghese JJ, Lafage R, et al. Sagittal alignment of the spine: what do you need to know? Clin Neurol Neurosurg 2015;139:295–301.)

discussed earlier, these patients are at higher risk than patients without a fracture history. Additionally, there is some evidence to support that additional and adjacent-level fractures are more likely to occur sooner after vertebral augmentation than with nonsurgical management, though the rate of adjacent-level fractures is similar.[24]

A systematic review by Papanastassiou et al[25] compared the available evidence, which showed that when comparing rates of additional or adjacent fracture, balloon kyphoplasty

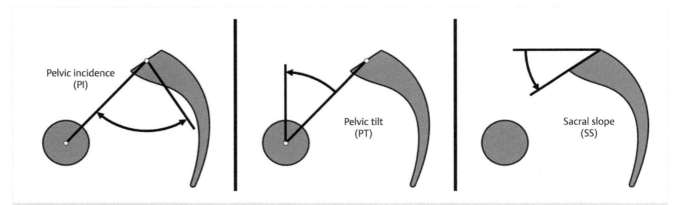

Fig. 17.3 Pelvic parameters also play a role in stresses on the spine and influence the risk of future fracture. (Reproduced with permission of Diebo BG, Varghese JJ, Lafage R, et al. Sagittal alignment of the spine: what do you need to know? Clin Neurol Neurosurg 2015;139:295–301.)

and vertebroplasty have rates of 11.7 and 11.5%, respectively, as compared with a rate of 22.7% for nonsurgical management. Additionally, fracture reduction, or increasing the height of a previously fractured vertebral body with kyphoplasty, does not increase the risk of adjacent-level fracture when compared with vertebroplasty.[26]

The data available suggest that the risk of additional and adjacent-level fractures is essentially the same whether or not the incident fracture has undergone vertebral augmentation.[26] However, certain factors associated with vertebral augmentation may increase the risk of fracture adjacent to the index fracture. In particular, the leakage of intradiskal cement during the procedure has been associated with an increased risk of fracture. Nieuwenhuijse et al[8] prospectively followed 115 patients with 216 VCFs for recurrent fracture after vertebroplasty. Both patient and vertebra-specific risk factors were assessed. While a number of risk factors of additional fracture were found, the only independent risk fracture related to vertebral augmentation was the presence of intradiskal cement leakage. This finding has been corroborated by other authors.[27–29]

References

[1] Edidin AA, Ong KL, Lau E, Kurtz SM. Life expectancy following diagnosis of a vertebral compression fracture. Osteoporos Int 2013;24(2):451–458

[2] Riggs BL, Melton LJ III. The worldwide problem of osteoporosis: insights afforded by epidemiology. Bone 1995;17(5, Suppl):505S–511S

[3] Hey HW, Tan JH, Tan CS, Tan HM, Lau PH, Hee HT. Subsequent vertebral fractures post cement augmentation of the thoracolumbar spine: does it correlate with level-specific bone mineral density scores? Spine 2015;40(24):1903–1909

[4] Lee BG, Choi JH, Kim DY, Choi WR, Lee SG, Kang CN. Risk factors for newly developed osteoporotic vertebral compression fractures following treatment for osteoporotic vertebral compression fractures. Spine J 2019;19(2):301–305

[5] Lee DG, Park CK, Park CJ, Lee DC, Hwang JH. Analysis of risk factors causing new symptomatic vertebral compression fractures after percutaneous vertebroplasty for painful osteoporotic vertebral compression fractures: a 4-year follow-up. J Spinal Disord Tech 2015;28(10):E578–E583

[6] Lu K, Liang CL, Hsieh CH, Tsai YD, Chen HJ, Liliang PC. Risk factors of subsequent vertebral compression fractures after vertebroplasty. Pain Med 2012;13(3):376–382

[7] Movrin I, Vengust R, Komadina R. Adjacent vertebral fractures after percutaneous vertebral augmentation of osteoporotic vertebral compression fracture: a comparison of balloon kyphoplasty and vertebroplasty. Arch Orthop Trauma Surg 2010;130(9):1157–1166

[8] Nieuwenhuijse MJ, Putter H, van Erkel AR, Dijkstra PD. New vertebral fractures after percutaneous vertebroplasty for painful osteoporotic vertebral compression fractures: a clustered analysis and the relevance of intradiskal cement leakage. Radiology 2013;266(3):862–870

[9] Ning L, Wan S, Liu C, Huang Z, Cai H, Fan S. new levels of vertebral compression fractures after percutaneous kyphoplasty: retrospective analysis of styles and risk factors. Pain Physician 2015;18(6):565–572

[10] Sun G, Tang H, Li M, Liu X, Jin P, Li L. Analysis of risk factors of subsequent fractures after vertebroplasty. Eur Spine J 2014;23(6):1339–1345

[11] Sun H, Sharma S, Li C. Cluster phenomenon of vertebral refractures after percutaneous vertebroplasty in a patient with glucocorticosteroid-induced osteoporosis: case report and review of the literature. Spine 2013;38(25):E1628–E1632

[12] Tseng YY, Yang TC, Tu PH, Lo YL, Yang ST. Repeated and multiple new vertebral compression fractures after percutaneous transpedicular vertebroplasty. Spine 2009;34(18):1917–1922

[13] Wang YT, Wu XT, Chen H, Wang C, Mao ZB. Adjacent-level symptomatic fracture after percutaneous vertebral augmentation of osteoporotic vertebral compression fracture: a retrospective analysis. J Orthop Sci 2014;19(6):868–876

[14] Yang S, Liu Y, Yang H, Zou J. Risk factors and correlation of secondary adjacent vertebral compression fracture in percutaneous kyphoplasty. Int J Surg 2016;36(Pt A):138–142

[15] Ross PD, Davis JW, Epstein RS, Wasnich RD. Pre-existing fractures and bone mass predict vertebral fracture incidence in women. Ann Intern Med 1991;114(11):919–923

[16] Marshall D, Johnell O, Wedel H. Meta-analysis of how well measures of bone mineral density predict occurrence of osteoporotic fractures. BMJ 1996;312(7041):1254–1259

[17] Tatsumi RL, Ching AC, Byrd GD, Hiratzka JR, Threlkeld JE, Hart RA. Predictors and prevalence of patients undergoing additional kyphoplasty procedures after an initial kyphoplasty procedure. Spine J 2010;10(11):979–986

[18] Lindsay R, Silverman SL, Cooper C, et al. Risk of new vertebral fracture in the year following a fracture. JAMA 2001;285(3):320–323

[19] Lunt M, O'Neill TW, Felsenberg D, et al; European Prospective Osteoporosis Study Group. Characteristics of a prevalent vertebral deformity predict subsequent vertebral fracture: results from the European Prospective Osteoporosis Study (EPOS). Bone 2003;33(4):505–513

[20] Tzermiadianos MN, Renner SM, Phillips FM, et al. Altered disc pressure profile after an osteoporotic vertebral fracture is a risk factor for adjacent vertebral body fracture. Eur Spine J 2008;17(11):1522–1530

[21] Song D, Meng B, Gan M, et al. The incidence of secondary vertebral fracture of vertebral augmentation techniques versus conservative treatment for painful osteoporotic vertebral fractures: a systematic review and meta-analysis. Acta Radiol 2015;56(8):970–979

[22] Baek SW, Kim C, Chang H. The relationship between the spinopelvic balance and the incidence of adjacent vertebral fractures following percutaneous vertebroplasty. Osteoporos Int 2015;26(5):1507–1513

[23] Jensen ME, Kallmes DF. Does filling the crack break more of the back? AJNR Am J Neuroradiol 2004;25(2):166–167

[24] Yi X, Lu H, Tian F, et al. Recompression in new levels after percutaneous vertebroplasty and kyphoplasty compared with conservative treatment. Arch Orthop Trauma Surg 2014;134(1):21–30

[25] Papanastassiou ID, Phillips FM, Van Meirhaeghe J, et al. Comparing effects of kyphoplasty, vertebroplasty, and non-surgical management in a systematic

review of randomized and non-randomized controlled studies. Eur Spine J 2012;21(9):1826–1843

[26] Xiao H, Yang J, Feng X, et al. Comparing complications of vertebroplasty and kyphoplasty for treating osteoporotic vertebral compression fractures: a meta-analysis of the randomized and non-randomized controlled studies. Eur J Orthop Surg Traumatol 2015;25(Suppl 1):S77–S85

[27] Jesse MK, Petersen B, Glueck D, Kriedler S. Effect of the location of endplate cement extravasation on adjacent level fracture in osteoporotic patients

undergoing vertebroplasty and kyphoplasty. Pain Physician 2015;18(5): E805–E814

[28] Zhong BY, He SC, Zhu HD, et al. Risk prediction of new adjacent vertebral fractures after PVP for patients with vertebral compression fractures: development of a prediction model. Cardiovasc Intervent Radiol 2017;40(2):277–284

[29] Lin EP, Ekholm S, Hiwatashi A, Westesson PL. Vertebroplasty: cement leakage into the disc increases the risk of new fracture of adjacent vertebral body. AJNR Am J Neuroradiol 2004;25(2):175–180

18 Predisposing Factors to Vertebral Fractures

Olivier Clerk-Lamalice

Summary

The risk factors for vertebral compression fractures (VCFs) include infection, trauma, and cancer but the vast majority of vertebral fractures are due to osteoporosis. There are contributing factors to osteoporosis that are modifiable including excessive alcohol and tobacco use, insufficient weight bearing activity, and low body mass. One of the predisposing fractures that is unmodifiable is a person's genetic predisposition to osteoporosis. There have been at least fifteen genes that have been confirmed as susceptibility genes and the number could be as high as thirty. After vertebral augmentation it appears that the primary risk factor associated with an additional vertebral fracture is the presence of osteoporosis and the treatment of that underlying disorder is important to limit or prevent additional fractures. Pathologic fractures due to metastatic disease may account for up to 25% of the Medicare patients treated for VCFs and the most common metastases to the spine include breast, kidney, prostate, lung, and, thyroid carcinomas. Given the relatively high prevalence of these lesions, a bone biopsy is indicated in focal lesions or with infiltrated bone marrow. Vertebral fractures due to infection should be treated with antibiotics and the infection eradicated before any additional structural support is provided by vertebral augmentation. The majority of vertebral fractures due to trauma happen in younger and healthier patients with a high energy fall being the most common cause. Most traumatic fractures are of the compression variety and involve the thoracolumbar junction. Traumatic fractures are most often not treated with vertebral augmentation but with the development of implant augmentation these fractures may commonly be treated by percutaneous implant augmentation in the future.

Keywords: vertebral compression fractures, osteoporosis, vertebral augmentation, metastatic disease, spondylodiskitis

18.1 Introduction

Approximately 1.5 million osteoporotic fractures occur each year in the United States, of which more than 50% are VCFs.[1] Osteoporosis is responsible for the vast majority of VCFs; however, trauma, infection, and neoplasm are also predisposing factors to fractures. The risk factors of osteoporotic VCFs are categorized as potentially modifiable and nonmodifiable. Nonmodifiable risk factors include being Caucasian of Northern European descent, female gender, advanced age, susceptibility to fall, presence of dementia, and history of fractures in a first-degree relative. On the other hand, potentially modifiable risk factors include estrogen deficiency, alcohol/tobacco use, frailty, impaired eyesight, insufficient physical activity, and low body weight. Pathologic vertebral fractures are surprisingly prevalent, responsible for up to 25% of the reported Medicare VCF volume. These fractures can be treated with vertebral augmentation especially when radiotherapy is considered. Traumatic vertebral fractures are the most prevalent in patients younger than 50 years. The most common causes of accidents responsible for those fractures are high-energy falls, followed by automobile accidents. Although vertebral augmentation has not been routinely adopted in treatment of traumatic VCFs, preliminary reports have concluded that such interventions could be performed in well-selected cases.

18.2 Current Information Based on Recent Literature and State-of-the-Art Practice

18.2.1 Osteoporosis

The World Health Organization has developed a definition of osteoporosis using dual-energy X-ray absorptiometry as a means of defining bone mass. The bone density is compared to the ideal peak bone mineral density (BMD) of a healthy 30-year-old adult. This comparison results in a T-score. A score of 0 means your BMD is equal to the norm for a healthy young adult. The bones are considered normal or healthy with a bone density from +1 to −1 standard deviation (SD). If the measurement reveals a bone mass between −1 and -2.5 SD, the patient is considered to have low bone mass. Individuals with measurements lower than −2.5 SD are considered osteoporotic. In addition, individuals with a T-score lower than −2.5 SD with an osteoporotic fragility fracture are considered to have severe osteoporosis (►Table 18.1).

The lifetime risk of all types of skeletal fractures for Caucasian women older than 50 years of age approaches 75%. In fact, the lifetime risk of a symptomatic vertebral fracture is 15.6% in white women and 5.0% in white men.[2] This fracture risk in postmenopausal woman increases sixfold[3] with 25% of additional risk increase in women with a history of prior vertebral fracture in the last 2 years.[4,5] Osteoporosis decreases the BMD, disrupts the bone microarchitecture, and alters the contents of noncollagenous proteins in the bone matrix.[6] This structural deterioration leads to fragile bones prone to fractures. It is estimated that approximately 44 million Americans have osteoporosis and an additional 34 million Americans have low bone mass.[7]

Table 18.1 World Health Organization definitions based on bone density levels

Level	Definition
Normal	Bone density is within 1 SD (+1 or −1) of the young adult mean
Low bone mass	Bone density is between 1 and 2.5 SD below the young adult mean (−1 to −2.5 SD)
Osteoporosis	Bone density is 2.5 SD or more below the young adult mean (−2.5 SD or lower)
Severe osteoporosis	**Bone density is more than 2.5 SD below the young adult mean, and** there have been one or more osteoporotic fractures

Genetic predisposition also has an important impact on VCF incidence within a studied population. There is indeed a threefold variation in VCF occurrence in Europe with higher rates seen in Scandinavian countries.[8] Also, at least 15 genes have been confirmed as susceptibility genes (i.e., RANKL, OPG, RANK, SOST, LRP5) and multiple others (at least 30) have been highlighted as promising genes. Those genes are regrouped in three biological pathways: the OPG/RANK/RANKL pathway, the Wnt/β-catenin pathway, and the estrogen, endocrine pathway.[9]

The typical risk factors associated with osteoporotic VCFs can be categorized as potentially modifiable and nonmodifiable. Nonmodifiable risk factors include being Caucasian of Northern European descent, female gender, advanced age, susceptibility to fall, presence of dementia, and history of fractures in a first-degree relative. Potentially modifiable risk factors include estrogen deficiency, alcohol/tobacco use, frailty, impaired eyesight, insufficient physical activity, and low body weight. Interestingly, age itself has been found to be a risk factor independent of bone density.[6]

The fracture risk is multifactorial but highly dependent on the peak bone mass achieved at 30 years of age. However, the peak bone mass is mainly determined by genetic factors, physical activity, endocrine status, nutrition, and health during growth. Health professionals recommend being active prior to this age to maximize the bone peak mass. Indeed, animal model and human studies suggest stress loading that is of high magnitude and is rapidly applied is effective in increasing bone density prior to 30 years of age along with continued regular exercise afterward.[10] Also, brief high-impact-jump training increases the BMD in premenopausal women.

The trunk muscles provide static equilibrium and appropriate response to changes in loading and displacement perturbations while ensuring stability of the vertebral column.[11] Unfortunately, the current understanding of the muscle/bone interaction in older patients remains limited. Studies report that prevalent VCFs are associated with lower trunk muscle density and/or increased fat accumulation in muscle.[12] It is also known that coactivation of antagonistic muscles can increase muscle stiffness and stability; however, this activation also increases spinal loads[13,14] and can contribute to VCFs.

After vertebral augmentation, the only risk factor significantly associated with subsequent compression fracture is the presence of osteoporosis (low T-score).[15] It has been thought and debated for many years that vertebral augmentation might predispose to adjacent-level fractures. However, meta-analyses demonstrated that there is no increase of adjacent-level fracture in patient treated with vertebral augmentation[16] and even a decrease of the incidence of subsequent fractures when comparing the vertebral augmentation arm to the conservative management arm.[17] This decrease in adjacent-level fractures is most likely related to corrected segmental kyphosis and decrease of the flexion moment introduced at the level of the functional spinal unit by the VCF.

18.2.2 Pathologic Fractures

The most common malignancies that metastasize to the bone and spine are breast, lung, kidney, prostate, and thyroid carcinomas. Spine metastases are 40 times more prevalent than all primary tumors combined and the vertebral body is 20 times more likely to be involved by a lesion in comparison to the posterior elements (▸Fig. 18.1). As a rule of thumb, most lesions involving the anterior column will be malignant (metastases, myeloma, lymphoma, chordoma) with the exception of hemangiomas and eosinophilic granuloma. On the other hand, lesions involving the posterior arc are typically benign such as osteoid osteoma, osteoblastoma, and aneurysmal bone cyst (benign but locally aggressive).

According to the Medicare data, up to approximately 25% of VCFs are neoplastic in origin.[18] Because of this high prevalence, a bone biopsy is indicated in patients with either a focal lesion or evidence of infiltrated bone marrow (characterized by a lower T1-weighted bone marrow signal when using the intervertebral disks or paraspinal muscles as a reference guide; ▸Fig. 18.2).

For cases of pathologic fracture with extraosseous soft-tissue component and/or multiple metastases, multidisciplinary

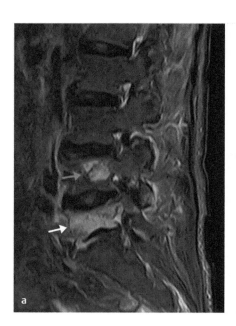
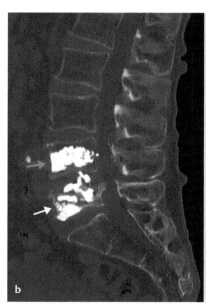

Fig. 18.1 **(a)** Sagittal STIR (short tau inversion recovery) MR image shows pathologic fractures secondary to prostate adenocarcinoma metastasis at L4 (*red arrow*) and L5 (*white arrow*). **(b)** Sagittal CT scan image after kyphoplasty of L4 and L5 demonstrates adequate PMMA (polymethyl methacrylate) filling of the vertebral bodies.

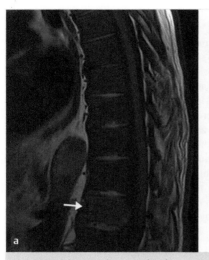 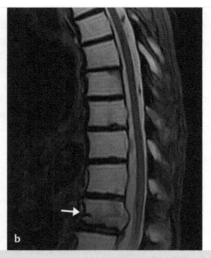 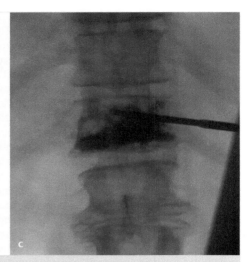

Fig. 18.2 (a) Sagittal T1-weighted sequence of the thoracic spine demonstrates diffuse metastatic infiltration of the bone marrow by a rectal mucinous adenocarcinoma (T1-weighted signal of the marrow significantly lower than the disk). (b) Sagittal T2-weighted sequence. *Arrows* in (a) and (b) show a T12 pathologic vertebral compression fracture. (c) Fluoroscopic image demonstrates adequate PMMA (polymethyl methacrylate) fill of the vertebral body from pedicle to pedicle and from end plate to end plate.

meetings are useful to optimize therapy approaches and patient outcomes. Indeed, discussions between the department of radiation oncology, neurosurgery, and interventional pain management help select candidates that might benefit from vertebral augmentation prior (or after) to radiation therapy. The goal of instilling polymethyl methacrylate (PMMA) in these patients is to provide anterior column support and reducing the risk of additional pathologic fractures related to the weakened trabecular bone due to radiation and tumor infiltration.

18.2.3 Fractures Secondary to Infection

VCF can be caused by underlying infection (spondylitis or spondylodiskitis). If an underlying infection is suspected, meticulous evaluation of the patient should be performed to make an adequate diagnosis and avoid catastrophic consequences related to instillation of PMMA within an infected nidus. It is important to recognize pyogenic spondylitis and to treat it accordingly with antibiotics. An infectious process is an absolute contraindication for an augmentation procedure, just like a suspected systemic infection.

The MR signal characteristics can sometimes be similar for both a metastasis and a spondylitis/spondylodiskitis. Both can have hypointense T1-wighted signal and hyperintense T2/short tau inversion recovery (STIR) weighted signal on MRI. However, in 95% of the infectious processes, the disk will be involved (▶ Fig. 18.3) and, due to its avascular characteristics, this anatomical location will be affected in only 1% of the neoplasm/metastasis.[19] Also, classic radiological findings can be useful to differentiate both entities (▶ Table 18.2). The patient history and clinical symptoms are also keys to differentiate both entities. The following points can provide arguments in favor of spondylitis/spondylodiskitis: history of intravenous (IV) drug usage, chronic preexisting disease, prior spinal surgery, and penetrating trauma.

With a suspected spondylitis, laboratory and microbiological tests should also be performed. An elevated C-reactive protein (CRP) will be highly suggestive of infection and will be seen in 90 to 98% of cases.[19] Blood sedimentation rate can also be helpful but is less specific than CRP. Elevated white cell count may or may not be present.

Aerobic and anaerobic cultures should also be obtained via blood culture (at least two blood culture pairs should be obtained). However, the pathogen is identified only in 25 to 60% of cases. A biopsy of the disk, end plate, or paravertebral soft tissue has a specificity close to 90% and should be considered whenever possible. Despite the high specificity, needle biopsies of the intervertebral disk may have a sensitivity of only 33%, so a negative culture result after a biopsy should not preclude empiric treatment for a suspected diskitis.[20]

Most commonly, spondylodiskitis occurs via hematogenous route. Typically, in adults, the bacteria will first affect the end plates and then will extend to the intervertebral disk. Another possible seeding mechanism is via direct extension, for instance in penetrating trauma or infection from instrumentation.

Spondylodiskitis is overwhelmingly caused by *Staphylococcus aureus* (50–70% of cases) in developed countries.[21,22] However, tuberculous spondylodiskitis, most commonly resulting from hematogenous spread, is the most common type worldwide.

Other gram-positive and gram-negative bacteria are responsible for spondylodiskitis such as the following: *Enterobacteriaceae* species such as *E. coli* (e.g., patients with active urinary tract infections); *P. aeruginosa* (e.g., patients with a history of IV drug abuse); *Brucellosis* (e.g., patients living in Mediterranean countries and in the Middle East); less commonly *Streptococcus pneumoniae* (e.g., patients with diabetes); and more rarely *Salmonella* species (e.g., patients with sickle cell disease or asplenia). *Brucella*, *fungi*, and *parasites* such as *hydatid disease* are other possible infectious pathogens, but are rarely seen.

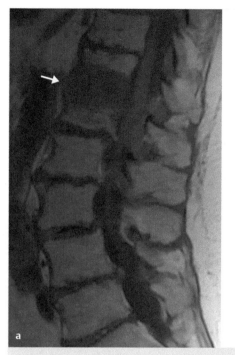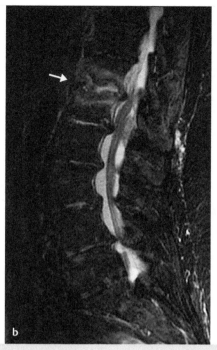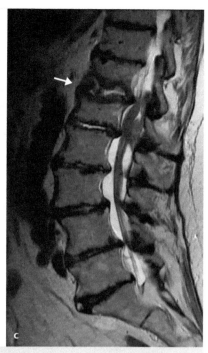

Fig. 18.3 Classic case of T12–L1 pyogenic spondylodiskitis. **(a)** T1-weighted, **(b)** STIR (short tau inversion recovery), and **(c)** T2-weighted sequences demonstrate a T1 hypointense focus with central T2 fluidlike signal centered on the disk space (*white arrows*).

Table 18.2 Radiological findings differentiating spondylitis/spondylodiskitis of metastases

MRI findings	In favor of spondylitis/ spondylodiskitis	In favor of metastases
Hyperintense T2/ STIR signal	X	X
Hypointense T1 signal	X	X
Disk involvement	X	
End plate erosion	X	
Paravertebral/ psoas/epidural inflammation or abscess	X	

Abbreviations: MRI, magnetic resonance imaging; STIR, short tau inversion recovery.

18.2.4 Traumatic Fractures

Traumatic spine fractures are more prevalent in the males, with a male-to-female ratio of 1.6:1.[23] In comparison to osteoporotic fractures that virtually happen all after 60 years of age, the majority of patients with traumatic vertebral fracture are between the age of 20 and 50 years. The most common cause of fracture is a high-energy fall (40%), followed by traffic accidents (25%). The fractures related to falls can happen anywhere along the spine, while fractures related to motor vehicle accident preferentially affect the thoracic and cervical spine. The majority of fractures, however, happen in the thoracolumbar region (L1: 29%; T12: 14%; L2: 12%).[23]

This high prevalence of fractures along the thoracolumbar region can be explained with underlying biomechanical reasons. The mid to upper thoracic region (T1–T8) is stabilized by the ribs. At T9–L2, there is a transition between the rigid/kyphotic midthoracic region and the flexible lordotic lumbar spine. Also, the positions of the center of gravity of the thoracic and lumbar spine are located completely opposite from one to the other; in the upper and midthoracic spine, the center of gravity is located anteriorly to the spine, while in the lumbar spine the center of gravity is located posteriorly. For these reasons, the thoracolumbar transitional region is susceptible to traumatic fractures.

The majority of traumatic spine fractures will be of compressive origin (55%); however, distraction (17%), rotation (18%), and fracture-dislocation (20%) are also prevalent mechanisms. Indeed, most of the fractures of the thoracic and lumbar region that have failure under axial compression without injury to the posterior ligamentous complex (PLC) are classified as Magerl or AO type A fractures. To date, only few studies have evaluated the use of vertebroplasty to treat traumatic vertebral fractures. This is mainly due to the younger age of the patients with traumatic fractures, uncertainties regarding the biomechanics alteration after PMMA cement instillation, and possible risk of cement leakage.[24] However, as discussed in prior chapters, these concerns have been addressed in multiple publications.

Our expectation is that more cases of vertebral augmentation will be performed in patients with vertebral traumatic fracture. However, it is worth noting that some of those cases require advanced expertise, and consultation between colleagues would be considered good practice, especially when younger patients are being treated. In the upcoming years, percutaneous implants will have an important role to play in traumatic vertebral fractures, both by ensuring an optimal correction of the kyphotic angle and by providing for decreased cement leakage.

18.3 Key Points

- VCFs are extremely prevalent, affecting close to 25% of the population of our society.
- Osteoporosis is responsible for the vast majority of VCFs; however, trauma, infection, and neoplasm are other predisposing factors to consider.
- Genetic predisposition has a significant impact on osteoporosis and VCF incidence. At least 15 genes have been confirmed as susceptibility genes.
- After vertebral augmentation, the only risk factor significantly associated with subsequent compression fracture is the presence of osteoporosis (low T-score).
- Spine metastases are 40 times more prevalent than all primary tumors.
- Spondylodiskitis is overwhelmingly caused by *S. aureus* (50–70% of cases) in developed countries
- Traumatic vertebral fractures happen in younger patients. The most common location of these fractures is at T9–L2 because of the transition between the rigid/kyphotic midthoracic region and the flexible lordotic lumbar spine.

References

[1] Melton LJ III, Thamer M, Ray NF, et al. Fractures attributable to osteoporosis: report from the National Osteoporosis Foundation. J Bone Miner Res 1997;12(1):16–23

[2] Melton LJ, Chrischilles EA, Cooper C, Lane AW, Riggs BL. How many women have osteoporosis? JBMR Anniversary Classic. JBMR, Volume 7, Number 9, 1992. J Bone Miner Res 2005;20(5):886–892

[3] Lane JM, Nydick M. Osteoporosis: current modes of prevention and treatment. J Am Acad Orthop Surg 1999;7(1):19–31

[4] Lindsay R, Silverman SL, Cooper C, et al. Risk of new vertebral fracture in the year following a fracture. JAMA 2001;285(3):320–323

[5] Roux C, Fechtenbaum J, Kolta S, Briot K, Girard M. Mild prevalent and incident vertebral fractures are risk factors for new fractures. Osteoporos Int 2007;18(12):1617–1624

[6] Kim DH, Vaccaro AR. Osteoporotic compression fractures of the spine; current options and considerations for treatment. Spine J 2006;6(5):479–487

[7] Qaseem A, Wilt TJ, McLean RM, Forciea MA; Clinical Guidelines Committee of the American College of Physicians. Noninvasive treatments for acute, subacute, and chronic low back pain: a clinical practice guideline from the American College of Physicians. Ann Intern Med 2017;166(7):514–530

[8] O'Neill TW, Felsenberg D, Varlow J, Cooper C, Kanis JA, Silman AJ. The prevalence of vertebral deformity in european men and women: the European Vertebral Osteoporosis Study. J Bone Miner Res 1996;11(7):1010–1018

[9] Ralston SH. Genetics of osteoporosis. Proc Nutr Soc 2007;66(2):158–165

[10] Bailey CA, Brooke-Wavell K. Exercise for optimising peak bone mass in women. Proc Nutr Soc 2008;67(1):9–18

[11] Stokes IA, Gardner-Morse M, Henry SM, Badger GJ. Decrease in trunk muscular response to perturbation with preactivation of lumbar spinal musculature. Spine 2000;25(15):1957–1964

[12] Mokhtarzadeh H, Anderson DE. The role of trunk musculature in osteoporotic vertebral fractures: implications for prediction, prevention, and management. Curr Osteoporos Rep 2016;14(3):67–76

[13] Granata KP, Marras WS. The influence of trunk muscle coactivity on dynamic spinal loads. Spine 1995;20(8):913–919

[14] Gardner-Morse MG, Stokes IA. The effects of abdominal muscle coactivation on lumbar spine stability. Spine 1998;23(1):86–91, discussion 91–92

[15] Lu K, Liang C-L, Hsieh C-H, Tsai Y-D, Chen H-J, Liliang P-C. Risk factors of subsequent vertebral compression fractures after vertebroplasty. Pain Med 2012;13(3):376–382

[16] Fan B, Wei Z, Zhou X, et al. Does vertebral augmentation lead to an increasing incidence of adjacent vertebral failure? A systematic review and meta-analysis. Int J Surg 2016;36(Pt A):369–376

[17] Papanastassiou ID, Phillips FM, Van Meirhaeghe J, et al. Comparing effects of kyphoplasty, vertebroplasty, and non-surgical management in a systematic review of randomized and non-randomized controlled studies. Eur Spine J 2012;21(9):1826–1843

[18] Curtis JR, Taylor AJ, Matthews RS, et al. "Pathologic" fractures: should these be included in epidemiologic studies of osteoporotic fractures? Osteoporos Int 2009;20(11):1969–1972

[19] Herren C, Jung N, Pishnamaz M, Breuninger M, Siewe J, Sobottke R. Spondylodiscitis: diagnosis and treatment options. Dtsch Arztebl Int 2017;114(51–52):875–882

[20] Nam KH, Song GS, Han IH, Choi BK, Cha SH. Diagnostic value of biopsy techniques in lumbar spondylodiscitis: percutaneous needle biopsy and open biopsy. Korean J Spine 2011;8(4):267–271

[21] Waldvogel FA, Medoff G, Swartz MN. Osteomyelitis: a review of clinical features, therapeutic considerations and unusual aspects. N Engl J Med 1970;282(4):198–206

[22] Patel AR, Alton TB, Bransford RJ, Lee MJ, Bellabarba CB, Chapman JR. Spinal epidural abscesses: risk factors, medical versus surgical management, a retrospective review of 128 cases. Spine J 2014;14(3):326–330

[23] Leucht P, Fischer K, Muhr G, Mueller EJ. Epidemiology of traumatic spine fractures. Injury 2009;40(2):166–172

[24] Knavel EM, Thielen KR, Kallmes DF. Vertebroplasty for the treatment of traumatic nonosteoporotic compression fractures. AJNR Am J Neuroradiol 2009;30(2):323–327

19 Bracing for Spinal Fractures

Aaron L. Cross and Andrew L. Sherman

Summary

Spine bracing has undergone extensive updates since the introduction of bracing in the 1930s and are now commonly recommended for patients undergoing rehabilitation from surgery or spine injury. Bracing is commonly employed after vertebral compression fractures but its effectiveness is still in question. The goal of bracing is to limit spine motion as much as possible and various types of braces exist for each anatomic segment of the spine. There are different types of cervical braces which are most commonly employed after a traumatic injury when nonsurgical management is the preferred method of treatment. Thoracic and lumbar braces are commonly used for compression fracture bracing. They can be either rigid or soft and provide varying degrees of spinal stability. Generally the spinal braces used for osteoporotic vertebral compression fractures (VCFs) have been shown to provide limited benefits in regard to pain and functional improvement or no benefit. Despite literature evidence supporting the use of bracing, it remains a common initial treatment for those patients with painful VCFs. There are also some potential complications of bracing that clinicians should be aware of including an increased risk of skin breakdown in the locations of the brace's pressure points. As opposed to osteoporotic VCFs, bracing is generally recommended in cases of traumatic VCFs where surgery is performed or as an adjunct to surgical fixation. While bracing may confer mild benefit in regard to patient comfort or slightly reduced healing time, additional investigation will need to be done to determine the effectiveness of spinal bracing in the treatment of patients with painful VCFs.

Keywords: bracing, spine brace, lumbosacral orthosis, TLSO, Jewett, lumbosacral orthosis

19.1 Introduction

Before the year 1931, spine braces were not patented and nor were they sold for use. Physicians would make them for specific patients. These early braces tended to be painful and not very functional and most of the bracing at that time was done to treat adolescent scoliosis. The Milwaukee brace, a removable cervicothoracolumbosacral orthosis (CTLSO) was invented in 1946.[1] The brace was cumbersome and the metal bars went from the neck down the lower lumbar spine. The result was that a person wearing the brace could not look down for balance and the brace could not be fitted under clothing. In 1972, an adolescent female in Boston diagnosed with idiopathic scoliosis refused to wear the Milwaukee brace because of the neck strap. Her father made some adjustments by cutting off the top part of the brace, changing the metal to plastic and adding padding at the pressure points. This was subsequently dubbed the Boston brace and since then, numerous adjustments and alterations have improved the comfort and functionality of the brace.[2]

Spine braces are routinely recommended for patients during rehabilitation from back injuries and surgeries either as the primary treatment method for a less severe spine fracture or after a surgical repair. For more serious fractures, bracing is felt to be an important adjunct to surgical management. Despite its acceptance, bracing is not without controversy; it is has not been shown that any back brace actually improves outcomes. This chapter will explore the main uses of braces and some of the published evidence regarding their use.

The goal of any brace, spine or otherwise, is immobilization. Immobilization allows for bone healing to occur. Some braces are better at immobilizing spines than others and custom-fitted "clamshell" braces that encompass your entire trunk in rigid plastic are more likely to reduce spinal movement, especially bending and twisting, than loose-fitting metal braces. Even the most aggressive braces, however, can probably only do so much to stabilize the spine and mitigate further vertebral compression or collapse of the vertebral body.

19.2 Cervical Fracture Bracing

Most fractures in the cervical spine are related to trauma and when neurological compromise or frank instability is present, surgery is usually the treatment of choice. When nonsurgical management (NSM) is the optimal course of treatment, a cervical orthosis is usually utilized. Johnson et al described four types of cervical braces: cervical collars, poster braces, cervical-thoracic braces, and the halo vest.[3] Each brace is utilized in specific situations as described below.

Most stable cervical spine fractures are placed in rigid or semirigid collars. The most common of these is the Philadelphia collar. The Philadelphia collar is a two-piece semirigid orthosis made of Plastazote and reinforced with anterior and posterior plastic struts. The Philadelphia collar restricts motion much better than a soft collar but is less comfortable. Other similar collars are the Miami J collar (▶ Fig. 19.1) and the Aspen collar. Despite their stiffness, the rigid collars lack the ability to effectively immobilize the lower cervical spine.[4]

The SOMI (Sterno-Occipito-Mandibular Immobilizer) orthosis provides better restriction of motion of the low-cervical spine and cervicothoracic junction compared to the collar option. The SOMI brace provides good restriction to flexion (93% restriction of motion), but is less beneficial for control of neck extension (42% restriction of motion), lateral bending (66% restriction of motion), and axial rotation (66% restriction of motion).[5,6] This brace is good for providing additional support to stable mid and lower cervical spine fractures.

For unstable upper cervical spine fractures, the orthosis most often utilized is the halo orthosis (▶ Fig. 19.2). The use of a halo vest is usually confined to injuries with limited displacement. The duration of treatment varies between 6 weeks and

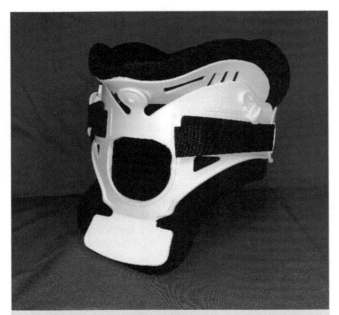

Fig. 19.1 Miami J orthosis. (This image is provided courtesy of Stephen R. Dsida, LP, CPO.)

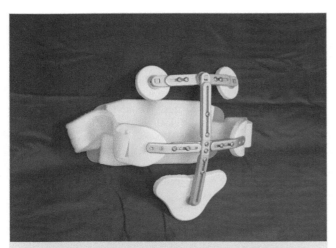

Fig. 19.3 Cruciform anterior spinal hyperextension (CASH) thoracolumbar orthosis. (This image is provided courtesy of Stephen R. Dsida, LP, CPO.)

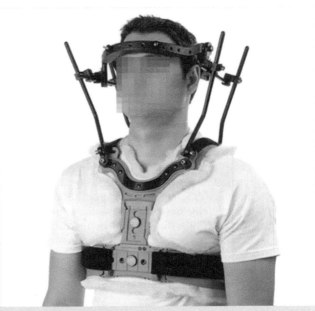

Fig. 19.2 Halo orthosis. (This image is provided courtesy of Össur.)

19.3 Lumbar and Thoracic Compression Fracture Bracing

19.3.1 Introduction

Spinal orthoses have been widely used in the management of thoracolumbar fractures. A large variety of braces are available as either prefabricated from numerous manufacturers or custom-fabricated units created with the assistance of a prosthetist/orthotist. The following is a review of the types of braces available and evidence regarding their efficacy in traumatic and osteoporotic fractures.

19.3.2 Types of Thoracolumbar Braces

Thoracolumbosacral Orthosis

TLSOs can be either rigid or soft. Both prefabricated and custom-fabricated options are available. The rigid-type design controls extension, flexion, lateral bending, and rotation. The TLSOs are primarily used in the management of VCFs with significant deformity or stable burst fractures from T6 to L4 that do not require surgical intervention.[10] Examples of TLSOs in order of increasing immobilization include the dorsal lumbar corset, the Jewett hyperextension brace, the cruciform anterior sternal hyperextension (CASH) brace (▶ Fig. 19.3), and the custom-molded thermoplastic TLSO (▶ Fig. 19.4).

Lumbosacral Orthosis

Lumbosacral-type orthoses can also be either rigid or soft. Both prefabricated and custom-fabricated options are available. A rigid lumbosacral orthosis (LSO) provides the most restriction of motion and is typically used to immobilize the lumbar spine at the L3 segment and below. If there is a need to provide significantly more immobilization to the L4–L5 and

4 months.[6] A halo vest is the most rigid external immobilizer, especially for the upper cervical spine. It restricts up to 75% of flexion–extension at C1–C2, and offers superior control of lateral bending and rotation compared to other cervical braces.[7] As effective as the halo vest is at immobilizing the cervical spine, it can limit pulmonary function. Taitsman et al found that the halo vest leads to increased risk of pulmonary complications including pneumonia.[8]

Bracing treatment of lower cervical and upper thoracic spine fractures may also be done by using the Minerva brace, a cervical collar jacket.[9] Sharpe et al found that for cervical fractures, except for above C1, the Minerva provided "improvement in control of flexion/extension of the upper cervical spine and in control of rotation."[9]

L5–S1 segments, a unilateral thigh extension can be added.[11] The lumbosacral corset is a typically made from cloth and is most often used as an adjunctive support for individuals with low back pain (▶ Fig. 19.5). The lumbosacral chairback orthoses (▶ Fig. 19.6) are designed with a circumferential band that typically starts at the lower thoracic levels and extends down midway between the iliac crest and the greater trochanter. Chairback orthoses are also often used to provide support for those with low back pain or postoperatively following lumbar fusion surgery.

Garment Orthoses

Garment-type orthoses are semirigid or flexible, prefabricated braces designed to fit closely to the body with shoulder straps and a pelvic band to prevent migration.[12] Examples include the SpinoMed (▶ Fig. 19.7) and OsteoMed orthoses. They have been used primarily in women with osteoporosis for long-term

management of osteoporotic compression fractures. In general, they have been shown to provide small and limited benefits by reducing pain, improving strength, and improving posture or kyphosis.[13–15]

Kypho-Orthoses

Kypho-orthoses are semirigid or flexible, prefabricated braces that limit or counteract flexion. An example of this type of brace is the Posturex, a semirigid, backpack-style brace with adjustable paravertebral bars. This is a weighted kypho-orthosis that has a soft, backpack design with light weights suspended on the posterior aspect for the brace to encourage extension. Kypho-orthoses have primarily been used in women with subacute osteoporotic VCFs or in the long-term management of osteoporosis. A few small studies have evaluated their efficacy and found limited improvements primarily in balance and gait.[16–18]

19.3.3 Concepts on the Use of the TLSO Braces

Orthoses have been employed in the management of osteoporotic VCFs with the goal to provide stability to the fracture, reduce pain, and allow for earlier mobility. However, their overall effectiveness in these areas is uncertain and there are

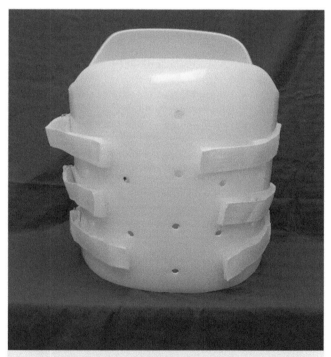

Fig. 19.4 Custom-fabricated thoracolumbar sacral orthosis (TLSO). (This image is provided courtesy of Stephen R. Dsida, LP, CPO.)

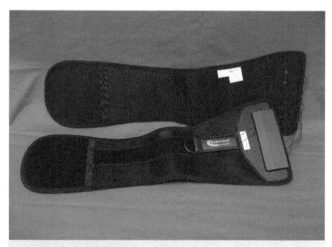

Fig. 19.5 Lumbosacral corset. (This image is provided courtesy of Stephen R. Dsida, LP, CPO.)

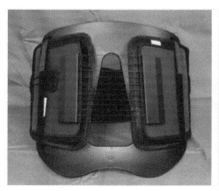

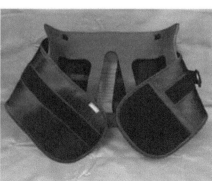

Fig. 19.6 Lumbosacral chairback orthosis. (This image is provided courtesy of Stephen R. Dsida, LP, CPO.)

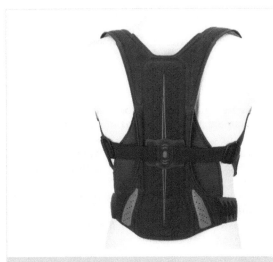

Fig. 19.7 SpinoMed orthosis. (This image is provided courtesy of Stephen R. Dsida, LP, CPO.)

no compelling data to support their use as an effective method of adjunctive treatment in patients with osteoporotic VCFs.[19,20] A number of studies have examined the role of bracing in osteoporotic compression fractures or for osteoporosis with and without compression fractures. These efforts have varied widely in the types of orthoses evaluated, time after injury that bracing was applied, the duration of treatment, and the outcomes accessed. The heterogeneity and overall paucity of these data have resulted in a confusing picture of what role bracing should have in the management of osteoporotic VCFs. Some current guidelines provide conflicting recommendations with some recommending for the use of back braces in patients with painful VCFs and some guidelines recommending against their use.[21,22] Despite evidence supporting spinal bracing, it remains a common first-line treatment in the NSM of VCFs in most cases. A brief review of recent data may provide some guidance as to the use of bracing in patients with painful VCFs.

One of the best studies evaluating the outcomes of patients with acute osteoporotic compression fractures without neurologic injury is a randomized controlled trial comparing types of braces and no bracing. These patients were either treated using a rigid TLSO, a soft brace or no brace within 3 days after injury. After 12 weeks, the baseline-adjusted Oswestry Disability Index for the no brace group was not inferior to the rigid TLSO or soft brace groups. All groups had statistically significant improved adjusted Oswestry Disability Index, visual analog scores, and improvement in anterior vertebral body compression.[20] The lack of difference between the braced groups and the group without the brace along with the overall improvement in all groups is important to consider when evaluating studies comparing one brace to another due to the fact that any overall improvement of the patient discomfort of functional capacity may be due to the improvement of their condition apart from their use of a brace.

The rates of radiographic fracture union with use of a TLSO following osteoporotic compression fracture were investigated by Murata et al with approximately 54% of fractures achieving union after 2 months, 80% at 3 months, and 89% at 6 months.[23] In comparison, the authors report approximately 60% of osteoporotic compression fractures treated with a soft corset exhibited dynamic radiographic union at an average of 20 months. The authors conclude that a plastic TLSO plays a biomechanical role in the healing of osteoporotic VCFs but acknowledge that when comparing the two groups clinically there was no significant difference between the groups at 6 months.

Several studies specifically investigated the effectiveness of the garment-type SpinoMed orthosis in female subjects. When treatment was initiated 1 week following the fracture for a total treatment time of 3 weeks, the SpinoMed was no better in reducing pain or improving function compared with a soft lumbar orthosis.[13] However, wearing the orthosis for 6 months following acute fracture was associated with increased back extensor strength, increased abdominal flexor strength, decreased kyphotic angle, increased vital capacity, less pain, and improved function when compared with no brace controls (A14, A23). Further, in a study designed to evaluate the long-term effect of using the SpinoMed orthosis in the setting of osteoporosis and prior compression fractures of indeterminate age, females who used the orthosis for at least 2 hours a day for 6 months had significantly decreased back pain and increased isometric trunk muscle strength.[24] Finally, a study that compared the SpinoMed brace with a three-point orthosis in both males and females found a statistically significant improvement in pain, disability, and forced expiratory volume in the SpinoMed group.[25] These small studies point to favorable outcomes following long-term use of the SpinoMed orthoses but have looked at fractures of indeterminate age, have compared one type of brace to another, and have compared bracing to treatments with calcium and bisphosphonates, none of which is optimal NSM for patients with acute or subacute VCFs.

The treatment of patients with bracing is also not without potential complications. A single small trial found 11% of patients immobilized with plaster corset for an average of 2.3 months had skin breakdown requiring plaster corset removal compared with no skin changes seen in patients treated with other orthoses for an average of 2.9 months.[26]

Plaster corsets have been out of favor for quite some time and thoracic and lumbar fractures are currently treated with the Jewett brace or the CASH brace because of their hyperextension properties. The Jewett brace is a three-point pressure system with two anterior pads that place pressure over the sternum and pubic symphysis, and one posterior pad to produce an opposing pressure in the midthoracic region. Although the Jewett and CASH braces provide excellent sagittal hyperextension and limit flexion–extension motion, they are not able to prominently reduce the motion in the coronal and transverse planes. A new design of brace known as the Knight–Taylor brace is less effective for preventing flexion and extension but is much better in preventing lateral bending. Similar to the Jewett and CASH braces, the Knight–Taylor brace is ineffective in restricting axial rotation.[27] The movement that is allowed in the Knight–Taylor brace, however, has been shown to allow patients to maintain static and dynamic motor balance.[28]

19.3.4 Bracing for Traumatic Burst Fractures of the Lumbar and Thoracic Spine

A traumatic burst fracture is a spinal fracture where the vertebra fractures from immediate and severe axial loading. Acute trauma such as a car accident or a fall from a height is the leading cause for burst fractures. Often there are pieces of the vertebra that are displaced into the surrounding tissues and sometimes the spinal canal. For fractures that are unstable (three-column fractures) or associated with neurological injury, surgical intervention is typically the treatment of choice with TLSO bracing used postoperatively as an adjunctive treatment. For relatively stable fractures as defined by less than 25- to 30-degree kyphosis, less than 50% loss of vertebral body height, and less than 50% retropulsion of bone into the spinal canal, bracing is recommend.[29] A TLSO is typically worn for 8 to 12 weeks after the injury and the patient is monitored with serial radiographs. Wood et al reported that while early analysis (4 years) revealed few significant differences between the two groups, the long-term follow-up (between 16 and 22 years), those with relatively stable burst fracture who were treated nonoperatively reported less pain, no worse kyphosis, and had better function compared with those who were treated surgically.[30]

Another group of studies showed that while surgical stabilization and possible decompression may result in earlier mobilization, reduced time to hospital discharge, and faster return to work, surgical intervention may also expose patients to more complications and increased risk for subsequent revision surgery and may end up as a more expensive treatment associated with greater overall health care costs.[31,32] The conclusion of one major study was that: "Non-operative management including symptomatic pain control, early mobilization, and perhaps a brace may be an acceptable alternative in properly selected patients."[33]

19.4 Osteoporotic Lumbar and Thoracic Fractures

Compared with evidence of bracing in traumatic fractures, the available evidence regarding bracing for patient with osteoporotic VCFs is limited.[34] There are not many high-quality studies in this patient population that have been performed or published. The origin of brace use after osteoporotic spinal fracture is largely empiric and extrapolated from the use of bracing in higher velocity traumatic fractures. The theory is immobilization and reduction of compressive forces that would cause additional compression of the vertebrae. The success of bracing to prevent further deformity and allow healing relies on the supposition that the spinal braces actually immobilize the spine.

One prospective randomized study used TLSO to manage osteoporotic VCFs and found no difference in outcome whether a brace was used or not.[20] Another study looked at 62 patients with such fractures. When comparing one brace to another, there was increased trunk muscle strength, improved posture, and improved vertebral height in the braced group using a brace that allowed more movement.[14]

A second randomized control trial evaluated the outcomes of patients with acute osteoporotic compression fractures without neurologic injury. These patients were treated using either a rigid brace or no brace within 3 days after injury. The primary outcome was the patient function as measured by the Roland–Morris Disability Questionnaire at 3 months post-injury and secondary outcomes were assessed until 2 years after the injury. They found no significant difference between the treatment groups for any outcome measured at any time point throughout the entire study.[35] The authors concluded that treatment without bracing was equivalent to treatment with a TLSO brace for severely comminuted type A3 fractures and the influence of the brace on early pain control and late function remains yet to be determined. They also concluded that even comminuted burst fractures, in the absence of an associated posterior ligamentous complex injury, are a very stable injury and may not require a brace.

A separate question when the treating clinician elects to use a brace is what the best orthosis is for thoracic and lumbar osteoporotic VCFs. One study found that plaster corsets gave better stability and patients had more mobility but were less compliant. Another study found that compared to three-point orthoses, patients treated with a dynamic orthosis had a greater reduction in pain and a greater improvement in quality of life and respiratory function, with equal effectiveness in stabilizing the fracture, and fewer complications.[25] An additional study found that a lower profile LSO was less effective than a full TLSO for restricting motion not only in the upper lumbar but in the lower lumbar spine as well.[12,35,36]

In summary, despite the widespread acceptance of spinal bracing in treating osteoporotic VCFs, evidence proving the effectiveness of these orthoses in treating patients with VCFs is lacking and much of the better quality studies show no differences in patient outcomes whether a brace is used or not. There may be a benefit of increased patient comfort or reduced healing time when a TLSO is used, but this has not been reliably shown and further investigations are needed. In patients with subacute fractures, there is some evidence that garment-type and kyphosis-limiting orthoses may be of benefit by decreasing pain and improving core strength, but it is unknown if this increase in strength has any clinical significance.[20,37] The efficacy for bracing in osteoporotic compression fracture remains inconclusive. In the future, additional studies are needed with standardized outcome measures to demonstrate the benefit of bracing in the setting of vertebral fracture.

What is conspicuously absent is a study comparing vertebral augmentation to bracing, which is a decision commonly encountered by clinicians on a daily basis throughout the country. Based on current literature information, bracing would likely be far inferior to vertebral augmentation, but this study has yet to be done.

References

[1] Fayssoux RS, Cho RH, Herman MJ. A history of bracing for idiopathic scoliosis in North America. Clin Orthop Relat Res 2010;468(3):654–664

[2] Périé D, Aubin CE, Petit Y, Beauséjour M, Dansereau J, Labelle H. Boston brace correction in idiopathic scoliosis: a biomechanical study. Spine 2003;28(15):1672–1677

[3] Johnson RM, Hart DL, Simmons EF, Ramsby GR, Southwick WO. Cervical orthoses. A study comparing their effectiveness in restricting cervical motion in normal subjects. J Bone Joint Surg Am 1977;59(3):332–339

[4] Lauweryns P. Role of conservative treatment of cervical spine injuries. Eur Spine J 2010;19(Suppl 1):S23–S26

[5] Basu S, Chatterjee S, Bhattacharya MK, Seal K. Injuries of the upper cervical spine: A series of 28 cases. Indian J Orthop 2007;41(4):305–311

[6] Fisher SV. Proper fitting of the cervical orthosis. Arch Phys Med Rehabil 1978;59(11):505–507

[7] Richter D, Latta LL, Milne EL, et al. The stabilizing effects of different orthoses in the intact and unstable upper cervical spine: a cadaver study. J Trauma 2001;50(5):848–854

[8] Taitsman LA, Altman DT, Hecht AC, Pedlow FX. Complications of cervical halo-vest orthoses in elderly patients. Orthopedics 2008;31(5):446

[9] Sharpe KP, Rao S, Ziogas A. Evaluation of the effectiveness of the Minerva cervicothoracic orthosis. Spine 1995;20(13):1475–1479

[10] Agabegi SS, Asghar FA, Herkowitz HN. Spinal orthoses. J Am Acad Orthop Surg 2010;18(11):657–667

[11] Fidler MW, Plasmans CM. The effect of four types of support on the segmental mobility of the lumbosacral spine. J Bone Joint Surg Am 1983;65(7):943–947

[12] Newman M, Minns Lowe C, Barker K. Spinal orthoses for vertebral osteoporosis and osteoporotic vertebral fracture: a systematic review. Arch Phys Med Rehabil 2016;97(6):1013–1025

[13] Li M, Law SW, Cheng J, Kee HM, Wong MS. A comparison study on the efficacy of SpinoMed and soft lumbar orthosis for osteoporotic vertebral fracture. Prosthet Orthot Int 2015;39(4):270–276

[14] Pfeifer M, Kohlwey L, Begerow B, Minne HW. Effects of two newly developed spinal orthoses on trunk muscle strength, posture, and quality-of-life in women with postmenopausal osteoporosis: a randomized trial. Am J Phys Med Rehabil 2011;90(10):805–815

[15] Vogt L, Hübscher M, Brettmann K, Banzer W, Fink M. Postural correction by osteoporosis orthosis (Osteo-med): a randomized, placebo-controlled trial. Prosthet Orthot Int 2008;32(1):103–110

[16] Gündoğdu M, Oncel S, Sahin E, Baydar M, Dilek B. The effect of posture support corset on balance, quality of life, dorsal kyphosis in patients with kyphosis due to osteoporosis. Turk Geriatri Derg 2013;16:253–259

[17] Sinaki M, Brey RH, Hughes CA, Larson DR, Kaufman KR. Significant reduction in risk of falls and back pain in osteoporotic-kyphotic women through a Spinal Proprioceptive Extension Exercise Dynamic (SPEED) program. Mayo Clin Proc 2005;80(7):849–855

[18] Raeissadat SA, Sedighipour L, Pournajaf S, Vahab Kashani R, Sadeghi S. Effect of posture training with weighted kypho-orthosis (WKO) on improving balance in women with osteoporosis. J Aging Res 2014;2014:427–903

[19] Dionyssiotis Y, Trovas G, Thoma S, Lyritis G, Papaioannou N. Prospective study of spinal orthoses in women. Prosthet Orthot Int 2015;39(6):487–495

[20] Kim HJ, Yi JM, Cho HG, et al. Comparative study of the treatment outcomes of osteoporotic compression fractures without neurologic injury using a rigid brace, a soft brace, and no brace: a prospective randomized controlled noninferiority trial. J Bone Joint Surg Am 2014;96(23):1959–1966

[21] Faciszewski T, McKiernan F. Calling all vertebral fractures classification of vertebral compression fractures: a consensus for comparison of treatment and outcome. J Bone Miner Res 2002;17(2):185–191

[22] Esses SI, McGuire R, Jenkins J, et al. American Academy of Orthopaedic Surgeons clinical practice guideline on: the treatment of osteoporotic spinal compression fractures. J Bone Joint Surg Am 2011;93(20):1934–1936

[23] Murata K, Watanabe G, Kawaguchi S, et al. Union rates and prognostic variables of osteoporotic vertebral fractures treated with a rigid external support. J Neurosurg Spine 2012;17(5):469–475

[24] Pfeifer M, Begerow B, Minne HW. Effects of a new spinal orthosis on posture, trunk strength, and quality of life in women with postmenopausal osteoporosis: a randomized trial. Am J Phys Med Rehabil 2004;83(3):177–186

[25] Meccariello L, Muzii VF, Falzarano G, et al. Dynamic corset versus three-point brace in the treatment of osteoporotic compression fractures of the thoracic and lumbar spine: a prospective, comparative study. Aging Clin Exp Res 2017;29(3):443–449

[26] Talic A, Kapetanovic J, Dizdar A. Effects of conservative treatment for osteoporotic thoracolumbal spine fractures. Mater Sociomed 2012;24(1):16–20

[27] Patwardhan AG, Li SP, Gavin T, Lorenz M, Meade KP, Zindrick M. Orthotic stabilization of thoracolumbar injuries. A biomechanical analysis of the Jewett hyperextension orthosis. Spine 1990;15(7):654–661

[28] Liaw MY, Chen CL, Chen JF, Tang FT, Wong AM, Ho HH. Effects of Knight-Taylor brace on balance performance in osteoporotic patients with vertebral compression fracture. J Back Musculoskeletal Rehabil 2009;22(2):75–81

[29] Rajasekaran S. Thoracolumbar burst fractures without neurological deficit: the role for conservative treatment. Eur Spine J 2010;19(Suppl 1):S40–S47

[30] Wood KB, Butterman GR, Phukan R, et al. Operative compared with nonoperative treatment of a thoracolumbar burst fracture without neurological deficit a prospective randomized study with follow-up at sixteen to twenty-two years. J Bone Joint Surg Am 2015;97(1):3–9

[31] Thomas KC, Bailey CS, Dvorak MF, Kwon B, Fisher C. Comparison of operative and nonoperative treatment for thoracolumbar burst fractures in patients without neurological deficit: a systematic review. J Neurosurg Spine 2006;4(5):351–358

[32] Aleem IS, Nassr A. Cochrane in CORR: surgical versus non-surgical treatment for thoracolumbar burst fractures without neurological deficit. Clin Orthop Relat Res 2016;474(3):619–624

[33] Abudou M, Chen X, Kong X, Wu T. Surgical versus non-surgical treatment for thoracolumbar burst fractures without neurological deficit. Cochrane Database Syst Rev 2013;(6):CD005079

[34] Longo UG, Loppini M, Denaro L, Brandi ML, Maffulli N, Denaro V. The effectiveness and safety of vertebroplasty for osteoporotic vertebral compression fractures. A double blind, prospective, randomized, controlled study. Clinical Cases in Mineral and Bone Metabolism 2010;7(2):109–113

[35] Bailey CS, Dvorak MF, Thomas KC, et al. Comparison of thoracolumbosacral orthosis and no orthosis for the treatment of thoracolumbar burst fractures: interim analysis of a multicenter randomized clinical equivalence trial. J Neurosurg Spine 2009;11(3):295–303

[36] Tuong NH, Dansereau J, Maurais G, Herrera R. Three-dimensional evaluation of lumbar orthosis effects on spinal behavior. J Rehabil Res Dev 1998;35(1):34–42

[37] Chang V, Holly LT. Bracing for thoracolumbar fractures. Neurosurg Focus 2014;37(1):E3

20 Amount of Cement or Vertebral Fill Material for Optimal Treatment and Pain Relief

Kieran Murphy and Susannah Ryan

Summary

Vertebral augmentation with injection stabilizing material results in renewed stability of the vertebral body and has been shown to be one of the most effective of all spine procedures in alleviating pain and restoring function. It is presumably the restoration of the structural integrity that results in the prominent decrease in patient pain and this result can be seen in both benign and malignant causes of vertebral instability. The amount of fill material necessary to re-establish the strength of the vertebral body and to be durable over time has evolved over the last decade as new information has indicated that the single most important and modifiable strategy that can be employed for the best and most durable results in vertebral augmentation is the injection of an optimal amount of bone cement. The amount necessary is more than was traditionally thought and is between 15 and 25% of the volume of the uncompressed vertebral level. This will provide optimal strength and stiffness to the vertebral body as well as relieving the patient's pain. The greater amount of cement appears to more optimally stabilize the vertebral body and the results seem to last longer than injecting smaller cement amounts. In addition to injecting an optimal amount of bone cement, other features of the vertebral body that can lead to instability should be taken into consideration. Any nonunion clefts seen on preoperative imaging or on intraoperative fluoroscopy should be filled to ensure an optimal response to vertebral augmentation.

In addition to pain provoking instability within the vertebral body, degenerative end plate changes can give rise to back pain and prominent disability when present. The pathway of pain transmission through the basivertebral nerve (BVN) can be disrupted using BVN ablation. This technique ablates the BVN and can decrease the patients' pain and improve their function with a minimally invasive outpatient needle procedure. The type of degenerative end plate changes is important as Modic type 1 and 2 changes are associated more commonly with back pain than type 3 changes. Modic type 1 changes may have some instability associated with them and it has been shown that injection of bioactive resorbable bone cement can result in significantly decreased pain and significant functional improvements in patients with back pain and type 1 degenerative end plate changes.

Keywords: polymethylmethacrylate, Modic changes, degenerative end plate changes, basivertebral nerve ablation, bone cement fracture cleft

20.1 Introduction

Vertebral augmentation with cement results in stabilization of fracture fragments in a structurally destabilized vertebral body. The loss of mechanical integrity can be due to benign or malignant disease. In benign disease, a failure point is reached that causes a loss of weight-bearing ability. Failure occurs at a lower force in more severely osteoporotic patients. The force necessary to cause fracture is proportional to the degree of bone density and the quality of the bone. In malignant disease with lytic destructive resorption of cortex and trabecula, weight-bearing ability is also lost. The nature of the fracture or that pain that results from it is dependent on the irregular and random distribution of the metastatic disease. The instability caused by an osteoporotic fracture or a neoplasm can be restabilized with vertebral augmentation, and the pain transmission through the BVN complex that innervates the vertebral body can be subsequently decreased after this procedure.[1] An adequate amount of bone cement must be injected to get optimal and durable pain relief and more recent data have further categorized the amount most commonly necessary to establish adequate pain relief.[2]

In addition to an optimal amount of bone cements, other portions of the vertebral body such as nonunion clefts should be filled to ensure optimal stability and response to vertebral augmentation.[3] Within an ostensibly stable vertebral body, there can be pain transmission from the end plate at the junction between a degenerated intervertebral disk and the cartilaginous end plate that gives rise to degenerative end plate changes. This pain transmission through the BVN can be disrupted from ablating the nerve itself prior to its primary point of arborization.[4] *Alternatively, degenerative end plate changes, specifically Modic type 1 degenerative changes can be treated with resorbable bone cement, thereby providing improvement in pain and function in patients with pain originating from this condition.*[5] Whether the symptomatic improvement is a function of increased stability of the vertebral body or ablation of some of the pain transmitting nerve fibers within the vertebral body will be a topic of further investigation.

20.2 What are the Mechanisms of Pain Relief in Vertebral Augmentation?

The mechanism of pain relief in vertebral augmentation is mechanical stabilization of the vertebral body and possibly, to a lesser degree, the denervation of the basivertebral nerve and its C fibers.

20.2.1 Mechanical Stability

Cement Distribution

Tohmeh et al[6] and Belkoff et al[7] published in 1999 and 2002, respectively, that cement injection into fractured cadaveric vertebral specimens could increase the compressive strength of vertebral bodies. Belkoff et al also showed that unilateral cement injection could increase compressive strength of a vertebral body almost as much as a bilateral injection provided the injection was done with the correct technique placing it in the center of the vertebral body. Injection of 6 mL of cement via a unilateral approach was almost as effective as an injection of 5 mL of cement bilaterally.

Get Cement into the Fracture Clefts

While Belkoff et al's work in cadaver spines showed that unilateral cement injection in an isolated vertebral body has almost the same compression strength as a bilateral injection (as measured by an Instron strain gauge), this may not translate into living human experience. Clinically we know that unless clefts and fracture plains in a vertebra are filled with cement fracture, pain may persist after a vertebral augmentation (▶Fig. 20.1).[3] In fact, a second procedure is sometimes needed to selectively fill fractures that were not successfully injected initially (▶Fig. 20.2).[8,9]

Careful analysis of preprocedural imaging is strongly suggested, as this will predict for you where cement extravasation may occur due to areas of cortical disruption and it is important to visualize clefts or areas void of cancellous bone within the vertebral body and to make sure these are filled during the vertebral augmentation procedure. It is especially important to recognize and fill clefts and fractures adjacent to the end plate as they will commonly occur in this location and the cement may not extend to the areas adjacent to the end plate even with a large-volume injection. Magnetic resonance (MR) imaging can allow for visualization of the clefts, but computed tomography (CT) scanning can give excellent bone detail and can provide a high level of cortical definition, thereby aiding in the preprocedure planning.

Volume

An Australian group led by William Clark et al published the vertebroplasty for acute painful osteoporotic fractures (VAPOUR) trial[10] with fascinating results. They deliberately treated patients in severe pain (7/10 or higher on visual analog scale [VAS]), within 6 weeks after fracture, and aimed for a high-volume vertebral cement fill from the superior end plate to the inferior endplate in the center of the vertebral body through a bilateral fill technique. At every time point, the treated arm patients did better than the placebo group.

Registry data from Switzerland showed that cement volume was a significant predictor for pain relief after vertebral augmentation and that cement volumes greater than 4.5 mL were recommended for achieving optimal pain relief and durability of the results.[11] The authors found that cement volume was not only an important predictor for pain relief in patients treated with balloon kyphoplasty (BKP) but also the third most important covariate (behind the sex of the patient and the location of the fracture); however, it was the only modifiable factor. They reported a clear dose–outcome relationship between filling volumes of cement and pain relief.

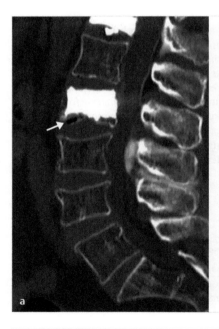
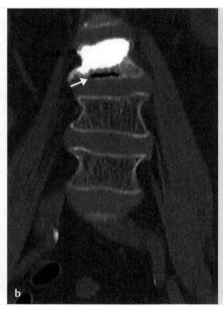

Fig. 20.1 Sagittal (a) and coronal (b) computed tomography reconstruction images show an air-filled cleft (*white arrows* in both images) just inferior to the cement in the L2 vertebral body. The air-filled cleft indicates a focal region of nonunion within the vertebral body and can be associated with persistent pain and discomfort.

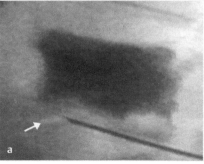
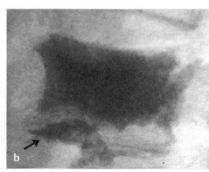

Fig. 20.2 Lateral fluoroscopic images (a, b) showing a needle approaching an air-filled cleft (*white arrow* in a) via a transdiskal approach. The *arrow* in (b) shows successful injection of bone cement into the previously air-filled cleft. This procedure was associated with significant relief of the patient's back pain.

A manuscript by Boszczyk et al, discussing the two vertebroplasty versus sham trials published in 2009 in the New England Journal of Medicine (NEJM), noted that only one of the studies reported the volume of fill material and that was reported to be 2.8 mL.[12] It was the authors' observation that in order to fill the minimum fill volume of an average thoracolumbar vertebral body, it would require a minimum volume of 4 mL. They derived this amount by referencing an average volume of a thoracolumbar vertebral body, which is 30 mL, and using previously reported minimum fill volumes of 13 to 16% that would be necessary to achieve an adequate biomechanical effect regarding restoring the vertebral body strength.[2,13,14] The authors also pointed out that there are many lumbar VCFs and the volumes required to adequately fill the vertebral body increases toward the lower lumbar spine. They concluded that based on the available information regarding the minimum amount of fill material the reported average volume of 2.8 mL would only be enough to treat the mid to upper thoracic VCFs and that the available data strongly illustrate that patients treated with vertebral augmentation were not treated in an effective manner.

The minimum volume necessary to provide adequate stabilization to the vertebral body has been studied by many different authors. Nieuwenhuijse et al[14] published a prospective study of 106 patients with 196 osteoporotic VCFs and followed the pain response over the course of a year and compared the pain response to the cemented volume of the vertebral body as determined from a postoperative CT scan of the treated levels. Out of all of the patients treated, they reported that 27.3% or 29 patients were nonresponders. This group had a significantly lower mean cemented vertebral body volume or fraction than the patients that were responsive to the procedure (0.15 vs. 0.21, $p = 0.002$). The mean volume of cement in all of the treated levels was 3.94 mL. Using this information, they concluded that a vertebral body fraction of 24% was the most optimal amount to inject to optimize the patient's pain response. This fraction was calculated to correspond to a 93 to 100% specificity for providing pain relief. This amount was based on the observation that there were few to no cases that did not have pain relief and were balanced with the need to keep the risk of cement leakage and adjacent-level fractures to a minimum.

In 2015, Martinčič et al published a study with the stated intent of finding the optimal amount of cement to inject into the vertebral body to restore the vertebral stiffness and adjacent intradiskal pressure without causing an undue amount of cement extravasation.[2] This investigation was done on cadavers in the thoracolumbar spine after having loaded the vertebral bodies sufficiently to cause a fracture. Subsequently, vertebroplasty was performed, four times in the same vertebral body and the cement volume injected ranged from 5 to 20%. Biomechanical testing performed before and after the fracture and after each of the cement injections showed that after a vertebral fracture the compressive stiffness was reduce to just under half that of the prefractured vertebral body and was restored to 61% after a 10% cement injection. The measured intradiskal pressure gradually increased to 71% at a 15% cement fill or the point where no significant increase in compressive stiffness or intradiskal pressure could be detected. Based on these observations, they concluded that 15% was the target amount for a minimum cement fill volume. Based on typical vertebral bodies, this would amount to at least 4 to

6 mL or more of cement to attain the minimum fill amount that would be necessary to reestablish the compressive stiffness of the vertebral body.

The key issue here is the concept of adequate filling of the vertebral body. The VAPOUR trial revealed a fundamental philosophical difference on filling between his study and previous two randomized studies, the Vertoss II study comparing vertebroplasty and nonsurgical management[15] and the Kallmes trial comparing vertebroplasty versus sham treatment.[16] The treating physicians in the VAPOUR trial injected a higher polymethyl methacrylate (PMMA) volume than reported in previous randomized control trials, and used a higher viscosity PMMA cement. Their mean PMMA volume used to treat the fracture in the VAPOUR trial was 7.5 mL and in Vertoss II, the average cement volume was 4.1 mL. In the trial comparing vertebroplasty versus sham by Buchbinder et al, the average cement volume amount was a mere 2·8 mL.[17] Molloy et al reported that pain relief happened first and prior to the reestablishment of the strength and stiffness of the vertebral body.[13] This observation may serve to explain why some practitioners conclude that a lesser amount of cement is preferable to more cement when treating vertebral fractures. As we have seen from the above clinical and biomechanical studies, it is necessary to inject between 15 and 25% of the uncompressed vertebral volume to adequately restore the biomechanical properties of the vertebral body.

T Spine versus L Spine Augmentation

In the VAPOUR study,[10] benefits from vertebroplasty were concentrated in the thoracolumbar fracture subgroup, where 48% more patients in the vertebroplasty group met the primary endpoint than in the placebo group. Conversely, there was no significant benefit from vertebroplasty over placebo group in the nonthoracolumbar subgroup, but there were also far fewer fractures in these groups with only 7 lumbar and 19 thoracic vertebroplasty levels representing just 39% of the total number of fractures. The thoracolumbar junction lies between the inflexible thoracic and flexible lumbar segments, subjecting it to increased dynamic load. Thoracolumbar fractures have the highest incidence of dynamic mobility and tend to be the site where VCFs occur the most, followed by the midthoracic spine.

20.2.2 Denervation of the Vertebra and the Role of C Fibers and the Basivertebral Nerve

The vertebral body and the end plates of the vertebra are supplied by the sinuvertebral nerve. This nerve also supplies the outer layers of the posterior and posterolateral portions of the intervertebral disk and the posterior longitudinal ligament. The BVN is an extension of the sinuvertebral nerve and extends into the vertebral body through the posterior nutrient foramen running parallel to the basivertebral vessels. The BVN arborizes as it branches superiorly and inferiorly and extends to the vertebral endplates. Its sensory fibers run back, along the same path as the vertebral venous plexus and synapse with the dorsal root ganglia bilaterally. Antonacci et al dissected the vertebral body and first found it was innervated by the BVN.[18] A few years following this discovery, Fras et al stained the BVN

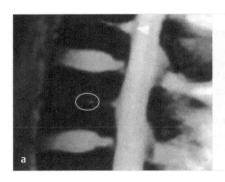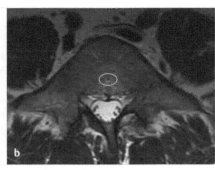

Fig. 20.3 (a, b) Target point of basivertebral nerve ablation is in the posterior portion of the center of the vertebral body (area within the *yellow circle*)

and revealed substance P nerve complex, which supported the underlying hypothesis that pain transmission was being carried through the BVN.

The pain transmission from vertebral fractures and discogenic pain from degenerated intervertebral disks is likely through the BVN complex. The pain relief from vertebral augmentation is likely due to the stabilization of the fracture itself but the thermal ablation of the BNV receptors in trabecular bone and vertebral periosteum likely has a contributory role in the degree of pain relief obtained. The temperatures achieved during the exothermic reaction of PMMA polymerization exceeds 45°C with most commercially available cements and this is adequate to ablate the sensory nerve tissue.

Radiofrequency (RF) ablation of the nerve can be performed of the BVN prior to its arborization. This point is located in the posterior portion of the center of the vertebral body (▶ Fig. 20.3). The intraosseous basivertebral nerve ablation for the treatment of chronic low back pain (SMART) study reported statistically significant reduction of pain and improvement of function in a level 1 prospective randomized double-blinded sham controlled study of RF ablation of the BVN in degenerative disk disease.[4] Although the ablation of the BVN within the vertebral body does produce significant pain relief in patients with discogenic back pain, degenerative end plate changes and an intact vertebral body low exothermic or nonexothermic bone cements can produce equivalent pain relief in patients with VCFs to that of cements with thermal neuroablation capability.[1,9] The pain relief in patients with VCFs, therefore, is much more likely or completely due to the reestablishment of the mechanical stability of the vertebral body rather than the ablative effects of the fill material on the vertebral body innervation. As mentioned previously, BVN ablation has been shown to effectively reduce pain and improve function in patients suffering from discogenic back pain[4]. It is a needle-based outpatient procedure designed to treat patients with stable discogenic back pain. The nerve ablation is done at the point of the BVN prior to its primary point of arborization (▶ Fig. 20.4) and the needles used to perform this ablation are very similar to needles used for bone augmentation procedures.

The pilot study for BVN ablation showed that 70% of patients had a clinically significant reduction of pain and the functional improvement ranged up to three times the minimal clinically important difference (MCID).[20] The SMART trial done later with 225 patients was a randomized double-blinded sham-controlled international investigational device exemption trial that followed the Oswestry Disability Index (ODI) as the primary endpoint and the VAS and SF-36 (36-item short form survey) as secondary endpoints.[4] The functional improvement was

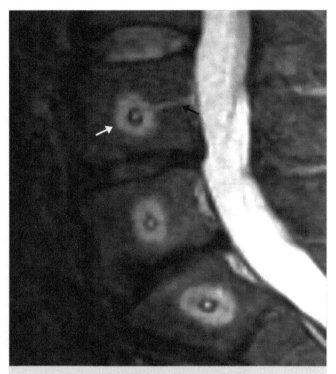

Fig. 20.4 Sagittal T2-weighted MR image showing the result of an intraosseous radiofrequency ablation of the basivertebral nerve (*rounded area* of increased signal indicated by the *white arrow*). The target area is at the anterior portion of the basivertebral vascular channel (*black arrow*) and prior to the primary arborization of the nerve within the vertebral body.

10 points or greater reduction in ODI in the patients in the active treatment arm, which was sustained throughout the trial and the patients who were treated with BVN ablation demonstrated a higher response rate. There were also no serious adverse device–related events and no unanticipated adverse events during the trial.

20.3 Treatment of Degenerative End Plate Changes with Osseous Augmentation

The presence of degenerative end plate changes has been shown to correlate with pain during discography[21] and the presence of abnormal end plates on MRI is associated with the clinical presence of back pain.[22] The type of degenerative end plate changes

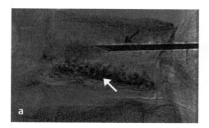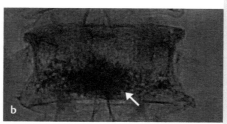

Fig. 20.5 Lateral (a) and posteroanterior (b) fluoroscopic images showing a needle accessing the vertebral body (*black arrow*) with injection of bone cement (*white arrow*) in a patient with Modic type 1 degenerative end plate changes on MR imaging (not shown). (Adapted from Masala S. Treatment of painful Modic type I changes by vertebral augmentation with bioactive resorbable bone cement. Neuroradiology 2014;56:637–645.)

is also important as Modic type 1 and 2 changes are associated far more often with pain during provocative discography.[23] Additionally, vertebral end plates that have degenerative end plate changes show increase end plate innervation.[24]

In an innovative study done by Masala et al, patients with painful Modic type 1 degenerative end plate changes were treated with vertebral augmentation (▶Fig. 20.5).[5]

Out of 1,124 patients with back pain and no radicular symptoms, they chose 218 patients to undergo vertebral augmentation with resorbable cement. Out of the 218 patient, 172 improved within 4 weeks and 42 patients improved over the course of 6 months. At 1 year, the pain level in both groups had significantly decreased with a corresponding increase in activities of daily living. They concluded that vertebral augmentation may be effective for treating patients with back pain and Modic type 1 degenerative end plate changes.

20.4 Conclusion

Vertebral augmentation with injection stabilizing material results in renewed stability of the vertebral body and has been shown to be one of the most effective of all spine procedures in alleviating pain and restoring function. It is presumably the restoration of the structural integrity that results in the prominent decrease in patient pain, and this result can be seen in both benign and malignant causes of vertebral instability. The amount of fill material necessary to reestablish the strength of the vertebral body and to be durable over time has evolved over the last decade as new information has indicated that the single most important and modifiable strategy that can be employed for the best and most durable results in vertebral augmentation is the injection of an optimal amount of bone cement. The amount necessary is more than was traditionally thought and between 15 and 25% of the uncompressed vertebral level. This will provide optimal strength and stiffness to the vertebral body as well as relieving the patient's pain. The greater amount of cement appears to more optimally stabilize the vertebral body and the results seem to last longer than injecting smaller cement amounts. In addition to injecting an optimal amount of bone cement, other features of the vertebral body that can lead to instability should be taken into consideration. Any non-union clefts seen on preoperative imaging or on intraoperative fluoroscopy should be filled to ensure an optimal response to vertebral augmentation.

In addition to pain provoking instability within the vertebral body, degenerative end plate changes can give rise to back pain and prominent disability when present. The pathway of pain transmission through the BVN can be disrupted using BVN ablation. This technique ablates the BVN and can decrease the patients' pain and improve their function with a minimally invasive outpatient needle procedure. The type of degenerative end plate changes is important as Modic type 1 and 2 changes are associated more commonly with back pain than type 3 changes. Modic type 1 changes may have some instability of the end plate associated with them and perhaps the instability can be treated or the distal basivertebral nerve may be ablated by cement as it has been shown that the injection of bioactive resorbable bone cement can result in significantly decreased back pain and significant functional improvements in patients with back pain and type 1 degenerative end plate changes.

Knowledge of the location of the pain generators within the vertebral body is important, as is how much cement to inject to provide not only pain relief but the optimal strength and stiffness to the augmented vertebral body. It should be understood that the lack of mechanical stability can give rise to severe pain that can be treated by re-establishing this stability and that this should be differentiated from the pain that is transmitted from the endplate through the vertebral body by the basivertebral nerve. This vertebrogenic pain is a different entity that can be treated with nerve ablation. This knowledge can hopefully refine and improve our techniques and ability to treat discogenic and vertebrogenic pain and to develop new minimally invasive techniques for treating patients with back pain. The underlying origin of what produces the symptomatic relief of pain and whether this is a result of increased vertebral integrity or an ablative process adversely affecting the vertebral sensory nerves is not currently well defined but will undoubtedly be better elucidated in the future.

20.5 Pearls

- The patient cares about the implant. That is what they have inside them.
- We care about the delivery system.
- It is about distribution. This is civil engineering.
- Extravasation is proportional to volume.
- Benign and malignant diseases need different cements.

References

[1] Beall DP, Chambers MF, Thomas SM, et al. Prospective and multicenter evaluation of outcomes for quality of life and activities of daily living for balloon kyphoplasty in the treatment of vertebral compression fractures: the EVOLVE trial. J Neurosurg 2019;84(1):169–178

[2] Martinčič D, Brojan M, Kosel F, et al. Minimum cement volume for vertebroplasty. Int Orthop 2015;39(4):727–733

[3] Jang JS, Kim DY, Lee SH. Efficacy of percutaneous vertebroplasty in the treatment of intravertebral pseudarthrosis associated with noninfected avascular necrosis of the vertebral body. Spine 2003;28(14):1588–1592

[4] Fischgrund JS, Rhyne A, Franke J, et al. Intraosseous basivertebral nerve ablation for the treatment of chronic low back pain: a prospective randomized double-blind sham-controlled multi-center study. Eur Spine J 2018;27(5): 1146–1156

[5] Masala S, Anselmetti GC, Marcia S, et al. Treatment of painful Modic type I changes by vertebral augmentation with bioactive resorbable bone cement. Neuroradiology 2014;56(8):637–645

[6] Tohmeh AG, Mathis JM, Fenton DC, Levine AM, Belkoff SM. Biomechanical efficacy of unipedicular versus bipedicular vertebroplasty for the management of osteoporotic compression fractures. Spine 1999;24(17):1772–1776

[7] Belkoff SM, Jasper LE, Stevens SS. An ex vivo evaluation of an inflatable bone tamp used to reduce fractures within vertebral bodies under load. Spine 2002;27(15):1640–1643

[8] Park SM, Park C, Kim H, et al. Is redo vertebroplasty an effective treatment on the same vertebra? Cardiovasc Intervent Radiol 2018;41(7):1058–1066

[9] Chen L-H, Hsieh M-K, Liao J-C, et al. Repeated percutaneous vertebroplasty for refracture of cemented vertebrae. Arch Orthop Trauma Surg 2011;131(7): 927–933

[10] Clark W, Bird P, Gonski P, et al. Safety and efficacy of vertebroplasty for acute painful osteoporotic fractures (VAPOUR): a multicentre, randomised, double-blind, placebo-controlled trial. Lancet 2016;388(10052):1408–1416

[11] Röder C, Boszczyk B, Perler G, Aghayev E, Külling F, Maestretti G. Cement volume is the most important modifiable predictor for pain relief in BKP: results from SWISSspine, a nationwide registry. Eur Spine J 2013;22(10): 2241–2248

[12] Boszczyk B. Volume matters: a review of procedural details of two randomised controlled vertebroplasty trials of 2009. Eur Spine J 2010;19(11): 1837–1840

[13] Molloy S, Riley LH III, Belkoff SM. Effect of cement volume and placement on mechanical-property restoration resulting from vertebroplasty. AJNR Am J Neuroradiol 2005;26(2):401–404

[14] Nieuwenhuijse MJ, Bollen L, van Erkel AR, Dijkstra PD. Optimal intravertebral cement volume in percutaneous vertebroplasty for painful osteoporotic vertebral compression fractures. Spine 2012;37(20):1747–1755

[15] Klazen CA, Verhaar HJ, Lampmann LE, et al. VERTOS II: percutaneous vertebroplasty versus conservative therapy in patients with painful osteoporotic vertebral compression fractures; rationale, objectives and design of a multicenter randomized controlled trial. Trials 2007;8:33

[16] Kallmes DF, Comstock BA, Heagerty PJ, et al. A randomized trial of vertebroplasty for osteoporotic spinal fractures. N Engl J Med 2009;361(6):569–579

[17] Buchbinder R, Osborne RH, Ebeling PR, et al. A randomized trial of vertebroplasty for painful osteoporotic vertebral fractures. N Engl J Med 2009;361(6):557–568

[18] Antonacci MD, Mody DR, Heggeness MH. Innervation of the human vertebral body: a histologic study. J Spinal Disord 1998;11(6):526–531

[19] Bae H, Hatten HP Jr, Linovitz R, et al. A prospective randomized FDA-IDE trial comparing Cortoss with PMMA for vertebroplasty: a comparative effectiveness research study with 24-month follow-up. Spine 2012;37(7): 544–550

[20] Becker S, Hadjipavlou A, Heggeness MH. Ablation of the basivertebral nerve for treatment of back pain: a clinical study. Spine J 2017;17(2):218–223

[21] Carragee EJ, Alamin TF, Miller JL, Carragee JM. Discographic, MRI and psychosocial determinants of low back pain disability and remission: a prospective study in subjects with benign persistent back pain. Spine J 2005;5(1):24–35. https ://doi. org/10.1016/j.spinee.2004.05.250

[22] Modic MT, Steinberg PM, Ross JS, Masaryk TJ, Carter JR. Degenerative disk disease: assessment of changes in vertebral body marrow with MR imaging. Radiology 1988;166(1 Pt 1):193–199

[23] Weishaupt D, Zanetti M, Hodler J, Min K, Fuchs B, Pfirrmann CWA, Boos N. Painful lumbar disk derangement: relevance of endplate abnormalities at MR imaging. Radiology 2001;218(2):420–427

[24] Ohtori S, Inoue G, Ito T, et al. Tumor necrosis factor-immunoreactive cells and PGP 9.5-immunoreactive nerve fibers in vertebral endplates of patients with discogenic low back pain and Modic type 1 or type 2 changes on MRI. Spine 2006;31(9):1026–1031

21 Clinical Presentation and the Response to Vertebral Augmentation

Alexios Kelekis and Dimitrios K. Filippiadis

Summary

The presence of a vertebral compression fracture (VCF) can be defined anatomically as an objective loss in vertebral body height or by imaging criteria including increased signal on the fluid sensitive magnetic resonance (MR) imaging sequences. There are a number of clinical scenarios that may produce symptomatic VCFs including neoplasia, trauma, and osteoporosis. Vertebral fractures are common and have adverse effects on mobility and pulmonary function and can lead to prominently increased rates of morbidity and mortality. The kyphosis produced by the fracture also places increased strain on the adjacent vertebral bodies and increases the risk of an adjacent or additional vertebral fracture. Patients with VCFs complain of pain when transitioning from one position to another and the physical examination techniques used to identify patients with VCFs include closed fist percussion and the inability for the patient to assume a supine position comfortably. Patients with vertebral compression fractures can be asymptomatic but can also present with severe pain and prominently limited function. Patients with persistently painful fractures also tend to not improve with nonsurgical management (NSM) and should undergo vertebral augmentation to treat their symptomatic fractures. Treatment of these fractures can produce both short term and long term benefits regardless of the underlying cause of the fracture and vertebral augmentation has been shown in multiple studies to significantly decrease patients' morbidity and mortality. The appropriate diagnosis and treatment of VCFs can produce better results and optimal outcomes for a large at risk patient population.

Keywords: clinical presentation, vertebral compression fracture, physical examination, morbidity, mortality

21.1 Clinical Presentation

VCF can be defined as the reduction in the height of the individual vertebral body by 20% over 10 to 20% of the vertebral body or a loss of vertebral height of at least 4 mm.[1] There are numerous pathophysiologic processes that contribute to VCFs including osteoporosis, neoplasms (e.g., myeloma, metastasis, lymphoma, and hemangioma), osteonecrosis, and trauma.[1] The burden of illness for VCFs results in a total annual hospitalization cost that is higher than the costs for myocardial infarction, cardiovascular arrest, and breast cancer.[2] VCFs result in both direct and indirect effects on the patients' quality of life and costs to the health care systems.[1] The typical clinical appearance in a patient with an acute VCF is severe back pain lasting for weeks to months or more. Additionally, apart from intractable pain, vertebral fractures negatively affect health status in a variety of ways including but not limited to progressive deformity, impaired mobility, reduced pulmonary function, sleep difficulty, eating disorders, weight loss, clinical depression, anxiety, and an overall decrease in the patient's quality of life. Additional symptoms may include sciatica or radiculopathy,

numbness, tingling, muscle spasm, weakness, and bowel or bladder changes. Neglected fractures can evolve to vertebra plana, retropulsion, and may even cause paralysis due to compression of the spinal cord or cauda equina.[3]

When compared to age-matched controls, patients with VCFs have a 40% lower survival rate, which is typically attributed to all the aforementioned clinical symptoms and biomechanical changes.[4] In these patients the resultant decreased mobility and bed rest are important predictors of adverse outcomes leading to complications such as functional decline and potentially deadly adverse events such as pneumonia or pulmonary embolism.[5]

Patients with VCFs suffering from severe pain will usually have mobility impairment which leads to increased morbidity and mortality rates.[4,5] Pain in these patients results both from the fracture itself as well as the vertebral body's instability with micro- or macro-movements (▶Video 21.1). The pain, in combination with the altered spinal biomechanics, the increased kyphotic angle, and the global spinal sagittal imbalance, creates a compensatory stance which in turn causes paraspinal muscular contraction that often results in chronic back pain. This imbalance plays an important role in increasing body sway, gait unsteadiness, and risk of falls in fragile patients who have already had an osteoporotic fracture.[6] Prior to vertebral augmentation and restabilization of the fracture (▶Video 21.2), the incident fracture disrupts the ability of the adjacent intervertebral disk to pressurize, and the resulting force transmitted to the adjacent vertebral body cortex is doubled, which produces an increased risk of future VCFs.[5] The change in the kyphotic angle also causes significant mechanical effects that result in decreased thoracic and abdominal space with subsequently decreased pulmonary function, decreased appetite, and a negative nutritional impact on an already frail patient.[7,8]

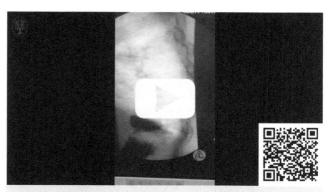

Video 21.1 Lateral thoracic fluoroscopic video of the thoracic spine showing a needle entering the posterior vertebral body of T9 and previous vertebral augmentation with PMMA at the T10 and T11 levels. The VCF at T9 is mobile and the superior end plate can be seen to move superoinferiorly with respiration. https://www.thieme.de/de/q.htm?p=opn/cs/19/11/10618073-85b5d5e3

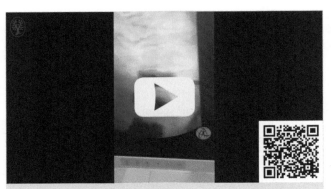

Video 21.2 Lateral thoracic fluoroscopic video of the thoracic spine taken after vertebral augmentation with PMMA at the T9 level shows two cannulas and bone fillers within the T9 vertebral body that is now stable. No movement of the superior end plate is seen with respiration. https://www.thieme.de/de/q.htm?p=opn/cs/19/11/10618072-eaf53de7

During clinical examination, the entire spinal length should be examined for physical signs and symptoms that are reliable for diagnosing the presence of a vertebral fracture. On using a firm, closed-fist percussion, the patient will complain of a sharp, sudden, fracture pain.[9] This is typically an effective physical exam maneuver in patients with VCFs as it has been shown to have a sensitivity and specificity for detecting symptomatic VCFs of 87.5 and 90%, respectively. Patients with vertebral fractures also complain of pain during rotation and positional changes (turning while lying or standing) and Postacchini et al found that pain-related behaviors such as grimacing, sighing, and requesting help with position changes were correlated with the presence of a VCF as confirmed by MR imaging and were not present in the control patients without fractures.[19] A useful physical examination sign is the presence of back pain when lying supine.[9] The patient is asked to lie supine on the examination couch with only one pillow. The clinical sign is positive when a patient is unable to lie supine due to severe pain in their spine.[9] Despite the presence of some reliable signs of a painful VCF, clinical examination cannot stand alone for the diagnosis of a vertebral fracture as preoperative imaging will provide valuable information to confirm the diagnosis as well as to assess the fracture anatomy including the posterior vertebral body wall integrity and can exclude other causes of back pain that can mimic a VCF.[1] Radiographs of the spine in anteroposterior and lateral projections still remain the simplest and most direct approach and can provide basic information. The absence of a fracture on a radiograph, however, does not exclude the presence of a fracture, especially in the osteoporotic patient population. MR imaging with Short TI Inversion Recovery (STIR) and T1-weighted sequences are the most sensitive for fracture detection and should always be used in case of clinical suspicion. It can be useful to assess the fracture's age and healing status (acute vs. chronic, incompletely healed vs. consolidated).[1] Tanigawa et al reported that the improvement postvertebral augmentation is closely related to the bone edema pattern illustrated in the pretherapeutic MR imaging.[10] The authors showed that patients with an extensive bone marrow edema pattern involving more than 50% of the vertebral body reported significantly greater clinical improvement than either patients with fractures that had no bone marrow edema.[10]

Apart from the clinical signs and symptoms directly caused by a VCF, there is a long list of indirect effects. Immobility of patients with VCFs results in loss of bone density and muscle strength as well as muscular contractures and pressure sores.[11] In the acute phase the bone mineral density loss can be as high as 2% per week, which not only predisposes the patient to additional VCFs but the loss can only be reversed by either high impact exercise or anabolic bone agents.[11] The muscle strength loss is also rapid, declining approximately 10 to 15% per week and roughly half of the patient's strength is lost within four to five weeks after the fracture.[11] VCFs are also associated with decreased cardiac performance (including increased heart rate, shorter diastolic times, reduced coronary blood flow, decreased stroke volume, and left ventricular function with lower cardiac output), deep venous thrombosis, and pulmonary compromise (with average of 9% decrease in forced vital capacity, 25–50% decrease in respiratory capacity, deconditioning of respiratory muscles, and increased risk of pneumonia).[11] Indirect effects of VCFs are also reported in the gastrointestinal system (loss of appetite, constipation, fecal impaction, and glucose intolerance), in the urinary tract (infection, sepsis, and calculus formation), and in the central nervous system (imbalance, increase sensitivity, and intolerance to pain, anxiety, depression, and insomnia).[11,12]

21.2 Response to Vertebral Augmentation

One of the confusing aspects of patients with VCFs is the dichotomy of how these patients present. On one hand VCFs are common in the general population with a population-based study by Sanfélix-Genovés et al confirming that one in three women over the age of 50 has osteoporosis and one in five will have a VCF.[20] Additionally, one in ten fractures will be classified as moderate to severe. Out of all the patients that had the fractures, only 1.5% were aware of their fractures. This situation exemplifies the dichotomous situation that asymptomatic VCFs are quite common and don't need treatment but symptomatic fractures are less common and when the symptoms from the fractures are severe the patients need treatment.

In a study by Suzuki et al the authors treated patients with NSM in patients who had a 7 out of 10 level of pain for one year.[21] After a full year of NSM, only 10% of the patients reported little or no pain whereas 76% of the patients still had pain that they regarded as severe and averaged a 6 out of 10 level of pain. In another study by Bornemann et al, the authors treated patient with painful VCFs with NSM for 6 weeks then offered the patients an additional 6 weeks of NSM or vertebral augmentation.[22] They defined clinical success as a decreased amount of pain on the Visual Analog Scale (VAS) and no functional worsening on the Oswestry Disability Index (ODI) scale. After the initial 6 weeks of NSM only one patient met the criteria for clinical success and only five patients met the clinical criteria for success after an additional 6 weeks of NSM. The authors concluded that for the majority of patients with a pain level of a 5 out of 10 or more, NSM provides no clinical improvement but nearly all patients undergoing vertebral augmentation had rapid and substantial improvement. The authors went on to say that surgery was clearly much more effective than NSM and should be offered to patients much sooner.[22]

The dichotomy for VCFs is that while most fractures are asymptomatic and do not need treatment there are a subset that are painful and cause prominent disability that tend not to improve with NSM and should be treated promptly. The clinical care pathway for treating VCFs, discussed in detail in Chapter 14, reflects the current recommendation which focuses more on the patients' clinical symptoms to determine the appropriate treatment rather than on an arbitrary requirement for NSM.

After vertebral augmentation there is significant and immediate pain reduction and functional improvement. In patients with acute or subacute osteoporotic fractures, the pain reduction amount after vertebral augmentation is 90% as opposed to approximately 80% for chronic osteoporotic fractures and hemangiomas and 60 to 85% in fractures due to neoplastic involvement.[1] Tsoumakidou et al has reported the reduction in the requirement for analgesics to be 91% after vertebral augmentation and improved mobility is 84 to 93% and 50 to 88% after treatment for acute and chronic osteoporotic fractures, respectively.[1] After vertebral augmentation there are short- and long-term benefits. The improvement in pain is the greatest potential short-term benefit, whereas prevention of recurrent pain due to fracture at the treated levels, limitation or reversal of height loss, and spinal deformity as well as improved functional capability are included in the potential long-term benefits.[12]

It has been reported by Mailli et al that vertebral augmentation is efficient and safe for symptomatic vertebral fractures independently of the number of vertebrae treated per session. Additionally the underlying cause of the vertebral fracture (benign or malignant) does not affect the technique's safety and efficacy when treating a single VCF or multiple levels during a single session.[13] Kelekis et al in a comparative prospective study among patients with VCFs treated with percutaneous vertebroplasty and a control group of healthy volunteers reported that patients prior to their vertebroplasty procedure had a statistically significant difference in load distribution variation as compared to the control group.[14] After treatment this difference normalized in a statistically significant way showing the efficacy of vertebral augmentation in restoring equilibrium in load distribution.[14] There is also a very significant reduction in mortality and morbidity after vertebral augmentation (see Chapter 22), with rates of mortality reduction after vertebral augmentation ranging from 11 to 55% and statistically significant reductions in morbidities.[15,23]

During follow-up, patients should be examined for pain that is both related and unrelated to the previous vertebral augmentation procedure. Immediate pain after treatment usually relates to soft tissue discomfort or a hematoma at the puncture site(s). Bracing after treatment is not mandatory although it can be helpful to provide additional support and increase patient comfort and should be considered in especially frail patients. The usual follow-up includes a patient visit and clinical examination within 7 to 14 days. This visit can include radiographs or cross-sectional imaging to assess the prior vertebral augmentation and/or look for additional fractures if the patient's symptoms have returned. In case of pain or aches that seem unrelated to the previous vertebral augmentation procedure or an additional VCF, clinical examination and laboratory exams may be necessary to verify the origin of the pain. Most of the time the pain is of a benign origin and due to the changes in sagittal balance and altered loading of the intervertebral disks and facets and changes in muscle function.[16] In those cases targeted treatment by image-guided injections should be explored.[17] If there is recalcitrant pain and/or neurological symptoms during follow-up the patient should be examined thoroughly, including new MR imaging, as there is always the risk of infection, tumor growth, or additional fracture, either at the treated level or at another level.[18]

In conclusion, when patients are treated after a spinal fracture, whether it is due to benign or malignant disease they should be examined and the vertebral augmentation treatment planned for optimal patient outcomes. Vertebral augmentation is just one treatment among others for back pain and in many occasions the VCF will be just one of many pain generators especially in the patient population where VCFs commonly occur. Finding and attributing the pain to the appropriate pathology and treating the culprit that is producing the patient's pain and discomfort are our responsibilities as physicians.

References

[1] Tsoumakidou G, Too CW, Koch G, et al. CIRSE guidelines on percutaneous vertebral augmentation. Cardiovasc Intervent Radiol 2017;40(3):331–342

[2] Singer A, Exuzides A, Spangler L, et al. Burden of illness for osteoporotic fractures compared with other serious diseases among postmenopausal women in the United States. Mayo Clin Proc 2015;90(1):53–62

[3] Clark W, Bird P, Gonski P, et al. Safety and efficacy of vertebroplasty for acute painful osteoporotic fractures (VAPOUR): a multicentre, randomised, double-blind, placebo-controlled trial. Lancet 2016;388(10052):1408–1416

[4] Lau E, Ong K, Kurtz S, Schmier J, Edidin A. Mortality following the diagnosis of a vertebral compression fracture in the Medicare population. J Bone Joint Surg Am 2008;90(7):1479–1486

[5] Brown CJ, Friedkin RJ, Inouye SK. Prevalence and outcomes of low mobility in hospitalized older patients. J Am Geriatr Soc 2004;52(8):1263–1270

[6] Sinaki M, Brey RH, Hughes CA, Larson DR, Kaufman KR. Balance disorder and increased risk of falls in osteoporosis and kyphosis: significance of kyphotic posture and muscle strength. Osteoporos Int 2005;16(8):1004–1010

[7] Yuan HA, Brown CW, Phillips FM. Osteoporotic spinal deformity: a biomechanical rationale for the clinical consequences and treatment of vertebral body compression fractures. J Spinal Disord Tech 2004;17(3):236–242

[8] Kado DM, Lui LY, Ensrud KE, Fink HA, Karlamangla AS, Cummings SR; Study of Osteoporotic Fractures. Hyperkyphosis predicts mortality independent of vertebral osteoporosis in older women. Ann Intern Med 2009;150(10): 681–687

[9] Langdon J, Way A, Heaton S, Bernard J, Molloy S. Vertebral compression fractures: new clinical signs to aid diagnosis. Ann R Coll Surg Engl 2010;92(2): 163–166

[10] Tanigawa N, Komemushi A, Kariya S, et al. Percutaneous vertebroplasty: relationship between vertebral body bone marrow edema pattern on MR images and initial clinical response. Radiology 2006;239(1):195–200

[11] Babayev M, Lachmann E, Nagler W. The controversy surrounding sacral insufficiency fractures: to ambulate or not to ambulate? Am J Phys Med Rehabil 2000;79(4):404–409

[12] Beall DP, McRoberts WP, Berven SH, Ledlie JT, Tutton SM, Parsons BP. Critique of the analysis of UpToDate.com on the treatment of painful vertebral compression fractures: time to update UpToDate. AJNR Am J Neuroradiol 2015;36(4):631–636

[13] Mailli L, Filippiadis DK, Brountzos EN, Alexopoulou E, Kelekis N, Kelekis A. Clinical outcome and safety of multilevel vertebroplasty: clinical experience and results. Cardiovasc Intervent Radiol 2013;36(1):183–191

[14] Kelekis A, Filippiadis DK, Vergadis C, et al. Comparative prospective study of load distribution projection among patients with vertebral fractures treated with percutaneous vertebroplasty and a control group of healthy volunteers. Cardiovasc Intervent Radiol 2014;37(1):186–192

[15] Bolland MJ, Grey AB, Gamble GD, Reid IR. Effect of osteoporosis treatment on mortality: a meta-analysis. J Clin Endocrinol Metab 2010;95(3): 1174–1181

[16] Capozzi A, Scambia G, Pedicelli A, Evangelista M, Sorge R, Lello S. Clinical management of osteoporotic vertebral fracture treated with percutaneous vertebroplasty. Clin Cases Miner Bone Metab 2017;14(2):161–166

[17] Hofmann UK, Keller RL, Walter C, Mittag F. Predictability of the effects of facet joint infiltration in the degenerate lumbar spine when assessing MRI scans. J Orthop Surg Res 2017;12(1):180

[18] Beall DP, Coe JD, McIlduff M, et al. Serious adverse events associated with readmission through one year after vertebral augmentation with either a polyetheretherketone implant or balloon kyphoplasty. Pain Physician 2017;20(6):521–528

[19] Postacchini R, Paolino M, Faraglia S, Cinotti G, Postacchini F. Assessment of patient's pain-related behavior at physical examination may allow diagnosis of recent osteoporotic vertebral fracture. Spine J 2013;13(9):1126–1133

[20] Sanfélix-Genovés J, Reig-Molla B, Sanfélix-Gimeno G, et al. The population-based prevalence of osteoporotic vertebral fracture and densitometric osteoporosis in postmenopausal women over 50 in Valencia, Spain (the FRAVO study). Bone 2010;47(3):610–616

[21] Suzuki N, Ogikubo O, Hansson T. The course of the acute vertebral body fragility fracture: its effect on pain, disability and quality of life during 12 months. Eur Spine J 2008;17(10):1380–1390

[22] Bornemann R, Hanna M, Kabir K, Goost H, Wirtz DC, Pflugmacher R. Continuing conservative care versus crossover to radiofrequency kyphoplasty: a comparative effectiveness study on the treatment of vertebral body fractures. Eur Spine J 2012;21(5):930–936

[23] Ong KL, Beall DP, Frohbergh M, Lau E, Hirsch JA. Reply to "At what price decreased mortality risk?" Osteoporos Int 2018;29(8):1929–1930

22 Effect of Vertebral Augmentation on Morbidity and Mortality

Jae Hun Kim and Yong-Chul Kim

Summary

Vertebral compression fractures (VCFs) are common and are typically managed with either nonsurgical management (NSM) or vertebral augmentation including vertebroplasty and kyphoplasty. The different treatment types will also have different outcomes in regard to patient morbidity and mortality. The presence of a painful VCF will cause a significant increase in mortality due to complications such as pneumonia and pulmonary embolism caused by the patient's deconditioned status. Many studies from many countries have shown a consistent mortality benefit of vertebroplasty over NSM and of kyphoplasty over vertebroplasty. As a result of the downward trend in treating VCFs resulting from the negative vertebroplasty versus sham articles published in 2009 patient mortality rates associated with VCFs have increased. Many review articles and meta-analyses have reported the safety of vertebral augmentation and have reported a very similar amount of pain relief with both vertebroplasty and kyphoplasty but better vertebral height restoration and lower cement extravasation rates with kyphoplasty. Patients with moderate to severe pain who undergo NSM rather than vertebral augmentation tend to have persistent and severe pain, functional impairments, and increased rates of mortality. This increased mortality rate can be reduced by vertebral augmentation which not only reduces the risk of death for the patient but can demonstrably prolong their life expectancy as well. The presence of a VCF is an important marker for the increased risk of another VCF and should be looked upon as a possible indication to treat the patient. In general, vertebral augmentation will provide optimal clinical outcomes in improving patients' pain, function and quality of life and has been shown to significantly decrease morbidity and mortality.

Keywords: morbidity, mortality, vertebral compression fracture, pneumonia, pulmonary embolism, nonsurgical management

22.1 Introduction

The VCF is the most common type of osteoporotic fracture and occurs in approximately 20% of the individuals older than 70 years and in 40% of women over the age of 80.[1,2] Despite being common, only about one-third of the VCF patients present with pain. A VCF may cause acute pain, disability, and increased mortality, especially in elderly patients.[1] There are various treatments for VCF and the goals of these treatments are reducing pain, restoring mobility, and stabilizing the vertebra.[2] NSM includes medications such as NSAIDs or opioids, bed rest, or external bracing. These treatments, however, can give rise to undesirable adverse effects or fail in preventing kyphotic deformity and alleviating pain.[3,4] Vertebral augmentation including vertebroplasty and kyphoplasty is an effective treatment for pain related to VCFs. Vertebral augmentation procedures are minimally invasive surgical treatments that contribute to the objectives of decreasing pain, restoring vertebral height, and improving mobility.[5]

22.2 Nonsurgical Management vs. Vertebral Augmentation

There are several treatment modalities for VCFs. In general, two sets of treatments are identified, the surgical and the NSM treatments. Some patients undergo vertebroplasty or kyphoplasty and other patients are prescribed medications and/or use orthostatic braces for the treatment of their VCFs. In this chapter, a review and the description of the effect of morbidity and mortality of vertebral augmentation versus the NSM of VCFs will be discussed.

Although the etiology of increased mortality is not directly tied to the pathophysiology of the acute VCF itself, several studies report that painful VCF increases the mortality of the affected patients.[6–11] This high incidence of the mortality is not the direct consequence of the fracture but is related to deconditioning and the elderly patient's poor health status, weight loss, and physical frailty. Additionally, the patients undergoing NSM for a compression fracture have increased pulmonary impairment.[6–8] Moreover, the risk of death related to pulmonary problems is higher in patients who have severe thoracic kyphosis, and the risk of pneumonia is significantly higher in patients not undergoing vertebroplasty.[6,9] In a cohort study, when comparing nonvertebroplasty patients to vertebroplasty patients, a hazard ratio of 1.39 related to death after 1 year was observed.[6] The results showed that aged patients who did not receive vertebroplasty within 3 months had higher risks of death and respiratory failure than those patients who received vertebroplasty within the first 3 months. The increased risk of death and respiratory failure in nonvertebroplasty patients remained even after 12 years.[6] According to these results, vertebroplasty was recommended for older (≥ 70 years old) patients with severe pain.

Edidin et al[12] investigated the morbidity and mortality after VCFs in a US Medicare population (a total 1,038,956 VCF patients). According to this study, the NSM cohort had a 55% higher adjusted risk of mortality than kyphoplasty cohort and 25% higher adjusted risk of mortality than the vertebroplasty cohort. The kyphoplasty cohort had a 19% lower adjusted risk of mortality than the vertebroplasty cohort. Additionally, the kyphoplasty cohort had significantly lower risks of morbidity than the NSM cohort, with those patients undergoing NSM having increased risks for deep venous thrombosis, infection, myocardial infarction, and cardiac complications.[12]

In the United States, the number of vertebral augmentation procedures began decreasing after 2009, probably related to the publications in the *New England Journal of Medicine* that reported no significant difference between vertebroplasty and a sham procedure.[13,14] The majority of the medical societies continued to recommend vertebroplasty as a safe and effective procedure for treating VCFs but there was opposition from some societies and some health technology assessments.[15–17] The reduction in vertebroplasty procedures amounted to a 10% decrease, from

24% of patients with painful VCFs receiving vertebral augmentation in 2008 to 10% in 2014.[18] This reduction was calculated from an analysis of the Medicare population of over two million VCF patients. The authors reported that in the 5-year time period following the publication of these articles an increased mortality rate was found in patients who presented with VCFs, presumably related to under-treatment of the fractures.[18] This increased mortality rate of patient treated with NSM was 55% more at 1 year and 24% more at 10 years than those patients treated with vertebral augmentation kyphoplasty.[18]

There are several comparative studies on the effectiveness and safety of NSM versus vertebroplasty, and kyphoplasty. These studies have collected various data, such as pain scores, short-form-36, EQ-5D, Roland Morris Disability Questionnaire (RDQ), QUALEFFO, Dallas Pain Questionnaire (DPQ), Oswestry Disability Index (ODI), Barthel scale, modified mini-mental state examination (MMSE), vertebral body height, kyphotic wedge angle, incidence of new fractures, cost-effectiveness, restricted activity days, and bed rest days. According to a recent meta-analysis, vertebroplasty was the more effective treatment for pain relief, quality of life, and daily function when compared to NSM.[2] Both vertebroplasty and kyphoplasty were more effective for improving quality of life and daily function than NSM. There were also no significant differences in the incidence of new fracture among the three treatments. They also analyzed the ranking probability and concluded that vertebroplasty was the most effective treatment for pain relief and kyphoplasty had the most beneficial effect on quality of life, daily function, and incidence of new fractures.[2]

Mattie et al[19] in a meta-analysis comparing vertebroplasty and NSM concluded that the pain reduction effect of vertebroplasty exceeded any pain relief obtained with NSM up to 1 year postoperatively. In other meta-analyses, there were controversies in the comparison between vertebroplasty and kyphoplasty about pain relief.[20-22] According to Zhao et al,[21] kyphoplasty was better than vertebroplasty in ODI and long-term pain relief but there were no significant differences in short-term visual analog scale (VAS), posterior vertebral body height, and adjacent level fractures. Ma et al[20] reported that kyphoplasty was superior to vertebroplasty in patients with a large kyphosis angle, vertebral fissures, fractures in the posterior edge of the vertebral body, or significant height loss in the fractured vertebrae. Finally, Xing et al[22] concluded that kyphoplasty had better outcomes than vertebroplasty in long-term kyphosis angle stability, improved the height of the vertebral body and reduced incidence of bone cement leakage. In these meta-analyses, vertebroplasty and kyphoplasty were safe and very effective surgical procedures for the treatment of painful VCFs.

A meta-analysis performed by Chen et al[23] regarding the efficacy and tolerability of NSM versus vertebroplasty and kyphoplasty found that the latter two significantly decreased pain compared with conservative treatment. In their ranking probabilities, vertebroplasty was the most effective treatment for pain relief but only kyphoplasty had a significantly lower risk of all-cause discontinuation compared with NSM. In this meta-analysis, there were no significant differences in the incidence of new fractures among the three different treatments,[23] and other meta-analyses have also showed no significant differences of new fractures between vertebroplasty and kyphoplasty[20-22] and between vertebroplasty and NSM.[24,25]

There are also several studies on the superiority of vertebroplasty over NSM in improving the daily function and quality of life.[24,25] Blasco et al[26] reported that vertebroplasty had higher QUALEFFO scores compared with NSM up to 6 months. The differences were mainly associated with difference in physical activity seen as the result of each treatment. Wardlaw et al[27] reported that kyphoplasty patients had a better quality of life (SF-36 PCS and EQ-5D) and RDQ scores than the NSM patients. Additionally, kyphoplasty decreased restricted activity days and bed rest about 2.9 days per 2 weeks at 1 month. However, after 12 months, there was no significant difference among NSM and kyphoplasty. Yang et al[28] reported that vertebroplasty yielded faster and better pain relief and improved function for up to 1 year. The results also showed fewer complications after vertebroplasty than NSM. Liu et al[29] found that kyphoplasty increased vertebral body height and decreased kyphotic wedge angle as compared with vertebroplasty.

According to a prospective multicenter international study, vertebroplasty produces rapid pain reduction at 1 day after treatment along with improvement in mobility and function.[30] Colangelo et al[31] reported that kyphoplasty allowed faster recovery and avoided the deformity in kyphosis related to VCFs compared with NSM. Interestingly, the risk of having a subsequent vertebral fracture was higher after kyphoplasty than NSM in this retrospective study, but, according to another meta-analysis, there were no differences in the incidence of secondary fractures between vertebral augmentation and NSM in the treatment of osteoporotic compression fractures.[32] A recent meta-analysis showed that there was no evidence of an increased risk of new fracture of vertebral bodies, especially those adjacent to the treated vertebrae following vertebral augmentation compared to conservative management.[33] Yi et al[34] in a prospective study containing 290 consecutive patients with 363 fractures found no increased risk of VCF for those patients treated with vertebral augmentation as compared to those patients treated with NSM, but they did find that the additional fractures occurred sooner in patients treated with vertebral augmentation. This differing temporal relationship of the appearance of subsequent VCFs may serve to explain why some analyses show differences in subsequent fractures while others don't. Finally, Masoudi et al[35] investigated the effect of kyphoplasty compared with conservative management in stable thoracolumbar fractures in parachute jumpers, and concluded that kyphoplasty in stable thoracolumbar fractures is related to decreased pain, better functional recovery, fewer days of absence from work, and a shorter duration in returning to parachuting. The outcomes of conservative management and vertebral augmentation have been discussed in ▶ Table 22.1.

22.3 Outcome of Patients with Vertebral Fractures Not Treated with Vertebral Augmentation

Many patients with VCFs are treated with NSM. Approximately two-thirds of all vertebral fractures are asymptomatic and the other one-third of vertebral fractures are symptomatic and painful. In most fractures the pain gradually decreases over time and patients return to activity or their work in about 6 to

Table 22.1 Outcomes of conservative management and vertebral augmentation

Study	Study design	No. of studies	No. of patients	Interventions	Outcome
Zhao et al[2]	Meta-analysis	16	2,046	NSM, VP, KP	Pain relief, daily function, quality of life: NSM < VP≈KP
					New fracture risk: NSM≈VP≈KP
					Rank probability of pain relief: NSM<KP<VP
					Rank probability of daily function, quality of life, decreasing new fracture: NSM<KP<VP
Edidin et al[12]	Retrospective cohort study		1,038,956	NSM, VP, KP	Risk of 4-year mortality: NSM>VP>KP
					Risk of pneumonia, myocardial infarction/cardiac complications, DVT, urinary tract infection: NSM>KP
					Urinary tract infection: NSM>VP
					Risk of pulmonary/respiratory complications, pulmonary embolism: NSM<VP
					Risk of pneumonia, pulmonary embolism, urinary tract infection: VP>KP
					Risk of infection, DVT, myocardial infarction/cardiac complication: VP≈KP
Mattie et al[19]	Meta-analysis	11	1,048	NSM, VP	Pain relief at 1 to 2 weeks, 2 to 3 months and 12 month: NSM<PV
Chen et al[23]	Meta-analysis	5	777	**NSM, VP, KP**	**Pain relief: NSM<VP≈KP**
					Rank probability of pain relief: NSM<KP<VP
					Risk of all cause discontinuation: NSM>KP
					Rank probability of all cause discontinuation: NSM>VP>KP
					Rank probability of new fracture: NSM<KP<VP
Anderson et al[24]	Meta-analysis	8		NSM, VP	Pain relief: NSM<VP
					Functional outcome: NSM<VP
					Health-related quality of life: NSM<VP
					New fractures: NSM≈VP
Yang et al[28]	RCT		135	NSM, VP	Pain relief and quality of life at 1 week, 1 month, 3 months, 6 months, and 1 year: NSM<VP
					Satisfaction: NSM<VP
					Complication: NSM<VP
Colangelo et al[31]	Case–control study		110	NSM, KP	Pain relief at 1 month: NSM<KP
					Quality of life at 1 month: NSM<KP
					Restoration of kyphosis: NSM<KP
Song et al[32]	Meta-analysis	13		NSM, VP, KP	Risk of secondary vertebral fracture: NSM≈VP/KP
Masoudi et al[35]	RCT		70	NSM, KP	Pain relief at 1 month, 3 months, 6 months, and 12 months: NSM<KP
					ODI score at 1 month, 3 months, 6 months, and 12 months: NSM>KP
					Shorter duration of absence from work: NSM<KP

Abbreviations: KP, kyphoplasty; NSM, nonsurgical management; ≈, no significant difference; RCT, randomized controlled trial; VP, vertebroplasty.

8 weeks. Some patients, however, have persistent pain and their VCF never heals or inadequately heals. Clinical VCFs have been related to pain but disability, and functional impairment can persist even though the pain resolves.[36,37] John A. Kanis et al[38] investigated the relationship between VCF and deaths in 16,051 men and women aged 50 years or more who required

hospitalization. The results showed 28% of all deaths were considered causally related to the VCF.

VCFs can have a prominent and persistent effect on quality of life. Additionally, patients without vertebral augmentation can have mobilization difficulty and various complications such as deep vein thrombosis, pulmonary embolism, pressure ulcers, progressive vertebral body collapse, kyphotic deformity, back pain, neurologic compression, sleep disturbances, depression, and worsening osteoporosis. Bed rest can exacerbate the osteoporosis because of loss of body mass and bone density. Conversely, asymptomatic vertebral fractures are not necessarily related to the impairment of quality of life as long as a new vertebral fracture does not develop.[37,39] In the case of a new VCF in a patient with an underlying asymptomatic vertebral fracture, the disability and functional impairment may be significantly increased.[39]

As mentioned above, VCFs can yield higher risks of morbidity and mortality, and vertebral augmentation may decrease these risks.[8,12,40,41] Mortality in the VCF patients is rarely caused directly by vertebral fracture but mostly related to cancer (in neoplastic fractures) or to pulmonary causes such as pneumonia or pulmonary embolism.[42–44] The adverse outcomes related to pulmonary causes are associated with impaired pulmonary function including a decrease in vital capacity and inspiratory time resulting from the VCF.[45–47] Therefore, the decreased risks of mortality after vertebral augmentation are very likely related to improved pulmonary function.[6,9,42,47] According to a population-based study, VCF is an independent risk factor for the future development of pneumonia, especially if the VCF is located in the thoracic region.[48] An investigation of the US Medicare population showed a higher mortality risk in the patients that did not undergo vertebral augmentation.[12] The NSM cohort had a 55% higher adjusted risk of mortality than kyphoplasty cohort and 25% higher adjusted risk of mortality than vertebroplasty cohort. Previously, Chen et al[49] reported that vertebroplasty improved adjusted survivorship by 15% and kyphoplasty by 32% compared with the NSM patients at 3 years of follow-up. The patients with VCFs not treated with vertebral augmentation had higher adjusted risks of pneumonia, myocardial infarction, cardiac complications, deep vein thrombosis, and urinary tract infections. Conclusively, the results of the US Medicare population asserted that the patients without spinal augmentation had a significantly higher adjusted risk of death most often associated with pneumonia and significantly higher rates of morbidities.[12] In an investigation outside the United States[6] a Taiwanese analysis of data from National Health Insurance Research Database after hospital admission of 10,785 painful VCF patients showed the risk of death was 39% higher in patients who received medical management (HR: 1.39, 95% CI: 1.09–1.78, $p = 0.008$) compared to those patients who underwent vertebroplasty.

The presence of a VCF along with increased age and low bone mineral density (BMD) is a known risk factor for the development of additional VCFs.[50,51] Therefore, previous vertebral fractures in combination with old age and low BMD are associated with a prominent increased vertebral fracture risk. Additionally, a recent vertebral fracture can increase the risk of a future fracture within 2 years, especially in year 1 after the initial fracture.[52,53] According to the investigation of Health Outcomes and Reduced Incidence with Zoledronic Acid Once Yearly (HORIZON) Pivotal Fracture Trial, prior vertebral fracture and vertebral fracture in the first year were independent predictors of subsequent vertebral fractures in years 2 and 3 (adjusted OR: 2.8, 95% CI 1.9–4.0 and 3.1, 95% CI 1.9–5.0, respectively).[51] In the long-term follow-up over 15 years, one prevalent fracture resulted in a 2.5-fold increased risk of incident fractures (95% CI: 1.8–3.4) and more than two prevalent vertebral fractures resulted in a 5.2-fold increased risk of fracture (95% CI: 3.5–7.8).[54]

Even though two-thirds of VCFs may be asymptomatic and not associated with functional impairment, the symptomatic VCF can increase the patient's risk of subsequent fractures and their associated risk of morbidity and mortality. Vertebral augmentation including vertebroplasty and kyphoplasty decreases the risks of morbidity and mortality and improves the patient's pain, mobilization, kyphotic angulation, and quality of life.

References

[1] Bliuc D, Nguyen ND, Milch VE, Nguyen TV, Eisman JA, Center JR. Mortality risk associated with low-trauma osteoporotic fracture and subsequent fracture in men and women. JAMA 2009;301(5):513–521

[2] Zhao S, Xu CY, Zhu AR, et al. Comparison of the efficacy and safety of 3 treatments for patients with osteoporotic vertebral compression fractures: A network meta-analysis. Medicine (Baltimore) 2017;96(26):e7328

[3] Goldstein CL, Chutkan NB, Choma TJ, Orr RD. Management of the elderly with vertebral compression fractures. Neurosurgery 2015;77(Suppl 4):S33–S45

[4] Reginster J, Minne HW, Sorensen OH, et al; Vertebral Efficacy with Risedronate Therapy (VERT) Study Group. Randomized trial of the effects of risedronate on vertebral fractures in women with established postmenopausal osteoporosis. Osteoporos Int 2000;11(1):83–91

[5] Teyssédou S, Saget M, Pries P. Kyphopasty and vertebroplasty. Orthop Traumatol Surg Res 2014;100(1, Suppl):S169–S179

[6] Lin JH, Chien LN, Tsai WL, Chen LY, Chiang YH, Hsieh YC. Early vertebroplasty associated with a lower risk of mortality and respiratory failure in aged patients with painful vertebral compression fractures: a population-based cohort study in Taiwan. Spine J 2017;17(9):1310–1318

[7] Melton LJ III. Excess mortality following vertebral fracture. J Am Geriatr Soc 2000;48(3):338–339

[8] Kado DM, Duong T, Stone KL, et al. Incident vertebral fractures and mortality in older women: a prospective study. Osteoporos Int 2003;14(7):589–594

[9] Kado DM, Browner WS, Palermo L, Nevitt MC, Genant HK, Cummings SR; Study of Osteoporotic Fractures Research Group. Vertebral fractures and mortality in older women: a prospective study. Arch Intern Med 1999;159(11):1215–1220

[10] Prather H, Watson JO, Gilula LA. Nonoperative management of osteoporotic vertebral compression fractures. Injury 2007;38(Suppl 3):S40–S48

[11] Johnell O, Kanis JA. An estimate of the worldwide prevalence and disability associated with osteoporotic fractures. Osteoporos Int 2006;17(12):1726–1733

[12] Edidin AA, Ong KL, Lau E, Kurtz SM. Morbidity and mortality after vertebral fractures: comparison of vertebral augmentation and nonoperative management in the medicare population. Spine 2015;40(15):1228–1241

[13] Buchbinder R, Osborne RH, Ebeling PR, et al. A randomized trial of vertebroplasty for painful osteoporotic vertebral fractures. N Engl J Med 2009;361(6):557–568

[14] Kallmes DF, Comstock BA, Heagerty PJ, et al. A randomized trial of vertebroplasty for osteoporotic spinal fractures. N Engl J Med 2009;361(6):569–579

[15] Barr JD, Jensen ME, Hirsch JA, et al; Society of Interventional Radiology. American Association of . Neurological Surgeons. Congress of Neurological Surgeons. American College of Radiology. American Society of Neuroradiology. American Society of Spine Radiology. Canadian Interventional Radiology Association. Society of Neurointerventional Surgery. Position statement on percutaneous vertebral augmentation: a consensus statement developed by the Society of Interventional Radiology (SIR), American Association of Neurological Surgeons (AANS) and the Congress of Neurological Surgeons (CNS), American College of Radiology (ACR), American Society of Neuroradiology (ASNR), American Society of Spine Radiology (ASSR), Canadian Interventional Radiology Association (CIRA), and the Society of NeuroInterventional Surgery (SNIS). J Vasc Interv Radiol 2014;25(2):171–181

[16] De Laet C, Thiry N, Holdt Henningsen K, Stordeur S, Camberlin C. (2015) Percutaneous vertebroplasty and balloon kyphoplasty—synthesis. Health Technology Assessment (HTA) Brussels: Belgian Health Care Knowledge Centre (KCE). KCE Reports 255Cs. https://kce.fgov.be/sites/default/files/page_documents/KCE_255C_Percutaneaous_vertebroplasty_Synthesis

[17] National Institute for Health and Care Excellence. (2013) Percutaneous vertebroplasty and percutaneous balloon kyphoplasty for treating osteoporotic vertebral compression fractures. nice.org.uk/guidance/ta279. Accessed May 26, 2017

[18] Ong KL, Beall DP, Frohbergh M, Lau E, Hirsch JA. Were VCF patients at higher risk of mortality following the 2009 publication of the vertebroplasty "sham" trials? Osteoporos Int 2018;29(2):375–383

[19] Mattie R, Laimi K, Yu S, Saltychev M. Comparing percutaneous vertebroplasty and conservative therapy for treating osteoporotic compression fractures in the thoracic and lumbar spine: a systematic review and meta-analysis. J Bone Joint Surg Am 2016;98(12):1041–1051

[20] Ma XL, Xing D, Ma JX, Xu WG, Wang J, Chen Y. Balloon kyphoplasty versus percutaneous vertebroplasty in treating osteoporotic vertebral compression fracture: grading the evidence through a systematic review and meta-analysis. Eur Spine J 2012;21(9):1844–1859

[21] Zhao G, Liu X, Li F. Balloon kyphoplasty versus percutaneous vertebroplasty for treatment of osteoporotic vertebral compression fractures (OVCFs). Osteoporos Int 2016;27(9):2823–2834

[22] Xing D, Ma JX, Ma XL, et al. A meta-analysis of balloon kyphoplasty compared to percutaneous vertebroplasty for treating osteoporotic vertebral compression fractures. J Clin Neurosci 2013;20(6):795–803

[23] Chen LX, Li YL, Ning GZ, et al. Comparative efficacy and tolerability of three treatments in old people with osteoporotic vertebral compression fracture: a network meta-analysis and systematic review. PLoS One 2015;10(4):e0123153

[24] Anderson PA, Froyshteter AB, Tontz WL Jr. Meta-analysis of vertebral augmentation compared with conservative treatment for osteoporotic spinal fractures. J Bone Miner Res 2013;28(2):372–382

[25] Shi MM, Cai XZ, Lin T, Wang W, Yan SG. Is there really no benefit of vertebroplasty for osteoporotic vertebral fractures? A meta-analysis. Clin Orthop Relat Res 2012;470(10):2785–2799

[26] Blasco J, Martinez-Ferrer A, Macho J, et al. Effect of vertebroplasty on pain relief, quality of life, and the incidence of new vertebral fractures: a 12-month randomized follow-up, controlled trial. J Bone Miner Res 2012;27(5):1159–1166

[27] Wardlaw D, Cummings SR, Van Meirhaeghe J, et al. Efficacy and safety of balloon kyphoplasty compared with non-surgical care for vertebral compression fracture (FREE): a randomised controlled trial. Lancet 2009;373(9668):1016–1024

[28] Yang EZ, Xu JG, Huang GZ, et al. Percutaneous vertebroplasty versus conservative treatment in aged patients with acute osteoporotic vertebral compression fractures: a prospective randomized controlled clinical study. Spine 2016;41(8):653–660

[29] Liu JT, Liao WJ, Tan WC, et al. Balloon kyphoplasty versus vertebroplasty for treatment of osteoporotic vertebral compression fracture: a prospective, comparative, and randomized clinical study. Osteoporos Int 2010;21(2):359–364

[30] Leali PT, Solla F, Maestretti G, Balsano M, Doria C. Safety and efficacy of vertebroplasty in the treatment of osteoporotic vertebral compression fractures: a prospective multicenter international randomized controlled study. Clin Cases Miner Bone Metab 2016;13(3):234–236

[31] Colangelo D, Nasto LA, Genitiempo M, et al. Kyphoplasty vs conservative treatment: a case-control study in 110 post-menopausal women population. Is kyphoplasty better than conservative treatment? Eur Rev Med Pharmacol Sci 2015;19(21):3998–4003

[32] Song D, Meng B, Gan M, et al. The incidence of secondary vertebral fracture of vertebral augmentation techniques versus conservative treatment for painful osteoporotic vertebral fractures: a systematic review and meta-analysis. Acta Radiol 2015;56(8):970–979

[33] Zhang H, Xu C, Zhang T, Gao Z, Zhang T. Does percutaneous vertebroplasty or balloon kyphoplasty for osteoporotic vertebral compression fractures increase the incidence of new vertebral fractures? A meta-analysis. Pain Physician 2017;20(1):E13–E28

[34] Yi X, Lu H, Tian F, et al. Recompression in new levels after percutaneous vertebroplasty and kyphoplasty compared with conservative treatment. Arch Orthop Trauma Surg 2014;134(1):21–30

[35] Masoudi MS, Haghnegahdar A, Ghaffarpasand F, Ilami G. Functional recovery following early kyphoplasty versus conservative management in stable thoracolumbar fractures in parachute jumpers: a randomized clinical trial. Clin Spine Surg 2017;30(8):E1066–E1073

[36] Hall SE, Criddle RA, Comito TL, Prince RL. A case-control study of quality of life and functional impairment in women with long-standing vertebral osteoporotic fracture. Osteoporos Int 1999;9(6):508–515

[37] Nevitt MC, Ettinger B, Black DM, et al. The association of radiographically detected vertebral fractures with back pain and function: a prospective study. Ann Intern Med 1998;128(10):793–800

[38] Kanis JA, Oden A, Johnell O, De Laet C, Jonsson B. Excess mortality after hospitalisation for vertebral fracture. Osteoporos Int 2004;15(2):108–112

[39] O'Neill TW, Cockerill W, Matthis C, et al. Back pain, disability, and radiographic vertebral fracture in European women: a prospective study. Osteoporos Int 2004;15(9):760–765

[40] Lau E, Ong K, Kurtz S, Schmier J, Edidin A. Mortality following the diagnosis of a vertebral compression fracture in the Medicare population. J Bone Joint Surg Am 2008;90(7):1479–1486

[41] Edidin AA, Ong KL, Lau E, Kurtz SM. Mortality risk for operated and nonoperated vertebral fracture patients in the medicare population. J Bone Miner Res 2011;26(7):1617–1626

[42] Hasserius R, Karlsson MK, Nilsson BE, Redlund-Johnell I, Johnell O; European Vertebral Osteoporosis Study. Prevalent vertebral deformities predict increased mortality and increased fracture rate in both men and women: a 10-year population-based study of 598 individuals from the Swedish cohort in the European Vertebral Osteoporosis Study. Osteoporos Int 2003;14(1):61–68

[43] Center JR, Nguyen TV, Schneider D, Sambrook PN, Eisman JA. Mortality after all major types of osteoporotic fracture in men and women: an observational study. Lancet 1999;353(9156):878–882

[44] Hasserius R, Karlsson MK, Jónsson B, Redlund-Johnell I, Johnell O. Long-term morbidity and mortality after a clinically diagnosed vertebral fracture in the elderly: a 12- and 22-year follow-up of 257 patients. Calcif Tissue Int 2005;76(4):235–242

[45] Krege JH, Kendler D, Krohn K, et al. Relationship between vertebral fracture burden, height loss, and pulmonary function in postmenopausal women with osteoporosis. J Clin Densitom 2015;18(4):506–511

[46] Harrison RA, Siminoski K, Vethanayagam D, Majumdar SR. Osteoporosis-related kyphosis and impairments in pulmonary function: a systematic review. J Bone Miner Res 2007;22(3):447–457

[47] Yang HL, Zhao L, Liu J, et al. Changes of pulmonary function for patients with osteoporotic vertebral compression fractures after kyphoplasty. J Spinal Disord Tech 2007;20(3):221–225

[48] Kim B, Kim J, Jo YH, et al. Risk of pneumonia after vertebral compression fracture in women with low bone density: a population based study. Spine 2018;43(14):E830–E835

[49] Chen AT, Cohen DB, Skolasky RL. Impact of nonoperative treatment, vertebroplasty, and kyphoplasty on survival and morbidity after vertebral compression fracture in the medicare population. J Bone Joint Surg Am 2013;95(19):1729–1736

[50] Weaver J, Sajjan S, Lewiecki EM, Harris ST, Marvos P. Prevalence and cost of subsequent fractures among U.S. patients with an incident fracture. J Manag Care Spec Pharm 2017;23(4):461–471

[51] Wustrack R, Seeman E, Bucci-Rechtweg C, Burch S, Palermo L, Black DM. Predictors of new and severe vertebral fractures: results from the HORIZON Pivotal Fracture Trial. Osteoporos Int 2012;23(1):53–58

[52] Lindsay R, Silverman SL, Cooper C, et al. Risk of new vertebral fracture in the year following a fracture. JAMA 2001;285(3):320–323

[53] Roux C, Fechtenbaum J, Kolta S, Briot K, Girard M. Mild prevalent and incident vertebral fractures are risk factors for new fractures. Osteoporos Int 2007;18(12):1617–1624

[54] Cauley JA, Hochberg MC, Lui LY, et al. Long-term risk of incident vertebral fractures. JAMA 2007;298(23):2761–2767

23 Number of Levels Appropriately Treated with Vertebral Augmentation

Pyung-Bok Lee and Yong-Chul Kim

Summary

Vertebral augmentation, such as vertebroplasty and kyphoplasty has been introduced as effective treatment options for vertebral compression fracture. Unfortunately, there are many multiple level fractures in both osteoporotic and metastatic compression fractures. There are also still some questions about the maximum number of levels that should undergo vertebral augmentation. Current guidelines indicate that complications of vertebral augmentation may be amplified when more than three vertebral levels are treated concurrently but this has not been reflected in numerous clinical trials, and some researchers have found that complications such as anemia and new compression fracture did not increase with multiple levels of augmentation. They also suggested that treating all the fractures at once might decrease the patients' morbidity. In conclusion although the number of compression fracture levels to treat with vertebral augmentation should be based on a meticulous analysis of each individual's circumstances and many levels can be treated in an attempt to decrease patient morbidity, a generally agreed upon maximum number of levels is three per augmentation session.

Keywords: complications, levels, multiple compression fractures, vertebral augmentation

23.1 Introduction

Vertebral compression fractures (VCFs) related to osteoporosis are very common in the elderly.[1,2] In recent years, minimally invasive percutaneous cement augmentation techniques, such as vertebroplasty and kyphoplasty, have been introduced as effective treatment options.[2–8] These techniques have demonstrated excellent clinical outcomes, restoring the collapsed body height and reducing pain both in the short- and long-term.[2,4] However, one of the difficulties of vertebral augmentation techniques is the treatment of multiple fractures.[3] In both osteoporosis and metastasis, it is common to find multiple fractures, and about 20 to 47% of the patients with a previously diagnosed compression fracture develop new ones.[5–7,9] Consequently, some authors suggest the prophylactic augmentation of decalcified vertebrae as a method to prevent subsequent fractures that may increase overall mortality.[8,10,11] Additionally, almost 4% of the fractures are a consequence of neoplastic disease, which can be sampled during the vertebral augmentation procedure via vertebral biopsy.[12–14] Pathological fractures due to malignant tumors of the vertebrae also have been found to be adequately treated with vertebroplasty, which can produce sufficient pain control and a better quality of life.[15,16]

23.2 Neoplastic Vertebral Fractures

From the retrospective analysis of cancer patients, most compression fractures occurred at the thoracolumbar junction, with T11, T12, L1, and L2 accounting for 69.4% of all treated levels. The distribution of compression fractures by type of cancer show that 88.2% of documented metastatic compression fractures and 71% of all compression fractures had multiple myeloma, breast cancer, or lung cancer. Unlike osteoporotic compression fractures, in cancer patients there was a fairly even distribution of all compression fractures and metastatic compression fractures between the two sexes.[17]

23.3 Risk Factors for Vertebral Compression Fractures

In a study with postmenopausal Japanese-American women, Ross et al[18] found a fivefold increase in the risk of a new vertebral fracture when a single vertebral fracture was present at baseline. This risk increased to 12-fold when there were two or more fractures at baseline. Lindsay et al[19] in a multicenter study involving 2,725 postmenopausal women with a mean age of 74 years found a cumulative incidence of 6.6% new fractures in the first year. Overall, 19.2% of the women with a confirmed incidental fracture had a second fracture within one year; 11.5% of the women with one previous fracture sustained a second fracture, whereas 24% of the women with two or more prevalent fractures at baseline had a new fracture within a year following the first observed fracture (▶ Fig. 23.1).

Bed rest or inactivity as a result of pain from VCFs accelerates bone loss, which may increase the risk of additional fractures. Increased kyphosis from previous fractures also predisposes the patient to recurrent fractures. Black et al[20] found that prevalent vertebral deformities from previous fractures were associated with a fivefold increase in the risk of new fractures. Moreover, the risk was higher as the number of preexisting fractures and the severity of the deformity increased. Additionally, the presence of multiple and severe VCFs was found to be a specific risk factor for sustaining femoral neck fractures.[21]

23.4 Number of Levels to Treat with Vertebral Augmentation

Although there is extensive information regarding the increased incidence of new vertebral fractures after an initial one, there is no firm consensus on how many levels should be treated with vertebral augmentation. Some authors have suggested that the augmentation of one vertebra can increase the probability of new fractures in the adjacent ones; thus, prophylactic augmentation of decalcified vertebrae should be considered.[8,10] Moreover, there are cases with multiple compression fractures, and as many as 16 levels of augmentations in a single patient have been reported (▶ Fig. 23.2).[22] However, there are still some questions about the number of levels that should undergo vertebral augmentation. Should all the compressed levels be treated

First year of study

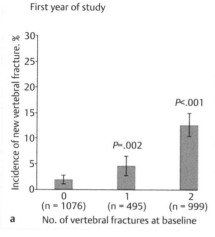

First year after vertebral fracture during study

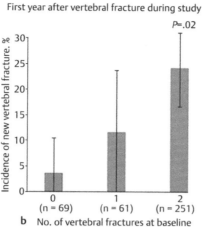

Fig. 23.1 (a, b) Incidence of vertebral fracture by number of baseline vertebral fractures. New compression fractures happened more in previous multilevel fractures at 1-year follow-up.

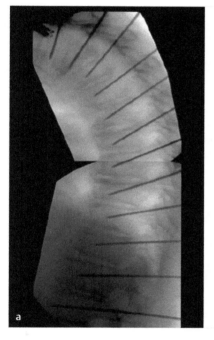

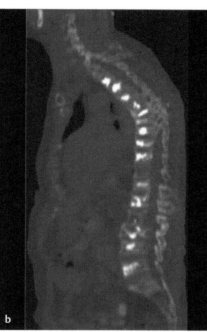

Fig. 23.2 (a, b) Multilevel vertebral augmentation. As many as 16 levels were treated with vertebral augmentation.

with augmentation? If not, which level(s) should be chosen to perform the vertebral augmentation? Finally, in the case of a single-level compression, is it better to perform an additional augmentation to the adjacent decalcified vertebrae?

23.5 Diagnosis of Painful Vertebral Compression Fractures

First of all, attention must be centered in the accurate diagnosis of the compressed fracture level that is contributing to the recent pain escalation. Lyritis et al[23] attempted to determine the clinical outcomes based on the initial radiographic appearance of the vertebral fractures. In their study, patients with an obvious wedge fracture had severe, sharp pain, which gradually decreased within 4 to 8 weeks (▶ Fig. 23.3). Conversely, patients with minimal superior end-plate discontinuity tended to have a gradual progression to complete collapse of the vertebral body and had dull, less severe, and recurrent pain. Conclusively, before considering a vertebral augmentation, a thoughtful, cautious,

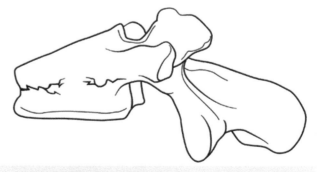

Fig. 23.3 Wedge shape compression fracture. Wedge fractures can have severe, sharp pain.

and accurate physical examination must be performed. In the patients with a possible VCF, the key physical examination signs are the presence of severe concordant pain with palpation or percussion on the suspected fractured spinous process, deep tenderness of paravertebral muscle pain, and facet joint

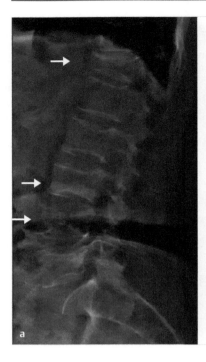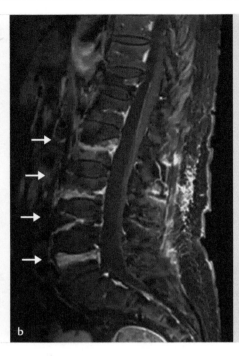

Fig. 23.4 (a, b) Hidden multiple compression fracture. MRI revealed the hidden acute fractures (*arrows*).

compression. Langdon et al[24] found that closed-fist percussion had sensitivity and specificity of 87.5 and 90%, respectively, for detecting VCFs. These authors also described a supine sign test that was 81.25% sensitive and 93.33% specific for detecting VCFs when the patient was unable to lie supine without prominent discomfort. Finally, when both physical and radiographic image examinations are positive for vertebral fracture, performing vertebral augmentation at one or two levels is often enough to successfully control the acute pain.

In cases with multiple compression fractures, Wang and Fahim[16] concluded that the patients treated with vertebral augmentation at once had better pain control than the ones treated in two different sessions, the first to repair a portion of the fractured vertebral bodies and a second to repair the remaining fractures. The patients with two procedures remained bed bound due to the persistent pain, had an increased hospice stay, and suffered additional morbidities. Additionally, there may be hidden neoplastic lesions or fractures despite the interrogation by experienced physical examinations and conventional radiography. Bone scanning plays a role in identifying osteoporotic fractures in patients who have negative findings on plain radiographs and in identifying additional fractures at other levels. Magnetic resonance imaging (MRI) of the spine is one of the most useful tests for determining fracture age, ruling out a malignant tumor, and selecting the appropriate treatment. Park et al[25] suggested that MRI with STIR sequencing exhibited a multitude of benefits in the exact identification of both acute and hidden lesions. In this study, MRI with STIR sequencing revealed that 23% of the single fracture group and 65% of the multiple fracture group had additional acute lesions that were not identified on a CT scan (▶Fig. 23.4). Therefore, as suggested in previous studies, the determination of the appropriate level is critical to achieving better clinical outcomes after vertebral augmentation. Additionally, 31 of their cases had multiple hidden lesions. They concluded that if the hidden lessons are not treated and the cement augmentation is performed at a single

level only, undesirable clinical outcomes may arise as a consequence of the missed and untreated lesion(s) which may further deteriorate after the initial procedure. In neoplastic lesions bone SPECT may be comparable for differentiating malignant from benign VCFs, especially, in the case of VCFs with a complete replacement of the normal fatty marrow. This means it is possible to use bone single-photon emission tomography (SPECT) as a substitute for MRI for differentiating malignant from benign VCFs.[26]

23.6 Safety of Treating Multiple Vertebral Compression Fractures

Other authors and published guidelines on vertebral augmentation consider a safe practice not to perform more than three levels in a single session to avoid major complications. This is a somewhat arbitrary rule that limits amount of pulmonary flow of marrow material and nearly always provides a safe limit on the patient's exposure to the potential hazards of the procedure especially if the operators are not extensively experienced in vertebral augmentation.[27–31]

Current guidelines indicate that complications of vertebral augmentation may be amplified when more than three vertebral levels are treated concurrently. There is purported increased risk of infection, bleeding, local trauma (pneumothorax, fracture of ribs, and adjacent vertebra), cement leakage (radiculopathy, canal stenosis, paralysis), pulmonary embolism, and death. Additionally, there is a theoretical increased risk of anemia, especially in elderly patients, due to the role of the vertebrae in hematopoiesis. Lee et al[32] analyzed the complications of percutaneous vertebral augmentation. They reviewed the procedural complications rate per the number of levels treated and found that vertebroplasty had a significantly increased rate of complications compared with kyphoplasty in all the prospective studies included in

Table 23.1 Osteoporotic vs. pathologic fractures per number of levels treated

	Procedure type	No. of levels	Cement leak (Total)	Symptomatic cement leak
Pathologic fractures	KP	214	6.07% (13/214)	0.00% (0/214)
	VP	760	79.07% (601/760) $P < 0.05$	0.26% (21/760) $P < 0.05$
Osteoporotic fractures	KP	1901	6.89% (131/1901)	0.05% (1/1901)
	VP	5260	20.79% (1094/5260) $P < 0.05$	0.03% (21/5260) $P < 0.05$

Table 23.2 Complications rate per number of levels treated

	Procedure type	Procedure-related complications	Medical complications
All Studies	KP (per no. levels treated)	0.30% (9/2731)	0.90% (24/2731)
	VP (per no. levels treated)	2.80% (215/7771) $P < 0.001$	0.30% (22/7771) $P < 0.001$
Prospective	KP (per no. levels treated)	0.40% (3/1290)	0.70% (9/1290)
	VP (per no. levels treated)	2.40% (3/1727) $P < 0.001$	0.30% (5/1727) $P < 0.005$

the meta-analysis (▶ Table 23.1). Additionally, the ratio of total cement leaks per number of levels treated were significantly higher for vertebroplasty, after isolating pathologic and osteoporotic fractures (▶ Table 23.2).

Although early vertebral augmentation procedures focused on the complete fill of the vertebral body, it is now evident that somewhat smaller volumes may restore the biomechanical properties of the vertebral body appropriately. Moreover, the volume of cement injected into the vertebral body is directly related to the stiffness and strength that is achieved.[33] Therefore, a lesser amount of approximately 15 to 25% volume fraction may be adequate to restore the stiffness of the vertebral body to its prefractured level. Additionally, if the vertebral body is filled preferentially on one side the stiffness of the nonaugmented side may be lower than the augmented side, which might lead to an imbalance of stress on the vertebral body in the unilaterally filled vertebral body. However, when cement crosses the midline, stiffness of both sides increase comparatively and biomechanical balance is thus achieved.[34] For this reason, a significant number of clinicians tend to hesitate to perform multiple vertebral augmentation, especially if the cement fill per vertebral bodies is relatively replete.

In order to decrease the complications such as anemia after multilevel vertebral vertebroplasty and kyphoplasty, some clinicians reduced the amount of cement injected. There are two approaches for the cement filling, a bipedicular approach that requires the cannulation of both sides of the vertebral body for cement injection and the unipedicular technique that accesses one side to inject the polymethylmethacrylate (PMMA).[35,36] The latter theoretically reduces the risks involved with cannulation by 50% and also potentially reduces procedure time and radiation exposure. The PMMA is cytotoxic due to its chemical and thermal effects during polymerization, and the temperature during polymerization is high enough to produce coagulation of tumoral cells. Therefore, care should be taken when deciding the amount of cement. There should be enough to fill the center of the vertebral body and have the cement extend from superior end plate to the inferior end plate. In regard to fill material, PMMA has been used successfully, and almost exclusively, for vertebroplasty and kyphoplasty. The advantages of this product are that: (1) surgeons and proceduralists are familiar with it, (2) it is easy to handle, (3) radiopaque materials can be added to it, (4) it provides the necessary strength and stiffness to be

durable, and (5) it is inexpensive. Conversely, the disadvantages are that: (1) it has no osteoinductive properties, (2) high polymerization temperatures can occasionally result in damage to surrounding tissues, (3) unreacted monomer has systemic cardiopulmonary side effects, and (4) it is not remodeled by creeping substitution over time. Although several investigators have reported promising results of vertebral augmentation with the use of biodegradable products, such as calcium phosphate, hydroxyapatite, or coral granules in vitro, there is insufficient evidence in clinical practice for the use of most of these alternative fill materials.[37]

Nieto-Iglesias et al[38] investigated the occurrence of new vertebral fractures after percutaneous vertebroplasty and reported that adjacent vertebral procedure and intradiskal cement leakage were risk factors for new fractures. Additionally, the incidence of new compression fractures tended to increase when more levels of vertebroplasty were performed (▶ Table 23.3). In a prospective study containing 290 consecutive patients with 363 fractures, Yi et al found no increased risk of VCF for those patients treated with vertebral augmentation as compared to those patients treated with NSM but they did find that the additional fractures occurred sooner in patients treated with vertebral augmentation.[39] This may serve to explain the impression that more fractures occur after vertebral augmentation despite clear evidence that this is not the case.[40]

Some particular causes of compression fracture, such as multiple myeloma, secondary osteoporosis, and metastases, where the patients have more than three painful vertebral collapses, are recommended to undergo multilevel treatment to achieve back-pain regression and to improve their quality of life. In these cases, if a mini-invasive technique is employed by a skilled operator, multilevel vertebroplasty could be feasible, safe, and successful. Hussein et al[41] declared in the international myeloma working group consensus statement in 2008 that multiple augmentation procedures for multiple myeloma may be necessary and appropriate. In general, three to four vertebrae per intervention is considered reasonable and feasible during a single procedure when needed. Additionally, they recommended that vertebral augmentation for adjacent or suspicious vertebrae without fracture may be necessary. The prophylactic augmentation may be considered in cases of fracture with kyphosis in the thoracolumbar region because the stress resultant from the deformity in this region is very high.[8,10]

Table 23.3 Occurrence of new compression fracture in the first year after vertebral augmentation

Characteristic	All vertebrae		Adjacent vertebrae only	
	HR	PValue	HR	PValue
No. of OVCFs treated				
1	1	—	1	—
2	0.49 (0.16, 1.47)	.200	0.44 (0.14, 1.31)	.140
≥3	0.77 (0.21, 2.85)	.690	0.64 (0.19, 2.17)	.470
Distance to treated level				
Adjacent	3.53 (1.52, 8.19)	.003*	—	—
One level	2.98 (1.35, 6.58)	.007*	—	—
Two or more levels	1	—	—	—
Intradiskal cement leakage present	8.21 (3.47, 19.4)	<.001*	5.47 (2.35, 12.7)	—

Another consideration for prophylactic augmentation is the cases when the vertebra is located between two fractured vertebrae such as T11 and L1, in which T12 requires treatment to avoid postprocedure collapse.

Wang and Fahim[16] evaluated the complications after multilevel (above four levels) kyphoplasty which was performed in 19 patients to a total of 189 levels. Unexpectedly, none of the patients developed anemia after multilevel kyphoplasty, but 13 (68.4%) of the 19 patients had anemia before the procedure and continued to have anemia after the surgery. The authors concluded that there are no absolute contraindications to multilevel kyphoplasty, and they disagree with the recommended maximum number of vertebrae that may be treated at one time. Conversely, patients with untreated levels of fracture spent more days in bed, which results in increased risks of deep venous thrombosis (DVT), decubitus ulcers, atelectasis, pneumonia, loss of muscle mass, loss of bone density, and other health detriments associated with immobility. Therefore, treating all the fractures at once in the same anesthetic time, regardless of their location in the thoracic or the lumbar spine, may decrease the morbidity associated with delaying ambulation and, conversely, leaving some painful fractures untreated may increase the risk of such complications. Nonetheless, the decision should be taken case by case, according to each patient's circumstances including the precise level, the biomechanical properties, the patient's general conditions, premedical history, and the physician's experience, among others.

23.7 Conclusion

In conclusion, the number of compression fracture levels to treat with vertebral augmentation should be based on a meticulous analysis of the individual's circumstances and according to technical modulations. However, it is evident that complications such as anemia and new compression fractures after vertebral augmentation might not be serious and are preventable for experienced physicians.

References

[1] Farrokhi MR, Alibai E, Maghami Z. Randomized controlled trial of percutaneous vertebroplasty versus optimal medical management for the relief of pain and disability in acute osteoporotic vertebral compression fractures. J Neurosurg Spine 2011;14(5):561–569

[2] Genev IK, Tobin MK, Zaidi SP, Khan SR, Amirouche FML, Mehta AI. Spinal compression fracture management: a review of current treatment strategies and possible future avenues. Global Spine J 2017;7(1):71–82

[3] Watts NB. Is percutaneous vertebral augmentation (vertebroplasty) effective treatment for painful vertebral fractures? Am J Med 2003;114(4):326–328

[4] Li L, Ren J, Liu J, et al. Wang X, Liu Z, Sun T. Results of vertebral augmentation treatment for patients of painful osteoporotic vertebral compression fractures; A meta-analysis of eight randomized controlled trials. PLoS One 2015;10(9):e0138126

[5] Longo UG, Loppini M, Denaro L, Maffulli N, Denaro V. Osteoporotic vertebral fractures: current concepts of conservative care. Br Med Bull 2012;102:171–189

[6] Hsieh MK, Chen LH, Chen WJ. Current concepts of percutaneous balloon kyphoplasty for the treatment of osteoporotic vertebral compression fractures: evidence-based review. Biomed J 2013;36(4):154–161

[7] Taylor RS, Taylor RJ, Fritzell P. Balloon kyphoplasty and vertebroplasty for vertebral compression fractures: a comparative systematic review of efficacy and safety. Spine 2006;31(23):2747–2755

[8] Chiang CK, Wang YH, Yang CY, Yang BD, Wang JL. Prophylactic vertebroplasty may reduce the risk of adjacent intact vertebra from fatigue injury: an ex vivo biomechanical study. Spine 2009;34(4):356–364

[9] Beall DP, Chambers MF, Thomas SM, et al. Prospective and multicenter evaluation of outcomes for quality of life and activities of daily living for balloon kyphoplasty in the treatment of vertebral compression fractures: the EVOLVE trial. J Neurosurg 2018;0:1–11

[10] Kulcsár Z, Marosfoi M, Berentei Z, Veres R, Nyáry I, Szikora I. [Frequency of adjacent vertebral fractures following percutaneous vertebroplasty] Orv Hetil 2009;150(37):1744–1748

[11] Ong KL, Beall DP, Frohbergh M, Lau E, Hirsch J. Were VCF patients at higher risk of mortality following the 2009 publication of the vertebroplasty "sham" trials? Osteoporos Int 2017;doi:10.1007/s00198-017-4281-z

[12] Saracen A, Kotwica Z. Treatment of multiple osteoporotic vertebral compression fractures by percutaneous cement augmentation. Int Orthop 2014;38(11):2309–2312

[13] Tseng YY, Yang TC, Tu PH, Lo YL, Yang ST. Repeated and multiple new vertebral compression fractures after percutaneous transpedicular vertebroplasty. Spine 2009;34(18):1917–1922

[14] Cosar M, Sasani M, Oktenoglu T, et al. The major complications of transpedicular vertebroplasty. J Neurosurg Spine 2009;11(5):607–613

[15] Kotwica Z, Saracen A. Early and long-term outcomes of vertebroplasty for single osteoporotic fractures. Neurol Neurochir Pol 2011;45(5):431–435

[16] Wang AC, Fahim DK. Safety and efficacy of balloon kyphoplasty at 4 or more levels in a single anesthetic session. J Neurosurg Spine 2018;28(4):372–378

[17] Jha RM, Hirsch AE, Yoo AJ, Ozonoff A, Growney M, Hirsch JA. Palliation of compression fractures in cancer patients by vertebral augmentation: a retrospective analysis. J Neurointerv Surg 2010;2(3):221–228

[18] Ross PD, Davis JW, Epstein RS, Wasnich RD. Pre-existing fractures and bone mass predict vertebral fracture incidence in women. Ann Intern Med 1991;114(11):919–923

[19] Lindsay R, Silverman SL, Cooper C, et al. Risk of new vertebral fracture in the year following a fracture. JAMA 2001;285(3):320–323

[20] Black DM, Arden NK, Palermo L, Pearson J, Cummings SR; Study of Osteoporotic Fractures Research Group. Prevalent vertebral deformities predict hip fractures and new vertebral deformities but not wrist fractures. J Bone Miner Res 1999;14(5):821–828

[21] Kinoshita T, Ebara S, Kamimura M, et al. Nontraumatic lumbar vertebral compression fracture as a risk factor for femoral neck fractures in involutional osteoporotic patients. J Bone Miner Metab 1999;17(3):201–205

[22] Erdem E, Samant R, Malak SF, et al. Vertebral augmentation in the treatment of pathologic compression fractures in 792 patients with multiple myeloma. Leukemia 2013;27(12):2391–2393

[23] Lyritis GP, Mayasis B, Tsakalakos N, et al. The natural history of the osteoporotic vertebral fracture. Clin Rheumatol 1989;8(Suppl 2):66–69

[24] Langdon J, Way A, Heaton S, Bernard J, Molloy S. Vertebral compression fractures: new clinical signs to aid diagnosis. Ann R Coll Surg Engl 2010;92:163–166

[25] Park SY, Lee SH, Suh SW, Park JH, Kim TG. Usefulness of MRI in determining the appropriate level of cement augmentation for acute osteoporotic vertebral compression fractures. J Spinal Disord Tech 2013;26(3):E80–E85

[26] Tokuda O, Harada Y, Ueda T, Ohishi Y, Matsunaga N. Malignant versus benign vertebral compression fractures: can we use bone SPECT as a substitute for MR imaging? Nucl Med Commun 2011;32(3):192–198

[27] Anselmetti GC, Bonaldi G, Carpeggiani P, Manfrè L, Masala S, Muto M. Vertebral augmentation: 7 years experience. Acta Neurochir Suppl (Wien) 2011;108:147–161

[28] Gangi A, Guth S, Imbert JP, Marin H, Dietemann JL. Percutaneous vertebroplasty: indications, technique, and results. Radiographics 2003;23(2):e10

[29] Kallmes DF, Jensen ME. Percutaneous vertebroplasty. Radiology 2003;229(1):27–36

[30] McGraw JK, Cardella J, Barr JD, et al; Society of Interventional Radiology Standards of Practice Committee. Society of Interventional Radiology quality improvement guidelines for percutaneous vertebroplasty. J Vasc Interv Radiol 2003;14(9 Pt 2):S311–S315

[31] Peh WC, Gilula LA. Percutaneous vertebroplasty: indications, contraindications, and technique. Br J Radiol 2003;76(901):69–75

[32] Lee MJ, Dumonski M, Cahill P, Stanley T, Park D, Singh K. Percutaneous treatment of vertebral compression fractures: a meta-analysis of complications. Spine 2009;34(11):1228–1232

[33] Nieuwenhuijse MJ, Putter H, van Erkel AR, Dijkstra PD. New vertebral fractures after percutaneous vertebroplasty for painful osteoporotic vertebral compression fractures: a clustered analysis and the relevance of intradiskal cement leakage. Radiology 2013;266(3):862–870

[34] Jacobson RE, Palea O, Granville M. Progression of vertebral compression fractures after previous vertebral augmentation: technical reasons for recurrent fractures in a previously treated vertebra. Cureus 2017;9(10):e1776

[35] Lee DG, Park CK, Park CJ, Lee DC, Hwang JH. Analysis of Risk Factors Causing New Symptomatic Vertebral Compression Fractures After Percutaneous Vertebroplasty for Painful Osteoporotic Vertebral Compression Fractures: A 4-year Follow-up. J Spinal Disord Tech 2015;28(10):E578–E583

[36] Rao RD, Singrakhia MD. Painful osteoporotic vertebral fracture. Pathogenesis, evaluation, and roles of vertebroplasty and kyphoplasty in its management. J Bone Joint Surg Am 2003;85(10):2010–2022

[37] Yuan WH, Hsu HC, Lai KL. Vertebroplasty and balloon kyphoplasty versus conservative treatment for osteoporotic vertebral compression fractures: A meta-analysis. Medicine (Baltimore) 2016;95(31):e4491

[38] Nieto-Iglesias C, Andrés-Nieto I, Peces-García E, et al. Vertebroplasty and kyphoplasty: techniques, complications, and troubleshooting. Tech Reg Anesth Pain Manage 2014;18:40–48

[39] Yi X, Lu H, Tian F, et al. Recompression in new levels after percutaneous vertebroplasty and kyphoplasty compared with conservative treatment. Arch Orthop Trauma Surg 2014;134(1):21–30

[40] Papanastassiou ID, Phillips FM, Van Meirhaeghe J, et al. Comparing effects of kyphoplasty, vertebroplasty, and non-surgical management in a systematic review of randomized and non-randomized controlled studies. Eur Spine J 2012;21(9):1826–1843

[41] Hussein MA, Vrionis FD, Allison R, et al; International Myeloma Working Group. The role of vertebral augmentation in multiple myeloma: International Myeloma Working Group Consensus Statement. Leukemia 2008;22(8):1479–1484

24 Pain after Vertebral Augmentation

Scott Kreiner

Summary

Vertebral augmentation is a very effective procedure for relieving pain from a vertebral compression fracture (VCF). If pain persists after vertebral augmentation, the temporal relationship of the pain to the procedure is the most important factor in determining the cause of the pain. Pain immediately after the augmentation procedure is most commonly due to inadequate treatment of the fracture, complications associated with the procedure or an unrepaired additional fracture. Pain present before the fracture that returns or is perceived as worse is likely related to a degenerative or neoplastic process depending on the particular patient's underlying condition. The most common cause of pain is an additional vertebral fracture and when this is suspected additional imaging should be obtained. Additional imaging should be obtained when infection or procedural complications are suspected. Any additional treatment will depend on the underlying disorder but can include antibiotics for injection and decompression with or without stabilization for symptomatic cement extravasation. Recurrent fracture of the incident fracture level can occur and should be thought of in patients with recurrent pain after vertebral augmentation. Vertebral body collapse and intervertebral disk degeneration places additional stress on the posterior elements and facet joints. This additional stress can cause pain which can be substantially decreased by facet injection or medial branch blocks. Facet related pain is common after VCFs and should be considered in a patient with persistent pain. The kyphosis seen with VCFs creates a sagittal imbalance that places more stress on the paraspinal musculature and can give rise to increase energy expenditure to maintain an upright posture and can cause pain. If the sagittal imbalance is severe enough it may require the patient to use a cane or a walker to ambulate. Although vertebral augmentation cannot entirely prevent vertebral deformity it can improve it and optimal restoration of vertebral body height can serve to improve patient function and to minimize abnormal stresses on the spine caused by excessive kyphosis.

Keywords: postprocedure pain, vertebral augmentation, extravasation, recurrent fracture, kyphotic deformity, cone of economy, sagittal imbalance

24.1 Introduction

Vertebral augmentation is an effective treatment for pain caused by an acute compression fracture with 75 to 90% of patients obtaining good to excellent pain relief within 7 to 10 days after vertebral augmentation with or without cavity creation.[1-3] For this reason, when providing this treatment both the physician and the patient should have reasonable expectations of pain improvement fairly quickly following the procedure. However, on occasion, the patient's pain does not resolve, or they develop new pain at some point following the fracture.

Pain following vertebral augmentation, may or may not be associated with the compression fracture or the vertebral augmentation procedure. Most of the patients undergoing vertebral augmentation procedures have compression fractures related to osteoporosis or primary or secondary malignancy in the spine. These conditions are related to a host of comorbidities which are either directly or indirectly associated with other spine-related conditions that may cause pain.

The potential causes of spine pain after vertebral augmentation can be separated based on the timing of the pain in relation to the index procedure. For this reason, in patients who present with pain after the procedure, detailed questioning on exactly when the pain started, its quality, location, and aggravating/alleviating factors can help establish a diagnosis and develop an appropriate treatment plan.

In general, pain immediately surrounding the vertebral augmentation temporally is more likely related to the fracture, or complications of the procedure, or an adjacent level fracture. Pain that was present prior to the fracture is more likely related to degenerative changes that most often pre-date the presence of the VCF. Patients may also have preexisting conditions such as degenerative disk disease, facet arthropathy, or spinal stenosis that were painful and present prior to the fracture treatment but the more severe fracture pain overshadowed the secondary condition and following successful vertebral augmentation the pain from that secondary condition seemed to return or was, once again, noticed. Separating this from an additional fracture that was not seen on prior imaging or complications from the procedure itself is important.

24.2 Complications from Procedure

In the day or two following the procedure, it is reasonable to expect some postprocedural pain as a result of the incision and the needle traversing through the paraspinal soft tissue. In general, this pain should be limited to the first week following the procedure and usually within the first 3 to 4 days. If a patient returns to clinic with pain that is persisting over 10 days following the procedure, the most likely potential causes of the pain are inadequate treatment or refracture of the index fracture, and fractures at a level(s) other than the index level not identified prior to the procedure. There can also be some persistent pain at this time as the result of a fracture of a rib, pedicle, or transverse process during the procedure.

Patients who return to the office with complaints of persistent or worsening pain within the first 4 weeks after vertebral augmentation need assessment. If a thorough history and examination reveals severe, functionally limiting pain (≥7/10 on a numerical rating score), and/or the presence of "red flag" conditions, such as fever, chills, nausea, vomiting, inability to lie supine, new trauma, and/or pain with percussion to spinous process, then new imaging should be obtained.

Infection of the vertebral body and polymethyl methacrylate (PMMA) following vertebral augmentation (▶ Fig. 24.1) is rare to the point that it is case-reportable but there should at least be a consideration of this possibility as it can be life threatening in the frail and elderly patients that frequently

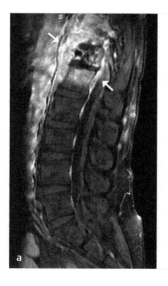
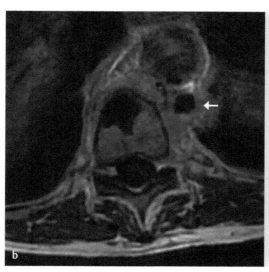

Fig. 24.1 Vertebral osteomyelitis after vertebral augmentation. **(a)** T1-weighted fat saturated MRI with gadolinium one week after vertebroplasty demonstrates anterior epidural and paraspinal enhancing soft tissue and vertebral enhancement involving L1, T12, T11, and T10 (*white arrows* in **a**) indicating vertebral osteomyelitis. T1-weighted post-gadolinium axial MRI of the T10 vertebrae obtained one week after vertebroplasty demonstrates enhancing paraspinal inflammation with a cystic structure (*white arrow* in **b**) representing a paraspinal abscess. The short interval of time after the procedure does not correspond with the wide range and advanced appearance of the infection indicating that the infection may have already been present at the time of vertebroplasty. (Reproduced with permission from Syed et al 2009.[5])

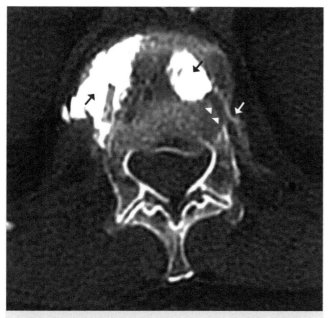

Fig. 24.2 Axial computed tomography (CT) image shows a fracture of the pedicle/vertebral body junction (*white arrow*). This was sustained during vertebral augmentation and the needle track through the lateral left pedicle can be seen (*white arrowheads*) along with the cement (*black arrows*).

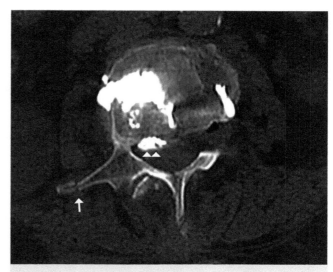

Fig. 24.3 Axial computed tomography (CT) image shows a fracture of the right transverse process (*white arrow*). This fracture occurred as a result of vertebral augmentation. Incidentally noted is extravasation of polymethyl methacrylate (PMMA) into the anterior epidural space (*white arrowheads*). This extravasation was asymptomatic.

get VCFs. In patients who present in the postoperative period with systemic complaints of infection (fever, chills, lethargy) work-up should include laboratory work-up complete blood count (CBC), erythrocyte sedimentation rate (ESR), C-reactive protein (CRP), and advanced imaging of the spine. Should this work-up be concerning for an infection, immediate aspiration/biopsy and culture of the area along with the long-term use of the appropriate antibiotics can be critical to the survival of the patient.[4] In the presence of neurologic deficit or spinal instability, prompt surgical treatment should be considered.

There are direct, procedure-related complications that can cause back pain and/or radicular pain after vertebral augmentation. These complications include fracture of the rib, pedicle, or transverse process, and extravasation of PMMA into locations where it is not desired (▶Fig. 24.2 and ▶Fig. 24.3). Some of the locations of extravasation that can cause symptoms include the neural foramen or spinal canal (▶Fig. 24.4 and ▶Fig. 24.5). Most if not all of these complications can be avoided if proper technique is used during the procedure. These technical aspects include not applying substantial torque by levering the needle once in the pedicle, carefully observing and managing the flow of the PMMA during its administration, and replacing the stylet into the introducer needle cannula once administration of the PMMA is complete.

Treatment of these complications varies. Pedicle fracture occurs about 1% of the time,[7–9] and usually it does not require treatment if it is unilateral. It occurs most commonly in the thoracic spine where the pedicles are smaller, as compared with

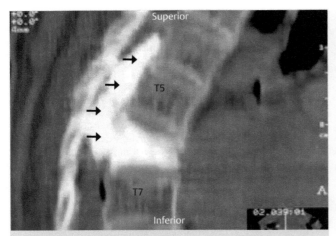

Fig. 24.4 Sagittal computed tomography (CT) scan of the thoracic spine showing polymethyl methacrylate (PMMA) leak into the epidural space (*black arrows*). (Adapted from Lopes and Lopes 2004.[6])

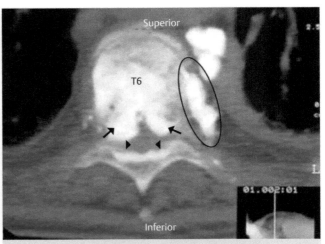

Fig. 24.5 Axial computed tomography (CT) scan of the thoracic spine showing extravasation of polymethyl methacrylate (PMMA) into the vertebral canal (*black arrows*) with compression of the spinal cord (*black arrowheads*) and nerve roots. Also note the presence of PMMA on the left side of the T6 vertebral body (area within black circle) which interfered with the lateral visualization of the PMMA injection. (Adapted from Lopes and Lopes 2004.[6])

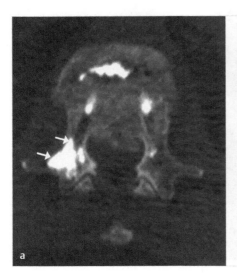
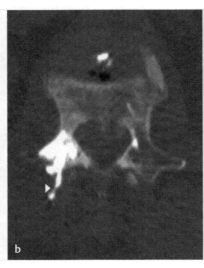

Fig. 24.6 Axial computed tomography (CT) image showing polymethyl methacrylate (PMMA) extending posteriorly into the right pedicle of T12 (*white arrows* in **a**). The PMMA extends into the soft tissues posterior to the pedicle (*white arrowhead* in **b**) forming a tail of PMMA.

the lumbar spine. If the pedicle fracture is symptomatic it can be stabilized by injecting cement into it, a technique known as pediculoplasty. This technique is discussed in detail in Chapter 10. Should the patient have a radiculopathy related to the presence of PMMA in the foramen, a selective nerve root or epidural injection can be performed in an attempt to improve or alleviate the radicular symptoms. If the symptoms persist or if there is weakness related to compression of the nerve, surgical intervention may be required. Treatment of a PMMA "tail" in the paraspinal musculature (▶Fig. 24.6) is also determined by the symptoms. The overwhelming majority of patients are not symptomatic when cement follows the needle track into the paraspinal soft tissues. In the rare circumstance that the patient has substantial pain or discomfort that the provider feels is related to the paraspinal cement, a block with local anesthetic of the paraspinal muscles/PMMA should be diagnostic. If so, removal of the cement can be done with a small incision and

fluoroscopic guidance. The cement can usually be identified under fluoro and removed with Ochsner-Kocher forceps or another type of clamping instrument.

24.3 Recurrent Fracture

Recurrent fracture at a level treated by vertebral augmentation is seen on an intermittent but regular basis, occurring in 1 to 2% of patients.[10–12] Chen et al have performed the largest study to date and report a 0.56% risk (10/1,800) of recurrent fracture after vertebroplasty.[13] When refracture occurs, it is typically painful with acute further compression of the vertebrae or increasing edema within the vertebral body occurring in the first 60 to 90 days postprocedure,[13,14] though these changes can occur at any time. Reasons for refracture include only partial filling of the fractured vertebral body, inadequately filling of the fracture site with cement, inadequate filling of a

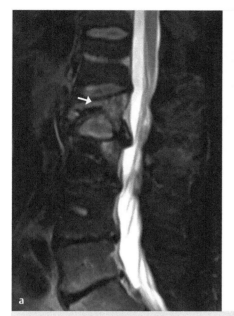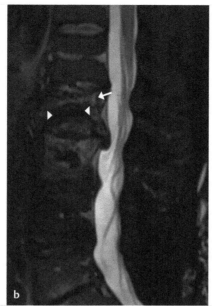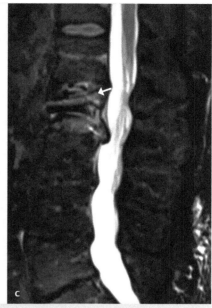

Fig. 24.7 Sagittal STIR magnetic resonance (MR) image demonstrating an acute vertebral fracture of the L2 vertebral body with prominent edema within the vertebral body (*white arrow* in **a**) that is substantially decreased after vertebral augmentation (*white arrow* in **b**) with polymethyl methacrylate (PMMA) (*white arrowheads* in **b**). The patient experienced increased pain in the region previously treated and a follow-up MRI obtained two-and-a-half months after the augmentation procedure showed increased edema within the L2 vertebral body (*white arrow* in **c**) relative to the previous MR imaging exam following treatment when the patient was asymptomatic from the fracture.

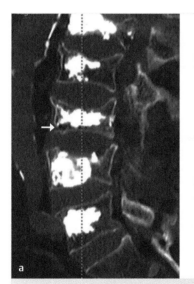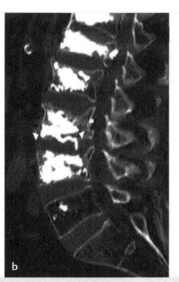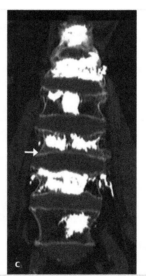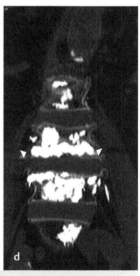

Fig. 24.8 Sagittal (**a** and **b**) and coronal (**c** and **d**) reconstructions of a lumbar computed tomography (CT) exam showing air within the inferior portion of a previously treated L3 vertebral body (*white arrow* in **a** and **c**) indicating refracture of the treated level. The vertebral fracture was reaugmented with 6 mL of additional bone cement which filled the cleft inferior to the existing cement (*white arrowheads* in **b** and **d**) and caused reduction in the fracture with increased vertebral body height.

known vertebral cleft, or development of cavitation around cement (▶ Fig. 24.7 and ▶ Fig. 24.8).[15]

In patients with a recurrent fracture, if severe, functionally limiting pain persists, it is reasonable to consider a repeat vertebral augmentation (▶ Fig. 24.8). Repeat vertebral augmentation in these patients can be difficult because the existing PMMA can interfere with vertebral body access but using additional approach techniques such as the parapedicular approach or the modified inferior end-plate extrapedicular approach can be helpful. These approaches are covered in detail in Chapter

6. Preprocedure planning with thorough analysis images (computed tomography [CT], magnetic resonance imaging [MRI]) can help plan an approach to maximize success. Treatment of a recurrent fracture has been shown to reduce pain.[10,13,16]

Progressive loss of vertebral height is common and should be separated from the phenomenon of a refracture of the incident vertebral level as this progressive height loss is often not painful. Studies show 10 to 15% gradual height loss in up to 30% of patients when followed up to 2 years after the procedure.[2,3,14]

24.4 Facet-Mediated Pain

The height loss of the vertebral body causes a biomechanical imbalance producing increased load on the posterior elements of the spine. In addition if the disk adjacent to the fractured vertebral body is degenerated, this can shift additional load posteriorly on to the facet joints.[17] This increased load, in addition to abnormal movement, can cause facet-joint overload, arthropathy, and pain. Imaging studies evaluating the facet joints have shown that facet-joint signal changes on MRI scan are higher in patients with acute and subacute compression fractures.[18] Further, Wilson et al[19] offered facet-joint injections to patients referred for vertebral augmentation procedures. Of the 61 patients in this cohort, 21 had a successful outcome as measured by a reduced VAS for pain requiring no further intervention, suggesting that at least in a portion of these patients, the posterior elements may be causing substantial pain. And, while it is clear that facet-joint injections are not a replacement for vertebral augmentation,[20–22] when patients return to the clinic with pain in the treated area, the facet joints should be considered as a source of that pain.

Facet-mediated pain, as compared with a recurrent fracture, is typically less severe, more gradual in onset and has different factors that reproduce or exacerbate the pain. The nature of this pain is typically dull, and patients classically describe symptoms frequently associated with osteoarthritis, such as stiffness, which worsen with rest and improve with heat and movement. Facet-joint pain is also characteristically elicited by lumbar extension, getting out of a chair or twisting movements. The facet joints are implicated as the source of pain in 27 to 80%[23,24] of patients with persistent pain after a fracture or having undergone vertebral augmentation. Facet-joint injections and medial branch blocks with radiofrequency neurotomy are effective treatments for this type of pain.[21,23–26]

24.5 Sagittal Imbalance

Dubousset first described the cone of economy in 1994[27] (▶Fig. 24.9). This theory describes the chain of balance starting at the support polygon (both feet), and progressing up the lower limbs, then pelvis, and then up the spinal segments terminating in the head. All of these elements work in concert to maintain a center of gravity through the middle of the body, requiring minimal energy expenditure to stand erect. Critical to this system are the spinal segments, making the normal lumbar and cervical lordosis and thoracic kyphosis, along with the pelvic incidence, the key players in the sagittal balance. When deviations of these curves occur, the center of gravity shifts from midline, increasing the energy expenditure required to maintain an erect posture. When the deviation becomes excessive, and the body falls outside the cone of economy, assistive devices such as a cane or walker are required to avoid falling.

VCFs, either in thoracic spine or at the thoracolumbar junction increase the kyphotic angle, directly influencing the sagittal balance of the spine. As the number and severity of the fractures increases, so does the kyphotic deformity.[28] This creates a positive sagittal balance with shifting of the superior spine anteriorly, resulting in increasing muscle effort, additional energy expenditure, and increased pain and disability.[29,30]

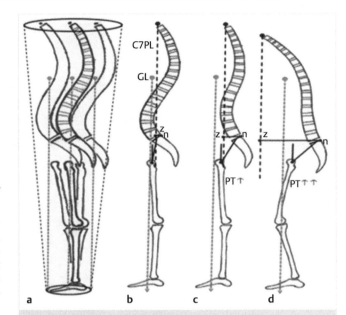

Fig. 24.9 Cone of economy. Diagram representation of the chain of balance with C7 plum line (C7PL) showing variation with changes in posture (*upper black circle* in **a**) and how this translates to the support polygon around the feet (*lower black circle* in **a**). The gravity line (*red dashed line* in **a** to **d**) varies with changes in posture (*red dashed lines* in **a**) and the presence of kyphosis shifts the C7PL anterior to the gravity line (*black dashed line* and *red dashed line* in **d**) and increases the pelvic tilt (PT angle in **c** and **d**). All of these elements work together to maintain a center of gravity through the center of the body and when the deviations above occur there is increased energy expenditure to maintain an erect posture (C7PL, C7 plumb line; PT, pelvic tilt; GL, gravity line).

The presence of an increased kyphotic deformity and positive sagittal balance has also been linked to increased risk of future fractures.[31]

While vertebral augmentation cannot entirely prevent deviation from normal sagittal balance, optimal height restoration during vertebral augmentation can help.[28,32–34] This is especially true with some of the implant-related technologies for VCF treatment that have the capability of restoring or nearly restoring the vertebral body to its original height. In addition, fixating the fractures, thereby reducing further collapse, also helps minimize this complication. Once positive sagittal balance has occurred, little can be done nonsurgically to correct this problem.

References

[1] Frankel BM, Monroe T, Wang C. Percutaneous vertebral augmentation: an elevation in adjacent-level fracture risk in kyphoplasty as compared with vertebroplasty. Spine J 2007;7(5):575–582

[2] Liu JT, Li CS, Chang CS, Liao WJ. Long-term follow-up study of osteoporotic vertebral compression fracture treated using balloon kyphoplasty and vertebroplasty. J Neurosurg Spine 2015;23(1):94–98

[3] Tsai YW, Hsiao FY, Wen YW, et al. Clinical outcomes of vertebroplasty or kyphoplasty for patients with vertebral compression fractures: a nationwide cohort study. J Am Med Dir Assoc 2013;14(1):41–47

[4] Park JW, Park SM, Lee HJ, Lee CK, Chang BS, Kim H. Infection following percutaneous vertebral augmentation with polymethylmethacrylate. Arch Osteoporos 2018;13(1):47

[5] Syed MI, Avutu B, Shaikh A, Sparks H, Mohammed MI, Morar K. Vertebral osteomyelitis following vertebroplasty: is acne a potential contraindication and are prophylactic antibiotics mandatory prior to vertebroplasty? Pain Physician 2009;12(4):E285–E290

[6] Lopes NM, Lopes VK. Paraplegia complicating percutaneous vertebroplasty for osteoporotic vertebral fracture: case report. Arq Neuropsiquiatr 2004;62(3B):879–881

[7] Kallmes DF, Schweickert PA, Marx WF, Jensen ME. Vertebroplasty in the mid- and upper thoracic spine. AJNR Am J Neuroradiol 2002;23(7):1117–1120

[8] Mehbod A, Aunoble S, Le Huec JC. Vertebroplasty for osteoporotic spine fracture: prevention and treatment. Eur Spine J 2003;12(Suppl 2):S155–S162

[9] Nussbaum DA, Gailloud P, Murphy K. A review of complications associated with vertebroplasty and kyphoplasty as reported to the Food and Drug Administration medical device related web site. J Vasc Interv Radiol 2004;15(11):1185–1192

[10] Gaughen JR Jr, Jensen ME, Schweickert PA, Marx WF, Kallmes DF. The therapeutic benefit of repeat percutaneous vertebroplasty at previously treated vertebral levels. AJNR Am J Neuroradiol 2002;23(10):1657–1661

[11] Lavelle WF, Cheney R. Recurrent fracture after vertebral kyphoplasty. Spine J 2006;6(5):488–493

[12] Wu AM, Chi YL, Ni WF. Vertebral compression fracture with intravertebral vacuum cleft sign: pathogenesis, image, and surgical intervention. Asian Spine J 2013;7(2):148–155

[13] Chen LH, Hsieh MK, Liao JC, et al. Repeated percutaneous vertebroplasty for refracture of cemented vertebrae. Arch Orthop Trauma Surg 2011;131(7):927–933

[14] Nieuwenhuijse MJ, Putter H, van Erkel AR, Dijkstra PD. New vertebral fractures after percutaneous vertebroplasty for painful osteoporotic vertebral compression fractures: a clustered analysis and the relevance of intradiskal cement leakage. Radiology 2013;266(3):862–870

[15] Jacobson RE, Palea O, Granville M. Progression of vertebral compression fractures after previous vertebral augmentation: technical reasons for recurrent fractures in a previously treated vertebra. Cureus 2017;9(10):e1776

[16] Lin CC, Chen IH, Yen PS, et al. Repeat percutaneous vertebroplasty at cemented vertebra with fluid sign and recurrent pain. Interv Neuroradiol 2008;14(Suppl 2):85–90

[17] Pollintine P, Dolan P, Tobias JH, Adams MA. Intervertebral disc degeneration can lead to "stress-shielding" of the anterior vertebral body: a cause of osteoporotic vertebral fracture? Spine 2004;29(7):774–782

[18] Lehman VT, Wood CP, Hunt CH, et al. Facet joint signal change on MRI at levels of acute/subacute lumbar compression fractures. AJNR Am J Neuroradiol 2013;34(7):1468–1473

[19] Wilson DJ, Owen S, Corkill RA. Facet joint injections as a means of reducing the need for vertebroplasty in insufficiency fractures of the spine. Eur Radiol 2011;21(8):1772–1778

[20] Im TS, Lee JW, Lee E, Kang Y, Ahn JM, Kang HS. Effects of facet joint injection reducing the need for percutaneous vertebroplasty in vertebral compression fractures. Cardiovasc Intervent Radiol 2016;39(5):740–745

[21] Solberg J, Copenhaver D, Fishman SM. Medial branch nerve block and ablation as a novel approach to pain related to vertebral compression fracture. Curr Opin Anaesthesiol 2016;29(5):596–599

[22] Wang B, Guo H, Yuan L, Huang D, Zhang H, Hao D. A prospective randomized controlled study comparing the pain relief in patients with osteoporotic vertebral compression fractures with the use of vertebroplasty or facet blocking. Eur Spine J 2016;25(11):3486–3494

[23] Kamalian S, Bordia R, Ortiz AO. Post-vertebral augmentation back pain: evaluation and management. AJNR Am J Neuroradiol 2012;33(2):370–375

[24] Park KD, Jee H, Nam HS, et al. Effect of medial branch block in chronic facet joint pain for osteoporotic compression fracture: one year retrospective study. Ann Rehabil Med 2013;37(2):191–201

[25] Georgy BA. Interventional techniques in managing persistent pain after vertebral augmentation procedures: a retrospective evaluation. Pain Physician 2007;10(5):673–676

[26] Hatgis J, Granville M, Jacobson RE. Evaluation and interventional management of pain after vertebral augmentation procedures. Cureus 2017;9(2):e1061

[27] Dubousset J. Three-dimensional analysis of scoliotic deformity. In: Weinstein S, ed. Pediatric Spine: Principles and Practice. New York, NY: Raven Press; 1994:479–483

[28] Zhang YL, Shi LT, Tang PF, Sun ZJ, Wang YH. Correlation analysis of osteoporotic vertebral compression fractures and spinal sagittal imbalance. Orthopade 2017;46(3):249–255

[29] Glassman SD, Bridwell K, Dimar JR, Horton W, Berven S, Schwab F. The impact of positive sagittal balance in adult spinal deformity. Spine 2005;30(18):2024–2029

[30] Wu SS, Lachmann E, Nagler W. Current medical, rehabilitation, and surgical management of vertebral compression fractures. J Womens Health (Larchmt) 2003;12(1):17–26

[31] Baek SW, Kim C, Chang H. The relationship between the spinopelvic balance and the incidence of adjacent vertebral fractures following percutaneous vertebroplasty. Osteoporos Int 2015;26(5):1507–1513

[32] Kanayama M, Oha F, Iwata A, Hashimoto T. Does balloon kyphoplasty improve the global spinal alignment in osteoporotic vertebral fracture? Int Orthop 2015;39(6):1137–1143

[33] Pradhan BB, Bae HW, Kropf MA, Patel VV, Delamarter RB. Kyphoplasty reduction of osteoporotic vertebral compression fractures: correction of local kyphosis versus overall sagittal alignment. Spine 2006;31(4):435–441

[34] Yokoyama K, Kawanishi M, Yamada M, et al. Postoperative change in sagittal balance after Kyphoplasty for the treatment of osteoporotic vertebral compression fracture. Eur Spine J 2015;24(4):744–749

25 Postural Fatigue Syndrome

Olivier Clerk-Lamalice

Summary

Postural fatigue syndrome (PFS) is one of the most common causes of postvertebral augmentation pain and is typically located in the thoracic spine and is seen more often in women. This pain is typically less severe than pain seen in patients with vertebral compression fractures (VCFs) and is worse when the patient is upright and better when they are recumbent or lying down. It is important to recognize PFS as a cause of pain to avoid misdiagnosing this persistent pain as some other type of pathology. It probably results from biomechanical alterations in spine after a VCF that places additional stress and strain on the posterior elements. The treatment for PFS is medial branch blocks or facet joint injections followed by radiofrequency rhizotomy if the pain relief from the initial injections meets or exceeds 80% but does not last beyond 12 weeks. A less invasive approach can also be taken as the pain from PFS usually goes away or decreases substantially in six to ten months after the vertebral augmentation. Physical therapy and bracing can be used as an alternative treatments to aid in the patient's recovery.

Keywords: postural fatigue syndrome, thoracic spine, posterior elements, pain, medial branch blocks, trauma, multiple myeloma, malignancy, kyphoplasty

25.1 Introduction

PFS is defined as persistent back pain after vertebral augmentation or other posture altering spine injury that worsens with upright posture and increased time standing and is relieved when sitting or lying recumbent. This syndrome most commonly affects the mid-thoracic and thoracolumbar junction regions. Being able to recognize this syndrome is extremely important for postprocedural patient care. Patients will present on follow-up with residual back pain that is not as severe as before the vertebral augmentation procedure but still bothersome to the patient. The characteristics of the pain are also different from VCF pain that worsens with patient movement and transition from one position to another. A lack of awareness of PFS can lead to misdiagnosing this syndrome and physicians labeling an otherwise well-performed vertebral augmentation as a "failed" intervention. More importantly, PFS was not diagnosed nor mentioned in three controversial randomized controlled trials.[1-3] The lack of assessment of this syndrome was a likely contributor to the absence of statistical superiority of the vertebroplasty arm in comparison to the sham group. Given the precarious statistical balance of the sham and vertebroplasty arms, it is possible that if this syndrome had been taken into consideration in those studies, different outcomes would have been published. This pathology can be easily and affectively treated by medial branch blocks, and most patients will do very well after a single medial branch block treatment. Even without treatment the pain typically decreases substantially within 6 to 10 months following vertebral augmentation.

25.2 Clinical Presentation

Patients with PFS most often present at approximately 2 to 6 weeks after vertebral augmentation with nonradicular back pain in the mid-thoracic and/or thoracolumbar junction region. This pain increases when standing upright and decreases when sitting down and typically increases the longer the patient stands or works with their arms extended out from the body. Most patients will have pain with a VAS intensity score of 3–5/10. Also, this pain is *categorically* different from a fracture pain and usually presents with a severity that is approximately half of what the original fracture pain was. The pain tends to fluctuate according to what position this patient is in but is not transitional pain that worsens during the change to different positions. Although *postural fatigue* pain is less intense than the initial VCF-related pain, the patient often considers it annoying enough to seek medical evaluation. This syndrome seems to occur less frequently with balloon kyphoplasty (or vertebral body implants) and more frequently with vertebroplasty, probably related to better correction of the vertebral body height, kyphotic angle, and realignment of the end plates seen with balloon kyphoplasty and implants. PFS can last up to 6 months before fading gradually with time. Since this is the first known description of this syndrome, the incidence of this pain disorder is not yet known but, according to our estimation, it is seen in approximately 5 to 10% of our vertebral augmentation patients at the time of follow-up.

25.3 Pathophysiology

After a VCF, nucleus pulposus pressure decreases,[4] with higher loads being redistributed toward the neural arch and facets when the patient stands upright. The *fracture mechanical instability* is corrected after adequate polymethyl methacrylate (PMMA) cement is injected. A subanatomic fracture restoration (i.e., incomplete correction of the kyphotic angle and/or vertebral body height restoration and/or end-plate realignment), however, leads to residual functional spinal unit (FSU) instability and persistent increase in stress on the posterior arch and facet joints when the patient stands upright (Chapter 18). This phenomenon is supported by previous studies that suggest that the ability to restore vertebral body height and the kyphotic deformity of the fractured end plate should be the ideal end point to normalized load transmission across the FSU and fractured level.[4,5] In brief, in a patient with a subanatomic VCF restoration, when a patient stands upright the facet loading increases, and when the patient sits or is in flexed position, the load is transferred toward the anterior column resulting in relief for the patient.[6,7] It can take a few months before the patient accommodates to their altered biomechanics and experiences a subsequent decrease in pain.

25.4 Treatment

Treating patients with PFS consist of bracing, physical therapy, or performing medial branch blocks at the VCF-PMMA-treated level in addition to one or two levels above the fracture and one or two levels below the fracture. Typically, the *postural fatigue* pain fades within 6 to 10 months following the vertebral augmentation. Most patients do very well after a single medial branch block; however, in some cases a second medial branch block or even thoracic radiofrequency rhizotomy might be required.

25.5 Key Points

- PFS is defined as persistent pain after vertebral augmentation that worsens with upright posture, working with the arms and hands extended, and is relieved when the patient sits down or lies down.
- This syndrome affects most frequently the mid-thoracic and thoracolumbar junction region.
- The PFS pain is *categorically* different from a fracture pain by being significantly less intense and fluctuates according to what position the patient is in (standing vs. sitting).
- This syndrome is more frequently seen in patients treated with vertebroplasty and less frequently in patients treated with balloon kyphoplasty, vertebral body implants, or other modalities that can optimally restore the vertebral body height and improve the kyphotic angle.
- Typically, the pain fades within 6 to 10 months following vertebral augmentation.
- Treatment of PFS consists of bracing, physical therapy, and performing medial branch blocks or thoracic radiofrequency rhizotomy at the painful levels.

References

[1] Kallmes DF, Comstock BA, Heagerty PJ, et al. A randomized trial of vertebroplasty for osteoporotic spinal fractures. N Engl J Med 2009;361(6):569–579

[2] Buchbinder R, Osborne RH, Ebeling PR, et al. A randomized trial of vertebroplasty for painful osteoporotic vertebral fractures. N Engl J Med 2009;361(6):557–568

[3] Firanescu CE, de Vries J, Lodder P, et al. Vertebroplasty versus sham procedure for painful acute osteoporotic vertebral compression fractures (VERTOS IV): randomised sham controlled clinical trial. BMJ 2018;361:k1551

[4] Tzermiadianos MN, Renner SM, Phillips FM, et al. Altered disc pressure profile after an osteoporotic vertebral fracture is a risk factor for adjacent vertebral body fracture. Eur Spine J 2008;17(11):1522–1530

[5] Renner SM, Tsitsopoulos PP, Dimitriadis AT, et al. Restoration of spinal alignment and disk mechanics following polyetheretherketone wafer kyphoplasty with StaXx FX. AJNR Am J Neuroradiol 2011;32(7):1295–1300

[6] Pollintine P, Przybyla AS, Dolan P, Adams MA. Neural arch load-bearing in old and degenerated spines. J Biomech 2004;37(2):197–204

[7] Pollintine P, Dolan P, Tobias JH, Adams MA. Intervertebral disc degeneration can lead to "stress-shielding" of the anterior vertebral body: a cause of osteoporotic vertebral fracture? Spine 2004;29(7):774–782

26 Physical Therapy after Vertebral Augmentation

Murray Echt, Andrew I. Gitkind, and Allan L. Brook

Summary

Vertebral compression fractures (VCFs) carry with them a known adverse effect on the patient's abilities to carry out their normal activities of daily life. The morbidities associated with VCFs are well known and have been recorded in several different publications. Most of these morbidities result from immobility and prolonged periods of bed rest. The goal of vertebral augmentation and the therapy that follows is pain control and prompt return to more normal physical activity. Treatment of painful VCFs with vertebral augmentation has been shown to reduce morbidity and mortality and an appropriate rehabilitation care plan can improve the patient's strength, posture, and balance and enhance the chances of an optimal treatment outcome. Physical exercise programs have been shown to maintain hip and spine bone mineral density and to reduce the frequency of falls. Certain rehabilitation regimens have been developed to optimize reduce falls, decrease pain from VCFs, and to reduce the chances of getting additional VCFs. These programs use a combination of weight-bearing exercise, extensor muscle strengthening, and balance training to accomplish the desired outcomes. It is important to begin the rehabilitation program as soon as possible after vertebral augmentation and a life-long adherence to an exercise program can, and has been shown to, be beneficial for increasing bone mineral density and for preventing additional VCFs.

Keywords: rehabilitation, morbidity, physical therapy, exercise program, core muscle strengthening, extensor training

26.1 Introduction

VCFs due to osteoporosis are associated with pain, loss of function, impaired quality of life, and increased morbidity and mortality.[1-4] Multiple studies published over the past decades have provided insight into the population-level morbidity associated with VCF in the United States.[5] These include large reviews of the Nationwide Inpatient Sample, reviews of data from the Centers for Medicare and Medicaid Services, and data from the American College of Surgeons National Surgical Quality Improvement Program database.[6-10] These investigations have identified significant rates of deep vein thrombosis (0.7–6.6%), pulmonary embolism (0.4–1.9%), pneumonia (3.1–13.0%), and decubitus ulcers (1.1–4.4%), regardless of treatment type. Most of these complications are in part a result of prolonged periods of bed rest. Thus, the importance of mobilizing the patient is paramount and must not be overlooked.

The goals of management with vertebroplasty and balloon kyphoplasty are pain control, prevention of spinal deformity, and functional restoration. Vertebral augmentation reduces pain without reliance on narcotics alone, allowing for early and increased mobility.[11,12] It has been shown to reduce morbidity and mortality with conservative care.[1,6] Management does not cease here, as the patient still needs to improve strength, correct posture, and enhance balance to increase independence and prevent further progression. This is accomplished through physical therapy and rehabilitation.

26.2 Rehabilitation as Part of Routine Anti-Osteoporosis Care

The protective effects of stronger back muscles on the spine has been highlighted as necessary in a guideline on the management of osteoporosis and postmenopausal women at risk for osteoporosis.[13] Several studies have demonstrated that physical exercise programs maintain spine and hip bone mineral density (BMD) as well as decrease the frequency of falls.[14-16] Recent consensus guidelines recommend that individuals with vertebral osteoporosis should engage in a multicomponent exercise program that includes progressive resistance training, in combination with mobility and balance training, and guidance on safe movements.[15,17,18] High-risk individuals benefit from improved muscle strength in the back, legs, upper arms and core, and enhanced posture, balance, and coordination.[19] Exercises for lower extremity muscles should focus on every major group around each joint. Back strengthening and postural exercises will reduce forward head posture, improve shoulder range of motion and trunk stability, and reduce vertebral fractures over time.[20] Elbow extensor strength also facilitates transfers by moving the body with their arms and is related to reduced risk of nursing home admission after hip fracture.[21]

If an exercise program is to be prescribed for patients with spinal osteoporosis, a cautious approach is recommended. Regular weight-bearing exercise (e.g., walking 30–40 minutes per session, plus back and posture exercises for a few minutes, 3–4 days per week) should be advocated throughout life.[20,22-24] Extension or isometric back and abdominal strengthening exercises seem most appropriate.[25] ▶Fig. 26.1 demonstrates these exercises.

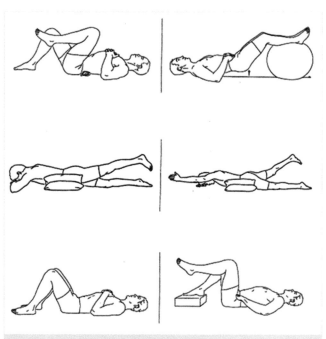

Fig. 26.1 Extension back and core strengthening exercises.

Table 26.1 Potential risks of prescribed exercise and preventive strategies

Potential risk	Preventive strategy
Fall	Focus on balance training and progressive resistance training over walking or aerobic activity Close observation or monitoring during exercise program Optimize lighting and removing excess clutter in environment Review medications that may pose an increased risk for falls
New spinal compression fracture	Avoid forward flexion exercises Avoid excess weight-bearing or twisting movements of the spine (e.g., yoga) Avoid sports/activities involving spinal flexion (e.g., biking, gardening/yard work) Bend knees rather than spine to pick up objects
Pain from osteoarthritis	Use low-impact exercises Brief loading of bones with rest periods
Pain from old compression fracture	Rule out new fracture or progression of deformity if present Brace during exercise Adequate analgesia or local pain-relieving techniques (e.g., massage)

Source: Adapted from Fiatarone 2014.[53]

Not all types of exercise are appropriate for these patients because of the fragility of their vertebrae. Potential risks of prescribed exercise and preventive strategies are summarized in ▶ Table 26.1. Exercises that place flexion forces on the vertebrae tend to cause an increased number of vertebral fractures in these patients. Excess weight and side bending exercises similarly need to be avoided. Yoga exercises have become a concern due to the extreme spinal flexions performed, including several patients in whom VCFs developed as a direct result of participating in this activity.[26] Similarly, rowing, lifting weights with a flexed spine, bowling, sit-ups, house and yard work must also be avoided due to increased risk of vertebral wedge fractures.[17,18] Additionally, high-impact activities and exercises that require rapid and/or loaded twisting, and explosive or abrupt actions, such as golf and racquet sports, are contraindicated for high-risk individuals.

Prolonged aerobic training, such as swimming and cycling, is beneficial to cardiovascular health but does not provide a stimulus to bone growth. Regular walking has also been shown in two meta-analyses as a single intervention having minimal or no effect on BMD in the lumbar spine.[27,28] Trials have also found that prescription of fast or brisk walking programs may actually increase the rate of falls.[29] The inclusion of walking training may not be a crucial feature of program design and therefore recommend that walking training be included in a program as long as it is not at the expense of balance training.[30] The addition of a weighted vest would seem to add a missing component to walking as an intervention; however, a study did not find significant improvement in strength, physical function, bone turn-over, or health-related quality of life.[31] Thus, despite the benefits of aerobic fitness, walking is insufficient to optimize bone health, has little or no effect on balance, and may increase risk of falls.

Studies on early postmenopausal women have shown that strength training leads to small yet significant changes in BMD. A meta-analysis of 16 trials including 699 subjects showed a 2% improvement in lumbar spine BMD in the group that exercised compared with the group that did not.[14] Effects of exercise on BMD are modest, but a meta-analysis estimated that exercise reduces the 20-year risk of osteoporotic fracture in the lumbar spine by 10%.[15] One study of the effect of strengthening exercises for back extensor muscles in healthy postmenopausal women demonstrated a significant increase in back extensor muscle strength and improvement of posture with reduction in kyphosis without association with BMD.[32] Others depicted improvement in muscle strength and BMD of the lumbar spine in estrogen-deficient women.[18,33]

Subject compliance with prescribed exercise interventions presents a challenge. In 2- to 3-year controlled, randomized studies, the dropout rate was 34 to 41% in the exercise groups.[29,34] Subjects who are not self-motivated may not continue with prescribed exercise programs. Sinaki et al[20] looked at the long-term protective effect of stronger back muscles on the spine in 50 healthy white postmenopausal women, aged 58 to 75 years, 8 years after they had completed a 2-year randomized, controlled trial. In the trial, 27 subjects had performed progressive, resistive back-strengthening exercises for 2 years and 23 had served as controls. BMD, spine radiographs, back extensor strength, biochemical marker values, and level of physical activity were obtained for all subjects at baseline, at 2 years, and at 10 years. The difference in BMD, which was not significant between the two groups at baseline and 2-year follow-up, was significant at the 10-year follow-up. They also found that the relative risk for compression fracture was 2.7 times greater in the control group than in the back-exercise group at 10 years. This emphasizes the importance of life-long adherence to an exercise program.

26.3 Rehabilitation after Osteoporotic Vertebral Compression Fractures

The consensus seems to be that an exercise regimen is most beneficial if osteoporosis has been caused by a lack of physical activity.[35] The concurrent decline in bone and muscle mass with aging is compounded with inactivity after a VCF.[36] Likewise, there are varying degrees of fat infiltration and paraspinal muscle atrophy in other degenerative lumbar diseases.[37-40] Thus, exercise is an integral part of both nonsurgical and postinterventional treatments for osteoporotic VCFs.

The rehabilitation process following a VCF is sequential from the acute to the subacute phase followed by long-term care.[41] During the acute stage, evidence shows that the patient should be mobilized out of bed as soon as possible.[42,43] The clinician may begin with educating the patient on the correct positions to maintain in bed. Patients can begin doing exercises of the limbs that don't require any mobilization to avoid rigidity and to reduce the muscular atrophy. Next, focus on gradually advancing to sitting on the edge of the bed, transferring, and ultimately different degrees of weight-bearing either in a chair or standing with or without aid of a walker. Further advancement is done through ambulation with either one- or two-person assistance or with different assistive devices. This stage is where the use of a brace may be beneficial. During the 2 months after the acute vertebral fracture, exercises should avoid intensive muscular strengthening and instead focus on relaxing exercises, maintaining mobility of the major joints, and breathing exercises.

More intensive rehabilitation can start generally during 8 to 12 weeks from the acute event depending on patient's level of pain and their imaging findings. The rehabilitation program includes back-extensor muscle exercises, which decrease the kyphotic posture that can predispose to back pain and to a higher risk of falls with subsequent fractures,[44] and proprioceptive training to improve patient balance.[45] The re-conditioning phase starts with removal of the vertebral brace, resumption of normal activities, and with the establishment of life-long regular weight-bearing exercise.[46]

26.4 Rehabilitation as Part of Postinterventional Care

Rehabilitation after vertebral augmentation for compression fractures should be employed to improve the patient's strength and to reduce their pain, as well as to establish an optimized routine care habit. Data shows that 41 to 67% of new vertebral fractures occur at level adjacent to the augmented vertebra.[47-50] Subsequent VCFs in patients affected by osteoporosis may not be a complication of the procedure itself but rather is part of the natural history. Physical therapy not only aids in patient recovery from the vertebral fracture, but also helps in deterring the long-term progression of the disease.

In a retrospective study that looked specifically at rehabilitation following vertebroplasty, a reduced incidence of vertebral refracture rate was demonstrated.[51] Analysis of the refracture data showed that 75% of patients in the vertebroplasty group had a refracture within 12 months compared with 35% of patients in the vertebroplasty plus rehabilitation program. The median time before refracture also differed significantly between vertebroplasty only and vertebroplasty plus rehab groups with time to refracture of 4.5 months and 20.4 months, respectively.

Another study involved a single center that performed a prospective randomized control trial looking at the clinical benefit of a 2-year systematic exercise program following vertebroplasty.[52] Systematic back muscle exercises resulted in a significant advantage in both the Oswestry Disability Index (ODI) as well as the visual analogue scale (VAS). The first significant difference was discovered 6 months postoperatively using the ODI. From then on, the clinical outcomes between the two groups were observed to gradually separate with the patients on the exercise program doing progressively better. There were increasingly significant differences of both VAS and ODI at 1 and 2-year follow-ups. These findings suggested that short-term clinical outcomes are not only maintained but enhanced in the long-term by adherence to a supplementary physical therapy intervention. By adopting systematic back muscle exercise, patients enjoyed a more favorable daily life and tended to have fewer problems while sitting and walking and had less back pain. Although it is time consuming, a systematic back muscle exercise program should be recognized as an important therapy for patients after vertebral augmentation.

26.5 Conclusion

Physical therapy and rehabilitation are indispensable to patients as part of routine anti-osteoporosis care, following a VCF, as well as postvertebral augmentation. Guidelines agree that regular weight-bearing and back-extensor exercises are optimal to increase strength and improve posture, and balance training is important to reduce falls. A cautious approach is required in high-risk individuals, and certain exercises such as flexion against resistance should be avoided. Walking programs and aerobic activities do not provide the same benefit as weight-bearing workouts and may increase the risk of falls especially in otherwise sedentary patients. Mobilization is key to prevent the morbidity and mortality associated with prolonged bed rest, and improved mobility is commonly the scenario for any patient after undergoing vertebral augmentation for a painful VCF. Physical therapy programs do not end with hospital discharge or with the completion of inpatient rehabilitation as benefits from regular exercise appear to increase over time and should be considered a life-long prescription.

References

[1] Edidin AA, Ong KL, Lau E, Kurtz SM. Morbidity and mortality after vertebral fractures: comparison of vertebral augmentation and nonoperative management in the medicare population. Spine 2015;40(15):1228–1241

[2] Edidin AA, Ong KL, Lau E, Kurtz SM. Life expectancy following diagnosis of a vertebral compression fracture. Osteoporos Int 2013;24(2):451–458

[3] Demers-Lavelle E, Cheney R, Lavelle W. Mortality prediction in a vertebral compression fracture population: the ASA physical status score versus the Charlson Comorbidity Index. Int J Spine Surg 2015;Cci:1–8

[4] Schlaich C, Minne HW, Bruckner T, et al. Reduced pulmonary function in patients with spinal osteoporotic fractures. Osteoporos Int 1998;8(3):261–267

[5] Goldstein CL, Chutkan NB, Choma TJ, Orr RD. Management of the elderly with vertebral compression fractures. Neurosurgery 2015;77(4, Suppl 4): S33–S45

[6] Chen AT, Cohen DB, Skolasky RL. Impact of nonoperative treatment, vertebroplasty, and kyphoplasty on survival and morbidity after vertebral compression fracture in the medicare population. J Bone Joint Surg Am 2013;95(19): 1729–1736

[7] McCullough BJ, Comstock BA, Deyo RA, Kreuter W, Jarvik JG. Major medical outcomes with spinal augmentation vs conservative therapy. JAMA Intern Med 2013;173(16):1514–1521

[8] Toy JO, Basques BA, Grauer JN. Morbidity, mortality, and readmission after vertebral augmentation: analysis of 850 patients from the American College of Surgeons National Surgical Quality Improvement Program database. Spine 2014;39(23):1943–1949

[9] Goz V, Errico TJ, Weinreb JH, et al. Vertebroplasty and kyphoplasty: national outcomes and trends in utilization from 2005 through 2010. Spine J 2015;15(5):959–965

[10] Zampini JM, White AP, McGuire KJ. Comparison of 5766 vertebral compression fractures treated with or without kyphoplasty. Clin Orthop Relat Res 2010;468(7):1773–1780

[11] Ledlie JT, Renfro M. Balloon kyphoplasty: one-year outcomes in vertebral body height restoration, chronic pain, and activity levels. J Neurosurg 2003;98(1, Suppl):36–42

[12] Klazen CAH, Lohle PNM, de Vries J, et al. Vertebroplasty versus conservative treatment in acute osteoporotic vertebral compression fractures (Vertos II): an open-label randomised trial. Lancet 2010;376(9746):1085–1092

[13] Camacho PM, Petak SM, Binkley N, et al. American Association of Clinical Endocrinologists and American College of Endocrinology Clinical Practice Guidelines for the diagnosis and treatment of postmenopausal osteoporosis—2016. Endocr Pract 2016;22(Suppl 4):1–42

[14] Kelley GA, Kelley KS, Tran ZV. Exercise and lumbar spine bone mineral density in postmenopausal women: a meta-analysis of individual patient data. J Gerontol A Biol Sci Med Sci 2002;57(9):M599–M604

[15] Kelley GA, Kelley KS. Efficacy of resistance exercise on lumbar spine and femoral neck bone mineral density in premenopausal women: a meta-analysis of individual patient data. J Womens Health (Larchmt) 2004;13(3):293–300

[16] Varahra A, Rodrigues IB, MacDermid JC, Bryant D, Birmingham T. Exercise to improve functional outcomes in persons with osteoporosis: a systematic review and meta-analysis. Osteoporos Int 2018;29(2):265–286

[17] Beck BR, Daly RM, Singh MAF, Taaffe DR. Exercise and Sports Science Australia (ESSA) position statement on exercise prescription for the prevention and management of osteoporosis. J Sci Med Sport 2017;20(5):438–445

[18] Nikander R, Sievänen H, Heinonen A, Daly RM, Uusi-Rasi K, Kannus P. Targeted exercise against osteoporosis: a systematic review and meta-analysis for optimising bone strength throughout life. BMC Med 2010;8(1):47

[19] de Kam D, Smulders E, Weerdesteyn V, Smits-Engelsman BCM. Exercise interventions to reduce fall-related fractures and their risk factors in individuals with low bone density: a systematic review of randomized controlled trials. Osteoporos Int 2009;20(12):2111–2125

[20] Sinaki M, Itoi E, Wahner HW, et al. Stronger back muscles reduce the incidence of vertebral fractures: a prospective 10 year follow-up of postmenopausal women. Bone 2002;30(6):836–841

[21] Singh NA, Quine S, Clemson LM, et al. Effects of high-intensity progressive resistance training and targeted multidisciplinary treatment of frailty on mortality and nursing home admissions after hip fracture: a randomized controlled trial. J Am Med Dir Assoc 2012;13(1):24–30

[22] Sinaki M, Wahner HW, Offord KP, Hodgson SF. Efficacy of nonloading exercises in prevention of vertebral bone loss in postmenopausal women: a controlled trial. Mayo Clin Proc 1989;64(7):762–769

[23] Sinaki M. Critical appraisal of physical rehabilitation measures after osteoporotic vertebral fracture. Osteoporos Int 2003;14(9):773–779

[24] Sinaki M. Musculoskeletal challenges of osteoporosis. Aging (Milano) 1998;10(3):249–262

[25] Sinaki M, Mikkelsen BA. Postmenopausal spinal osteoporosis: flexion versus extension exercises. Arch Phys Med Rehabil 1984;65(10):593–596

[26] Sinaki M. Yoga spinal flexion positions and vertebral compression fracture in osteopenia or osteoporosis of spine: case series. Pain Pract 2013;13(1):68–75

[27] Ma D, Wu L, He Z. Effects of walking on the preservation of bone mineral density in perimenopausal and postmenopausal women: a systematic review and meta-analysis. Menopause 2013;20(11):1216–1226

[28] Martyn-St James M, Carroll S. Meta-analysis of walking for preservation of bone mineral density in postmenopausal women. Bone 2008;43(3):521–531

[29] Ebrahim S, Thompson PW, Baskaran V, Evans K. Randomized placebo-controlled trial of brisk walking in the prevention of postmenopausal osteoporosis. Age Ageing 1997;26(4):253–260

[30] Sherrington C, Tiedemann A, Fairhall N, Close JCT, Lord SR. Exercise to prevent falls in older adults: an updated meta-analysis and best practice recommendations. N S W Public Health Bull 2011;22(3–4):78–83

[31] Greendale GA, Salem GJ, Young JT, et al. A randomized trial of weighted vest use in ambulatory older adults: strength, performance, and quality of life outcomes. J Am Geriatr Soc 2000;48(3):305–311

[32] Mika A, Unnithan VB, Mika P. Differences in thoracic kyphosis and in back muscle strength in women with bone loss due to osteoporosis. Spine 2005;30(2):241–246

[33] Nelson ME, Fiatarone MA, Morganti CM, Trice I, Greenberg RA, Evans WJ. Effects of high-intensity strength training on multiple risk factors for osteoporotic fractures: a randomized controlled trial. JAMA 1994;272(24):1909–1914

[34] Sinaki M, Wahner HW, Bergstralh EJ, et al. Three-year controlled, randomized trial of the effect of dose-specified loading and strengthening exercises on bone mineral density of spine and femur in nonathletic, physically active women. Bone 1996;19(3):233–244

[35] Giangregorio LM, McGill S, Wark JD, et al. Too fit to fracture: outcomes of a Delphi consensus process on physical activity and exercise recommendations for adults with osteoporosis with or without vertebral fractures. Osteoporos Int 2015;26(3):891–910

[36] Li Q, Sun J, Cui X, Jiang Z, Li T. Analysis of correlation between degeneration of lower lumbar paraspinal muscles and spinopelvic alignment in patients with osteoporotic vertebral compression fracture. J Back Musculoskeletal Rehabil 2017;30(6):1209–1214

[37] Ranson CA, Burnett AF, Kerslake R, Batt ME, O'Sullivan PB. An investigation into the use of MR imaging to determine the functional cross sectional area of lumbar paraspinal muscles. Eur Spine J 2006;15(6):764–773

[38] Mengiardi B, Schmid MR, Boos N, et al. Fat content of lumbar paraspinal muscles in patients with chronic low back pain and in asymptomatic volunteers: quantification with MR spectroscopy. Radiology 2006;240(3):786–792

[39] Lee JC, Cha J-G, Kim Y, Kim Y-I, Shin B-J. Quantitative analysis of back muscle degeneration in the patients with the degenerative lumbar flat back using a digital image analysis: comparison with the normal controls. Spine 2008;33(3):318–325

[40] Hyun S-J, Bae C-W, Lee S-H, Rhim S-C. Fatty degeneration of paraspinal muscle in patients with the degenerative lumbar kyphosis. J Spinal Disord Tech 2013;1

[41] Pratelli E, Cinotti I, Pasquetti P. Rehabilitation in osteoporotic vertebral fractures. Clin Cases Miner Bone Metab 2010;7(1):45–47

[42] Rapado A. General management of vertebral fractures. Bone 1996;18(3, Suppl):191S–196S

[43] Bonner FJ Jr, Sinaki M, Grabois M, et al. Health professional's guide to rehabilitation of the patient with osteoporosis. Osteoporos Int 2003;14(0, Suppl 2):S1–S22

[44] Itoi E, Sinaki M. Effect of back-strengthening exercise on posture in healthy women 49 to 65 years of age. Mayo Clin Proc 1994;69(11):1054–1059

[45] Sinaki M, Lynn SG. Reducing the risk of falls through proprioceptive dynamic posture training in osteoporotic women with kyphotic posturing: a randomized pilot study. Am J Phys Med Rehabil 2002;81(4):241–246

[46] Malmros B, Mortensen L, Jensen MB, Charles P. Positive effects of physiotherapy on chronic pain and performance in osteoporosis. Osteoporos Int 1998;8(3):215–221

[47] Sun G, Tang H, Li M, Liu X, Jin P, Li L. Analysis of risk factors of subsequent fractures after vertebroplasty. Eur Spine J 2014;23(6):1339–1345

[48] Trout AT, Kallmes DF, Kaufmann TJ. New fractures after vertebroplasty: adjacent fractures occur significantly sooner. AJNR Am J Neuroradiol 2006;27(1):217–223

[49] Hey HW, Tan JH, Tan CS, Tan HM, Lau PH, Hee HT. Subsequent vertebral fractures post cement augmentation of the thoracolumbar spine: does it correlate with level-specific bone mineral density scores? Spine 2015;40(24):1903–1909

[50] Lindsay R, Cooper C, Hanley DA, Barton I, Broy SB, Flowers K. Risk of new vertebral fracture. 2017;285(3):1–4

[51] Huntoon EA, Schmidt CK, Sinaki M. Significantly fewer refractures after vertebroplasty in patients who engage in back-extensor-strengthening exercises. Mayo Clin Proc 2008;83(1):54–57

[52] Chen B-L, Zhong Y, Huang Y-L, et al. Systematic back muscle exercise after percutaneous vertebroplasty for spinal osteoporotic compression fracture patients: a randomized controlled trial. Clin Rehabil 2012;26(6):483–492

[53] Fiatarone Singh MA. Exercise and bone health. In: Holick MF, Neeves JW, eds. Nutrition and Bone Health. 2nd ed. New York: Humana Press; 2014

27 Sham vs. Vertebral Augmentation

Laxmaiah Manchikanti and Joshua A. Hirsch

Summary

This chapter discusses the role of medical management, placebo, sham, or active control in vertebral augmentation trials and the role of real-world evidence with new perspectives and conceptualization. Randomized controlled trials (RCTs) continue to be in the forefront of decision-making process for therapeutic interventions. At the same time, negative RCTs have appeared questioning the effectiveness of vertebral augmentation. The vast majority of the extensive literature on vertebral augmentation procedures including RCTs, systematic reviews, guidelines, and development of appropriateness criteria have yielded support for the procedure but some negative RCTs have produced some discordant conclusions.

Among all the control modalities, various effects of sham controls have been described often with negative connotations. Two trials published in the *New England Journal of Medicine* showing lack of efficacy of augmentation procedures provided negative results, with resultant lack of access to augmentation procedures for many patients who meet the criteria, indications, and medical necessity. Only one true placebo control (VAPOUR) study has yielded appropriate results with significantly better results in treatment group with vertebroplasty. In addition, multiple RCTs and systematic reviews have provided basis for effectiveness of vertebral augmentation in managing acute or subacute osteoporotic fractures.

Thus, the emerging literature on placebo, nocebo, sham intervention, and active intervention with multiple conceptual factors including confluence of interest and intellectual bias provide overwhelming evidence of irregularities in interpretation of review of scientific literature. At the same time, this chapter also provides a perspective on utilization of therapeutic placebo in vertebral compression fractures along with robust development of real-world evidence.

Keywords: placebo, nocebo, sham, vertebral augmentation, randomized control trial, control group, evidence synthesis

27.1 Introduction

"It is simply no longer possible to believe much of the clinical research that is published, or to rely on the judgment of trusted physicians or authoritative medical guidelines. I take no pleasure in this conclusion, which I reached slowly and reluctantly over my two decades as an editor of The New England Journal of Medicine."

— *Marcia Angell,*
Former editor-in-chief of the New England Journal of Medicine

Numerous changes in medical, political, and economic spheres in health care, clinical evaluation of therapies, and the importance of randomized controlled trials (RCTs) in evidence synthesis continue to be in forefront of decision-making process for therapeutic interventions. However, over the last 30 years, negative RCTs have become the rule rather than exception, specifically in managing spinal pain with interventional techniques including vertebral augmentation procedures.[1,2]

Several attempts are made to overcome the present problem in evidence synthesis, based on various factors including understanding of the conduct of RCTs based on controlled design (active control vs. placebo control), outcomes assessments and implications of placebo and nocebo effects.[1] Beyond these factors, evidence synthesis has been done with discordant opinions due to intellectual bias, confluence of interest, and peer review bias, which extends beyond honest differences of professional opinions.[1-5] At the center of the controversy is a multitude of interventional techniques and surgical procedures including vertebral augmentation. Extensive literature on vertebral augmentation procedures in managing vertebral compression fractures (VCFs) has yielded not only discordant opinions,[6-19] but often emotional debate primarily initiated by two RCTs published in *New England Journal of Medicine* in 2009.[18,19] Despite numerous publications exceeding 3,000 manuscripts on vertebral augmentation, with multiple controlled trials[6-33] debate continues on whether it is effective and superior to sham intervention.[17,34,35] All of this has produced a significant decline in the utilization of vertebral augmentation procedures.[36] The present evidence indicates increased morbidity in patients treated with nonsurgical management (NSM) compared to those treated with vertebral augmentation.[8-37,38] In fact, a study by Ong et al[8] including more than 2 million patients showed 24% higher mortality risk for NSM compared to balloon kyphoplasty at 10 years and a 55% higher mortality rate at 1 year. In another study of over one million patients, with 4 years of follow-up,[9] the nonoperated patients also had a 55% higher propensity-adjusted mortality risk than balloon kyphoplasty patients and a 25% higher mortality risk than vertebroplasty patients. Similar results were also shown by McCullough et al, although McCullough attributed the longer term perceived benefits to artifact rather than actual benefit despite three of the four time points showing a significant mortality reduction.[10,37,38]

Even then, patients in need of vertebral augmentation procedures are facing reduced access based on RCTs and sham response. Consequently, in this chapter, we will discuss the role of placebo control or sham in vertebral augmentation trials and the role of real-world evidence with new perspectives and conceptualization.

27.2 Current Concepts of Controls in Trials

In the study of interventional or surgical trials, various types of controls are utilized, ranging from no treatment group, placebo control, to sham interventions. In RCTs for surgical or other interventions, any of the above controls may be utilized, but in most RCTs, treatments are typically tested by comparing the efficacy in an active treatment arm versus the efficacy in a placebo arm. The failure to detect significant differences between active treatments and placebos is one of the main sources of uncertainty in the RCTs, especially as "negative" RCTs continue to explode across spinal therapeutics. In fact, the failure rates of the active treatments were one of the highest in musculo-skeletal diseases.[2] Placebo response is most commonly provided explanation leading to a smaller difference between the effect of the intervention and placebo. The placebo-nocebo phenomenon is the subject of increasing debate, with extensive research often stoking the controversy.[39] A multitude of contextual factors of placebo and nocebo responses and definitions continue to evolve.[1]

Multiple related issues exist in control trials including placebo and nocebo response, masking, blinding, statistical analysis, and finally interpretation of the results and their application to clinical settings. Placebo control trials of pharmacological treatments are typically conducted in double-blind trials. In these studies, the process of masking the treatment assignment is considered ethically acceptable, provided that shared decision-making was made and the consent process established the nature of the study. However, in circumstances where a surgical or interventional procedure itself constitutes the treatment, a randomized, placebo-control trial raises different issues.[40] In these settings, only the patient is blinded, whereas the clinician can distinguish active from inactive treatment. Thus, the gold standard of clinical research, namely the double-blind randomized placebo-control trial, is challenging to make applicable in interventional settings. Consequently, in surgical and interventional techniques including vertebral augmentation procedures, instead of a placebo, a "sham" procedure is utilized. However, sham procedure itself is not same as placebo and creates a multitude of other issues.

Historically, it was long considered that there is no place for placebo in surgery and often any type of sham intervention was considered unethical.[40,41] However, in 1939 an Italian surgeon, Davide Fieschi tried a new technique for the treatment of patients with angina pectoris. The treatment increased blood flow to the heart, thereby alleviating the symptoms of angina, and this treatment was done by diverting chest arterial supply to the heart by ligating the internal mammary arteries. Approximately 75% of the patients showed improvement and 25% were considered as cured. Twenty years later, in 1959, Cobb et al tested this procedure in the way that one group of patients was treated using the Fieschi technique and the other group of patients just had incisions imitating real procedure. The results were shocking with no difference between the two groups.[42]

Similarly, Moseley et al[43] conducted a study to assess effectiveness of arthroscopy. In this trial, authors divided patients into three groups. In the first group, they peeled off the damaged cartilage, in the second group they washed the knee and that way removed possible causes of inflammation, and in the third group they made a false operation with only incisions. Results showed that there was no difference in the therapeutic success of the groups. A similar study by Kirkley et al[44] was also published in the New England Journal of Medicine by another group of investigators showing lack of additional benefit to arthroscopic debridement over NSM in patients with moderate-to-severe knee osteoarthritis. The results of these two publications in New England Journal of Medicine have resulted in extensive reductions in the utilization of arthroscopic procedures.[45,46]

27.3 Sham vs. Vertebroplasty

27.3.1 Similarities and Differences of Controls

In drug trials, a placebo is administered in a double-blind manner along with the concealment of allocation. Consequently, a placebo response has been defined as "the reduction in symptoms as a result of factors related to patient's perception of the therapeutic intervention."[1] However, with development of multiple modes of placebo intervention, the placebo has also been defined as a "psychobiology phenomenon occurring in the patient's brain after the administration of an inert substance, or of a sham physical treatment such as sham surgery, along with verbal suggestions (or any other cue of clinical benefit)."[1,47,48] Apart from placebo, there is also nocebo activity, which has been discussed extensively and is somewhat controversial.[1,49] The term was coined to denote negative repercussions from a treatment or a placebo, with description of worsening of the symptoms or reduction of the beneficial effect by the administration of an inactive or active treatment.[49] A patient's negative expectations regarding the treatment or an untoward effect from the sham treatment is thought to produce the nocebo response.

Placebo has been administered in interventional trials without appropriate forethought by administering an assumed inert substance, which may not be an inert substance into an active structure, or by administration of active substances into so-called inert structures that may not be inert. In contrast, conservative management groups receive no blinding, sham, or active treatment, thus avoiding the placebo effect that occurs by administration of a substance. On the other hand, placebo effect in these patients may occur due to education or other clinical cues. In sham surgery, typically an incision is made and procedure is carried out until the final intervention. The true placebo nature of such interventions is questionable due to induction of multiple psychological phenomenon.[47,48,50] Consequently, placebo and sham interventions may be similar to active interventions. Thus, placebo or sham interventions in studying efficacy of vertebral augmentation procedures are met with multiple flaws. Before the sham trials of vertebral augmentation there were multiple failures of placebo interventions with other interventional techniques due to injecting sodium chloride solution into the epidural space and facet joints.[3,4] Due to the potential to dilute or wash out inflammatory mediators in these locations, the possibility existed of converting the sham intervention into an active treatment. There is overwhelming evidence of effectiveness of local anesthetics of epidural injections and facet-joint nerve blocks, similar to the effectiveness of local anesthetics with steroids,[3,4,51] but the effectiveness may not be sufficient to show a significant difference when compared to a de facto active treatment but rendered as sham. The same disadvantages are present in a multiplied format when sham intervention is compared to vertebral augmentation.

Even if a placebo is a completely inert substance, its administration is done within a complex psychosocial context and in conjunction with the rituals of the therapeutic act. Sham intervention exceeds the magnitude of the placebo intervention and is provided not only within a complex psychosocial context, but also within physical and therapeutic contexts.

There is significant confusion between the definitions of placebo and placebo effect for clinicians, methodologists, and scientists. A clinician is interested in any improvement that may take place in the group of patients who either take the inert substance or receive a sham treatment, and this improvement may be attributed to a multitude of factors including spontaneous remission, regression toward the mean, and patients' expectation of the benefit. Contrary to the clinician, the scientist is typically more interested in the improvement that derives from the patients' expectations, namely, an active process occurring in the patient's brain. The methodologist is often mostly interested in assessing the difference in the statistical results without consideration of the clinical or scientific aspects.

In vertebral augmentation trials, a sham intervention is provided with injection of local anesthetic into the skin, followed by stab incisions at the level of the vertebral body, and local infiltration of periosteum and the pedicle with periosteal placement of bone needles. The difference between the augmentation group and the sham group is that augmentation group patients undergo needle placement via a transpedicular approach along with placement of the cement, and the sham patients undergo the first part of the procedure but do not have the cement injected.[18,19,33]

27.3.2 Sham vs. Vertebral Augmentation

In vertebral augmentation trials the simplest design is the one in which patients are prospectively followed after the intervention. This is followed by comparison of patients allocated into two groups, one with no treatment and the other group having undergone vertebral augmentation. These patients may have implied placebo effects because of contextual factors. The next category is the management of the patients with nonsurgical treatment that may also induce placebo effects. The third treatment group is patients receiving a placebo treatment with local infiltration of the skin with local anesthetic followed by a skin incision. This technique will induce both placebo and, to a lesser extent, nocebo effects. In contrast, sham intervention as defined originally by the NEJM trials is the procedure that is much more involved and includes the entire procedure with the exception of the placement of the cement. The rationale for this seeming unusual approach was originally intended to isolate the beneficial effect of PMMA.

27.4 Evidence Based on the Control and the Conduct of the Study

A systematic review performed by Hulme et al[6] in 2006 included a total of 69 clinical studies of which 25 were prospective. Overall, the results showed pain relief in a large proportion of patients in 87% with vertebroplasty and 92% with kyphoplasty.

In contrast, the evidence based on individual RCTs with sham controls including the 2009 NEJM articles as well as the 2018 VERTOS IV study[18,19,33] showed no significant difference between sham control and vertebroplasty. Apart from sham control being not a placebo treatment, it is very similar to an active control treatment. In fact, facet-joint injections as control group have shown significant effectiveness in decreasing patient's pain after osteoporotic VCFs at 1 month and 1 year after fracture in patients with severe pain due to vertebral fracture.[23] An author of the INVEST trial, Dr. David Wilson, published results in the *European Journal of Radiology* that reported 34% of patients with painful VCFs had immediate pain relief after facet-joint injections, and out of 75 patients included in his trial, 61 had facet injections.[52] There were 29 patients who failed facet injections and 24 of these patients underwent vertebroplasty. This study, along with the randomized control trial by Wang et al, shows the effectiveness of facet-joint injections in controlling the pain from VCFs. Compared to facet-joint injections, the sham intervention seen in the NEJM articles and VERTOS IV exceeds a facet-joint injection with a blockade of periosteum as well as the medial branch of the dorsal ramus. Depending on the volume of anesthetic injected (which was not controlled), the dorsal nerve root ganglion and ventral nerve root can be affected. Additionally, these studies utilizing sham control also have faced significant criticism.[17,35] Chandra et al[17] and Noonan[35] have eloquently described multiple flaws related to the initial two RCTs published in *New England Journal of Medicine*.[18,19] Apart from various issues related to the recruiting techniques, there were other shortcomings such as a low enrollment rate, selection bias, including worker's compensation patients, not having uniform diagnostic criteria for fractures, and not having a requirement for physical exam. There was a significantly higher rate of crossover within 3 months from the control group. Both studies were also supposed to be blinded, but the INVEST trial blinding was disrupted by patients receiving procedural bills following their vertebroplasty treatment.[18] Notably, there was also a trend toward a higher rate of clinically meaningful improvement in pain, with 30% reduction in the vertebroplasty group (64% vs. 48%) ($p = 0.6$). There were also a high proportion of patients with worker's compensation claims. Due to low recruitment, they resorted to a pain level of 3 as the criterion to be included, which is uncharacteristic of patients with painful VCFs. Sample size was very low even though the authors thought it to be enough patients to produce sufficient power to show a short-term treatment advantage. The final statistical analysis just barely showed any statistically significant difference between vertebroplasty and sham. If the same response rate were present for the originally intended 250 patients instead of the 131 patients that were enrolled, the p value would have been 0.01 in favor of vertebroplasty. Also, if a single patient had had a different response favoring vertebroplasty, the p value would have been 0.04, again a statistically significant result favoring vertebroplasty. The study by Buchbinder et al[19] also was met with multiple deficiencies, not the least of which was that the mean amount of cement injected in the vertebroplasty group was 2.8 mL. This amount was analyzed and determined to be an insufficient amount by Boszczyk et al who found that it "strongly indicates that the treatment arm includes patient who were not treated in a reasonably effective manner."[53] The VERTOS IV study provided similar results with similar issues related to the conduct of the study. Even though both groups showed no significant difference, pain scales in vertebroplasty group declined to a mean of 2.72 (2.18 to 3.26) from a baseline of 7.72 (7.21 to 8.24) with difference between baseline and 12 months of 5 (4.31 to 5.70) points which is typical of the pain reduction seen with vertebroplasty and is significant compared to the baseline. The sham intervention that they employed for this study, however, also profoundly reduced the pain levels from 7.9 to 3.17 with a prominent reduction of 4.75; thus, the vertebroplasty and the so-called sham treatments showed no significant difference. This lack of difference was not because the vertebroplasty difference was ineffective but because the sham response was profound with a pain decrease magnitude similar to that of very effective active pain treatments. When the VERTOS IV results are compared with the treatment and sham or NSM arms of other trials, the pain reduction curves clearly align with active

treatments and treatments that reflect the natural course of the VCF (▶Fig. 27.1 and ▶Fig. 27.2).

These differences cannot be explained on pure placebo response and are not seen in conservative management groups, nontreatment groups, or even in interventional placebo groups with local anesthetic infiltration and incision as shown in the VAPOUR study.[24] In fact, the VAPOUR study[24] utilized a placebo design without sham intervention as we have described above. In this trial, placebo procedure included subcutaneous lidocaine but not periosteal numbing. In addition, only a short needle was passed into the skin incision, but not as far as the periosteum. The results of this trial showed 24 or 44% of the patients in the vertebroplasty group and 12 or 21% in the control group had an NRS pain score below 4 out of 10 at 14 days. Authors of this study concluded that vertebroplasty was superior to placebo

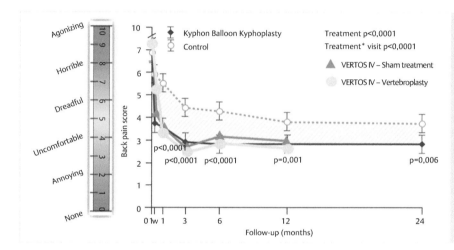

Fig. 27.1 Graph comparing the pain reduction results of the efficacy and safety of balloon kyphoplasty compared with nonsurgical care for vertebral compression fracture (FREE) trial which featured balloon kyphoplasty (*blue line*) and nonsurgical management (*orange dotted line*) as compared to the vertebroplasty vs. sham procedure for painful acute osteoporotic vertebral compression fractures (VERTOS) IV trial with vertebroplasty (*light blue line*) and sham treatment (*red line*). The sham treatment line of VERTOS IV paralleled the vertebroplasty arm of the same trial and had nearly identical pain reduction as the kyphoplasty patients in the FREE trial.[27,33]

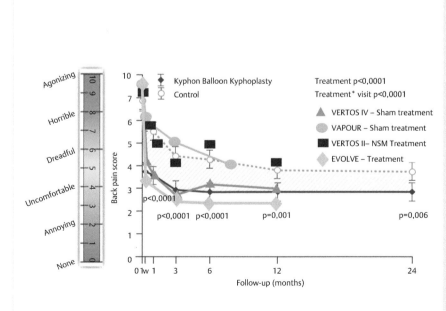

Fig. 27.2 Graph comparing the pain reduction results of the efficacy and safety of balloon kyphoplasty compared with nonsurgical care for vertebral compression fracture (FREE) trial which featured balloon kyphoplasty (*blue line*) and nonsurgical management (*orange dotted line*) as compared to the nonsurgical management arm of the vertebroplasty vs. sham procedure for painful acute osteoporotic vertebral compression fractures (VERTOS) II trial (*black line*) and the sham treatment arms of the VERTOS IV trial (*red line*) and the safety and efficacy of vertebroplasty for acute painful osteoporotic fractures (VAPOUR) trial (*green line*). These are compared with the post-market trial results of the prospective and multicenter evaluation of outcomes for quality of life and activities of daily living for balloon kyphoplasty in the treatment of vertebral compression fractures (EVOLVE) trial (*light blue line*). This graph illustrates that the sham treatment for VERTOS IV most closely resembles the pain reduction results for the FREE and EVOLVE trials and was distinctly different from the sham treatment group in the VAPOUR trial and the nonsurgical management group of the VERTOS II trial.[27,33]

intervention for pain reduction in patients with acute osteoporotic spinal fractures of less than 6 weeks duration. Results of this study at 6 months showed that proportion of patients with NRS pain score less than 4 was 69% in the vertebroplasty group and 47% in the control group. Analgesic use declined from 97% to 58% in vertebroplasty group and from 98% to 76% in the placebo group. The placebo used in the VAPOUR trial was representative of the typical placebo response instead of the active treatment response seen in the so-called sham arm of the VERTOS IV trial.

The next category with less rigorous placebo design is the augmentation compared to conservative treatment. Multiple RCTs were performed comparing augmentation with medical management.[26–32] These studies showed significant improvement with vertebroplasty and vertebral augmentation compared to NSM. Studies comparing kyphoplasty and vertebroplasty also showed similar outcomes.[21,22]

27.5 Conflicting Opinions

In a network meta-analysis of comparison of the efficacy and safety of three treatments for patients with osteoporotic VCFs,[13] 16 RCTs with 2,046 participants were included. The results of this meta-analysis showed that vertebral augmentation procedures were superior to conservative treatment in effectiveness and were safe. A comparative meta-analysis of the literature of percutaneous vertebroplasty and balloon kyphoplasty for the treatment of single-level VCFs[7] included eight RCTs with 845 patients. The results of this meta-analysis showed both procedures to be safe and effective in treating VCFs. Chandra et al[17] reviewed the latest data on effectiveness of vertebral augmentation procedures. They included analysis of multiple RCTs, including the most recent positive trials that followed initial negative trials in 2009 and multiple national claim datasets and recommendations of national organizations and medical societies. They concluded that patients with severe pain who are treated within 6 weeks are good candidates for vertebroplasty and elderly patients hospitalized with a VCF also benefit from the procedure. They also conclude that the recent data from the national datasets show that vertebroplasty results in lower hospital re-admission, sooner discharge, and decreased mortality.

Among multiple systematic reviews of robust data derived from large systematic reviews, a meta-analysis comparing vertebroplasty and kyphoplasty including 2,838 patients across 29 randomized, prospective nonrandomized, and retrospective comparative studies[50] showed equal effectiveness of vertebroplasty and kyphoplasty, along with optimal safety parameters for both.

27.6 Discussion

Discordance of clinical results and recommendations is based on inadequate study design and lack of consideration of what constitutes an active treatment by including a protocol that requires local periosteal infiltration of anesthetic and surgical placement of the needles. As described earlier, clinical trials are only aimed at establishing whether the patients who have the true treatment are better off than those who undergo a sham treatment. Some of the interesting, challenging, and debatable aspects of placebo research are related to the new emerging concepts that placebos are able to activate the same biochemical pathways that are activated by drugs,[54] which represent an interesting paradigm from an evolutionary and a neurobiological perspective. Endogenous systems are activated in the human body via a placebo response by way of positive expectations, therapeutic rituals, and social interactions combined with the physiologic release of endogenous opioids and endocannabinoids.[54] The endogenous opioids result in binding to opioid receptors and inhibition of pain transmission. In addition to the pharmacological effect of the drug, the ritual of its administration can induce activation of the same opioid receptors that involve a descending pain modulating network from the cerebral cortex to the spinal cord. In contrast to these placebos, nocebos provide a negative role that has been demonstrated to be highly prevalent in RCTs.[2] The literature is overwhelming in reinforcing the facts that placebo may provide relief, but rarely cure. Consequently, it has been presumed that therapeutic benefits associated with placebo effects do not alter the pathophysiology of the diseases beyond their symptomatic manifestations, and only address subjective and self-appraised symptomatology. In contrast to these assumptions, however, placebos have been shown to provide powerful innate healing mechanisms.[1] Multiple studies have demonstrated that placebo medication can improve objective measures including pulmonary function,[55,56] white blood cell count,[57] hepatic enzymes,[58] postprandial glucose,[59] carbon dioxide partial pressure (PCO2 levels),[60] and beta-2-adrenergic activity of the heart.[61]

There is also uncertainty of the placebo effect and the nocebo effect, complicating the main assumption underlying most RCTs that the total treatment effect is the sum of the placebo effect, plus the active drug effect. Thus, researchers tend to deduct the active drug effect by subtracting the placebo effect from the total treatment effect. It has been argued, however, that the assumptions of the additivity model of treatment and placebo may not be clinically applicable. Four implicit assumptions of the additivity model are (1) the drug effect and the placebo effect do not interact, (2) the placebo component is identical for both the placebo and the drug arms, (3) the total treatment effect is the sum of the drug effect plus the placebo effect, and (4) the active drug is not influenced by whether or not patients believe they have received the drug. As literature overwhelmingly shows, these assumptions are simply inaccurate. Since this model has been questioned in meta-analyses,[62,63] studies also have demonstrated differences in treatment effect with the "open-hidden approach."[64] In this effect the biochemical action of an active treatment is remarkably influenced by whether or not patients are aware of receiving an effective drug. This induces the nocebo effect that is in contrast to the placebo effect induced by sham treatment; thus, the difference between sham treatment and placebo treatment becomes less significant.

A double-blind procedure has been shown to reduce the bias inherent to active treatment. Due to the requirement of having an informed individual perform the procedure, however, double-blind procedures are not feasible to use in vertebral augmentation for overcoming the placebo response. Due to the increasing number of negative interventional trials, several designs and strategies have been developed to minimize the placebo response when conducting interventional trials. To achieve these goals, it is imperative to understand the differences between drug trials with placebos, sham interventions, and active control trials. Sham interventions often may also produce similar effects as interventions themselves. In fact, the simple placement of a needle described as dry needling has been shown to be effective in managing lumbar spinal stenosis.[65] In this report, 34 patients with lumbar spinal stenosis underwent fluoroscopically guided transforaminal epidural dry needling using a specifically designed flexed round needle. The needle was inserted 8 to 12 cm lateral to the midline at the level of the stenosis and advanced to a position between the anterior side of the facet joint and the pedicle just superior to the exiting nerve root at that level. The needle was advanced medially then back laterally a few millimeters along the anterosuperior portion of the foramen. The procedure was completed when a marked reduction in resistance was felt at the tip of the needle. The procedure was performed bilaterally at the level of the stenosis. The average follow-up time was 12 months and the procedure showed good-to-excellent response on the self-rated improvement scale in 65% of the patients. Effectiveness of dry needling was also reported in several other studies for multiple conditions including back pain.[66–70] Dry needling has also been utilized in managing cervical facet-joint pain and complex regional pain syndrome.[71]

In addition to dry needling, the effectiveness of injecting sodium chloride solution in the epidural space and facet joints has been shown along with the analogous success of injecting dextrose.[3] There are also studies that show equal effectiveness of local anesthetics compared with a combination of anesthetic and steroid when injected into the epidural space or around the nerve roots.[3]

To overcome these disadvantages, the development of real-world evidence is crucial.[72] The real-world evidence is widely used in the development of medical products and in generating evidence. The real-world evidence gathered by way of registries or phase 4 trials can provide information to further therapeutic development, outcomes research, patient care, research on health care systems, quality improvement, safety surveillance, and to help guide additional well-controlled effectiveness studies.[72] Additionally, major aspects of real-world evidence include that it can provide information on how factors such as clinical setting, provider, and health-system characteristics influence treatment effects and outcomes. This real-world evidence essentially removes some of the issues related to placebo effects, blinding, and misunderstandings of placebo controlled trials. Above all, real-world evidence provides clinically relevant data and pragmatic approaches, which is applicable in clinical settings in day-to-day life. Thus, real-world evidence can be viewed as a means of incorporating diverse types of evidence into information on health care, but the disadvantages include the uncertain quality of some large datasets, the use of analytic tools by nonexperts, and a shortage of researchers with adequate methodologic savvy, which may lead to poorly conceived study designs and inadequate experience to generate correct and reliable conclusions. In fact, the Food and Drug Administration (FDA) is laying groundwork that will play a major role in determining the future of real-world evidence. Further, real-world evidence has expanded dramatically in just a few years even though it has not yet established a clear role in the complex paradigm of evidence synthesis.

Also, some of the same factors that negatively influence some RCTs to produce falsely negative results can be present in real-world data including conflicts of interest and lack of understanding of the trial design. Although RCTs continue to be important especially in the development of clinical guidelines, real-world data such as claims databases and registries have improved dramatically. Real-world study designs continue to improve and produce more powerful analytic tools that can produce meaningful results. The 21st Century Cures Act, which was passed in 2016, has required the FDA to establish a program to evaluate the potential use of real-world evidence in approving new indications for existing drugs, as well as to help support postapproval safety and efficacy studies.[73] The Prescription Drug User Fee Act (PDUFA) has similar provisions and requires the FDA to engage the stakeholders in the process. These efforts have been added because of the need for credible information upon which to base regulatory decisions and a significant potential for real-world evidence to provide greater insight into the therapeutic benefit of certain medications and medical technologies.[74]

In addition to the development of a more optimized regulatory process, it is also crucial to understand the therapeutic role of placebo sham treatments that can actually provide durable therapeutic benefits while masquerading as a placebo as was seen with the infiltration of periosteal anesthetic in some of the vertebroplasty versus sham trials that had an outsized response to the sham treatment.

27.7 Conclusion

The emerging literature on placebos, nocebos, and sham interventions, along with demonstrations of intellectual bias, provides not only overwhelming evidence of irregularities in the interpretation of review of scientific literature, but also an updated clear perspective on utilization of therapeutic placebo in studies on the treatment of VCFs. Along with robust development of real-world evidence, the future of information synthesis depends on involvement of clinicians, robustness of real-world evidence, and application of appropriate placebos instead of therapeutic sham procedures.

References

[1] Manchikanti L, Boswell MV, Kaye AD, Helm Ii S, Hirsch JA. Therapeutic role of placebo: evolution of a new paradigm in understanding research and clinical practice. Pain Physician 2017;20(5):363–386

[2] Carlino E, Vase L. Can knowledge of placebo and nocebo mechanisms help improve randomized clinical trials? Int Rev Neurobiol 2018;138:329–357

[3] Manchikanti L, Knezevic NN, Boswell MV, Kaye AD, Hirsch JA. Epidural injections for lumbar radiculopathy and spinal stenosis: a comparative systematic review and meta-analysis. Pain Physician 2016;19(3):E365–E410

[4] Boswell MV, Manchikanti L. Appropriate design and methodologic quality assessment, clinically relevant outcomes are essential to determine the role of epidural corticosteroid injections. Commentary RE: Chou R, Hashimoto R, Friedly J, Fu R, Bougatsos C, Dana T, Sullivan SD, Jarvik J. Epidural corticosteroid injections for radiculopathy and spinal stenosis: a systematic review and meta-analysis. Ann Intern Med 2015;163:373–381. Evid Based Med 2016;21:89

[5] Manchikanti L, Kaye AD, Boswell MV, Hirsch JA. Medical journal peer review: process and bias. Pain Physician 2015;18(1):E1–E14

[6] Hulme PA, Krebs J, Ferguson SJ, Berlemann U. Vertebroplasty and kyphoplasty: a systematic review of 69 clinical studies. Spine 2006;31(17):1983–2001

[7] Wang H, Sribastav SS, Ye F, et al. Comparison of percutaneous vertebroplasty and balloon kyphoplasty for the treatment of single level vertebral compression fractures: a meta-analysis of the literature. Pain Physician 2015;18(3):209–222

[8] Ong KL, Beall DP, Frohbergh M, Lau E, Hirsch JA. Were VCF patients at higher risk of mortality following the 2009 publication of the vertebroplasty "sham" trials? Osteoporos Int 2018;29(2):375–383

[9] Edidin AA, Ong KL, Lau E, Kurtz SM. Morbidity and mortality after vertebral fractures: comparison of vertebral augmentation and nonoperative management in the Medicare population. Spine 2015;40(15):1228–1241

[10] McCullough BJ, Comstock BA, Deyo RA, Kreuter W, Jarvik JG. Major medical outcomes with spinal augmentation vs conservative therapy. JAMA Intern Med 2013;173(16):1514–1521

[11] Li L, Ren J, Liu J, et al. Results of vertebral augmentation treatment for patients of painful osteoporotic vertebral compression fractures: a meta-analysis of eight randomized controlled trials. PLoS One 2015;10(9):e0138126

[12] Chen LX, Li YL, Ning GZ, et al. Comparative efficacy and tolerability of three treatments in old people with osteoporotic vertebral compression fracture: a network meta-analysis and systematic review. PLoS One 2015;10(4):e0123153

[13] Zhao S, Xu CY, Zhu AR, et al. Comparison of the efficacy and safety of 3 treatments for patients with osteoporotic vertebral compression fractures: a network meta-analysis. Medicine (Baltimore) 2017;96(26):e7328

[14] Parreira PCS, Maher CG, Megale RZ, March L, Ferreira ML. An overview of clinical guidelines for the management of vertebral compression fracture: a systematic review. Spine J 2017;17(12):1932–1938

[15] Xie L, Zhao ZG, Zhang SJ, Hu YB. Percutaneous vertebroplasty versus conservative treatment for osteoporotic vertebral compression fractures: an updated meta-analysis of prospective randomized controlled trials. Int J Surg 2017;47:25–32

[16] Luthman S, Widén J, Borgström F. Appropriateness criteria for treatment of osteoporotic vertebral compression fractures. Osteoporos Int 2018;29(4):793–804

[17] Chandra RV, Maingard J, Asadi H, et al. Vertebroplasty and kyphoplasty for osteoporotic vertebral fractures: what are the latest data? AJNR Am J Neuroradiol 2018;39(5):798–806

[18] Kallmes DF, Comstock BA, Heagerty PJ, et al. A randomized trial of vertebroplasty for osteoporotic spinal fractures. N Engl J Med 2009;361(6):569–579

[19] Buchbinder R, Osborne RH, Ebeling PR, et al. A randomized trial of vertebroplasty for painful osteoporotic vertebral fractures. N Engl J Med 2009;361(6):557–568

[20] Tan HY, Wang LM, Zhao L, Liu YL, Song RP. A prospective study of percutaneous vertebroplasty for chronic painful osteoporotic vertebral compression fracture. Pain Res Manag 2015;20(1):e8–e11

[21] Li X, Yang H, Tang T, Qian Z, Chen L, Zhang Z. Comparison of kyphoplasty and vertebroplasty for treatment of painful osteoporotic vertebral compression fractures: twelve-month follow-up in a prospective nonrandomized comparative study. J Spinal Disord Tech 2012;25(3):142–149

[22] Dohm M, Black CM, Dacre A, Tillman JB, Fueredi G; KAVIAR investigators. A randomized trial comparing balloon kyphoplasty and vertebroplasty for vertebral compression fractures due to osteoporosis. AJNR Am J Neuroradiol 2014;35(12):2227–2236

[23] Wang B, Guo H, Yuan L, Huang D, Zhang H, Hao D. A prospective randomized controlled study comparing the pain relief in patients with osteoporotic vertebral compression fractures with the use of vertebroplasty or facet blocking. Eur Spine J 2016;25(11):3486–3494

[24] Clark W, Bird P, Gonski P, et al. Safety and efficacy of vertebroplasty for acute painful osteoporotic fractures (VAPOUR): a multicentre, randomised, double-blind, placebo-controlled trial. Lancet 2016;388(10052):1408–1416

[25] Tutton SM, Pflugmacher R, Davidian M, Beall DP, Facchini FR, Garfin SR. KAST study: The Kiva System as a vertebral augmentation treatment—a safety and effectiveness trial: a randomized, noninferiority trial comparing the kiva system with balloon kyphoplasty in treatment of osteoporotic vertebral compression fractures. Spine 2015;40(12):865–875

[26] Blasco J, Martinez-Ferrer A, Macho J, et al. Effect of vertebroplasty on pain relief, quality of life, and the incidence of new vertebral fractures: a 12-month randomized follow-up, controlled trial. J Bone Miner Res 2012;27(5):1159–1166

[27] Boonen S, Van Meirhaeghe J, Bastian L, et al. Balloon kyphoplasty for the treatment of acute vertebral compression fractures: 2-year results from a randomized trial. J Bone Miner Res 2011;26(7):1627–1637

[28] Farrokhi MR, Alibai E, Maghami Z. Randomized controlled trial of percutaneous vertebroplasty versus optimal medical management for the relief of pain and disability in acute osteoporotic vertebral compression fractures. J Neurosurg Spine 2011;14(5):561–569

[29] Klazen CA, Lohle PN, de Vries J, et al. Vertebroplasty versus conservative treatment in acute osteoporotic vertebral compression fractures (Vertos II): an open-label randomised trial. Lancet 2010;376(9746):1085–1092

[30] Rousing R, Hansen KL, Andersen MO, Jespersen SM, Thomsen K, Lauritsen JM. Twelve-months follow-up in forty-nine patients with acute/semiacute osteoporotic vertebral fractures treated conservatively or with percutaneous vertebroplasty: a clinical randomized study. Spine 2010;35(5):478–482

[31] Van Meirhaeghe J, Bastian L, Boonen S, Ranstam J, Tillman JB, Wardlaw D; FREE investigators. A randomized trial of balloon kyphoplasty and nonsurgical management for treating acute vertebral compression fractures: vertebral body kyphosis correction and surgical parameters. Spine 2013;38(12):971–983

[32] Yang EZ, Xu JG, Huang GZ, et al. Percutaneous vertebroplasty versus conservative treatment in aged patients with acute osteoporotic vertebral compression fractures: a prospective randomized controlled clinical study. Spine 2016;41(8):653–660

[33] Firanescu CE, de Vries J, Lodder P, et al. Vertebroplasty versus sham procedure for painful acute osteoporotic vertebral compression fractures (VERTOS IV): randomised sham controlled clinical trial. BMJ 2018;361:k1551

[34] Wali AR, Martin JR, Rennert R, et al. Vertebroplasty for vertebral compression fractures: placebo or effective? Surg Neurol Int 2017;8:81

[35] Noonan P. Randomized vertebroplasty trials: bad news or sham news? AJNR Am J Neuroradiol 2009;30(10):1808–1809

[36] Hirsch JA, Chandra RV, Pampati V, Barr JD, Brook AL, Manchikanti L. Analysis of vertebral augmentation practice patterns: a 2016 update. J Neurointerv Surg 2016;8(12):1299–1304

[37] Maravic M, Taupin P, Roux C. Hospital burden of vertebral fractures in France: influence of vertebroplasty. Osteoporos Int 2013;24(7):2001–2006

[38] Tsai YW, Hsiao FY, Wen YW, et al. Clinical outcomes of vertebroplasty or kyphoplasty for patients with vertebral compression fractures: a nationwide cohort study. J Am Med Dir Assoc 2013;14(1):41–47

[39] Jakovljevic M. The placebo-nocebo response: controversies and challenges from clinical and research perspective. Eur Neuropsychopharmacol 2014;24(3):333–341

[40] Miller FG, Kaptchuk TJ. Sham procedures and the ethics of clinical trials. J R Soc Med 2004;97(12):576–578

[41] Požgain I, Požgain Z, Degmečić D. Placebo and nocebo effect: a mini-review. Psychiatr Danub 2014;26(2):100–107

[42] Cobb LA, Thomas GI, Dillard DH, Merendino KA, Bruce RA. An evaluation of internal-mammary-artery ligation by a double-blind technic. N Engl J Med 1959;260(22):1115–1118

[43] Moseley JB, O'Malley K, Petersen NJ, et al. A controlled trial of arthroscopic surgery for osteoarthritis of the knee. N Engl J Med 2002;347(2):81–88

[44] Kirkley A, Birmingham TB, Litchfield RB, et al. A randomized trial of arthroscopic surgery for osteoarthritis of the knee. N Engl J Med 2008;359(11):1097–1107

[45] Ghomrawi HMK, Marx RG, Pan TJ, Conti M, Lyman S. The effect of negative randomized trials and surgeon volume on the rates of arthroscopy for patients with knee OA. Contemp Clin Trials Commun 2017;9:40–44

[46] Amin NH, Hussain W, Ryan J, Morrison S, Miniaci A, Jones MH. Changes within clinical practice after a randomized controlled trial of knee arthroscopy for osteoarthritis. Orthop J Sports Med 2017;5(4):2325967117698439

[47] Benedetti F, Carlino E, Pollo A. How placebos change the patient's brain. Neuropsychopharmacology 2011;36(1):339–354

[48] Price DD, Finniss DG, Benedetti F. A comprehensive review of the placebo effect: recent advances and current thought. Annu Rev Psychol 2008;59:565–590

[49] Kennedy WP. The nocebo reaction. Med World 1961;95:203–205

[50] Gu CN, Brinjikji W, Evans AJ, Murad MH, Kallmes DF. Outcomes of vertebroplasty compared with kyphoplasty: a systematic review and meta-analysis. J Neurointerv Surg 2016;8(6):636–642

[51] Manchikanti L, Kaye AD, Boswell MV, et al. A systematic review and best evidence synthesis of the effectiveness of therapeutic facet joint interventions in managing chronic spinal pain. Pain Physician 2015;18(4):E535–E582

[52] Wilson DJ, Owen S, Corkill RA. Facet joint injections as a means of reducing the need for vertebroplasty in insufficiency fractures of the spine. Eur Radiol 2011;21(8):1772–1778

[53] Boszczyk B. Volume matters: a review of procedural details of two randomised controlled vertebroplasty trials of 2009. Eur Spine J 2010;19(11):1837–1840

[54] Benedetti F, Frisaldi E, Shaibani A. Placebo effects: the need for a new perspective and conceptualization. Expert Rev Clin Pharmacol 2018;11(6):543–544

[55] Butler C, Steptoe A. Placebo responses: an experimental study of psycho-physiological processes in asthmatic volunteers. Br J Clin Psychol 1986;25 (Pt 3):173–183

[56] Kemeny ME, Rosenwasser LJ, Panettieri RA, Rose RM, Berg-Smith SM, Kline JN. Placebo response in asthma: a robust and objective phenomenon. J Allergy Clin Immunol 2007;119(6):1375–1381

[57] Giang DW, Goodman AD, Schiffer RB, et al. Conditioning of cyclophosphamide-induced leukopenia in humans. J Neuropsychiatry Clin Neurosci 1996;8(2):194–201

[58] Merz M, Seiberling M, Höxter G, Hölting M, Wortha HP. Elevation of liver enzymes in multiple dose trials during placebo treatment: are they predictable? J Clin Pharmacol 1997;37(9):791–798

[59] Sievenpiper JL, Ezatagha A, Dascalu A, Vuksan V. When a placebo is not a "placebo": a placebo effect on postprandial glycaemia. Br J Clin Pharmacol 2007;64(4):546–549

[60] van der Molen GM, van den Hout MA. Expectancy effects on respiration during lactate infusion. Psychosom Med 1988;50(4):439–443

[61] Benedetti F, Rainero I, Pollo A. New insights into placebo analgesia. Curr Opin Anaesthesiol 2003;16(5):515–519

[62] Boehm K, Berger B, Weger U, Heusser P. Does the model of additive effect in placebo research still hold true? A narrative review. JRSM Open 2017;8(3):2054270416681434

[63] Kube T, Rief W. Are placebo and drug-specific effects additive? Questioning basic assumptions of double-blinded randomized clinical trials and presenting novel study designs. Drug Discov Today 2017;22(4):729–735

[64] Benedetti F, Carlino E, Pollo A. Hidden administration of drugs. Clin Pharmacol Ther 2011;90(5):651–661

[65] Ahn K, Jhun HJ, Lim TK, Lee YS. Fluoroscopically guided transforaminal epidural dry needling for lumbar spinal stenosis using a specially designed needle. BMC Musculoskelet Disord 2010;11:180

[66] Ahn K, Lee YJ, Kim EH, et al. Interventional microadhesiolysis: a new nonsurgical release technique for adhesive capsulitis of the shoulder. BMC Musculoskelet Disord 2008;9:12

[67] Ahn K, Lee YJ, Lee SC, Lee CW, Lee YC. Clinical effect of fluoroscopy guided interventional muscle and nerve stimulation (IMNS) on intractable spinal origin pain. Korean J Anesthesiol 2004;47:96–100

[68] Kim EH. Clinical effects of fluoroscopy guided interventional microadhesiolysis and nerve stimulation (FIMS) on cervical zygapophyseal joints in patients with chronic cervical radicular pain. J Korean Pain Soc 2007;20: 31–39

[69] Vas L, Pai R, Geete D, Verma CV. Improvement in CRPS after deep dry needling suggests a role in myofascial pain. Pain Med 2018;19(1):208–212

[70] Pai RS, Vas L. Ultrasound-guided intra-articular injection of the radio-ulnar and radio-humeral joints and ultrasound-guided dry needling of the affected limb muscles to relieve fixed pronation deformity and myofascial issues around the shoulder, in a case of complex regional pain syndrome Type 1. Pain Pract 2018;18(2):273–282

[71] Shanmugam S, Mathias L. Immediate effects of paraspinal dry needling in patients with acute facet joint lock induced wry neck. J Clin Diagn Res 2017;11(6):YM01–YM03

[72] Sherman RE, Anderson SA, Dal Pan GJ, et al. Real-world evidence: what is it and what can it tell us? N Engl J Med 2016;375(23):2293–2297

[73] H.R. 34—21st Century Cures Act. P.L. 114–255, December 13, 2016

[74] The Prescription Drug User Fee Act of. PDUFA Public Law 1992:102–571

28 Treatment of Chronic Vertebral Compression Fractures

Alexios Kelekis and Dimitrios K. Filippiadis

Summary

Vertebral compression fractures (VCFs) can be persistently painful even past the acute or subacute phase. Chronic fractures are defined as fractures older than six months. Osteonecrosis of the vertebral body is one of the more common conditions that can lead to bone resorption and loss of mechanical integrity necessitating treatment with vertebral augmentation. Chronic fractures can be treated with either vertebroplasty or kyphoplasty and numerous studies have shown this to be effective and to produce significant pain relief provided the patient's pain is coming from the vertebral compression fracture. Although the presence of bone marrow edema tends to be predictive of pain relief after vertebral augmentation with a greater amount of bone marrow edema indicating the potential for greater pain relief, the absence of marrow edema does not mean that the patient will not improve after vertebral augmentation and patients have been shown to improve after treatment of chronic fractures irrespective of their appearance on magnetic resonance imaging (MRI).

Keywords: chronic, vertebral compression fractures, intravertebral cleft, bone marrow edema, osteonecrosis

28.1 Introduction

Depending upon the duration of fractures, all vertebral fractures can be defined as acute (<6 weeks), subacute (6–24 weeks), and chronic (>24 weeks).[1] The pathophysiology behind unhealed chronic, longer-lasting pain in these patients is multifactorial, including structural changes, nonunions, fibrous unions, osteoarthritis, and nerve irritation that results in chronic radiculopathy or complex regional pain syndrome.[2] In the early era of vertebral augmentation, treating older fractures was controversial; however, numerous literature publications have proven efficacy of cement injection in these unhealed fractures as well.[3-6] According to international reporting standards both painful chronic traumatic fracture with nonunion or internal cystic changes and painful fractures associated with osteonecrosis are included in the indications of vertebral augmentation.[7,8]

28.2 Preoperative Evaluation

Preoperative imaging evaluation is a pre-requisite in chronic cases as well. Radiographs of the spine in anteroposterior and lateral projections can provide initial information concerning the number and the extent of vertebral collapse, but defining the levels of treatment by standard radiographs is inaccurate in both acute and chronic lesions.[2,9] Similarly, in chronic vertebral fractures the usefulness of scintigraphy is controversial.[2] On the other hand, MRI is governed by high sensitivity for bone marrow edema indicating osseous activity at the fracture site, irrespective of the fracture's age. Timing of the fracture (acute or chronic) should not be confused with the presence of bone

edema in short TI inversion recovery (STIR) sequence of MR examination. Both acute and unhealed chronic fractures can show bone edema (illustrated as increased signal intensity on the STIR sequence) as a sign of bone marrow activity. MRI with STIR and T1-weighted sequences should be used to verify the fracture's age and healing status (acute vs. chronic, incompletely healed vs. consolidated) (▶Fig. 28.1).[8] Tanigawa et al reported that the improvement after vertebral augmentation is related to the bone edema pattern illustrated in the pretherapeutic MRI (▶Fig. 28.2). Specifically according to this study patients with an extensive bone marrow edema pattern

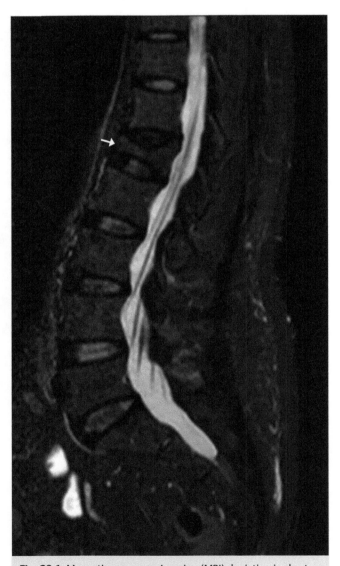

Fig. 28.1 Magnetic resonance imaging (MRI) depicting in short TI inversion recovery (STIR) sagittal sequence an L1 wedge vertebral fracture (*white arrow*), with no hyperintensity signal, hence no bone edema.

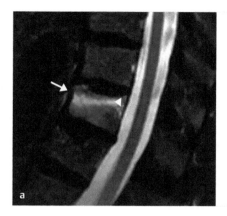
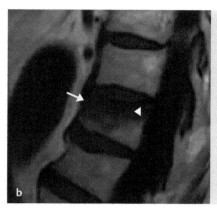

Fig. 28.2 Sagittal magnetic resonance (MR) image of vertebral body with short TI inversion recovery (STIR) (**a**) and T1W (**b**) sagittal sequences of a patient with T11 wedge fracture (*white arrow* in **a** and **b**). The vertebral edema (high in STIR and low signal in T1 as is indicated by *white arrowheads* in both images) extends through less than 50% of the vertebral body.

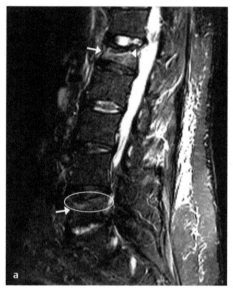
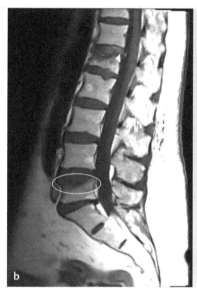

Fig. 28.3 Sagittal magnetic resonance imaging (MRI) of a patient consulting for low back pain. On short TI inversion recovery (STIR) there are two fractures of the upper end plate, one in L1 and one in L5 (*white arrows* in **a**). The L1 fracture has bone edema in more than 50% of the vertebral body (high signal in STIR and low in T1 as indicated by the *white arrowheads* in **a** and **b**) and may be clinically more painful than the L5 fracture, which has less than 50% bone edema (*white ovals* in **a** and **b**).

involving more than 50% of the vertebral body reported significantly greater clinical improvement than those without this pattern[10] (▶Fig. 28.3).

28.3 Vertebral Osteonecrosis

Vertebral body osteonecrosis is characterized by cellular death and bone resorption that result in mechanical insufficiency and vertebral collapse (▶Fig. 28.4). It can be idiopathic or secondary to trauma, cytotoxicity, and genetic factors.[11–13] The process of osteonecrosis and subsequent rapid collapse of a vertebral body has been given the eponymous name Kummell disease after the German surgeon Hermann Kummell who first described this condition in 1891. The pathognomonic sign of vertebral osteonecrosis is the intravertebral vacuum sign that may contain gas, fluid, or both.[13] MRI cannot easily distinguish between gas and compact bone, as both appear as low signal intensity areas. In case of suspicion of a gas pocket, CT imaging can easily detect the osteonecrotic gas cavity (▶Fig. 28.5). The literature examination of vertebral osteonecrosis is limited and inconsistent with substantial overlap with cases of nonunion, fibrous union, and pseudoarthrosis.[14] The most common reported risk factors include low bone density and the use of glucocorticoids but many factors may work in combination. Recently, vertebral

osteonecrosis was classified into four stages based upon radiological findings and sagittal alignment:[13]

- 0: Theoretical phase.
- 1: Early phase.
- 2: Instability phase.
- 3: Fixed deformity phase.

According to this classification proposed by Formica et al, stage 1 is managed with nonsurgical management (NSM) as opposed to stages 2 and 3 which require different therapeutic approaches according to local and global sagittal alignment.[13] It is evident that the treatment of vertebral osteonecrosis should be adjusted according to symptoms and disability, neurological status, comorbidities, and surgical risk.

28.4 Sequela of Chronic Fractures

A chronic fracture can affect a whole spine segment by creating a degenerative cascade phenomenon which implicates all adjacent structures. This includes disk degeneration and herniation, facet osteoarthritis, nerve irritation associated with foraminal stenosis, muscle atrophy, ligament strain and sprain, Baastrup disease, scoliosis, and spinal stenosis. These secondary effects from the initial deformity can also be pain

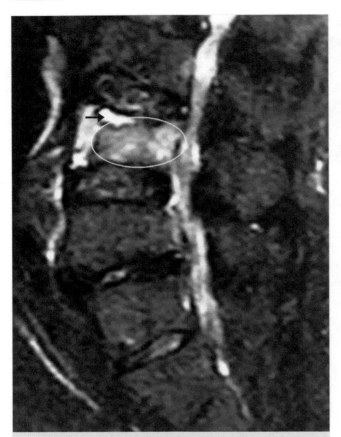

Fig. 28.4 L3 vertebral fracture in short TI inversion recovery (STIR) sagittal sequence illustrating a fluid-filled cleft (*black arrow*), just below the superior end plate. The edema (high signal in STIR as indicated by *white oval*) extends through the middle third to the anterior third of the vertebral body. Notice the bone marrow edema, which is characterized by its high intensity on STIR, has a lower signal than the fluid seen in the cleft (*black arrow*).

generators, thus creating a situation with complex pain symptoms. Augmentation techniques aim to provide structural support by forming an intraosseous cast and as such can help the pain and the structural deformity associated with the fracture. In order therefore to have a clinically successful treatment it is very important to differentiate the pain associated with the nonhealing fracture from the pain related to the secondary pathology. Treating a complex pain syndrome, although outside of the scope of this book, is as critical as treating the painful fracture itself and in most cases multiple treatments will work in a complementary manner.

28.5 The Treatment of Chronic VCFs

Numerous studies in the literature have proven the safety and efficacy of different vertebral augmentation techniques in the treatment of painful chronic fractures and vertebral osteonecrosis.[15-23] Vertebroplasty has been reported to be an effective therapeutic technique for these cases but has also been reported to have an increased risk cement leakage and recurrent kyphosis.[15-18] Balloon kyphoplasty has been similarly reported to be an effective technique for symptomatic chronic and osteonecrotic vertebrae with no reports of increased cement leakage or recurrent kyphosis.[19,20] Comparative studies between these two techniques for vertebral osteonecrosis report similar clinical and radiological results as well as similar incidence of cement leakage.[21,22] Recently, vertebral implants have been used with promising results for the treatment of vertebral osteonecrosis specifically an intravertebral expandable jack consisting of a central screw and of two deployable plates. This jack device known as the SpineJack has been applied in 19 patients with significant pain reduction and no complications.[23]

Studies have also reported the effectiveness of the treatment of chronic VCFs even with imaging findings showing no bone marrow edema or evidence of an unhealed fracture.[2] Brown

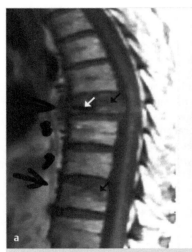
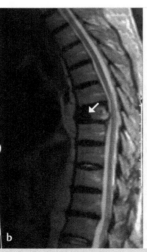
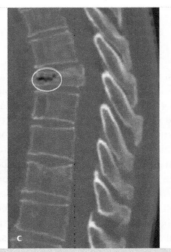
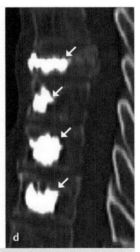

Fig. 28.5 Thoracic spine imaging showing a hypointense area in T7 and T10 vertebral bodies (*black arrows* in **a**) as noted on the T1-weighted sagittal magnetic resonance (MR) image. The decreased signal in the T7 vertebral body remains hypointense on the T2-weighted image (*white arrows* in **a** and **b**). This area of decreased T1 and T2 signal was shown to be an air-filled cleft on a CT exam (area within the *white circle* in **c**). Four vertebral levels were augmented, to treat the two fractures, as well as to augment the osteoporotic vertebral bodies in between. The augmentation (*white arrows* in **d**) is best seen on the post-treatment CT.

et al studied the outcomes of vertebroplasty in patients with chronic VCFs of more than 1 year old.[2] They reported on 45 patients and recorded the imaging findings, changes in pain, and improvements in mobility up to 28 months and found that two-thirds of the patients did not have marrow edema on their preprocedural MRI examination. This preprocedure MRI exam results were correlated with the procedure outcomes and it was found that all of the 15 patients that had edema on their preprocedure MRI examination received clinical benefit with 40% of these patients achieving complete pain relief and the remainder experiencing substantial clinical improvement. Of the patients with no marrow edema 17% had complete resolution of pain, 63% were improved, and 20% were unchanged. None of these patients had worsening of their symptoms, and mobility was improved in 57%. Overall they found that 87% of the patients with VCFs older than 1 year received clinical benefit from vertebroplasty irrespective of the preprocedure MRI findings, and although all of the patients with bone marrow edema had clinical benefit, no direct correlation was seen between symptom resolution and the presence of edema on preprocedural MRI. They went on to conclude that the absence of abnormal marrow signal does not definitively predict the outcome of vertebroplasty in chronic fractures.[2]

In a study to analyze and compare the outcomes of vertebroplasty with unipedicular and bipedicular kyphoplasty for the treatment of VCFs, Bozkurt et al examined the changes in pain, function, and height restoration rates in 296 patients.[24] There were 433 fractures treated with vertebral augmentation, with an average fracture age of 23.4 months from the onset of symptoms to the time of treatment. In this patient population with the mean fracture age of nearly 2 years, the mean height restoration was slightly over 24% in the vertebroplasty group and 37% in the bilateral kyphoplasty group, with pain and functional scores improving in all of the groups. In this patient population with chronic VCFs, the authors concluded that both vertebroplasty and kyphoplasty were effective in providing pain relief and improvement in functional capacity and showed a substantial amount of restoration in vertebral body height.[24]

28.6 Conclusion

In conclusion, vertebral augmentation techniques including vertebroplasty, balloon kyphoplasty, and vertebral implants can be considered safe and efficacious techniques for the treatment of symptomatic chronic vertebral fractures. The diagnostic criteria for the treatment of chronic vertebral fractures are no different than the criteria for treatment of acute or subacute fractures with the patient presenting with substantial pain and/or functional debilitation and the presence of a vertebral fracture by imaging that corresponds with the pain generator on physical exam. The goals for the treatment of all fractures regardless of acuity are pain reduction and improvement of functional capacity and quality of life by restoring the vertebral body stability and correcting structural spine deformities with the least invasive technique available.

References

[1] Rad AE, Kallmes DF. Correlation between preoperative pain duration and percutaneous vertebroplasty outcome. AJNR Am J Neuroradiol 2011;32 (10):1842–1845

[2] Brown DB, Glaiberman CB, Gilula LA, Shimony JS. Correlation between preprocedural MRI findings and clinical outcomes in the treatment of chronic symptomatic vertebral compression fractures with percutaneous vertebroplasty. AJR Am J Roentgenol 2005;184(6):1951–1955

[3] Kaufmann TJ, Jensen ME, Schweickert PA, Marx WF, Kallmes DF. Age of fracture and clinical outcomes of percutaneous vertebroplasty. AJNR Am J Neuroradiol 2001;22(10):1860–1863

[4] Brown DB, Gilula LA, Sehgal M, Shimony JS. Treatment of chronic symptomatic vertebral compression fractures with percutaneous vertebroplasty. AJR Am J Roentgenol 2004;182(2):319–322

[5] Maynard AS, Jensen ME, Schweickert PA, Marx WF, Short JG, Kallmes DF. Value of bone scan imaging in predicting pain relief from percutaneous vertebroplasty in osteoporotic vertebral fractures. AJNR Am J Neuroradiol 2000;21(10):1807–1812

[6] Jensen ME, Dion JE. Percutaneous vertebroplasty in the treatment of osteoporotic compression fractures. Neuroimaging Clin N Am 2000;10(3):547–568

[7] Baerlocher MO, Saad WE, Dariushnia S, Barr JD, McGraw JK, Nikolic B; Society of Interventional Radiology Standards of Practice Committee. Quality improvement guidelines for percutaneous vertebroplasty. J Vasc Interv Radiol 2014;25(2):165–170

[8] Tsoumakidou G, Too CW, Koch G, et al. CIRSE guidelines on percutaneous vertebral augmentation. Cardiovasc Intervent Radiol 2017;40(3):331–342

[9] Stallmeyer MJB, Zoarski GH, Obuchowski AM. Optimizing patient selection in percutaneous vertebroplasty. J Vasc Interv Radiol 2003;14(6):683–696

[10] Tanigawa N, Komemushi A, Kariya S, et al. Percutaneous vertebroplasty: relationship between vertebral body bone marrow edema pattern on MR images and initial clinical response. Radiology 2006;239(1):195–200

[11] Shah KN, Racine J, Jones LC, Aaron RK. Pathophysiology and risk factors for osteonecrosis. Curr Rev Musculoskelet Med 2015;8(3):201–209

[12] Lafforgue P. Pathophysiology and natural history of avascular necrosis of bone. Joint Bone Spine 2006;73(5):500–507

[13] Formica M, Zanirato A, Cavagnaro L, et al. Vertebral body osteonecrosis: proposal of a treatment-oriented classification system. Eur Spine J 2018;27(Suppl 2): 190–197

[14] Formica M, Zanirato A, Cavagnaro L, et al. What is the current evidence on vertebral body osteonecrosis?: a systematic review of the literature. Asian Spine J 2018;12(3):586–599

[15] Hirsch JA, Reddy AS, Linfante I, Rachlin JR. Pseudo-Kümmel's disease: a unique application for vertebroplasty. Pain Physician 2003;6(2):207–211

[16] Kim DY, Lee SH, Jang JS, Chung SK, Lee HY. Intravertebral vacuum phenomenon in osteoporotic compression fracture: report of 67 cases with quantitative evaluation of intravertebral instability. J Neurosurg 2004;100(1, Suppl Spine):24–31

[17] Cho SM, Heo DH, Cho YJ. Spontaneous migration of a polymethylmethacrylate mass after vertebroplasty in osteoporotic lumbar compression fracture with avascular osteonecrosis: a case report. Joint Bone Spine 2011;78(1):98–99

[18] Fang X, Yu F, Fu S, Song H. Intravertebral clefts in osteoporotic compression fractures of the spine: incidence, characteristics, and therapeutic efficacy. Int J Clin Exp Med 2015;8(9):16960–16968

[19] Huang Y, Peng M, He S, Tang X, Dai M, Tang C. Clinical efficacy of percutaneous kyphoplasty at the hyperextension position for the treatment of osteoporotic Kummell disease. Clin Spine Surg 2016;29(4):161–166

[20] Chen GD, Lu Q, Wang GL, et al. Percutaneous kyphoplasty for Kummell disease with severe spinal canal stenosis. Pain Physician 2015;18(6):E1021–E1028

[21] Zhang GQ, Gao YZ, Chen SL, Ding S, Gao K, Wang HQ. Comparison of percutaneous vertebroplasty and percutaneous kyphoplasty for the management of Kümmell's disease: a retrospective study. Indian J Orthop 2015;49(6):577–582

[22] Wu AM, Ni WF, Weng W, Chi YL, Xu HZ, Wang XY. Outcomes of percutaneous kyphoplasty in patients with intravertebral vacuum cleft. Acta Orthop Belg 2012;78(6):790–795

[23] Premat K, Vande Perre S, Cormier É, et al. Vertebral augmentation with the SpineJack in chronic vertebral compression fractures with major kyphosis. Eur Radiol 2018;28(12):4985–4991

[24] Bozkurt M, Kahilogullari G, Ozdemir M, et al. Comparative analysis of vertebroplasty and kyphoplasty for osteoporotic vertebral compression fractures. Asian Spine J 2014;8(1):27–34

29 Treatment of Neoplastic Vertebral Compression Fractures

Kyung-Hoon Kim

Summary

The spine is the most frequently involved bony structure in cancer metastasis, the order of frequency being the thoracic (70%), lumbosacral (20%), and cervical (10%) spine. The spine metastasis usually originates from a cancer of the adjacent organs: the thoracic spine from the lung and breast; the lumbosacral spine from the colon, prostate, urinary bladder, and uterine cervix; the cervical spine from the thyroid or lung.

Diagnosis is rendered by a history of weight-bearing pain, tenderness in the supraspinous area with or without adjacent facet area tenderness on physical examination, loss of a pedicle on a plain film x-ray with or without vertebral height loss on the lateral view, active bone lesions on bone scans, and posterior wall destruction of the compressed vertebral body on computed tomography (CT) or magnetic resonance imaging (MRI).

Treatment for painful osteolytic and osteoblastic metastatic fractures, such as percutaneous vertebroplasty (PVP) or kyphoplasty, may start with performing facet-joint injections to determine the exact painful level in patients with multilevel spine metastases. This is done with the patient in the prone position with care taken to minimize facet-mediated pain. The levels are localized so as to minimize obscuration of the underlying anatomy by the potentially overlying radio-opaque bone cement.

A vertebral needle should be placed at the anterior one-third to one-fourth of the vertebral body to prevent leakage of bone cement into the anterior epidural space through the damaged posterior wall of the vertebral body. Injecting bone cement equal to 20 to 25% of the volume of the vertebral body is sufficient.

The mechanism of pain relief is not only augmentation by bone cement that provides pain relief by stabilizing the vertebral body but also denervation (by both thermal and chemical means) of basivertebral nerve branches that carry pain from the end plates through the vertebral. If leakage of bone cement is avoided, the result of PVP is similar to that of percutaneous kyphoplasty.

PVP for the treatment of painful metastatic osteolytic or osteoblastic compression fractures provides immediate pain relief and allows for early ambulation.

Keywords: augmentation, bone cement, denervation, kyphoplasty, neoplasm, metastasis, spine, vertebroplasty, zygapophyseal joint

29.1 Introduction

Percutaneous vertebroplasty (PVP) was first reported for the treatment of painful benign vertebral angioma in 1987.[1] The procedure has been widely used to treat painful osteoporotic compression fractures, commonly in the thoracolumbar junction.

Increased life expectancy after cancer diagnoses and a higher prevalence of bony metastases has increased the number of cases of painful metastatic vertebral compression fractures (VCFs). As with osteoporosis, metastatic vertebral fractures mainly occur in the thoracic spine, followed in frequency by the lumbosacral and cervical spines.[2]

Spinal metastases usually develop from cancers of the adjacent organs, and most common types of spinal metastases (60%) originate from breast, lung, or prostate, and far less frequently from the kidney, urinary bladder, and thyroid.[2] The segment of the spine involved with metastatic disease is usually the portion of the spine nearest to the affected organ. For example, the thoracic spine is usually affected by cancers of the lung and breast; the lumbosacral spine by cancers from the colon, prostate, urinary bladder, and uterine cervix; the cervical spine by cancers from the thyroid or lung.

Spinal metastases from breast cancer are common in women in their forties and fifties but spinal metastases from lung cancer are more common in men in their sixties and seventies. About 10% of all cancers eventually metastasize to the spine.[2]

29.2 Diagnosis

29.2.1 History

Patients who have painful metastatic osteolytic or osteoblastic fractures are more frequently referred from the oncology department, rather than from a pain or spine clinic. In patients with spine metastases, it is easier to find the metastasis to the spine if there are red flags, such as recent sudden weight loss, combined motor deficits, or if the patient is less than 40 years old and has severe unremitting back pain.

On the contrary, in cases referred by way of findings on cross-sectional imaging usually come to the physician's attention after an emergency room visit or following a scan obtained after surgery, chemotherapy, or radiotherapy. The typical complaints are of sudden and severe back pain that is exacerbated with the patient changing position or in transition. Many times the patient is debilitated to the point where they are unable to sit and stand by themselves and are relegated to lying on their back.

29.2.2 Physical Examination

It is important to check combined motor deficits in a supine position and it is especially important for both doctors and patients to recognize existing motor deficits that may be present prior to the procedure. After discovery of any motor deficits, the doctor should inform the patient as to their presence. The motor deficits may eventually progress, whether or not the PVP is performed and it is optimal to document this prior to performing any intervention. The initial examination must include palpation of the paraspinal region and overlying the posterior superior iliac spine keeping in mind that it may not be easy to put the patient in the prone in order to be able to examine them.[3]

If the metastatic vertebral fractures are combined with diskogenic back pain or facet-joint pain, it may be very difficult to determine the exact region that is producing the pain.

In this case it may be better to perform intradiskal or facet-joint injections prior to the PVP to be able to further localize the pain generator. The merits of performing injections prior to the PVP are (1) after relieving pain from the painful disk or facet joint, the residual presence of supraspinous tenderness has a value in choosing the correct level for the PVP among the multiple metastatic levels, (2) after relieving the patients' degenerative back pain, they can lie in a prone position and better cooperate with the augmentation procedure, and (3) if the PVP is performed prior to the injections, the cement may obscure the injection targets, making it difficult to perform the appropriate injections.[3]

29.2.3 Imaging Diagnosis

- Plain film X-rays: It is difficult to diagnose neoplastic VCFs until they are prominent or even severe. However, if there is a loss of the pedicle on the anteroposterior view, this provides strong evidence of spinal metastasis. This is in contradistinction to a vertebra with intact pedicles but a compressed vertebral body. This type of compression fracture can be difficult to determine whether the fracture is a result of osteoporosis or tumor (▶Fig. 29.1).
- Bone scans: Nuclear medicine bone scanning tends to be an optimal diagnostic tool if the lesions detected are in the posterior wall of the vertebral body or pedicle. In the sacrum and pelvis, a signature sign of a benign sacral insufficient fracture is classically seen as a 'Honda sign' on bone scan, composed of vertically oriented fractures primarily through S1 and S2 vertebral bodies and a horizontally oriented fracture through S2 (▶Fig. 29.2a).
- Computed tomography (CT): It is helpful to reveal whether the posterior wall of the vertebral body is intact or not and where the exact fracture lines in the vertebrae are located.
- Positron emission computed tomography (PET/CT): Is effective in evaluating the status of both the primary focus of the cancer and spinal metastasis and when combined with CT or MRI scanning can be highly accurate at localizing the exact anatomic location of the neoplastic involvement.
- Magnetic resonance imaging (MRI): The soft tissues such as the intervertebral disks, spinal cord, cauda equina, and dorsal nerve root ganglion are seen clearly, as well as other areas of interest such as the anterior epidural space and the cerebral spinal fluid. The extent of the tumor or metastasis involvement is typically well characterized by MRI.

29.2.4 Valuable Scoring Systems for Evaluation of the Patients with Metastatic Bone Lesions

- Karnofsky performance status (KPS) scale (▶Table 29.1): It is very helpful to evaluate patients' physical performance status before and after PVP. If the score is 50% or higher, patients can be discharged from the hospital.[4]
- Tokuhashi revised scoring system for preoperative evaluation of metastatic spine tumor prognosis (▶Table 29.2): It is important to predict the prognosis of a metastatic spine tumor before the PVP.[5]

29.3 Treatment

29.3.1 Thoracic and Lumbar Vertebrae

In a typical vertebra of the thoracic or lumbar spine, a transpedicular approach is a common method for accessing the painful vertebral bodies. However, if there is metastatic destruction on one side of the pedicle, it may be difficult to choose between accessing the involved or uninvolved pedicle and deciding between a transpedicular, peripedicular, or extrapedicular approach.

In most of the cases, if the needle can be placed in the anterior one-third or one-fourth of the vertebral body there is confidence that leakage into the anterior epidural space can be avoided. It is okay to access the vertebral body through an involved pedicle and not necessary to have bone cement completely filling the entire anteroposterior extent of the vertebral body. Pain relief by PVP is obtained not only by augmentation of the structure of the vertebral body, but also by thermal and chemical ablation of the ingrown nerves and in-dwelling tumor.

29.3.2 Sacrum

The sacral body and sacral ala are connected but are separate anatomic structures (▶Fig. 29.2b). It is not difficult, however, to place the needle(s) into both anatomic locations during one sacroplasty session and to fill two to three or more adjacent levels of the sacral ala with bone cement at one time, due to the fused structure of the sacral segments (▶Fig. 29.2c).

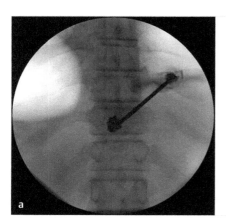
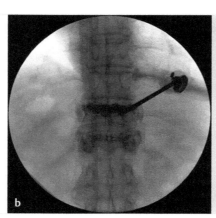

Fig. 29.1 (a) Osteolytic metastatic fracture at T11. The right pedicle cannot be seen, but the height of the vertebral body is preserved. (b) Osteoporotic compression fracture at T11. Both pedicles can be seen clearly, but the height of the body is reduced.

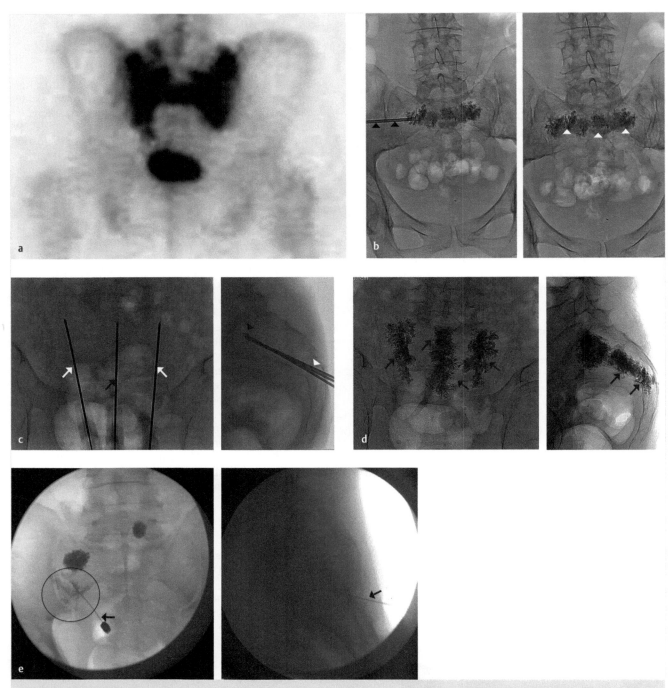

Fig. 29.2 Sacral insufficiency fractures. (**a**) A "Honda sign," which is composed of the fractured sacral body with the two vertically oriented fracture lines through the sacral ala, is apparent in the posterior view on the nuclear medicine bone scan. (**b**) A needle (*black arrowheads*) is positioned through the patient's left sacroiliac joint into the left sacral ala after having been placed through the sacral body and into the right sacral ala where bone cement was injected (*white arrowheads*) to treat the patients' sacral fractures. (**c**) Anteroposterior (left image) and lateral (right image) views show needles placed into the sacral ala (*white arrows*). A single needle is placed into the center of the sacral body (*black arrow*) from an inferior position. The lateral view shows the needles entering the sacrum at the mid-portion of S3 (*white arrowhead*) and extending to the superior portion of S1 (*black arrowhead*). (**d**) Anteroposterior (left) and lateral (right) views show bone cement injected into the sacral ala and sacral body (*black arrows*). (**e**) Anteroposterior (left) and lateral (right) fluoroscopic images show a 22-gauge needle (*black arrows*) entering the sacroiliac joint. The contrast within the joint is best seen on the anteroposterior view (within the *circle* on the AP view).

When performing sacral augmentation, caution should be taken not to pierce or penetrate the sacral foramina when the needle is advanced into the sacral body or ala. A safe insertion of a needle into the sacral ala involves placing it halfway between the lateral border of the sacral foramina and the medial border of the sacroiliac joint. If the sacral foramina are difficult to visualize, contrast can be injected into the epidural space via the sacral hiatus to highlight the foramina. A sacroiliac joint injection may also be performed to outline the anatomy of the sacroiliac joint (▶Fig. 29.2e).

Table 29.1 Karnofsky performance status (%)

100	Normal to no complaints	No evidence of disease	Able to carry on normal activity and to work; no special care needed
90	Able to carry on normal activity	Minor signs or symptoms of disease	
80	Normal activity with effort	Some signs or symptoms of disease	
70	Cares for self	Unable to carry on normal activity or to do active work	Unable to work; able to live at home and care for most personal needs; varying amount of assistance needed
60	Requires occasional assistance	Able to care for most of their personal needs	
50	Requires considerable assistance	Frequent medical care	
40	Disabled	Requires special care and assistance	Unable to care for self; requires equivalent of institutional or hospital care; disease may be progressing rapidly
30	Severely disabled	Hospital admission is indicated although death not imminent	
20	Very sick	Hospital admission necessary; active supportive treatment necessary	
10	Moribund	Fatal processes progressing rapidly	
0	Dead		

Table 29.2 Tokuhashi revised scoring system for preoperative evaluation of metastatic spine tumor prognosis

Characteristic	Score
1. General condition (performance scale)	
Poor (10–40%)	0
Moderate (50–70%)	1
Good (80–100%)	2
2. Number of extraspinal bone metastases foci	
≥3	0
1–2	1
0	2
3. Number of metastases in the vertebral body	
≥3	0
1–2	1
0	2
4. Metastases to the major internal organs	
Lung, osteosarcoma, stomach, bladder, esophagus, pancreas	0
Liver, gall bladder, unidentified	1
Others	2
Kidney, uterus	3
Rectum	4
Thyroid, breast, prostate, carcinoid tumor	5
5. Palsy	
Complete (Frankel A, B)	0
Incomplete (Frankel C, D)	1
None (Frankel E)	2
Criteria of predicted prognosis	
Total score 0–8 < 6 months	
Total score 9–11 ≥ 6 months	
Total score 12–15 ≥ 1 year	

29.3.3 Cervical vertebrae

C1 Vertebra (The Atlas)

The atlas or C1 vertebra is composed of the anterior arch, posterior arch, lateral masses with superior and inferior articular facets, vertebral foramen, and transverse processes with the transverse foramina. The superior facets of the lateral masses become weight-bearing units articulating at the occiput of the head. When the structural integrity of the lateral masses is compromised, cement augmentation may be performed to re-establish the weight-bearing capability of the lateral masses of the atlas.

Cement augmentation on atypical vertebrae, including C1 and C2, should be performed while paying appropriate attention to avoid injury to the internal carotid artery, internal jugular vein, vertebral artery, and nerve roots (▶Fig. 29.3). An ultrasound guided or a manual compression anterolateral approach technique with or without using a blocking needle provides safe guidance for a larger gauge vertebral needle.

C2 Vertebra (The Axis)

The other atypical cervical vertebra, the C2, or atlas, also has specific anatomic features. The anterior structures include the vertebral body and dens (odontoid process) and lateral masses with superior and inferior articular facets. Laterally there are transverse processes with foramina called the foramina transversarium. Posteriorly the structures include the laminae and spinous process.

The odontoid process of the axis is one of the more commonly injured vertebral structures. There are three types of the C2 fractures: type I (an oblique fracture through the upper part of the dens) which is least common type of dens injury and has the potential to be unstable; type II (a fracture across the base of the dens at the dens-body junction) which is unstable and has a high risk of non-union; type III (a fracture through the dens that extends into the vertebral body and lateral masses). The type III dens fracture has the best prognosis for healing.[6] Metastatic osteolytic fractures at C2 show similar patterns to the three types of fractures from trauma.

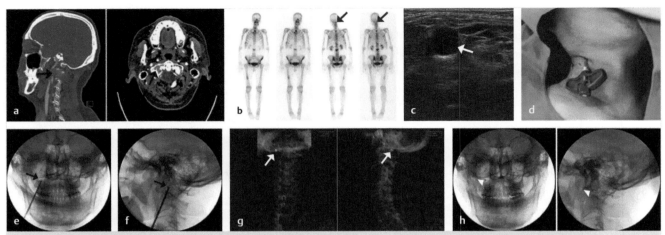

Fig. 29.3 Percutaneous osteoplasty (POP) of the right lateral mass of the atlas (C1). **(a)** An osteolytic lesion is present in the right lateral mass as seen on sagittal reconstruction and axial computed tomography (CT) images (*black arrows*). **(b)** Nuclear medicine bone scan images show an active lesion in the location of the right lateral mass. **(c)** An ultrasound-guided approach can reduce the risk of piercing the major vessels and nerves in the neck. An axial ultrasound image shows the internal carotid neurovascular bundle with the internal jugular vein as the most prominent hypoechoic structure (*white arrow*). **(d)** A vertebral needle is placed into the right lateral mass from a right paravertebral and submental approach. **(e)** AP and **(f)** lateral fluoroscopic images show the trajectory of the needle and the needle tip within the right lateral mass of C1 (*black arrows*). **(g)** Three-dimensional CT reconstruction images show a bright purple-colored bone cement located in the destroyed right lateral mass of C1 (*white arrows*). **(h)** The cement is seen as a black dot on AP and lateral fluoroscopic images (*white arrowheads*).

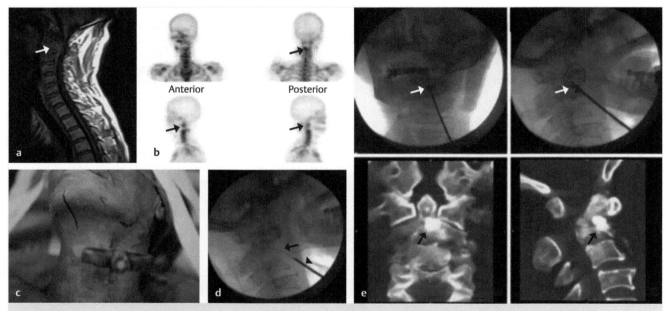

Fig. 29.4 Percutaneous osteoplasty (POP) in the dens and body of the axis. **(a)** Sagittal T1-weighted image shows an osteolytic lesion in the left dens and body (*white arrow*). **(b)** Anteroposterior, posteroanterior, and oblique views of a nuclear medicine bone scan shows an active lesion in the body and dens of C2 (*black arrows*). **(c)** A vertebral needle with an anteromedial approach is inserted into the body and dens of the C2 verte-brae (*black arrow* in **d**) with the guidance of a blocking needle (*black arrowhead* in **d**). **(e)** Anteroposterior and lateral fluoroscopic views show a needle injecting bone cement into the junction between the dens and body of C2 (*white arrows* on the upper images). Anteroposterior and lateral CT images demonstrate the cement at the dens/body junction (*black arrows* on the lower images).

As with C1, percutaneous osteoplasty (POP) of C2 can be performed with fluoroscopic or ultrasound guidance approach and the body of C2 may be accessed via anterolateral, postero-lateral, or transoral approaches (▶Fig. 29.4).[7]

Typical Vertebrae (C3–C7)

The anatomic components of the typical cervical vertebrae from C3 to C7 consist of the vertebral body with the uncinate processes, the transverse processes with the foramen transver-sarium (for the vertebral artery), superior and inferior articular facets, the vertebral arch composed of the pedicles and lamina, and the spinous process.

In an anterior approach to the vertebral body it is important to avoid damage to the tracheoesophageal complex, internal carotid artery, internal jugular vein, spinal cord, dorsal nerve root ganglion, and spinal nerves. A vertebral needle may be inserted into the cervical vertebral body using an anteromedial

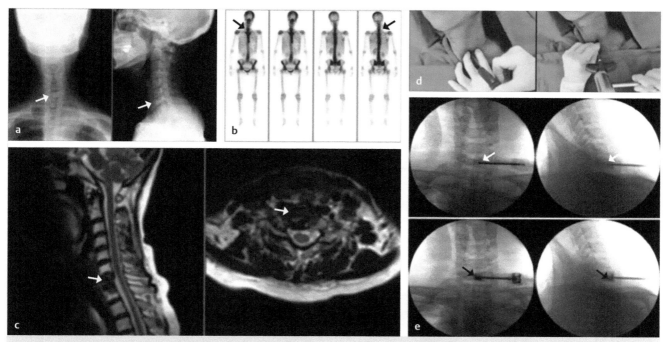

Fig. 29.5 Percutaneous vertebroplasty (PVP) at C7. (**a**) An osteoblastic lesion is observed in a minimally compressed C7 vertebral body on the anteroposterior and lateral X-ray views of the cervical spine (*white arrows*). (**b**) The nuclear medicine bone scan shows an active lesion in the C7 vertebral body (*black arrows*). (**c**) The metastatic lesion is seen on sagittal and axial T2-weighted MR images (*white arrows*). (**d**) A vertebral needle, using an anteromedial approach, is inserted into the vertebral body while pushing aside the tracheoesophageal complex and major vessels with the second and third fingers (left image). (**e**) The vertebral needle is placed into the center and anterior portion of the C7 vertebrae (*white arrows* on the upper AP and lateral fluoroscopic images) followed by injection of bone cement into the vertebral body (*black arrows* on the lower AP and lateral fluoroscopic images).

approach by pushing aside the tracheoesophageal complex and major vessels with one's second and third fingers. The needle should be placed in the center or anterior one-third of the vertebral body (▶Fig. 29.5).[8]

Extraspinal Percutaneous Osteoplasty (POP)

PVP is performed on the vertebral body whereas POP is a general term that describes osteoplasty with the injection of bone cement into various types of osseous structures including flat bones, long bones, and extravertebral axial skeletal bones.[9] Although the most frequent site of bony metastasis is known to be the spine and vertebroplasty is commonly performed in painful osteolytic or osteoblastic metastases or VCFs associated with osseous metastases, the treatment for painful extraspinal bony metastasis is also a challenging field of palliative care that can involve osteoplasty of the affected area.

There are precautions to be taken when inserting a needle into the targeted bone to avoid predictable complications. The most important thing is to choose an appropriately sized needle with a suitable bevel, in order to be able to direct the needle to the correct position while avoiding over-penetrating or falling short of the target area. It is also important to avoid major vessels and nerves. Additionally, it is better to choose the shortest available route to the targeted bone, which can reduce patient pain and procedure time.

The most common sites for the origin of the metastatic disease, in order of decreasing frequency, are the lung, liver, breast,

colon, and kidney.[10] The sites where extraspinal POP is most frequently performed include the rib, scapula, ilium, humeral head, ischium, femur, and sternum, in that order (▶Fig. 29.6). Injections into the joints adjacent to the extraspinal POP may also be necessary.[11,12]

29.4 Controversies

29.4.1 Vertebroplasty versus Kyphoplasty

- Even though the merits of the reduced risk of cement leakage using balloon kyphoplasty for the treatment of osteolytic metastatic compression fracture has been much emphasized,[13] augmentation using only a vertebral needle may be sufficient because (1) the target point of cement insertion is the anterior one-third or one-fourth of the vertebral body, (2) the insertion of slices of gelatin sponge after detection of leakage using an injection of a contrast medium prior to cement injection prevents cement leakage into the disrupted posterior wall of the vertebral body, and (3) vertebral body cement fill equal to 15 to 25% of the thoracolumbar vertebrae is a sufficient amount to treat the pain from the neoplasm as well as to re-establish the strength and stiffness of the vertebral body.[14–16]
- On the contrary, if not performed correctly with incorporation of cement into the surrounding interstices of the bone and/or neoplasm, balloon kyphoplasty sometimes produces a separated cement ball within the void. It may also be difficult to expand the balloon in case of an osteoblastic

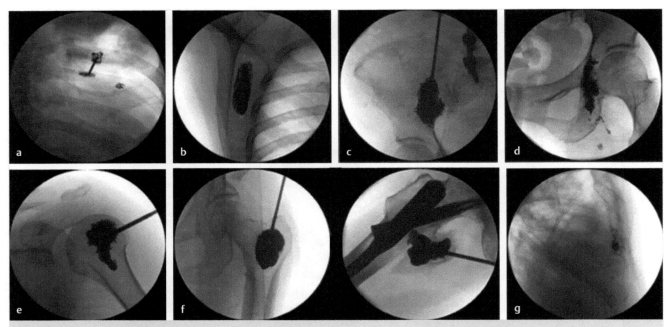

Fig. 29.6 Extraspinal percutaneous osteoplasties (POPs). **(a)** Cosoplasty, **(b)** scapuloplasty, **(c)** ilioplasty, **(d)** ischioplasty, **(e)** humeroplasty, **(f)** femoroplasty (greater trochanter and lesser trochanter), and **(g)** sternoplasty.

lesion from prostate, liver, or breast cancers. Displacement of metastatic foci may also theoretically contribute to tumor spread into the adjacent tissue during expansion of the inflatable bone tamp.[17]

29.4.2 Increased Risk of VCFs after Radiotherapy

- Even though an increased risk of VCFs, ranging from 11 to 39%, after radiotherapy has been observed,[18,19] radiotherapy along with PVP is a standard regimen for painful metastatic vertebrae. It is supposed that radiation damages the (organic) collagen rather than mineral (hydroxyapatite) components, and produces osteoradionecrosis. In cases using ≥20 Gy/fraction in patients with a lytic tumor or spinal misalignment and a baseline VCF, caution should be used.[19]
- The spinal instability neoplastic score (SINS) (▶Table 29.3)[18–20] was developed for assessing patients with spinal neoplasia and it identifies patients who may be at risk for spinal instability and would therefore benefit from surgical intervention to stabilize the spine. This scoring system is an objective measurement tool to predict the degree of stability of the metastatic spine.

29.5 Conclusion

The spine is the most common osseous structure for bony metastases. The thoracic vertebrae are the most common site of metastatic disease, followed by the lumbosacral and cervical vertebrae.

A common feature of painful metastatic compression fractures is the presence of intractable pain when the patient is in a weight-bearing position or transitional pain when changing positions from standing to sitting or sitting to laying down. Access to diagnostic imaging modalities such as conventional X-rays, bone scans, CT, PET-CT, and MRI is essential.

Vertebral body cement fill equal to 15 to 25% of the thoracolumbar vertebrae (approximately 3.5–6.0 mL) is a sufficient amount to treat the pain from the neoplasm as well as to reestablish the strength and stiffness of the vertebral body.[14,15] Pain relief from PVP originates from not only the stabilization provided by the augmentation but also the thermal and chemical ablation from the polymethyl methacrylate (PMMA). Due to its strength, resistance to compression, and exothermic reaction, PMMA is preferred to calcium phosphate for painful metastatic compression fractures.

It is important when treating the cervical and sacral vertebrae to understand their anatomy and adjacent major neurovascular structures. Technical accuracy and knowledge of important surrounding structures are essential when performing cervical PVP, especially at C1 and C2, to avoid unnecessary complications or injury to the cervical neurovascular structures. Cervical procedures may require multiple imaging modalities for guidance, including ultrasound, fluoroscopy, and CT.

In conclusion, PVP provides immediate and durable pain relief in patients with painful metastatic VCFs. The pain relief from stabilizing the vertebral body is substantial and cannot be provided by analgesics, including opioids and nonsteroidal anti-inflammatory drugs. Medications rendered unnecessary by PVP, especially sensorium altering medications, may be reduced or eliminated following a successful vertebroplasty.

Table 29.3 Spinal instability neoplastic score (SINS)

1. Patient specific	
Pain	
Mechanical pain	3
Occasional pain but not mechanical	1
Pain free	0
2. Spine specific	
(1) Location	
Junctional spine: occiput-C2, C7–T2, T11–L1, L5–S1	3
Mobile spine: C3–C6	2
Semi-rigid spine: T3–T10	1
Rigid spine: S2–S5	0
(2) Spinal alignment	
Subluxation/translation	4
Kyphosis/scoliosis	2
Normal	0
(3) Presence of vertebral compression fracture	
≥ 50% collapse	3
< 50% collapse	2
No collapse with ≥ 50% body involved	1
None of the above	0
3. Tumor specific	
(1) Type of lesion	
Osteolytic	2
Mixed	1
Osteosclerotic	0
(2) Posterolateral involvement of spinal elements	
Bilateral	3
Unilateral	1
None	0
Total SINS	
0–6	Stable
7–12	Potentially unstable
13–18	Unstable

References

[1] Galibert P, Deramond H, Rosat P, Le Gars D. Preliminary note on the treatment of vertebral angioma by percutaneous acrylic vertebroplasty Neurochirurgie 1987;33(2):166–168

[2] Aebi M. Spinal metastasis in the elderly. Eur Spine J 2003;12(Suppl 2): S202–S213

[3] Kim TK, Kim KH, Kim CH, et al. Percutaneous vertebroplasty and facet joint block. J Korean Med Sci 2005;20(6):1023–1028

[4] Hollen PJ, Gralla RJ, Kris MG, et al. Measurement of quality of life in patients with lung cancer in multicenter trials of new therapies: psychometric assessment of the Lung Cancer Symptom Scale. Cancer 1994;73(8):2087–2098

[5] Tokuhashi Y, Matsuzaki H, Oda H, Oshima M, Ryu J. A revised scoring system for preoperative evaluation of metastatic spine tumor prognosis. Spine 2005;30(19):2186–2191

[6] Anderson LD, D'Alonzo RT. Fractures of the odontoid process of the axis. 1974. J Bone Joint Surg Am 2004;86(9):2081

[7] Yoon JY, Kim TK, Kim KH. Anterolateral percutaneous vertebroplasty at C2 for lung cancer metastasis and upper cervical facet joint block. Clin J Pain 2008;24(7):641–646

[8] Seo SS, Lee DH, Kim HJ, Yoon JW, Kwon OS, Kim KH. Percutaneous vertebroplasty at C7 for the treatment of painful metastases: a case report. Korean J Anesthesiol 2013;64(3):276–279

[9] Kim KH. Preoperative motion-related pain in cancer patients with extraspinal metastases treated by percutaneous osteoplasty. J Anesthe Clinic Rec 2011;S1:004

[10] Smith HS, Mohsin I. Painful boney metastases. Korean J Pain 2013;26(3): 223–241

[11] Yi YR, Lee NR, Kwon YS, Jang JS, Lim SY. Pulsed radiofrequency application for the treatment of pain secondary to sacroiliac joint metastases. Korean J Pain 2016;29(1):53–56

[12] Lee JH, Kim SY, Ok HG, Kim TK, Kim KH. Extraspinal percutaneous osteoplasty for the treatment of painful bony metastasis. J Korean Med Sci 2018;33(8):e61

[13] Berenson J, Pflugmacher R, Jarzem P, et al; Cancer Patient Fracture Evaluation (CAFE) Investigators. Balloon kyphoplasty versus non-surgical fracture management for treatment of painful vertebral body compression fractures in patients with cancer: a multicentre, randomised controlled trial. Lancet Oncol 2011;12(3):225–235

[14] Martinčič D, Brojan M, Kosel F, et al. Minimum cement volume for vertebroplasty. Int Orthop 2015;39(4):727–733

[15] Luo J, Daines L, Charalambous A, Adams MA, Annesley-Williams DJ, Dolan P. Vertebroplasty: only small cement volumes are required to normalize stress distributions on the vertebral bodies. Spine 2009;34(26):2865–2873

[16] Ma XL, Xing D, Ma JX, Xu WG, Wang J, Chen Y. Balloon kyphoplasty versus percutaneous vertebroplasty in treating osteoporotic vertebral compression fracture: grading the evidence through a systematic review and meta-analysis. Eur Spine J 2012;21(9):1844–1859

[17] Cruz JP, Sahgal A, Whyne C, Fehlings MG, Smith R. Tumor extravasation following a cement augmentation procedure for vertebral compression fracture in metastatic spinal disease. J Neurosurg Spine 2014;21(3):372–377

[18] Sahgal A, Whyne CM, Ma L, Larson DA, Fehlings MG. Vertebral compression fracture after stereotactic body radiotherapy for spinal metastases. Lancet Oncol 2013;14(8):e310–e320

[19] Sahgal A, Atenafu EG, Chao S, et al. Vertebral compression fracture after spine stereotactic body radiotherapy: a multi-institutional analysis with a focus on radiation dose and the spinal instability neoplastic score. J Clin Oncol 2013;31(27):3426–3431

[20] Fisher CG, Schouten R, Versteeg AL, et al. Reliability of the spinal instability neoplastic score (SINS) among radiation oncologists: an assessment of instability secondary to spinal metastases. Radiat Oncol 2014;9:69

30 Vertebral Augmentation in Instrumented Spinal Fusions

John W. Amburgy, Patrick R. Pritchard, Steven M. Theiss, James Mooney, D. Mitchell Self, and M. R. Chambers

Summary

Vertebral augmentation is a minimally invasive treatment known to reduce pain and disability and improve the quality of life in patients with painful vertebral fractures. In addition to its applications across a wide range of etiologies, it offers promise in select patients when used in combination with instrumented fixation to help alleviate spinal instability. These patients often have elevated risks of hardware failure, collapse of constructs, and junctional fractures. Supplemental vertebral augmentation of pedicle screw fixation may mitigate these risks. Biomechanical studies demonstrate improved pullout strength of augmented screws placed into osteoporotic bone.

Keywords: vertebral augmentation, spinal fusion, pedicle screws, spinal fixation, burst fracture, osteopenia, osteoporosis

30.1 Introduction

The utility of vertebral augmentation is quite broad with applications ranging from the treatment of complications of benign disease such as osteoporosis to primary malignancies and metastatic disease. An important application is its use in combination with instrumented fixation in patients with spinal instability. These patients are a heterogeneous population but they have in common the need for bony vertebral fusion. They often have elevated risks of hardware failure, collapse of constructs, and junctional fractures. Supplemental vertebral augmentation of pedicle screw fixation offers the spine surgeon intraoperative options to mitigate these risks.

30.2 Instrumentation in Spinal Fusion

Roy-Camille is credited with the first description of posterior plates with screws positioned sagittally through the pedicles and articular processes with a system that he and Judet had been using since 1963.[1] This became the foundation for pedicle screw fixation. Harrington and Tullos described the first transpedicular screw placement in the United States in 1969. Subsequent pedicle screw systems and modifications came from Louis, Steffee, Magerl, Luque, Wiltse, and others. Design modifications continue today in an effort to improve purchase, strength, and fusion outcomes.[2–5]

In 1991, Lorenz et al prospectively evaluated 68 patients with at least 6 months of disabling back pain who had failed conservative care to compare single-level posterolateral lumbar fusions (PLF) with and without pedicle screws. Twenty-nine patients were fused without hardware and 39 were fused with variable screw placement (VSP) fixation. An improved fusion rate was reported for patients undergoing pedicle screw fixation with pseudarthrosis seen in 58.6% of the non-instrumented group and no pseudarthrosis in instrumented patients. Pain improvement was better in the instrumented group (76.9 vs. 41.4%) and the rate of return to work was higher in the instrumented patients (72 vs. 31%) compared to the non-instrumented patients.[6]

In a report to the contrary, Thomsen et al suggested that pedicle screw fixation did not affect functional improvement or fusion rates long-term.[7] Despite this controversy, pedicle screw fixation has become routine in posterolateral fusions. Guidelines for the performance of fusion procedures for degenerative disease of the lumbar spine were published in the *Journal of Neurosurgery Spine* in 2014. An association, but no direct correlation, was reported between increased fusion rates and pedicle screw and rod fixation as assessed with dynamic radiographs. Despite the routine nature of this practice, the guidelines recommend "the use of pedicle screw fixation as a supplement to PLF (posterolateral fusion) be reserved for those patients in whom there is an increased risk of nonunion when treated with only PLF."[8]

Although an in-depth analysis of the addition of pedicle screw fixation to fusion constructs is not the focus of this chapter, one must understand that attempts to further stabilize the pedicle screw may be inextricably linked to data correlating pedicle screw fixation to improve the stability of the fusion and therefore the functional and radiographic outcomes. As seen in the examples above, results are not definitive.

30.3 Vertebral Augmentation in Spinal Fusion

Data supporting vertebral augmentation and its benefit to spinal fusion date back over 30 years. In 1986, Zindrick et al[18] assessed various biomechanical performances of sacral screw fixation, including fixation augmented with polymethyl methacrylate (PMMA). The authors reported that placement of PMMA around a loosened screw restored fixation and doubled its pullout force. This was reproduced in osteoporotic models of the lumbar spine by Soshi et al[9] who measured the pullout force of a 7-mm pedicle screw on normal cadaveric lumbar vertebrae compared to those with mild and severely osteoporotic bone. A pullout force of 1,056.4 N was required in the normal, non-osteoporotic group, 495.6 N in the mildly osteoporotic group, and 269.5 N in the severely osteoporotic group. The use of bone cement for augmentation reduced the risk of screw pullout in the osteoporotic vertebrae by a twofold increase in pullout strength.[9]

Mermelstein et al further categorized the bending moments of pedicle screws augmented with calcium phosphate (CP) cement. The bending moment was reduced by 59% in flexion and 38% in extension, and the mean stiffness was increased by 40%.[10] Sarzier et al reported in 2002 that augmentation of osteoporotic vertebrae increased pedicle screw pullout forces. The maximum attainable force was approximately twice the pullout force of the non-augmented pedicle screws for each osteoporotic (Jikei scale) grade. The mean increase in pullout force in osteoporotic spines was 181% for Grade I, 206% for Grade II, and 213% for Grade III.[11]

30.4 Indications

Vertebral augmentation is used to treat vertebral compression fractures (VCFs) across a wide range of etiologies. Augmentation of spinal instrumentation may be indicated for a select patient population, including osteoporotic patients, those requiring revision surgery, especially those high-risk patients who may not tolerate lengthy general anesthesia and surgery, and adults with spinal deformity. In osteoporotic patients, augmentation may reduce the risk of screw pullout. In addition, patients who require revision of their instrumented spinal fusion should benefit from augmentation as it increases the stiffness and pullout strength of the replacement screws. Augmentation in high-risk patients can be used to provide construct stability and prolonged pain relief. Finally, augmentation has been shown to decrease the need for revisions and reduce the risk of proximal junctional fractures (PJFs) following instrumentation in adults with spinal deformities.[12,13] See ▶ Fig. 30.1.

30.5 Outcomes and Variables

Many variables affect outcomes following instrumented fusion, with or without augmentation. Here, we review outcomes of fusions with vertebral augmentation as they relate to etiology, method of delivery, instrumentation, cement composition, volume, and timing.

30.5.1 Osteoporosis

Significant risk of screw pullout and fractures exist in osteoporotic patients as coercive attempts at deformity correction are made with instrumentation. The risk of hardware failure

is proportional to corrective forces applied. In osteoporotic patients, bone quality becomes most important in determining outcomes and the axiom, "bone holds metal; metal doesn't hold bone" applies. Pedicle screw augmentation with PMMA improves the initial fixation strength and fatigue strength of instrumentation in osteoporotic vertebrae. Numerous studies of the lumbar and thoracic spine, ilium, and sacrum demonstrate a 1.5- to 2-fold increase in pullout strength of augmented screws compared to non-augmented screws.[9,11,14–16] This benefit may be realized only in low-quality bone of osteopenic and osteoporotic patients.[17]

30.5.2 Revision Surgery

Similar to results in osteoporotic patients, PMMA or other cements can salvage screw fixation and increase the force required for pullout twofold.[18] The pullout strength of augmented replacement screws in thoracolumbar vertebrae returned to baseline or increased above baseline in these revision cases.[19,20] Initial and final stiffness of the larger diameter screws was also increased with the addition of the cement augmentation.[21]

30.5.3 Select High-Risk Patients

Comorbid disease or poor general health may preclude internal fixation and fusion surgery. In these select patients, vertebral augmentation may provide an alternative. For example, Puri and Erdem[22] described two patients with multiple myeloma who had failed posterior spinal interbody fusions and had significant pain, but were felt to be at high risk of complications from general anesthesia due to their multiple comorbidities. Rather than lengthy construct revisions under general anesthesia, unilateral

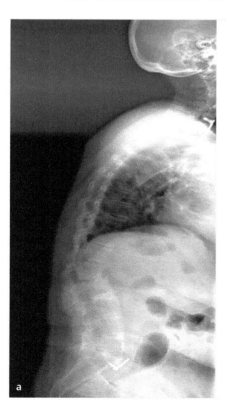
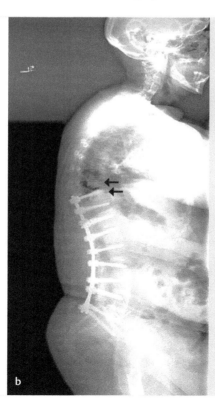

Fig. 30.1 (a, b) Sixty-five-year old female who underwent an instrumented fusion from T10 to the pelvis with a Smith Peterson osteotomy at L1–L2. Along with the instrumentation, she had polymethyl methacrylate (PMMA) placed in the upper instrumented vertebra (UIV) and the vertebra immediately cephalad to the construct (UIV+1) (*black arrows* in **b**). (This image is provided courtesy of Dr. Steven M. Theiss, MD.)

transpedicular vertebroplasties were performed under intravenous conscious sedation.

The first patient had previously undergone thoracic vertebrectomy with interbody device placement and dorsal internal fixation from T6 to T10. Six months later, when recurrent pain prompted MR and CT imaging, construct failure and apparent loosening of the interbody device was identified. Believing that constant micromotion by the cage might be causing the pain, the authors performed transpedicular vertebroplasty with a diamond-tipped needle placed in the anterior third of the T9 vertebral body. With real-time fluoroscopic guidance, PMMA cement was deliberately directed upward toward the cage at T6–T8. The cement crossed several disk spaces and surrounded the cage anteriorly with some minor filling of the cage.

The second patient had undergone partial corpectomy at L3 with placement of a left paracentral interbody device and dorsal fixation from L2 and L4. Pain recurred approximately 7 months after surgery. MR and CT imaging demonstrated a new compression fracture at L1 and lucencies around the L2–L4 construct. After vertebroplasty was performed at L1, attention was turned to L3. A right parapedicular injection was used to deliver PMMA cement across the midline to the left side anterior to the cage, then a transpedicular injection delivered additional cement to the right side of remaining L3 vertebral body, also anterior to the cage.

Both patients had significant reductions in pain and at 18 months, the constructs demonstrated stability and patients had continued pain relief.[22]

30.5.4 Adult Spinal Deformity

Adult patients with spinal deformity and long-segment (>5 levels) instrumented fusions are at high risk of proximal junctional kyphosis (PJK), PJFs, and hardware failure (▶Fig. 30.2). This is particularly true in patients with deformity in the sagittal plane. While the specific etiology of these junctional problems is often multifactorial, they are generally due to the stress riser that naturally occurs at the junction of the instrumented and uninstrumented spine.

This is particularly true at the upper instrumented vertebra (UIV) and the vertebra immediately cephalad to the construct (UIV+1). Junctional kyphosis is differentiated into PJK and PJF. PJK is defined as kyphosis of greater than 10 degrees in the segment above a long construct compared with preoperative measurements, while PJF is defined as a structural failure of the spinal column with vertebral body fracture, failure of the posterior ligamentous complex, screw pullout, and vertebral subluxation. Vertebral augmentation is used to prevent both PJK and PJF and has been shown to be effective.[23] Hart et al[24] revealed a 15% reduction in the incidence of PJF following kyphoplasty cranial to the UIV. Martin et al[25] reported that only 5% of patients who underwent vertebral augmentation at UIV and UIV+1 had PJF, much lower than the historic rate without vertebral augmentation. Theologis and Burch[12] went further to report that patients with UIV and UIV+1 augmentation had fewer revisions due to fractures (0 vs. 19), better functional outcomes, and significantly less disability. Patients without augmentation were 9.2 times more likely to undergo revision surgery than those with prophylactic UIV and UIV+1 augmentation. Ghobrial et al[13] reported a decreased incidence (23.7 vs. 36%)

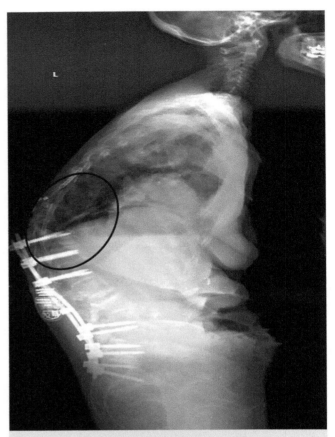

Fig. 30.2 Proximal junctional kyphosis (PJK) (area within *black oval*) following a lengthy instrumented fusion. (This image is provided courtesy of Dr. Steven M. Theiss, MD.)

and magnitude (5.65 vs. 9.36 degrees) of PJK in patients with UIV and UIV+1 kyphoplasties. In addition to the early clinical studies examining the effectiveness of vertebral augmentation in the prevention of junctional kyphosis, biomechanical studies have been done as well. Cadaveric analyses of augmentation at UIV and UIV+1 (▶Fig. 30.1) demonstrated fewer PJFs (17%) than those with only a single-level vertebroplasty (that was not at the UIV or UIV+1 level) (67%) or spines without cement (100%)[26] (▶Fig. 30.3).

30.5.5 Method of Delivery

Cement delivery may be made through standard transpedicular delivery with injection directly into the cancellous bone or via balloon kyphoplasty techniques with augmentation prior to the placement of pedicle screws. This allows the cement to cure or harden around the screws. Pedicle screws placed in osteoporotic vertebrae had higher pullout loads when augmented with the kyphoplasty technique compared to vertebroplasty augmentation (1414 +/– 338 vs. 756 +/– 300 N, respectively; $p < 0.001$).[27] In addition, an unpaired t-test showed that fatigued pedicle screws in osteoporotic vertebrae augmented by kyphoplasty showed higher pullout resistance than those placed in healthy control vertebrae ($p = 0.002$).[27] Both kyphoplasty-type augmentation ($p = 0.007$) and vertebroplasty augmentation ($p = 0.02$) increased pullout loads compared to pedicle screws

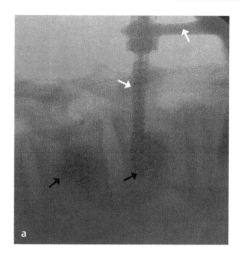
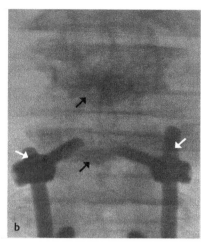

Fig. 30.3 Lateral (**a**) and anteroposterior (**b**) fluoroscopic views show vertebral augmentation with polymethyl methacrylate (PMMA) at upper instrumented vertebra (UIV) and UIV+1 (*black arrows*) in a patient who has previously undergone pedicle screw and rod augmentation (*white arrows*). (This image is provided courtesy of Fred Parsons, RT.)

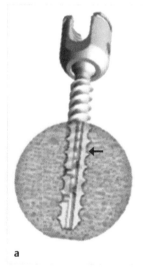
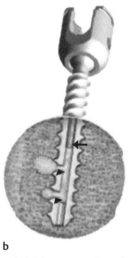
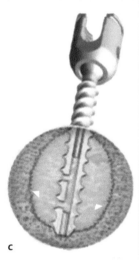

Fig. 30.4 Examples of fenestrated pedicle screw used for polymethyl methacrylate (PMMA) delivery to cancellous bone.[29] The screw (*black arrow* in **a**) has a central channel (*black arrow* in **b**) with fenestrations (*black arrowheads*) through which PMMA can be injected (*white arrowheads* in **c**).

placed in non-augmented osteoporotic vertebrae when tested after fatigue cycling.[27]

Alternatively, cannulated or fenestrated pedicle screws may be placed and then cement injected through the screws. Cement injected through a cannulated screw is injected into the vertebral body while cement injected into a fenestrated screw surrounds the screw by the PMMA flowing through the fenestrations within the pedicle screw[28] (▶ Fig. 30.4).

During PMMA delivery through screws with different numbers of side holes (fenestrations), Chen et al[30] noted (1) a large amount of PMMA flowed out from the oppositely arranged proximal side holes, whereas almost no PMMA was observed in the distal holes; and (2) the nearer the proximal side hole was to the screw head the greater the risk of cement leakage.[30] Published results comparing the conventional needle injection of cement technique around the pedicle screws to delivery of the cement via cannulated screws indicate that although the pullout strength and screw backout torque was significantly higher in the needle injection group (234.1 vs. 187.8 N, 1119.6 vs. 836.7 N mm, respectively), the operation time was shorter and the cement leakage rate was less in the cannulated pedicle screw group (211.4 vs. 296.3 min, 14.05 vs. 26.2%, respectively).[31,32]

The number, design, and specific layout of the fenestrations of the screw may affect pullout strength.[33] Based on the biomechanical performance of various cement-augmented cannulated screw designs, Tolunay et al[32] declared in 2015 that the unilateral, sequential, three-radial hole, drilled, cannulated screw was the optimal alternative when considering pullout and torsional strength as criteria. In the same year, Dai et al[34] described "a new approach for the application of PMMA augmentation of bone cement-injectable cannulated pedicle screws." Forty-three consecutive patients with osteoporosis and a degenerative disk disease who had failed at least 6 months of conservative therapy underwent fusion with a novel bone cement-injectable cannulated pedicle screw (CICPS) (Kanghui Medical Devices Co., Ltd., Jiangsu, China). All patients were followed for a mean of 15.7±5.6 months (range: 6–35 months). The Visual Analog Scale and Oswestry Disability Index scores showed a significant reduction in back pain ($p = 0.018$) and an improvement in lower extremity function ($p = 0.025$) in patients who underwent lumbar fusion using the novel screw. Intraoperative cement leakage occurred in four patients, but no neurological complications were observed. Radiological observation indicated no loosening or pulling out of the novel screw, and the bone fusion was excellent.

30.5.6 Thoracolumbar Burst Fractures

While cement augmentation of pedicle screw instrumentation can improve the fixation of the screws as described above, other methods of improving fixation in traumatic burst fractures (▶ Fig. 30.5 and ▶ Fig. 30.6) have been investigated. Norton et al[35] performed a biomechanical analysis of treatment for thoracolumbar burst fractures, comparing a four-screw construct (instrumentation immediately above and below the fracture site) to a six-screw construct (pedicle instrumentation of the burst fracture and one level above and one level below). The authors noted a high rate of failure of fixation and early loss of reduction following the four-screw posterior short-segment instrumentation technique. Additional pedicle screws at the level of the fracture (six-screw construct) provided results superior to those utilizing only a four-screw construct. As the additional fixation at the level of the fracture was hypothesized to increase stiffness and reduce the stress on other pedicle screws, a more recent evaluation examined the addition of vertebral augmentation to the four-screw construct compared to the six-screw construct without cement. Clinical outcomes were similar but the traditional six-screw construct was advantageous in terms of shorter operating times, lower blood loss, and lower failure rates.[36] However, finite element analysis (FEA) demonstrated that short-segment fixation with two intermediate pedicle screws (the six-screw construct) together with cement at the fractured vertebrae may provide a stiffer construct and less stress on the pedicle screws and rods as compared to other types of short-segment fixation.[37] This has yet to be clinically demonstrated. The ability of augmentation of the fractured vertebrae to aid in reduction of traumatic deformity has been investigated. Oner et al[38] showed in a cadaveric burst model that balloon-assisted end-plate reduction resulted in predictable reduction of the end plate and kyphosis when combined with vertebral augmentation.[38] However, vertebral augmentation combined with posterior instrumentation does not necessarily prevent kyphosis recurrence. Aono et al[39] showed that kyphosis recurrence following four-screw constructs can occur even when combined with vertebral augmentation. This is not a result of collapse of the fractured vertebral body, but rather collapse of the adjacent disk, which is injured at the time of the traumatic episode. End-plate reduction and vertebral augmentation though does not affect ultimate disk space collapse.[39]

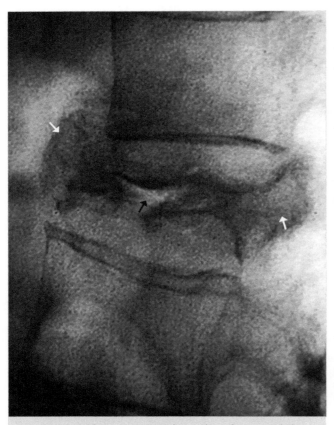

Fig. 30.5 Lateral fluoroscopic view shows a burst fracture with the anterior and posterior portions of the vertebral body wider in the anteroposterior dimension than the vertebral body above (*white arrows*). The image also shows air within the vertebral body (*black arrow*).

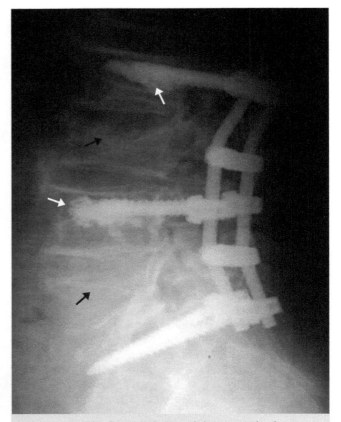

Fig. 30.6 Lateral radiograph shows pedicle screw and rod construct stabilized with polymethyl methacrylate (PMMA) at the level above the L3 fracture and at L4 below the upper fracture (*white arrows*) and the vertebral compression fractures (VCFs) (*black arrows*) that are spanned by the construct.

30.5.7 Cement

In vitro data have suggested that augmentation of pedicle screws with PMMA redistributes the pullout forces from the interface of the bone and screw alone to the entire augmented vertebral body and surrounding cortex.[11]

Cement Composition

Chapter 7 provides a detailed discussion of the various cements and fill materials. PMMA is the most popular bone cement used in vertebral augmentation. The development of PMMA began in 1928 and was first used in orthopaedic surgery in the mid-1950s. It was FDA-approved for treating VCFs in 2004. PMMA is inexpensive, has excellent biocompatibility, and has been associated with minimal long-term complications. However, cardiovascular complications including unpredictable hypotension can occur with its use,[28,40] and it may aggravate cardiovascular deterioration in the event of pulmonary cement embolism by stimulating coagulation.[41]

Other less commonly used bone cements include calcium phosphate (CP), calcium sulfate (CS), calcium triglyceride (CT), and magnesium phosphate (MP). Calcium-based cements typically require 24 hours for curing and thus do not enhance fixation at the time of surgery. They have a lower viscosity and therefore a higher potential for extravasation, although clinical relevance has not been demonstrated.[28] In biomechanical analyses, PMMA may have a higher pullout strength and resistance to failure.[20,42,43]

Cement Volume

While most studies of vertebroplasty describe cement volumes between 2 and 5 mL, many reports note that cement volumes ranging between 2 and 3 mL maximize the initial pullout strength of the screws and that higher volumes may increase the likelihood of cement extravasation.[19,44] In a biomechanical analysis comparing pullout strength after standard transpedicular vertebroplasty vs. kyphoplasty, higher volumes of cement were correlated with increased pullout strength.[27,33] In 2016, Tan et al[33] investigated the optimum injection volume of PMMA to augment a then-novel fenestrated pedicle screw with diameter-tapered perforations. They evaluated how the distribution of cement affected the biomechanical performance of the screw. Study results indicated 1.5 mL of PMMA was a conservative volume for augmentation and that more cement would significantly increase the risk of cement leakage.

Timing of Cement Placement

Based on the in vitro data suggesting that augmentation of pedicle screws with PMMA redistributes the corrective pullout forces from the interface of the bone and screw alone to the entire augmented vertebral body and surrounding cortex, and the theory that screw failure occurs at the bone-cement interface when screws are placed in "soft" cement, it has been suggested that allowing the cement to partially cure prior to screw placement may improve outcomes.[11,20] CP cement takes up to 24 hours to harden and therefore does not allow for placement of screws into "hardened" cement, but PMMA, which cures more quickly, may be the best cement for pedicle screw augmentation.[28]

Regarding the order of screw placement and augmentation, Zapałowicz et al described the ease and benefits of performing vertebral augmentation *after* the placement of screws with good outcomes.[45] Screw placement was followed by extrapedicular vertebroplasty in 22 vertebrae. Radiographically, 73% of the cement was placed centrally and 95% of the vertebral bodies were filled to greater than 70% of their height. There was only a single screw that was not at least partially surrounded by cement. There was a 45% rate of extravasation, but none were symptomatic or clinically relevant.

30.6 Conclusion

Instrumentation has long been used to treat spinal instability. Decades of design modifications have led to improved screw purchase, shorter construct strength, and better fusion outcomes. Vertebral augmentation following instrumentation may further improve outcomes in select patients. Used in combination with pedicle screw fixation, vertebral augmentation offers special promise treating pain and spinal instability in osteoporotic and cancer patients. These patients have elevated risks of hardware failure, collapse of constructs, and junctional fractures.

Outcomes of fusions with vertebral augmentation may vary by etiology, instrumentation, and cement. The cement composition, volume, timing, and method of delivery may all affect success. Biomechanical studies demonstrate improved pullout strength of augmented pedicle screws compared to non-augmented screws in the lumbar and thoracic spine, ilium, and sacrum of osteoporotic patients. Augmentation has been shown to decrease the need for revisions and reduce the risk of PJFs following instrumentation in adults with spinal deformities.

Numerous investigators have correlated outcomes with volumes and methods of cement delivery as well as the biochemical and mechanical properties of available bone cements. PMMA is the most commonly used bone cement and, based on its physical properties, may be the best cement for pedicle screw augmentation. The volume of cement delivered is limited by the risk of leakage. Cement delivery may be made using standard vertebroplasty or balloon kyphoplasty techniques prior to the placement of pedicle screws or via cannulated and/or fenestrated screws. Although there are reports noting the ease and benefit of performing vertebral augmentation after the placement of screws, placement of cement prior to the screws allows the cement to cure or harden around the screws. This may facilitate redistribution of the corrective pullout forces from the interface of the bone and screw alone to the entire augmented vertebral body and surrounding cortex.

Vertebral augmentation is known to reduce pain and disability and improve the quality of life in patients with painful vertebral fractures. In addition to its applications across a wide range of etiologies, it offers promise in select patients when used in combination with instrumented fixation for spinal instability.

References

[1] Roy-Camille R, Saillant G, Berteaux D, Salgado V. Osteosynthesis of thoraco-lumbar spine fractures with metal plates screwed through the vertebral pedicles. Reconstr Surg Traumatol 1976;15(15):2–16

[2] Roy-Camille R, Sailant G, Bisserie M. Surgical treatment of spinal metastatic tumors by posterior plating and laminectomy. In: Proceedings of the 51st Annual Meeting of the American Academy of Orthopaedic Surgeons; 1984

[3] Roy-Camille R, Sailant G, Lapresle P, et al. A secret in spine surgery: the pedicle. In: Proceedings of the 51st Annual Meeting of the American Academy of Orthopaedic Surgeons; 1984

[4] Roy-Camille R, Saillant G, Mazel C. Internal fixation of the lumbar spine with pedicle screw plating. Clin Orthop Relat Res 1986(203):7–17

[5] Kabins M, Weinstein J. The history of vertebral screw and pedicle screw fixation. Iowa Orthop J 1991;11:127–136

[6] Lorenz M, Zindrick M, Schwaeger P, et al. A comparison of single-level fusions with and without hardware. Spine 1991;16(8, Suppl):S455–S458

[7] Thomsen K, Christensen FB, Eiskjaer SP, Hansen ES, Fruensgaard S, Bünger CE. 1997 Volvo Award winner in clinical studies. The effect of pedicle screw instrumentation on functional outcome and fusion rates in posterolateral lumbar spinal fusion: a prospective, randomized clinical study. Spine 1997;22(24):2813–2822

[8] Groff MW. Introduction: guideline update for the performance of fusion procedures for degenerative disease of the lumbar spine. J Neurosurg Spine 2014;21(1):1

[9] Soshi S, Shiba R, Kondo H, Murota K. An experimental study on transpedicular screw fixation in relation to osteoporosis of the lumbar spine. Spine 1991;16(11):1335–1341

[10] Mermelstein LE, McLain RF, Yerby SA. Reinforcement of thoracolumbar burst fractures with calcium phosphate cement: a biomechanical study. Spine 1998;23(6):664–670, discussion 670–671

[11] Sarzier JS, Evans AJ, Cahill DW. Increased pedicle screw pullout strength with vertebroplasty augmentation in osteoporotic spines. J Neurosurg 2002;96(3, Suppl):309–312

[12] Theologis AA, Burch S. Prevention of acute proximal junctional fractures after long thoracolumbar posterior fusions for adult spinal deformity using 2-level cement augmentation at the upper instrumented vertebra and the vertebra 1 level proximal to the upper instrumented vertebra. Spine 2015;40(19):1516–1526

[13] Ghobrial GM, Eichberg DG, Kolcun JPG, et al. Prophylactic vertebral cement augmentation at the uppermost instrumented vertebra and rostral adjacent vertebra for the prevention of proximal junctional kyphosis and failure following long-segment fusion for adult spinal deformity. Spine J 2017;17(10):1499–1505

[14] Liu D, Wu ZX, Pan XM, et al. Biomechanical comparison of different techniques in primary spinal surgery in osteoporotic cadaveric lumbar vertebrae: expansive pedicle screw versus polymethylmethacrylate-augmented pedicle screw. Arch Orthop Trauma Surg 2011;131(9):1227–1232

[15] Yu BS, Li ZM, Zhou ZY, et al. Biomechanical effects of insertion location and bone cement augmentation on the anchoring strength of iliac screw. Clin Biomech (Bristol, Avon) 2011;26(6):556–561

[16] Yu BS, Zhuang XM, Zheng ZM, Zhang JF, Li ZM, Lu WW. Biomechanical comparison of 4 fixation techniques of sacral pedicle screw in osteoporotic condition. J Spinal Disord Tech 2010;23(6):404–409

[17] Hoppe S, Loosli Y, Baumgartner D, Heini P, Benneker L. Influence of screw augmentation in posterior dynamic and rigid stabilization systems in osteoporotic lumbar vertebrae: a biomechanical cadaveric study. Spine 2014;39(6):E384–E389

[18] Zindrick MR, Wiltse LL, Widell EH, et al. A biomechanical study of intrapeduncular screw fixation in the lumbosacral spine. Clin Orthop Relat Res 1986(203):99–112

[19] Frankel BM, D'Agostino S, Wang C. A biomechanical cadaveric analysis of polymethylmethacrylate-augmented pedicle screw fixation. J Neurosurg Spine 2007;7(1):47–53

[20] Renner SM, Lim TH, Kim WJ, Katolik L, An HS, Andersson GB. Augmentation of pedicle screw fixation strength using an injectable calcium phosphate cement as a function of injection timing and method. Spine 2004;29(11):E212–E216

[21] Kiner DW, Wybo CD, Sterba W, Yeni YN, Bartol SW, Vaidya R. Biomechanical analysis of different techniques in revision spinal instrumentation: larger diameter screws versus cement augmentation. Spine 2008;33(24):2618–2622

[22] Puri AS, Erdem E. Salvage percutaneous vertebral augmentation in failed spinal interbody fusions associated with multiple myeloma. Spine J 2010;10(8):e5–e10

[23] Hyun SJ, Lee BH, Park JH, Kim KJ, Jahng TA, Kim HJ. Proximal junctional kyphosis and proximal junctional failure following adult spinal deformity surgery. Korean J Spine 2017;14(4):126–132

[24] Hart RA, Prendergast MA, Roberts WG, Nesbit GM, Barnwell SL. Proximal junctional acute collapse cranial to multi-level lumbar fusion: a cost analysis of prophylactic vertebral augmentation. Spine J 2008;8(6):875–881

[25] Martin CT, Skolasky RL, Mohamed AS, Kebaish KM. Preliminary results of the effect of prophylactic vertebroplasty on the incidence of proximal junctional complications after posterior spinal fusion to the low thoracic spine. Spine Deform 2013;1(2):132–138

[26] Kebaish KM, Martin CT, O'Brien JR, LaMotta IE, Voros GD, Belkoff SM. Use of vertebroplasty to prevent proximal junctional fractures in adult deformity surgery: a biomechanical cadaveric study. Spine J 2013;13(12):1897–1903

[27] Burval DJ, McLain RF, Milks R, Inceoglu S. Primary pedicle screw augmentation in osteoporotic lumbar vertebrae: biomechanical analysis of pedicle fixation strength. Spine 2007;32(10):1077–1083

[28] Hoppe S, Keel MJ. Pedicle screw augmentation in osteoporotic spine: indications, limitations and technical aspects. Eur J Trauma Emerg Surg 2017;43(1):3–8

[29] Lubansu A, Rynkowski M, Abeloos L, Appelboom G, Dewitte O. Minimally invasive spinal arthrodesis in osteoporotic population using a cannulated and fenestrated augmented screw: technical description and clinical experience. Minim Invasive Surg 2012;2012:507826

[30] Chen LH, Tai CL, Lai PL, et al. Pullout strength for cannulated pedicle screws with bone cement augmentation in severely osteoporotic bone: influences of radial hole and pilot hole tapping. Clin Biomech (Bristol, Avon) 2009;24(8):613–618

[31] Chang MC, Kao HC, Ying SH, Liu CL. Polymethylmethacrylate augmentation of cannulated pedicle screws for fixation in osteoporotic spines and comparison of its clinical results and biomechanical characteristics with the needle injection method. J Spinal Disord Tech 2013;26(6):305–315

[32] Tolunay T, Arslan K, Yaman O, Dalbayrak S, Demir T. Biomechanical performance of various cement-augmented cannulated pedicle screw designs for osteoporotic bones. Spine Deform 2015;3(3):205–210

[33] Tan QC, Wu JW, Peng F, et al. Augmented PMMA distribution: improvement of mechanical property and reduction of leakage rate of a fenestrated pedicle screw with diameter-tapered perforations. J Neurosurg Spine 2016;24(6):971–977

[34] Dai F, Liu Y, Zhang F, et al. Surgical treatment of the osteoporotic spine with bone cement-injectable cannulated pedicle screw fixation: technical description and preliminary application in 43 patients. Clinics (São Paulo) 2015;70(2):114–119

[35] Norton RP, Milne EL, Kaimrajh DN, Eismont FJ, Latta LL, Williams SK. Biomechanical analysis of four- versus six-screw constructs for short-segment pedicle screw and rod instrumentation of unstable thoracolumbar fractures. Spine J 2014;14(8):1734–1739

[36] Liao JC, Fan KF. Posterior short-segment fixation in thoracolumbar unstable burst fractures: transpedicular grafting or six-screw construct? Clin Neurol Neurosurg 2017;153(153):56–63

[37] Liao JC, Chen WP, Wang H. Treatment of thoracolumbar burst fractures by short-segment pedicle screw fixation using a combination of two additional pedicle screws and vertebroplasty at the level of the fracture: a finite element analysis. BMC Musculoskelet Disord 2017;18(1):262

[38] Oner FC, Verlaan JJ, Verbout AJ, Dhert WJ. Cement augmentation techniques in traumatic thoracolumbar spine fractures. Spine 2006;31(11, Suppl):S89–S95, discussion S104

[39] Aono H, Ishii K, Tobimatsu H, et al. Temporary short-segment pedicle screw fixation for thoracolumbar burst fractures: comparative study with or without vertebroplasty. Spine J 2017;17(8):1113–1119

[40] Shridhar P, Chen Y, Khalil R, et al. A review of PMMA bone cement and intra-cardiac embolism. Materials (Basel) 2016;9(10)

[41] Ding T, Yang H, Maltenfort M, Xie R. Silk fibroin added to calcium phosphate cement to prevent severe cardiovascular complications. Med Sci Monit 2010;16(9):HY23–HY26

[42] McLachlin SD, Al Saleh K, Gurr KR, Bailey SI, Bailey CS, Dunning CE. Comparative assessment of sacral screw loosening augmented with PMMA versus a calcium triglyceride bone cement. Spine 2011;36(11):E699–E704

[43] Moore DC, Maitra RS, Farjo LA, Graziano GP, Goldstein SA. Restoration of pedicle screw fixation with an in situ setting calcium phosphate cement. Spine 1997;22(15):1696–1705

[44] Fölsch C, Goost H, Figiel J, Paletta JR, Schultz W, Lakemeier S. Correlation of pull-out strength of cement-augmented pedicle screws with CT-volumetric measurement of cement. Biomed Tech (Berl) 2012;57(6):473–480

[45] Zapałowicz K, Godlewski B, Jekimov R, Grochal M. Augmentation of transpedicular screws by intraoperative vertebroplasty. Neurol Neurochir Pol 2012;46(6):560–568

31 Biomechanical Changes after Vertebral Compression Fractures

Olivier Clerk-Lamalice

Summary

Spine biomechanics are important to know as the function of the spine plays a direct role in understanding how to treat various types of vertebral compression fractures (VCFs). The degree of stability or instability, the function of the spinal unit, the sagittal balance, and the degree of kyphosis; are all important factors to optimize to ensure adequate stability and function after a vertebral compression fracture. The degree and anatomy of the fracture compression are important elements that can have an effect on the risk of future vertebral fractures. Additionally, the spine can be divided into functional spine units composed of two adjacent vertebrae, the intervertebral disk, the facet joints, and the intervening ligaments. Most of the axial load of the spine is transmitted through the vertebral bodies. The load through the lumbar spine varies dramatically will differences in posture and weight bearing with the greatest amount of spinal local being present when the patient is in the flexed standing position. This concept explains why some people are at risk of vertebral fracture when performing certain common activities of daily life. As the intervertebral disk degenerates, it places more load on the adjacent vertebral bodies and shifts the overall load more posteriorly. As the load shifts posteriorly there is less stress on the vertebral bodies resulting in less bone density and less bone strength. The combination of disk degeneration, less vertebral body strength, and a flexion neutral posture can prominently predispose the patient to a VCF.

Keywords: vertebral compression fractures, biomechanical, sagittal balance, functional spinal unit, compression force, Magerl, fracture mechanical instability

31.1 Introduction

Spine biomechanics has gained significant interest in the past few years. Key concepts such as the functional spinal unit (FSU), mechanical stability, sagittal balance, and correction of the kyphotic angle have been increasingly studied in patients with VCFs. These concepts are of paramount importance to determine the amount and location of polymethyl methacrylate (PMMA) cement or other fill material to be injected within a fractured vertebral body and to understand the importance of correcting of the end-plate deformity/kyphotic angle. By optimizing these parameters, mechanical stability and pain control can be maximized in addition to lessening the risk of adjacent-level fractures. Thus, this chapter contains some of the core knowledge of this book justifying the "How" and the "Why" for every single vertebral augmentation procedure.

An inappropriate application of these principles has previously contributed to studies that failed to demonstrate the superiority of vertebral augmentation versus a sham arm[1–3] and caused significant collateral damage in our field by decreasing therapy access while increasing the morbidity and mortality of VCF patients.[4] On the other hand, when biomechanical factors are carefully considered, optimal results can be obtained, resulting in significant and long-term improvement of the patient's pain, function, and quality of life.[5] Spine biomechanics also helps understand why vertebral augmentation decreases the risks of recurrent/adjacent-level fractures and helps determine which patient may benefit from prophylactic vertebral augmentation. We will review here the key biomechanical concepts that spine interventionists should carefully consider prior to vertebral augmentation.

31.2 Current Information based on Recent Literature and State-of-the-Art Practice

31.2.1 Physiologic Loads on the Vertebral Body

When placed under dynamic loading, the spine allows multi-directional movements that can be analyzed with a six-degree-of-freedom biomechanical model. To analyze the spine and its biomechanical characteristics, this structure is often subdivided in smaller physiological motion units called FSUs. The FSU is composed of two adjacent vertebrae, the intervertebral disk and the ligaments providing support and stability. According to a purist's definition, the FSU does not include muscles or other connecting tissues. Each vertebra of the FSU can move in space according to orthogonal X, Y, Z axes in addition to rotations along each axis. Because of the musculoligamentous apparatus and the orientation of the facet joints, physical limitations are exerted on FSUs. Furthermore, these limitations fluctuate depending on the region of the spine studied (i.e., cervical, thoracic, or lumbar). At the thoracolumbar level (where most of the VCFs happen), the forces applied on the FSU can be simplified in four main categories: compression forces (axial forces), shear forces, bending moment, and axial torque (▶ Fig. 31.1).

In the thoracolumbar spine, the majority of the axial load is borne by the vertebral bodies. Each vertebral body is composed of two structural constituents that sustain that load: the cancellous core and the cortical shell. First, the cancellous core is a dense network of inner trabeculae oriented vertically and horizontally. The vertical trabeculae support the vertebral body thin cortex (measuring approximately 0.4 mm) and resist to the axial loading by transmitting forces from the upper to the lower end plate. On the other hand, the horizontal trabeculae reinforce and provide support to the vertical trabeculae by preventing sideway displacement under compressive loading with and without shear forces. Although the thickness of the cortical bone is not substantial (approximately 0.4 mm), the bone mass attributable to the cortical shell is surprisingly large when

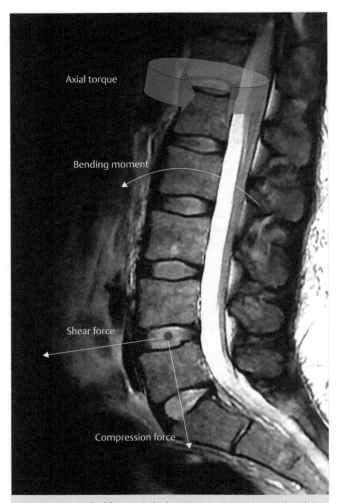

Fig. 31.1 Simplified forces applied on the spine: axial torque, bending moment, shear force, and compression force.

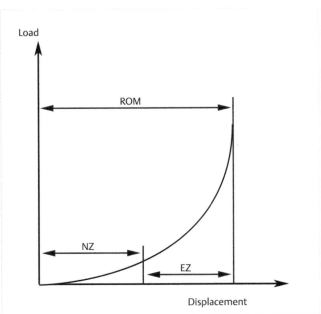

Fig. 31.2 Functional spinal unit (FSU) load-displacement curve. The relation between the load applied on the FSU and the displacement is not linear. The range of motion (ROM) of the spinal joints includes an initial neutral zone (NZ) with relatively large displacements at low load. Because of the tension provided by the ligaments and capsule, the elastic zone (EZ) has more resistance to movement leading to increased load per unit of displacement.

compared to the rest of the vertebral body, estimated to be up to ~40% of the total bone mass and providing approximately 45% of the structural support.[6] Also, the cortical shell allows less plastic deformity than the cancellous core before fracture (~2 vs. ~10%). Thus, it is unlikely to have a fracture of the core of the vertebral body without a fracture of the shell.

The physiologic range of motion (ROM) of an FSU consists of a neutral zone (NZ) and an elastic zone (EZ) (►Fig. 31.2). These characteristics (NZ and EZ) are intrinsic to any two consecutive vertebra[7] and have very different biomechanical behaviors. In the NZ, the spine undergoes relatively large motions with minimal force loading due to the laxity of ligaments and capsule. In the EZ, there is resistance to movement leading to increase load per unit of displacement[8] until failure. Several studies have demonstrated that the NZ increases with injury, muscle weakness, and degeneration. This increase in the NZ tends to lead to FSU instability. The NZ may be brought within a physiological limit with osteophyte formation, surgical fixation/fusion, and muscle strengthening.[8]

When a person stands upright, the mass of the trunk, head, and arms presses vertically on the lower lumbar spine with a force of approximately 55% of the body weight, corresponding to 385 N for a 70 kg man.[9] The measurements of the various components of spinal loads are complex and vary depending on the region of the spine evaluated, the posture (flexion vs. extension), and the angulation of the motion segment. Sato et al[10] measured in vivo spinal loads at the L4–L5 level with intradiskal pressure measurement. Those pressures were of 91 kPa in the prone position, 151 kPa in the lateral position, 539 kPa in the upright standing position, and 623 kPa in the upright sitting position. The maximum intradiskal pressure in the flexed standing position was more than twice the upright standing position with a value of 1,324 kPa. The spinal load calculated for healthy 73 kg subjects were then: 144 N prone, 240 N in lateral decubitus, 800 N upright standing, and 996 N upright sitting.[10] These results demonstrate that the vertebral body loads fluctuate significantly according to the position of the patient. This concept explains well why patients with severe osteoporosis are at risk of developing VCFs when performing simple daily tasks, such as walking, getting down the stairs, or holding groceries.

31.2.2 Impact of Disk Degeneration on the FSU

The role of the disk is to sustain compressive forces in addition to supporting shear and tensile forces.[11] The disk is an important component of the FSU as it redistributes loads from the inferior end plate of the superior vertebra to the superior end plate of the inferior vertebra. As disk degeneration increases, the intradiskal pressure measurements decrease[10] and higher loads are transmitted from one vertebral body to the other (creating peak loads) including to a posterior load redistribution that results in a greater load placed on the facet joints and vertebral arch (►Fig. 31.3). The loss of normal nucleus

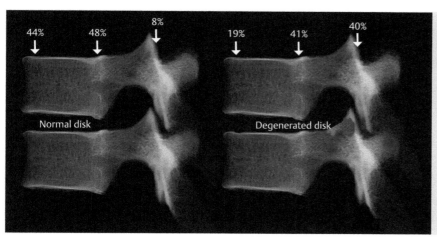

Fig. 31.3 Load redistribution in a functional spinal unit (FSU) with a normal disk and with a degenerated disk. Degenerative disk disease alters the compression loads on the vertebrae resulting in increased load toward the posterior portion of the vertebral body and neural arch. Adapted from Pollintine et al.[12]

Table 31.1 Modified Pfirrmann grading system for lumbar disk degeneration

Grade	Signal from nucleus and inner fibers of annulus	Distinction between inner and outer fibers of annulus at posterior aspect of disk	Height of disk
1	Uniformly hyperintense, equal to CSF	Distinct	Normal
2	Hyperintense (>presacral fat and <CSF) ± hypointense intranuclear cleft	Distinct	Normal
3	Hyperintense though <presacral fat	Distinct	Normal
4	Mildly hyperintense (slightly > outer fibers of annulus)	Indistinct	Normal
5	Hypointense (= outer fibers of annulus)	Indistinct	Normal
6	Hypointense	Indistinct	>30% reduction in disk height
7	Hypointense	Indistinct	30–60% reduction in disk height
8	Hypointense	Indistinct	>60% reduction in disk height

Source: Adapted from Griffith et al.[13]

pulposus microarchitecture can first be appreciated on MRI by a T2-weighted signal intensity drop of the nucleus pulposus of the disk which can be quantified with the modified Pfirrmann grading system (▶ Table 31.1).

As compressive load within a normal disk increases, the hydrostatic pressure within the nucleus pulposus also increases, and some of the inner pressure (horizontal pressure) is transferred to the annulus fibrosus by circumferential stress (hoop stress). The end-plate forces are normally evenly distributed on the anterior column with less forces transmitted to the posterior elements and facet joints. With increased disk degeneration, there is less load bearing on the ventral end plates (decreasing from 44 to 19%) and more stress on the neural arch, specifically on the facet joints (increasing from 8 to 40%) (▶ Fig. 31.3).[12] Load redistribution can be further exaggerated with extension maneuvers (in that context, up to 90% of the compressive forces can occur on the facets).

This anterior-to-posterior redistribution due to disk degeneration gives rise to *Stress Shielding*. As the load switches posteriorly, *as per* Wolff's law, there is less trabecular turnover and remodeling in the anterior vertebral body, resulting in decrease of up to 20% in the trabecular volume and increase of up to 28% in intertrabecular spacing.[14] As discussed earlier, upright flexion results in higher stress on the disk. In patients with disk degeneration, the load delta on the anterior portion of the FSU is even further increased. For example, in flexion versus neutral

position, the loads applied to the FSU can increase by up to 300%,[12] further predisposing osteoporotic patients to VCFs.

31.2.3 Biomechanical Changes after Vertebral Compression Fractures

The vertebral end plate itself or its trabecular support is the most common region of the vertebral body to fracture under stress (AO-type A1 or Magerl-type A1.1).[15–18] Because of numerous vascular channels transferring metabolites to the nucleus pulposus, the end plates represent areas of weakness within the vertebral body that are even more pronounced in osteoporotic patients.[19] Once an end-plate fracture happens, the disk loses its inner pressure.[20] This loss of internal pressure results in increased compressive loading of the anterior wall during active flexion predisposing to adjacent-level fracture[20] but also, when the patient is upright, there is an increase in the compressive stress along the posterior vertebral body, posterior annulus fibrosus, and neural arc.[21,22] These changes further contribute to the downward spiral of *Stress Shielding* seen with disk degeneration, thereby predisposing the patient to adjacent-level VCFs.

In wedge-type compression fracture (AO-type A1 or Magerl-type A1.2), segmental kyphosis contributes to stress shift toward the posterior arc of the affected and adjacent levels. This kyphosis amplifies the *Stress Shielding* of the adjacent level and also contributes to the adjacent-level fracture risk ranging from

12 to 20%.[23–26] In summary, untreated fractures result in altered FSU biomechanics that predispose to adjacent-level fracture both by creating altered peak loads amplified with flexion of the spine and with increased *Stress Shielding*, resulting in a VCF "domino" effect.

31.2.4 Technical Considerations during Vertebral Augmentation: Correcting Fracture and FSU-Related Instability

As just mentioned, after a VCF the FSU loads are displaced posteriorly (similar to degeneration of the intervertebral disk). For this reason, whenever possible, PMMA cement should be instilled within the posterior third of the vertebral body to provide further structural support and avoid collapse of the middle column (▶ Fig. 31.4). To avoid this collapse, experts in interventional pain management pay great attention to correct the kyphotic angle, realign end plates, and instill cement uniformly within the vertebral body from pedicle to pedicle, superior end plate to the inferior end plate, and the anterior cortex of the vertebral body to the posterior cortex. This process is also referred in our practice as "Civil Engineering of the Spine."

It is commonly taught in academic centers that PMMA cement should be instilled only in the anterior two-thirds of the vertebral body. The latest biomechanical data argue against this teaching since more posteriorly located structural support is required to avoid posterior wall collapse. However, additional experience and care is required to reliably perform this technique and avoid extravasation in the ventral epidural space. The degree of comminution, the Magerl fracture type and the experience of the interventionist should all be taken into consideration before attempting to more aggressively fill the vertebral body. This adequate PMMA filling will help correct the motion segment instability.

Indeed, after a VCF there are two types of instability that can be improved with vertebral augmentation:
• Fracture mechanical instability.
• FSU instability.

Fracture mechanical instability is when the FSU loading results in microscopic or macroscopic trabecular/bony displacements within the vertebral body. These displacements result in painful nociceptors stimuli transmitted via the basivertebral nerve. Mechanical stability of the fracture can only be achieved when the fracture/cleft is completely filled with PMMA cement, avoiding then all painful stimuli generated from abnormal movement. New bone will be able to grow within the cement porosity and around the cement to heal the fracture.

FSU instability is when a compression fracture alters the mechanical characteristics of the building blocks of the FSU. For instance, a compression fracture will result in decompression of the intradiskal pressure and impairs the ability of the disk to distribute load evenly to the adjacent vertebral body. Also there is an increase in the NZ,[8] resulting in increased ROM that further facilitates peak loads (for instance with flexion maneuvers). Previous studies suggest that in addition to restoring spinal sagittal alignment, the ability to restore height and kyphosis of the fractured end plate should be the ideal end point to normalized load transmission across the fractured level.[20,27]

Furthermore, other mechanical changes are noticed after VCF, such as decreased strength and stiffness. Restoring biomechanical characteristics of the FSU is highly dependent on the volume of PMMA injected. At least 16% of the vertebral body volume needs to be filled with cement to restore strength and 29% of the vertebral body volume needs to be filled to restore stiffness.[28] Interestingly, even after injection of 8 mL of PMMA at the lumbar level, the vertebral body still had not reached the prefracture stiffness level. Stiffness of the vertebral body is important to obtain after vertebral augmentation to restore intradiskal pressure and normalize the FSU load distribution. However, if the disk nucleus pulposus is severely degenerated (i.e., modified Pfirrmann grades 7 and 8), axial loading will be transferred directly to the next vertebral body end plate without being dampened by hoop stress propagating the force from the nucleus pulposus to

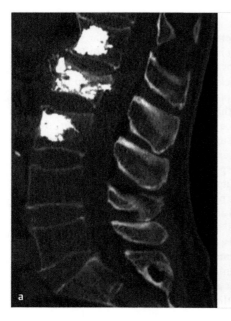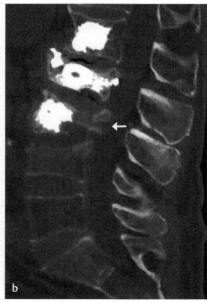

Fig. 31.4 Follow-up after polymethyl methacrylate (PMMA) vertebral augmentation. **(a)** Sagittal CT-scan reformat demonstrates PMMA vertebral augmentation of L1, L2, L3. **(b)** Sagittal CT-scan reformat shows fracture of the posterior portion of the vertebral body with retropulsion of the bone fragments (*white arrow*) resulting in symptomatic moderate spinal canal stenosis.

the annulus fibrosus. In those cases, prophylactic vertebroplasty can selectively be performed to reduce the risk of adjacent-level fracture.[29]

31.2.5 Technical Considerations during Vertebral Augmentation: Quantity of Cement to Inject

This topic is discussed in greater detail in Chapter 20 of this book but the amount of cement injected within a vertebral body is not only the most important predictor of pain relief in balloon kyphoplasty[30,31] but it is also of paramount importance in restoring the FSU stability. The recommended amount of cement to be injected varies significantly in the literature and in clinical studies. The vast majority of vertebral augmentation publications use insufficient cement amount according to the biomechanical data standards. For instance, in the 2009 Buchbinder NEJM study, an average of 2.8 ± 1.2 mL of PMMA cement was injected to treat patients. Considering that the L4 and L5 vertebral bodies have a volume of approximately 45 mL in men and 30 mL in women,[32] to restore the vertebral body stiffness after a fracture 29% of the vertebral body volume should be filled, corresponding to a *minimum* cement volume of 13 mL in men and 8.7 mL in women.

By injecting more cement, the risk of PMMA leakage also increases. Cement leakage within the ventral epidural space is the most feared type of extravasation as it may result in paralysis, radiculopathy, or cauda equine syndrome. Cement leakage into the disk should also be avoided whenever possible. This leakage is not dangerous per se, but if large enough, it will create an axial load vector from the treated vertebral body to the adjacent end plate. Cement extravasation within the nucleus pulposus is a predictor of adjacent vertebral body fracture with an odds ratio of 4.633.[33]

Patients with severe disk degeneration (Pfirrmann grades 7 and 8) are particularly at risk to have nucleus pulposus PMMA cement leakage, especially when the vertebral fracture is highly comminuted. Fluid hyper-pressurization technique of the disk with saline or anesthetic diskogram (mixture of dexamethasone and lidocaine) is the one technique used to reduce adjacent-level fracture[33] and can be performed whenever necessary to avoid cement leakage.

31.2.6 Biomechanics after Vertebral Augmentation: Adjacent-Level Fracture Risk

The correlation between vertebral augmentation and adjacent level fracture has been debated for many years. Computer-based finite element models initially suggested that the axial loading necessary to cause an adjacent-level fracture was lower in patient with vertebral augmentation.[34-36] However, these computer studies did not put much emphasis on the intervertebral disk. The intervertebral disk is an extremely important building block of the FSU and has a critical role in the risk of adjacent-level fracture after a VCF. Indeed, the fractured end plate alters the pressure profile of the damaged disk (decompresses the disk) resulting in increased compressive

loading of the anterior vertebral body wall during active flexion predisposing to adjacent-level fracture.[20]

Luo et al[37] demonstrated a threefold increase in creep deformation within the anterior column of the vertebra adjacent to a VCF. In their study, vertebroplasty was a protective factor of adjacent levels by reversing adjacent-level creep deformations by 52%. Also, the intradiskal pressure was normalized after vertebroplasty, measuring 76% of the baseline intradiskal pressure.[37] Other recent biomechanical cadaver studies supported the protective role of vertebroplasty.[38-40] In fact many studies have demonstrated that the instillation of cement within a vertebral body increases the nucleus pulposus pressure but never above baseline.[21,37,39-41] Furthermore, these studies supported that injecting a larger volume of cement (at least 7 mL) was shown to restore the compressive stiffness of the spine and significantly decrease the stress on the neural arch.[39]

Clinical trials further demonstrate that vertebroplasty did not increase the rate of adjacent-level fracture and is even a protective factor. Trout et al[42] evaluated 432 patients and of all the new fractures that occurred, only 40% of new fractures were adjacent to the level augmented; in other words, most new fractures happened in nonadjacent levels and are related to the underlying osteoporosis. Finally, systematic reviews of the published literature to date done by two meta-analyses demonstrated no adjacent-level fracture risk increase in one study,[43] while a decrease of the risk in adjacent-level fracture was demonstrated in other study.[44]

31.3 Key Points

- The FSU is used to analyze spine biomechanics. This unit is composed of two adjacent vertebrae, the intervertebral disk, and the ligaments providing additional stability while excluding muscles or other connecting tissues.
- The maximum loading on the FSU happens in the flexed standing position corresponding to more than twice the upright standing position.
- With increased disk degeneration and nucleus pulposus microarchitectural disturbances, there is less load bearing on the ventral end plates (decreasing from 44 to 19%) and more stress on the neural arch, and facet joints (increasing from 8 to 40%).
- After a VCF, the fractured end plate alters the pressure profile of the damaged disk (decompresses the disk) resulting in increased compressive loading of the anterior vertebral body wall during active flexion, thereby predisposing to adjacent-level fracture(s).
- Vertebral augmentation improves both the fracture mechanical instability and the FSU instability.
- Adequate vertebral augmentation includes correction of the kyphotic angle, restoration of the height of the depressed end plate, and complete filling of the vertebral body (pedicle to pedicle, end plate to end plate, and from the anterior cortex to the posterior cortex).
- To restore the vertebral body stiffness after a VCF, 29% of the vertebral body volume should be filled.
- Biomechanical data and clinical studies demonstrate that vertebral augmentation decreases the stress on the adjacent level and can even reduce the incidence of adjacent-level fractures.

References

[1] Kallmes DF, Comstock BA, Heagerty PJ, et al. A randomized trial of vertebroplasty for osteoporotic spinal fractures. N Engl J Med 2009;361(6):569–579

[2] Buchbinder R, Osborne RH, Ebeling PR, et al. A randomized trial of vertebroplasty for painful osteoporotic vertebral fractures. N Engl J Med 2009;361(6):557–568

[3] Firanescu CE, de Vries J, Lodder P, et al. Vertebroplasty versus sham procedure for painful acute osteoporotic vertebral compression fractures (VERTOS IV): randomised sham controlled clinical trial. BMJ 2018;361:k1551

[4] Ong KL, Beall DP, Frohbergh M, Lau E, Hirsch JA. Were VCF patients at higher risk of mortality following the 2009 publication of the vertebroplasty "sham" trials? Osteoporos Int 2018;29(2):375–383

[5] Beall D, Chambers M, Thomas S, et al. EVOLVE: a prospective and multicenter evaluation of outcomes for quality of life, pain and activities of daily living for balloon kyphoplasty in the treatment of Medicare-eligible subjects with vertebral compression fractures. J Vasc Interv Radiol 2017;28(2, Suppl):S25

[6] Eswaran SK, Gupta A, Adams MF, Keaveny TM. Cortical and trabecular load sharing in the human vertebral body. J Bone Miner Res 2006;21(2):307–314

[7] Panjabi MM. The stabilizing system of the spine. Part I. Function, dysfunction, adaptation, and enhancement. J Spinal Disord 1992;5(4):383–389, discussion 397

[8] Panjabi MM. The stabilizing system of the spine. Part II. Neutral zone and instability hypothesis. J Spinal Disord 1992;5(4):390–396, discussion 397

[9] Adams MA, Burton K, Bogduk N. The Biomechanics of Back Pain. Elsevier Health Sciences; 2006

[10] Sato K, Kikuchi S, Yonezawa T. In vivo intradiscal pressure measurement in healthy individuals and in patients with ongoing back problems. Spine 1999;24(23):2468–2474

[11] Inoue N, Espinoza Orías AA. Biomechanics of intervertebral disc degeneration. Orthop Clin North Am 2011;42(4):487–499, vii

[12] Pollintine P, Dolan P, Tobias JH, Adams MA. Intervertebral disc degeneration can lead to "stress-shielding" of the anterior vertebral body: a cause of osteoporotic vertebral fracture? Spine 2004;29(7):774–782

[13] Griffith JF, Wang Y-XJ, Antonio GE, et al. Modified Pfirrmann grading system for lumbar intervertebral disc degeneration. Spine 2007;32(24):E708–E712

[14] Adams MA, Pollintine P, Tobias JH, Wakley GK, Dolan P. Intervertebral disc degeneration can predispose to anterior vertebral fractures in the thoracolumbar spine. J Bone Miner Res 2006;21(9):1409–1416

[15] Yoganandan N, Larson SJ, Gallagher M, Pintar FA, Reinartz J, Droese K. Correlation of microtrauma in the lumbar spine with intraosseous pressures. Spine 1994;19(4):435–440

[16] Brinckmann P, Biggemann M, Hilweg D. Prediction of the compressive strength of human lumbar vertebrae. Spine 1989;14(6):606–610

[17] Hutton WC, Adams MA. Can the lumbar spine be crushed in heavy lifting? Spine 1982;7(6):586–590

[18] Curry WH, Pintar FA, Doan NB, et al. Lumbar spine endplate fractures: biomechanical evaluation and clinical considerations through experimental induction of injury. J Orthop Res 2016;34(6):1084–1091

[19] Brown MF, Hukkanen MV, McCarthy ID, et al. Sensory and sympathetic innervation of the vertebral endplate in patients with degenerative disc disease. J Bone Joint Surg Br 1997;79(1):147–153

[20] Tzermiadianos MN, Renner SM, Phillips FM, et al. Altered disc pressure profile after an osteoporotic vertebral fracture is a risk factor for adjacent vertebral body fracture. Eur Spine J 2008;17(11):1522–1530

[21] Luo J, Skrzypiec DM, Pollintine P, Adams MA, Annesley-Williams DJ, Dolan P. Mechanical efficacy of vertebroplasty: influence of cement type, BMD, fracture severity, and disc degeneration. Bone 2007;40(4):1110–1119

[22] Adams MA, Freeman BJ, Morrison HP, Nelson IW, Dolan P. Mechanical initiation of intervertebral disc degeneration. Spine 2000;25(13):1625–1636

[23] Silverman SL. The clinical consequences of vertebral compression fracture. Bone 1992;13(Suppl 2):S27–S31

[24] Klotzbuecher CM, Ross PD, Landsman PB, Abbott TA III, Berger M. Patients with prior fractures have an increased risk of future fractures: a summary of the literature and statistical synthesis. J Bone Miner Res 2000;15(4):721–739

[25] Melton LJ III, Atkinson EJ, Cooper C, O'Fallon WM, Riggs BL. Vertebral fractures predict subsequent fractures. Osteoporos Int 1999;10(3):214–221

[26] Lindsay R, Silverman SL, Cooper C, et al. Risk of new vertebral fracture in the year following a fracture. JAMA 2001;285(3):320–323

[27] Renner SM, Tsitsopoulos PP, Dimitriadis AT, et al. Restoration of spinal alignment and disc mechanics following polyetheretherketone wafer kyphoplasty with StaXx FX. AJNR Am J Neuroradiol 2011;32(7):1295–1300

[28] Molloy S, Mathis JM, Belkoff SM. The effect of vertebral body percentage fill on mechanical behavior during percutaneous vertebroplasty. Spine 2003;28(14):1549–1554

[29] Kobayashi N, Numaguchi Y, Fuwa S, et al. Prophylactic vertebroplasty: cement injection into non-fractured vertebral bodies during percutaneous vertebroplasty. Acad Radiol 2009;16(2):136–143

[30] Röder C, Boszczyk B, Perler G, Aghayev E, Külling F, Maestretti G. Cement volume is the most important modifiable predictor for pain relief in BKP: results from SWISSspine, a nationwide registry. Eur Spine J 2013;22(10):2241–2248

[31] Nieuwenhuijse MJ, Bollen L, van Erkel AR, Dijkstra PDS. Optimal intravertebral cement volume in percutaneous vertebroplasty for painful osteoporotic vertebral compression fractures. Spine 2012;37(20):1747–1755

[32] Limthongkul W, Karaikovic EE, Savage JW, Markovic A. Volumetric analysis of thoracic and lumbar vertebral bodies. Spine J 2010;10(2):153–158

[33] Komemushi A, Tanigawa N, Kariya S, et al. Percutaneous vertebroplasty for osteoporotic compression fracture: multivariate study of predictors of new vertebral body fracture. Cardiovasc Intervent Radiol 2006;29(4):580–585

[34] Berlemann U, Ferguson SJ, Nolte LP, Heini PF. Adjacent vertebral failure after vertebroplasty: a biomechanical investigation. J Bone Joint Surg Br 2002;84(5):748–752

[35] Fahim DK, Sun K, Tawackoli W, et al. Premature adjacent vertebral fracture after vertebroplasty: a biomechanical study. Neurosurgery 2011;69(3):733–744

[36] Wilcox RK. The biomechanical effect of vertebroplasty on the adjacent vertebral body: a finite element study. Proc Inst Mech Eng H 2006;220(4):565–572

[37] Luo J, Annesley-Williams DJ, Adams MA, Dolan P. How are adjacent spinal levels affected by vertebral fracture and by vertebroplasty? A biomechanical study on cadaveric spines. Spine J 2017;17(6):863–874

[38] Aquarius R, van der Zijden AM, Homminga J, Verdonschot N, Tanck E. Does bone cement in percutaneous vertebroplasty act as a stress riser? Spine 2013;38(24):2092–2097

[39] Luo J, Daines L, Charalambous A, Adams MA, Annesley-Williams DJ, Dolan P. Vertebroplasty: only small cement volumes are required to normalize stress distributions on the vertebral bodies. Spine 2009;34(26):2865–2873

[40] Farooq N, Park JC, Pollintine P, Annesley-Williams DJ, Dolan P. Can vertebroplasty restore normal load-bearing to fractured vertebrae? Spine 2005;30(15):1723–1730

[41] Ananthakrishnan D, Berven S, Deviren V, et al. The effect on anterior column loading due to different vertebral augmentation techniques. Clin Biomech (Bristol, Avon) 2005;20(1):25–31

[42] Trout AT, Kallmes DF, Kaufmann TJ. New fractures after vertebroplasty: adjacent fractures occur significantly sooner. AJNR Am J Neuroradiol 2006;27(1):217–223

[43] Fan B, Wei Z, Zhou X, et al. Does vertebral augmentation lead to an increasing incidence of adjacent vertebral failure? A systematic review and meta-analysis. Int J Surg 2016;36(Pt A):369–376

[44] Papanastassiou ID, Phillips FM, Van Meirhaeghe J, et al. Comparing effects of kyphoplasty, vertebroplasty, and non-surgical management in a systematic review of randomized and non-randomized controlled studies. Eur Spine J 2012;21(9):1826–1843

32 Advanced Principles of Minimally Invasive Vertebral Body Stabilization in Severe Benign and Malignant Fractures: Stent-Screw Assisted Internal Fixation

Alessandro Cianfoni and Luigi La Barbera

Summary

The anterior and middle columns of the spine supports about 80% of the overall load across the spine. After vertebral augmentation the repaired vertebrae may refracture around the stabilizing cement or the refracture can involve the middle column of the vertebral body by fracturing posterior to the bone cement previously used in the augmentation procedure. The importance of the middle column has traditionally been underemphasized but is important to consider to maintain vertebral body stability given its weight bearing role and the fact that this area is typically not augmented with bone cement during most vertebral augmentation procedures. Osteolysis of the weight bearing portions of the vertebral bodies may be seen with osteolytic metastases. Although pedicle screw and rod fixation of the spine is commonly used in cases where the metastatic disease has compromised the stability of the spine, stand-alone vertebral augmentation may be another viable option to provide pain relief and stability to the spine. The technique of screw-assisted internal fixation (SAIF) was developed to address the limitations of stand-alone vertebral augmentation and is performed with a combination of vertebral body stents and percutaneous cannulated and fenestrated transpedicular screws. The vertebral body stent has advantages over balloon kyphoplasty in that the stent preserves the vertebral body height after the balloon that was used to expand it has been removed and the metallic mesh of the stent helps to control and confine the cement injection thereby making the stent more optimal for use in cases of severe fracturing or prominent osteolysis. In cases where additional support is necessary, such as with middle column fractures or fractures of the pedicles, the stents can be joined to screws placed using a transpedicular technique and cemented in place by injecting bone cement through the cannulated and fenestrated screw. The SAIF technique represents an image guided 360° fusion of the incident fracture level that is much less invasive and has even biomechanical stability than a traditional spanning pedicle screw and rod construct. The SAIF technique has also been shown to reduce the fracture risk of the superior endplate and the posterior vertebral body wall as compared to vertebral augmentation alone. The SAIF technique can be performed as a stand-alone construct or along with traditional spanning spine instrumentation and can be used to obviate or reduce the need for more invasive surgical techniques.

Keywords: screw assisted internal fixation, vertebral body stent, vertebral refracture, middle column, transpedicular screw

32.1 Introduction

Vertebral augmentation (VA) has been extensively used for pain palliation and stabilization of vertebral body (VB) fractures due to trauma, osteoporosis, and tumors.[1–3]

32.2 Osteoporotic Fractures

Osteoporotic vertebral fractures can occur spontaneously or due to trauma, generally a compressive load injury mechanism involving the VB.[4] Both the anterior and middle columns together support about 80% of the overall spinal load (i.e., muscle forces and body weight) and are most commonly affected. The spectrum of severity ranges from mild and stable compression fractures,[5] affecting the disk–end plate region and leading only to minor deformity to unstable fractures with a high-degree of osseous fragmentation, collapse deformity, middle-column involvement, pediculo-somatic junction fracture, and kyphotic deformity[6,7] (▶ Fig. 32.1a, b). The underlying poor bone quality surely represents a risk factor[8,9] and might prevent osseous healing, potentially evolving toward the creation of osteonecrotic clefts[10] and, together with the detrimental effect of the increased bending momentum due to kyphosis at the fracture level,[11] might be responsible for fracture progression (▶ Fig. 32.1c, d).

Cement VA is widely used to treat fragility fractures, palliate pain, restore axial load capability of the VB, and arrest fracture progression.[12]

Ideally, VB reconstruction, height restoration, and homogeneous cement augmentation should be obtained with bone cement filling the two anterior thirds of the VB from superior to inferior disk end plates on both sides of midline, especially for the most severe of these fractures.

In reality, vertebroplasty is not intended to restore VB structure or height, and balloon kyphoplasty (BKP) has not been proven to guarantee sufficient height restoration, either due to the fact that the balloon tamps expand following the path of least resistance, or due to the deflation effect between balloon removal and cement injection. Moreover, the polymethyl methacrylate (PMMA) cement does not have adhesive properties to ensure stability in highly fragmented osseous structures, and the cement might distribute into the fractured VB in a heterogeneous and unpredictable manner. The cement may extend around the trabeculae and into intra-osseous clefts and it is not always possible to safely augment the entire VB, especially the bone adjacent to the intervertebral disk and end plates. Cement injection, usually monitored with fluoroscopy or CT imaging, is halted if cement tends to leak outside the VB, into veins or if it approaches the posterior third of the VB. The termination of the cement injection is for the purpose of minimizing the risk of epidural leakage.

Following VA, refracture of the treated VB is a well-known and reported event.[13–17] The refracture usually implies subsidence of the non-augmented portions of the VB around the cement cast[18] (▶ Fig. 32.2). This occurrence might be asymptomatic or be accompanied by pain recurrence. The refracture may be simply a minimal remodeling of the VB around the cement augmentation or it may manifest as a more prominent collapse of the non-augmented portions of the VB.

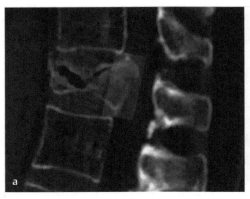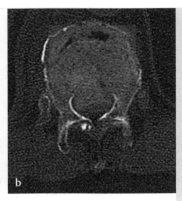

Fig. 32.1 Osteoporotic fracture: anterior and middle-column involvement—fracture progression. **(a, b)** An osteoporotic T12 compression fracture involving anterior (transparent red) and middle (transparent blue) columns, with gas-filled cleft. **(c)** A mild T8 compression fracture, with minimal height reduction, treated conservatively evolves into a higher degree of compression deformity and kyphosis **(d)**. *Arrowhead* in **d** points to a new distraction fracture of the spinous process.

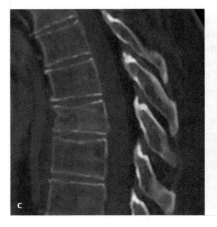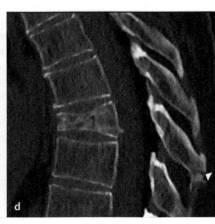

Fig. 32.2 Refracture of a treated vertebral body (VB). **(a, b)** An osteoporotic L1 compression fracture that has been treated with vertebral augmentation (VA) using the SpineJack shows an unfilled portion of the VB inferior to the implant and the cement (*white arrows* in a). A follow-up X-ray performed a few weeks later shows the unfilled portion in the inferior portion of the L1 VB has collapsed against the bone cement (*white arrows* in b).

A less frequent event is the refracture of the middle column, at the junction between middle and posterior third of the VB where most commonly the junction between cement-augmented and non-augmented VB is located.[19] These fractures are characterized by involvement and retropulsion of the posterior wall and eventually result in catastrophic splitting and separation between augmented anterior portion of the VB and middle column (▶ Fig. 32.3). This may also be accompanied by a kyphotic deformity at the incident level. Such fractures are not frequent and are largely unreported but when they do occur they pose a real therapeutic challenge.[20,21] These fractures may be repaired by surgical decompression of the central canal, corpectomy and grafting, and posterior stabilization, but this is a very invasive surgical procedure that is associated with significant morbidity and mortality risk, especially in elderly patients with scarce bone quality.[22]

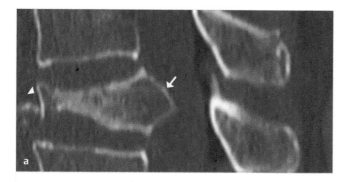

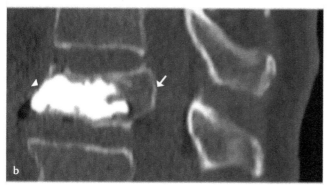

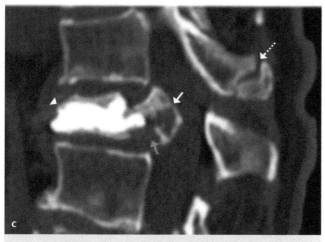

Fig. 32.3 Refracture of the middle column in a treated vertebral body (VB). Mid-sagittal sequential computed tomography (CT) images of an osteoporotic compression fracture **(a)**, with severe collapse of the anterior column (*arrowhead* in **a**) and involvement of the middle column with posterior wall retropulsion (*arrow* in **a**). After technically successful vertebral augmentation (VA) **(b)** there is height restoration of anterior column (*arrowhead* in **b**) and reduction of posterior wall retropulsion (*arrow* in **b**). The middle column remains non-augmented, as in almost all cases of VA. After 6 weeks the patient presented with recurrent severe back pain. The follow-up CT **(c)** shows maintained fracture reduction at the anterior column (*arrowhead* in **c**) but refracture of the middle column with cleavage at the junction between augmented of non-augmented portions of the VB (*red arrow* in **c**), and increased posterior wall retropulsion (*white arrow* in **c**). There is also focal kyphosis and spinous process fracture (*dashed arrow* in **c**) at the adjacent cranial level.

In our anecdotal experience these refractures occur mostly, although not exclusively, in the lumbar region, likely due to a combination of higher loads (both forces and bending moment)[23,24] that are accentuated by the kyphotic shape of the fractured vertebra.[11]

The importance of the middle-column stability might be indeed largely underestimated since the load-bearing capacity of the vertebra is usually referred to the anterior column as a whole structure, totally neglecting the important role of the middle column. Furthermore, the middle column, with the posterior third of the VB, the posterior wall, and the pediculo-somatic junctions, remains relatively non-augmented, even after satisfactory cement augmentation due to the safety measure to avoid cement dispersion too close to the posterior wall. The middle column, after cement augmentation, if observed on an axial post-procedure CT image, might be regarded as a "bare area," not reinforced, and therefore a potential point of weakness of the vertebra (▶ Fig. 32.4). Finally, some authors have reported the cement augmentation of the pedicles and pediculo-somatic junction, the so-called pediculoplasty,[25] but it should be considered that main stress forces at the level of the pedicles and pediculo-somatic junction are tensile, and PMMA is known to have optimal resistance to compressive loads rather than to tensile ones.[26]

Another aspect to consider is the transition between the augmented anterior portion of the vertebra that is completely filled with high-modulus bone cement, and the middle column, which is much weaker, particularly when osteoporosis is present. The result is a load intensification effect on the middle column, possibly explaining the collapse seen in clinical practice. Standard VA might therefore represent an under-treatment in osteoporotic fractures with middle-column involvement.

32.3 Neoplastic Osteolysis

Spinal osteolysis may cause severe instability, leading to fractures and neural compression.[27] Stability restoration is therefore of paramount importance in the treatment of lytic spinal tumors. To prevent or arrest vertebral collapse in patients with lesions affecting the weight-bearing portions of the vertebrae, posterior surgical fixation is widely used, but should be accompanied by anterior-column stabilization, either with corpectomy and grafting or with cement augmentation.[28,29] Posterior fixation, however, may not be feasible in patients with advanced disease, multilevel lesions, and poor bone quality and corpectomy, and grafting is highly invasive and carries significant morbidity risk especially in fragile neoplastic patients.[30]

Stand-alone VA is considered a viable option to achieve pain palliation and reinforce the anterior column,[2,3,31] but when the osteolysis causes extensive destruction of the cortical boundaries of the VB, the injection of cement may be challenging or impossible.[32,33] Cement distribution in these highly destroyed vertebral bodies might be unpredictable, uneven, or result in early extra-vertebral leaks leading to insufficient augmentation and stabilization or to clinical complications including vascular migration or neural compression.

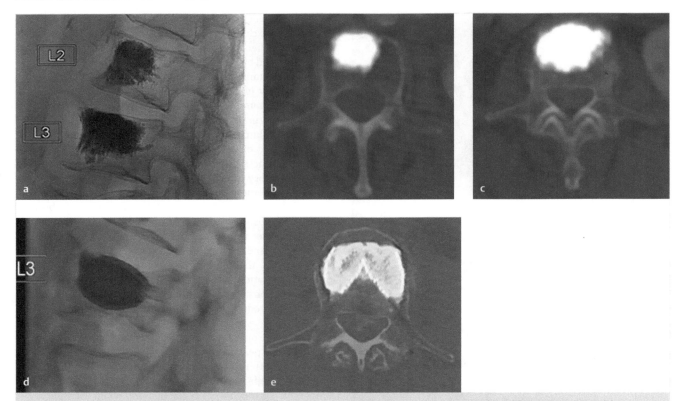

Fig. 32.4 "Bare area": non-augmented middle column following cement augmentation. In the upper row, lateral fluoroscopic image (**a**) post-augmentation of L2 and L3 with vertebroplasty technique. The augmentation result and cement distribution can be considered satisfactory but if the augmented vertebral bodies are seen on axial computed tomography (CT) images (**b, c**), the middle column (transparent red) remains non-augmented and therefore relatively unprotected. This "bare area" is highlighted with transparent red color in **b, c**, and **e**. Analogous findings in another case displayed on the lower row, (**d** and **e**) showing the result of a kyphoplasty performed with vertebral body stenting (VBS) technique. Even in this case, with larger amount of injected cement, the axial CT shows the "bare area" in the middle column (transparent red in **e**).

32.4 SAIF Technique

To address the limitations of standard VA in the most severe osteoporotic fractures and neoplastic lytic lesions, we have recently proposed the use of a new technique called "stent screw-assisted internal fixation (SAIF)."[34]

The SAIF is performed by combining the use of VB stent (VBS) (De Puy Synthes—Johnson & Johnson) augmentation and insertion of percutaneous cannulated fenestrated transpedicular screw (Injection pin—2B1, Milan, Italy).

The VBS is a balloon-expandable barrel-shaped metallic device, which is inserted unilaterally or bilaterally via a transpedicular access. Upon expansion, the VBS keeps the created cavity open after balloon-deflation until cement is injected. Introduced for treatment of vertebral compression fractures,[35–41] VBS has also been used in neoplastic fractures.[42] Most recently, it has been tested in cases of extensive osteolysis of the VB in order to reconstruct the anterior column.[43]

VB stenting has several potential advantages over traditional augmentation, including BKP, in that the rigid stent remains expanded after balloon-deflation thus maintaining the restored VB height.[38] The VBS metallic mesh guarantees a predictable and reasonably uniform barrel-shaped balloon-expansion, whereas a compliant balloon often follows the path of least resistance. The barrel shape of the VBS, with its large support surface, provides mechanical support, scaffolds the VB from within, and when necessary as in cases of fragmented cortical boundaries or osteolysis recreates VB walls. The metallic mesh helps confine the injected cement within the created cavity. These characteristics potentially favor the use of VBS in the most severe vertebral fractures, such as highly fragmented osteoporotic fractures, or neoplastic fractures with prominent cortical osteolysis.

Despite the advantages enumerated above, in the most severe osteolytic or neoplastic fractures the implanted VBS may only be partially contained by the nonintact cortical shell. In that situation, the VBS could potentially be expected to move[43] and possibly contribute to additional adverse events. In addition, VBS treatment alone would not be capable of addressing middle-column and pedicle fractures.

We have therefore implemented the VBS technique, combining the VBS implant with the insertion of percutaneous

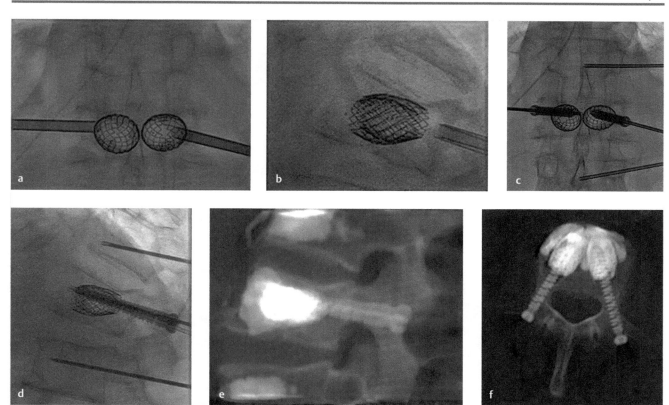

Fig. 32.5 Stent screw-assisted internal fixation (SAIF) technique. After bilateral transpedicular trocar placement at the pediculo-somatic junction, vertebral body (VB) stents are inserted into the VB and balloon-expanded **(a, b)**. The trocars are removed by exchanging them over k-wires and percutaneous fenestrated and cannulated pedicular screws are inserted inside the stents' lumen **(c, d)**. A thin 14 G trocar is inserted at the adjacent levels in this case to perform prophylactic augmentation. Polymethyl methacrylate (PMMA) bone cement is then injected through the fenestrated screws inside the stents and the cement interdigitates in the cancellous bone and around the stents, as seen on post-procedure computed tomography (CT) images **(e, f)**. The screws are fixed to the stents by the cement anchoring the stents to the posterior elements and bridging the middle column.

transpedicular cannulated fenestrated screws, followed by cement deposition through the screw (►Fig. 32.5). The intent is to anchor the VBS-cement implant to the posterior elements, thereby reducing the risk of VBS mobilization, bridging middle-column and pedicular fractures, and protecting the middle column of additional fracture.

This SAIF technique, as opposed to the standard surgical external fixation achieved with screws and bars bypassing the index level, might represent a minimally invasive image-guided 360° nonfusion form of vertebral reconstruction and stabilization that would be viable even in patients with severe osteoporotic or neoplastic thoracolumbar vertebral fractures (►Fig. 32.6).

32.4.1 Osteoporotic Fractures

To demonstrate the biomechanical advantages of the new SAIF technique in reducing the strains (i.e., fracture risk) on the bony structures of a representative osteoporotic spine, we conducted a biomechanical finite element analysis (FEA). The previously validated intact lumbar spine model[44,45] was modified to properly reflect osteoporosis[46] and the VB was filled with end-plate to end-plate cement (2.5 GPa).[46,47] The VB was then stressed to mimic standing and upper-body flexion.[48,49] VA, unilateral SAIF (1-SAIF), and bilateral SAIF (2-SAIF) techniques were equally effective in reducing the strains on the anterior column. VA and SAIF techniques effectively reduced the strains on the treated osteoporotic vertebra (►Fig. 32.7) but the bilateral SAIF technique was the most effective strategy to prevent the fracture risk on the superior EP and on the posterior wall, with significant reductions both over VA and 1-SAIF.

Our simulations also confirm the postoperative clinical CT images (►Fig. 32.8), demonstrating that refracture often occur in the weak middle column (the so-called "bare area") due to collapse and splitting. Our biomechanical analysis supports the effectiveness of SAIF technique.

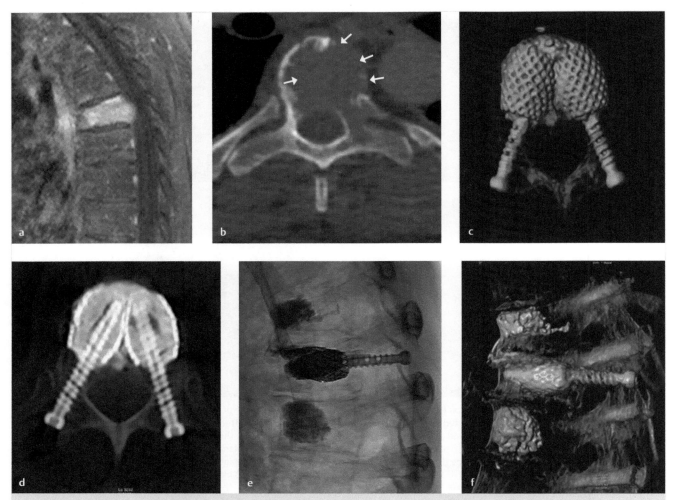

Fig. 32.6 Stent screw-assisted internal fixation (SAIF) technique in an extensively osteolytic metastasis. A T6 pathologic fracture as seen on magnetic resonance (MR) imaging with a sagittal T1-weighted image with fat saturation **(a)**. This lesion is characterized by prominent lytic changes and wide cortical erosion as seen on axial computed tomography (CT) (*white arrows* in **b**). Standard cement augmentation would be challenging, with high risk of cement leakage and insufficient stabilization. A SAIF technique was used to reconstruct the vertebral body (VB) from within, partially restoring height, scaffolding the VB, and preventing cement leakage through the stents' mesh. Post-procedure images **(c–f)** show the result of this nonfusion form of 360° internal fixation. Cement creates a bridge between the two stents and the screws anchor the cement-stent complex to the posterior elements.

32.4.2 Neoplastic Osteolysis

The biomechanical efficacy of SAIF technique was also investigated for the treatment of extreme osteolytic (EO) conditions by comparing this technique with standard posterior fixation.

A severe metastatic defect involving the entire L3 vertebra and one pedicle was created and described as a low-modulus region (5 MPa).[50] This lesion resulted in VB instability and a complete loss of capacity of the vertebra in supporting axil compressive loads[51] (▶ Fig. 32.9) and an increased fracture risk with standing and upper-body flexion.[48,49]

The SAIF technique (SAIF) with unilateral pin insertion and optimal end-plate to end-plate filling[47] with bone cement[46,52] was effective in recovering the stiffness of the treated vertebra to normal values while reducing the fracture risk on the superior EP and on the posterior wall. Posterior fixation coupled to SAIF technique (SAIF+FIX) had only very minor effects in further reducing the strain on the bony structures. As a stand-alone procedure, SAIF was much more effective than conventional posterior fixation (FIX) which only shielded the vertebra from supporting excessive compressive loads and was ineffective in decreasing the bony strain (▶ Fig. 32.9).

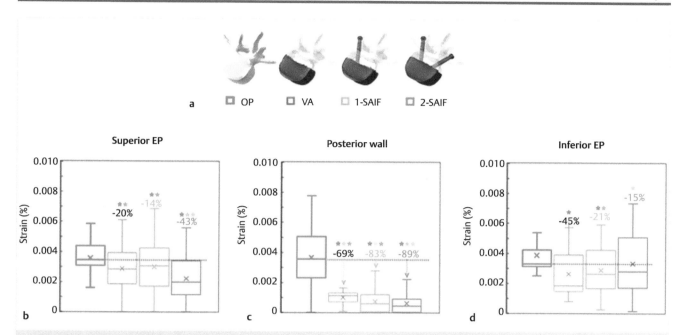

Fig. 32.7 Virtual models **(a)** of the osteoporotic L3 vertebra included in the biomechanical analysis: osteoporotic vertebra (OP), vertebral augmentation (VA), unilateral (1-SAIF) and bilateral (2-SAIF) screw-assisted internal fixation. The anterior two-thirds of the vertebral body (VB) is in shaded white, while screws and bone cement are depicted in black. Strain distributions on the superior end plate **(b)**, on the posterior cortical wall **(c)** and on the inferior end plate **(d)** of the middle column of L3 during simulated upper body bending. The median percentage values refer to OP model, while statistically significant differences on median values based on Wilcoxon paired-samples test are indicated (*).

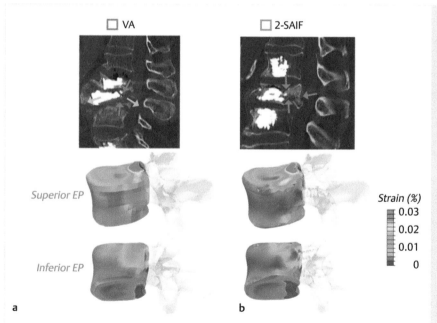

Fig. 32.8 Postoperative computed tomography (CT) images (sagittal slices) taken on lumbar vertebrae treated using vertebral augmentation (VA) and 2-SAIF (stent screw-assisted internal fixation). (This image is provided courtesy of A.C.) VA case **(a)**: the treated vertebra refractured with splitting of the anterior and middle column. A continuous fracture spreads from the superior to the inferior end plates (*red arrows* in **a**) with posterior cortical wall retropulsion (*yellow arrows* in **a**). 2-SAIF case **(b)**: the treated vertebra was found to have a new fracture involving a collapse of the superior and inferior end plate and the posterior wall as well (*red arrows* in **b**). In this case the fractured middle column does not split and there is less kyphotic deformity and posterior wall retropulsion. The principal strains' color maps calculated for standing simulations highlighted the strain intensification effect occurring on the superior and inferior end plates of each case. A correlation between these high-tensile strain regions and the fractured bony structures could be inferred.

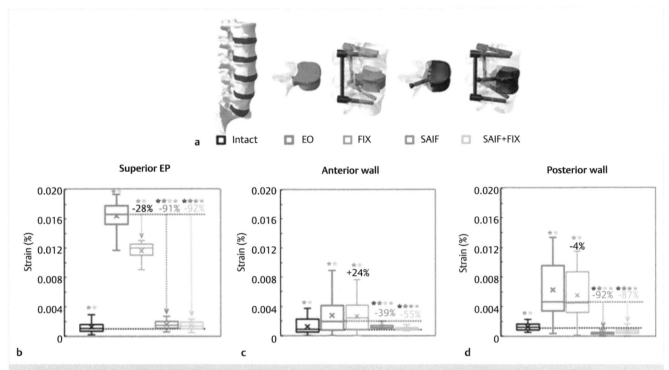

Fig. 32.9 Virtual scenarios **(a)** simulated in the biomechanical analysis modifying an intact L1–L5 model[48,52]: only the modified L3 vertebra is represented for the extreme osteolytic (EO) and stent screw-assisted internal fixation (SAIF) models, while only the L2–L4 segments are depicted for SAIF+conventional posterior fixation (FIX) and FIX scenarios. The metastasis and the injected bone cement are depicted in red and black, respectively. Strain distributions on the superior EP **(b)**, on the anterior **(c)** and posterior **(d)** cortical walls of L3 due to simulated upper body bending. The median percentage values refer to the EO model, while statistically significant differences on median values based on Wilcoxon paired-samples test are indicated (*).

32.5 Conclusion

SAIF can be performed as a stand-alone procedure or be combined with surgical posterior stabilization, potentially obviating the need for corpectomy and grafting or other invasive surgical procedures on the anterior column.

The SAIF technique remains a percutaneous minimally invasive image-guided procedure but ensures effective VB reconstruction via an internal VB prosthesis that allows a 360° nonfusion stabilization. This technique may be used in fractures in which height restoration, kyphosis correction, VB reconstruction, and middle-column protection are clinical concerns.

References

[1] Maestretti G, Sutter P, Monnard E, et al. A prospective study of percutaneous balloon kyphoplasty with calcium phosphate cement in traumatic vertebral fractures: 10-year results. Eur Spine J 2014;23(6):1354–1360

[2] Evans AJ, Kip KE, Brinjikji W, et al. Randomized controlled trial of vertebroplasty versus kyphoplasty in the treatment of vertebral compression fractures. J Neurointerv Surg 2016;8(7):756–763

[3] Berenson J, Pflugmacher R, Jarzem P, et al; Cancer Patient Fracture Evaluation (CAFE) Investigators. Balloon kyphoplasty versus non-surgical fracture management for treatment of painful vertebral body compression fractures in patients with cancer: a multicentre, randomised controlled trial. Lancet Oncol 2011;12(3):225–235

[4] Ensrud KE, Schousboe JT. Clinical practice: vertebral fractures. N Engl J Med 2011;364(17):1634–1642

[5] Denis F. The three column spine and its significance in the classification of acute thoracolumbar spinal injuries. Spine 1983;8(8):817–831

[6] Genant HK, Wu CY, van Kuijk C, Nevitt MC. Vertebral fracture assessment using a semiquantitative technique. J Bone Miner Res 1993;8(9):1137–1148

[7] McCormack T, Karaikovic E, Gaines RW. The load sharing classification of spine fractures. Spine 1994;19(15):1741–1744

[8] Nevitt MC, Cummings SR, Stone KL, et al. Risk factors for a first-incident radiographic vertebral fracture in women > or = 65 years of age: the study of osteoporotic fractures. J Bone Miner Res 2005;20(1):131–140

[9] Melton LJ III, Riggs BL, Keaveny TM, et al. Relation of vertebral deformities to bone density, structure, and strength. J Bone Miner Res 2010;25(9): 1922–1930

[10] Kim YC, Kim YH, Ha KY. Pathomechanism of intravertebral clefts in osteoporotic compression fractures of the spine. Spine J 2014;14(4):659–666

[11] Ottardi C, La Barbera L, Pietrogrande L, Villa T. Vertebroplasty and kyphoplasty for the treatment of thoracic fractures in osteoporotic patients: a finite element comparative analysis. J Appl Biomater Funct Mater 2016;14(2): e197–e204

[12] Filippiadis DK, Marcia S, Masala S, Deschamps F, Kelekis A. Percutaneous vertebroplasty and kyphoplasty: current status, new developments and old controversies. Cardiovasc Intervent Radiol 2017;40(12):1815–1823

[13] Fribourg D, Tang C, Sra P, Delamarter R, Bae H. Incidence of subsequent vertebral fracture after kyphoplasty. Spine 2004;29(20):2270–2276, discussion 2277

[14] Lindsay R, Silverman SL, Cooper C, et al. Risk of new vertebral fracture in the year following a fracture. JAMA 2001;285(3):320–323

[15] Villarraga ML, Bellezza AJ, Harrigan TP, Cripton PA, Kurtz SM, Edidin AA. The biomechanical effects of kyphoplasty on treated and adjacent nontreated vertebral bodies. J Spinal Disord Tech 2005;18(1):84–91

[16] Molloy S, Riley LH III, Belkoff SM. Effect of cement volume and placement on mechanical-property restoration resulting from vertebroplasty. AJNR Am J Neuroradiol 2005;26(2):401–404

[17] Uppin AA, Hirsch JA, Centenera LV, Pfiefer BA, Pazianos AG, Choi IS. Occurrence of new vertebral body fracture after percutaneous vertebroplasty in patients with osteoporosis. Radiology 2003;226(1):119–124

[18] Nagaraja S, Awada HK, Dreher ML, Bouck JT, Gupta S. Effects of vertebroplasty on endplate subsidence in elderly female spines. J Neurosurg Spine 2015;22(3):273–282

[19] Gan, et al. Balloon kyphoplasty for OP spinal fractures with middle column compromise. Injury 2014

[20] Abudou M, Chen X, Kong X, Wu T. Surgical versus non-surgical treatment for thoracolumbar burst fractures without neurological deficit. Cochrane Database Syst Rev 2013;6(6):CD005079

[21] Gonschorek O, Hauck S, Weiß T, Bühren V. Percutaneous vertebral augmentation in fragility fractures: indications and limitations. Eur J Trauma Emerg Surg 2017;43(1):9–17

[22] Winkler EA, Yue JK, Birk H, et al. Perioperative morbidity and mortality after lumbar trauma in the elderly. Neurosurg Focus 2015;39(4):E2

[23] Han KS, Rohlmann A, Zander T, Taylor WR. Lumbar spinal loads vary with body height and weight. Med Eng Phys 2013;35(7):969–977

[24] Cholewicki J, McGill SM. Mechanical stability of the in vivo lumbar spine: implications for injury and chronic low back pain. Clin Biomech (Bristol, Avon) 1996;11(1):1–15

[25] Eyheremendy EP, De Luca SE, Sanabria E. Percutaneous pediculoplasty in osteoporotic compression fractures. J Vasc Interv Radiol 2004;15(8):869–874

[26] Provenzano MJ, Murphy KP, Riley LH III. Bone cements: review of their physiochemical and biochemical properties in percutaneous vertebroplasty. AJNR Am J Neuroradiol 2004;25(7):1286–1290

[27] Coleman RE. Clinical features of metastatic bone disease and risk of skeletal morbidity. Clin Cancer Res 2006;12(20 Pt 2):6243s–6249s

[28] Moussazadeh N, Rubin DG, McLaughlin L, Lis E, Bilsky MH, Laufer I. Short-segment percutaneous pedicle screw fixation with cement augmentation for tumor-induced spinal instability. Spine J 2015;15(7):1609–1617

[29] Laufer I, Sciubba DM, Madera M, et al. Surgical management of metastatic spinal tumors. Cancer Contr 2012;19(2):122–128

[30] Yang Z, Yang Y, Zhang Y, et al. Minimal access versus open spinal surgery in treating painful spine metastasis: a systematic review. World J Surg Oncol 2015;13:68

[31] Yu W, Liang D, Jiang X, Yao Z, Qiu T, Ye L. Efficacy and safety of the target puncture technique for treatment of osteoporotic vertebral compression fractures with intravertebral clefts. J Neurointerv Surg 2017;9(11):1113–1117

[32] van der Linden E, Kroft LJ, Dijkstra PD. Treatment of vertebral tumor with posterior wall defect using image-guided radiofrequency ablation combined with vertebroplasty: preliminary results in 12 patients. J Vasc Interv Radiol 2007;18(6):741–747

[33] Chandra RV, Meyers PM, Hirsch JA, et al; Society of NeuroInterventional Surgery. Vertebral augmentation: report of the Standards and Guidelines Committee of the Society of NeuroInterventional Surgery. J Neurointerv Surg 2014;6(1):7–15

[34] Cianfoni A, Distefano D, Isalberti M, et al. J NeuroIntervent Surg :Epub ahead of print: [Dec 2018]

[35] Muto M, Greco B, Setola F, Vassallo P, Ambrosanio G, Guarnieri G. Vertebral body stenting system for the treatment of osteoporotic vertebral compression fracture: follow-up at 12 months in 20 cases. Neuroradiol J 2011;24(4):610–619

[36] Klezl Z, Majeed H, Bommireddy R, John J. Early results after vertebral body stenting for fractures of the anterior column of the thoracolumbar spine. Injury 2011;42(10):1038–1042

[37] Thaler M, Lechner R, Nogler M, Gstöttner M, Bach C. Surgical procedure and initial radiographic results of a new augmentation technique for vertebral compression fractures. Eur Spine J 2013;22(7):1608–1616

[38] Rotter R, Martin H, Fuerderer S, et al. Vertebral body stenting: a new method for vertebral augmentation versus kyphoplasty. Eur Spine J 2010;19(6):916–923

[39] Hartmann F, Griese M, Dietz SO, et al. Two-year results of VB stenting for the treatment of traumatic incomplete burst fractures. Minim Invasive Ther Allied Technol 2014;(9):1–6

[40] Diel P, Röder C, Perler G, et al. Radiographic and safety details of vertebral body stenting: results from a multicenter chart review. BMC Musculoskelet Disord 2013;14:233

[41] Werner CM, Osterhoff G, Schlickeiser J, et al. Vertebral body stenting versus kyphoplasty for the treatment of osteoporotic vertebral compression fractures: a randomized trial. J Bone Joint Surg Am 2013;95(7):577–584

[42] Mavrogenis AF, Papadopoulos EC, Starantzis K, Korres DS, Papagelopoulos PJ. Posterior decompression and stabilization, and surgical vertebroplasty with the vertebral body stenting for metastatic vertebral and epidural cauda equina compression. J Surg Oncol 2010;101(3):253–258

[43] Cianfoni A, Distefano D, Pravatà E, et al. Vertebral body stent augmentation to reconstruct the anterior column in neoplastic extreme osteolysis. J NeuroIntervent Surg :Epub ahead of print: [Aug 2018]

[44] Ottardi C, Galbusera F, Luca A, et al. Finite element analysis of the lumbar destabilization following pedicle subtraction osteotomy. Med Eng Phys 2016;38(5):506–509

[45] Luca A, Ottardi C, Sasso M, et al. Instrumentation failure following pedicle subtraction osteotomy: the role of rod material, diameter, and multi-rod constructs. Eur Spine J 2017;26(3):764–770

[46] Chae SW, Kang HD, Lee MK, Lee TS, Park JY. The effect of vertebral material description during vertebroplasty. Proc Inst Mech Eng H 2010;224(1):87–95

[47] Chevalier Y, Pahr D, Charlebois M, Heini P, Schneider E, Zysset P. Cement distribution, volume, and compliance in vertebroplasty: some answers from an anatomy-based nonlinear finite element study. Spine 2008;33(16):1722–1730

[48] La Barbera L, Galbusera F, Wilke H-J, Villa T. Preclinical evaluation of posterior spine stabilization devices: can the current standards represent basic everyday life activities? Eur Spine J 2016;25(9):2909–2918

[49] La Barbera L, Galbusera F, Wilke HJ, Villa T. Preclinical evaluation of posterior spine stabilization devices: can we compare in vitro and in vivo loads on the instrumentation? Eur Spine J 2017;26(1):200–209

[50] Whyne CM, Hu SS, Lotz JC. Parametric finite element analysis of vertebral bodies affected by tumors. J Biomech 2001;34(10):1317–1324

[51] Groenen KHJ, Janssen D, van der Linden YM, et al. Inducing targeted failure in cadaveric testing of 3-segment spinal units with and without simulated metastases. Med Eng Phys 2018;51:104–110

[52] Hansen D, Jensen JS. Mixing does not improve mechanical properties of all bone cements. Manual and centrifugation-vacuum mixing compared for 10 cement brands. Acta Orthop Scand 1992;63(1):13–18

33 Cementoplasty Outside the Spine

Peter L. Munk, Joshua A. Hirsch, Tyler M. Coupal, and Paul I. Mallinson

Summary

Metastatic disease to the skeletal system is a common occurrence that can be very painful and very debilitating. The metastatic tumors can weaken the bone leading to fracture or directly invade the bone and surrounding soft tissues. In addition to the conventional treatments for symptomatic metastases such as chemotherapy and radiation, percutaneous techniques such as tumor ablation and cementoplasty may be used to ameliorate symptoms produced by the metastases. While surgery may be appropriate for controlling symptoms produced by local invasion of tumor, patients who are significantly debilitated or those with a very short life expectancy may benefit from less invasive options such as percutaneous treatment. There are disadvantages to some of the conventional therapy including lack of structural stability after chemotherapy and radiation. Radiation is well known to cause regional osteoporosis and increase the risk of fracture in weight bearing bones. Cementoplasty also does not preclude the use of any of the other neoplastic treatments and can help provide structural stability to the axial and appendicular skeleton. Cementoplasty and the various ablative therapies can be effectively used alone or in combination with the conventional therapies for optimal local control of symptomatic metastatic disease. When utilizing the percutaneous therapies it is important to keep in mind the goals of providing adequate stabilization, ablating the interface between the tumor and normal bone, ablating the soft tissue component of the lesion that impinges on surrounding structures, and being mindful to not injure critical surrounding structures. When performing extraspinal cementoplasty and ablative therapies it is important to have adequate information prior to performing the procedure including adequate pre-procedure imaging and knowledge of the patient's most debilitating symptoms. Clear treatment goals should be established prior to the procedure and multiple sessions may be necessary to adequately treat the full extent of the tumor without putting the patient at undue risk. Computed tomography and fluoroscopy are the most commonly used imaging modalities to guide the treatment. The location of percutaneous treatments most often involves the pelvis and acetabulum and reinforcement of the acetabulum often produces profound pain relief by stabilizing this area of prominent weight bearing. In addition to bone cement, some interventionalists may also use percutaneous screws to supplement the strength of the construct especially when large metastases are treated. Although care should be taken to avoid cement extravasation into the normal anatomy surrounding the metastasis, small amounts of extravasation are surprisingly well tolerated even into such important structures such as weight bearing joints. Other axial and appendicular osseous areas are also responsive to cementoplasty including the inferior pubic ramus, pubis, ilium, and long bones of the upper and lower extremities. When using cement in any osseous structure it should be kept in mind that although bone cement offers excellent support and resistance to compression, it tends to break with tensile or rotational forces so its use in long bones and other areas undergoing these forces should be in combination with other supporting devices such as nails, screws, or wires. There have also been reports of cementoplasty in more unusual locations such as the sternum, scapula, and clavicle. Complications associated with cementoplasty are rare but care should be taken to avoid cement extravasation and large volume cement injections causing displacement of a large amount of bone marrow especially in patients with compromised pulmonary function. It is not known whether cement injection into metastases causes spread of the malignancy but the use of ablative treatments could serve to limit the potential tumor spread. A combination of ablative techniques and cementoplasty could also ablate the tumor all the way out to its margins and reduce the tumor volume thereby making the injection of cement into the tumor easier. Cryoablation can impede the inflow of cement and complete thawing of the ablation zone is necessary to adequately inject cement into the area previously ablated. There has been considerable experience demonstrating that cementoplasty of the pelvis is an important technique for improving patient's pain and quality of life in those patients suffering from painful pelvic metastases. Additional cementoplasty of metastatic disease outside the pelvis is limited but appears equally promising. The use of a combination of ablative treatments and cementoplasty can be a very effective way to manage patient with symptomatic metastases and should be considered in the appropriate clinical scenarios.

Keywords: cementoplasty, metastatic disease, tumor, radiation, chemotherapy, ablation, axial skeleton

33.1 Introduction

Metastatic bone disease is common in patients with certain types of neoplasms, and patients that die with metastatic disease often have metastatic bone deposits.[1,2] These can be intensely symptomatic, and significantly degrade the quality of their life. Successfully treating symptomatic bone disease can be challenging, often requiring coordinated multidisciplinary efforts. Bone pain can make even simple things such as patient transfer or rolling over in bed an excruciatingly painful ordeal.

Symptoms from metastatic bone deposits arise from a variety of different mechanisms. Weakening of the bone may result in a pathologic fracture. In addition, tumor can invade the periosteum, which is richly innervated, producing severe pain or cause bleeding and subsequent elevation of the periosteum. Even without a pathologic fracture, weakened bone placed under stress, as with weight bearing, can be painful, therefore inhibiting ambulation or use of an extremity. Tumors can also produce nociceptive factors that cause inflammation or that can be irritating to nerve fibers and thus result in pain. Associated soft tissue masses arising from the metastasis can cause compression of adjacent structures, such as neurovascular bundles and other organs (e.g., bowel or bladder).

Conventional methods for treating symptomatic metastases in the pelvis and extremities include surgery, radiation therapy, and chemotherapy. More recently, percutaneous techniques such as cementoplasty and ablative methods (e.g., radiofrequency ablation, microwave ablation, and cryoablation) have been introduced. Surgery can be highly efficacious, particularly in the treatment of pathologic fractures in long bones of the extremities. At times, excision of a metastasis can also be performed and, if surgery is successful, this can provide excellent and durable pain relief. Evaluation and management of acetabular metastases comparing patients treated with surgery versus those managed with percutaneous cementoplasty has been studied.[3-5] Surgical treatment may have some advantages in patients that are candidates for this type of surgery, in that symptom control and mobility may be better than with cementoplasty alone. There are several disadvantages inherent to surgery, including the fact that patients are often in such debilitated condition that they are poor surgical candidates for anesthesia and major resection. Prolonged period of convalescence may be required after surgery, which may be undesirable in an individual with a restricted lifespan. These debilitated patients are often difficult to rehabilitate. It has been argued that percutaneous imaging-guided cement injections may provide a less invasive, less expensive, but still highly effective treatment that decreases pain, and improves mobility and quality of life and stabilizes the skeletal area of interest particularly in those with limited projected survival.[3,4,6]

Radiation is an extremely useful tool and extensive experience with this modality exists. This technique is noninvasive and often provides excellent pain control but, unfortunately, up to 30% of patients do not receive satisfactory improvement in their symptoms.[6] In addition, although radiation is useful in treatment of tumor, it does not provide mechanical reinforcement of bone so patients with symptoms on weight bearing may find that their symptom improvement after radiation is limited.[7] Partial reconstitution of bone with healing can sometimes occur but may take months and the previously applied radiation may promote regional osteoporosis, thereby further increasing the risk of fracture.[6,8] Chemotherapy can be a useful adjunct but a significant portion of patients may show incomplete or no response. Chemotherapy toxicity can be significant. Often the appropriate treatment approach uses multiple modalities, making multidisciplinary treatment decisions crucial. It is important to remember that cementoplasty does not preclude use of other treatment modalities. Subsequent radiotherapy can be performed in the presence of cement, and indeed may allow radiation to be held in reserve for future use if needed.

33.2 Anatomic Sites

This chapter will focus principally on cementoplasty within the pelvis, exclusive of the sacrum as this is covered elsewhere in this textbook. Pelvic cementoplasty procedures were first performed in the mid-1990s but have gained considerable popularity in the last 10 years.[9-11] This technique is still not uniformly available, even in major medical centers, but is gaining in acceptance. More recently, some experience with cementoplasty of long bones and other sites have also been reported.[1]

33.2.1 Pelvic Cementoplasty

The pelvis is a large osseous structure that contains a substantial amount of cancellous bone and is an extremely common site

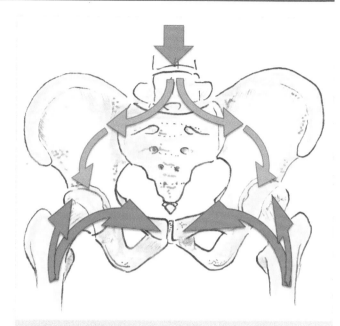

Fig. 33.1 Schematic of the transmission of forces through the lumbar spine via the pelvis into the lower limbs. Force is transmitted down from the spine into the pelvic ring (*blue arrows*), while force from the lower extremity is transmitted cranially (*red arrows*).

of metastatic bone disease. Considerable force is transmitted through the pelvic ring, particularly in the upright position and on ambulation. Force is transmitted through the spine through the sacroiliac joints toward the acetabular roof and superior pubic ramus or from the lower extremity in the upright position (►Fig. 33.1). Destruction of osseous integrity along this pathway can produce symptoms, particularly on ambulation and/or weight bearing.[6]

Regrettably patients may present with large metastatic deposits. Large lesions can be challenging to treat, as it may not be practical or reasonable to treat the entirety of the tumor particularly if a considerable soft tissue component is present. In this situation it is helpful to devise a plan of treatment whereby the areas most likely to provide symptom relief are targeted. Several principles should be considered in choosing the regions of the tumor to treat:

- Reinforcement of weight- or stress-bearing bone with cement or other stabilizing material.
- Cementation +/− ablation or ablation alone of the interface between tumor and normal bone.
- Ablation of soft tissue components of the lesion which impinge on adjacent structures.
- It is important to be aware of adjacent important structures, such as neurovascular bundles, bowel, bladder, and joints to minimize the possibility of leakage into the surrounding structures.

At present these procedures are relatively uncommon with only modest experience having been accrued. Both patients and referring doctors may know very little about them. Before embarking on a cementoplasty procedure in the pelvis, it is important to have clear goals as to what is hoped to be achieved. Moreover, it is crucial that the patient be aware of the potential risks and benefits and be involved in the decision making regarding the treatment goals and potential outcomes. Recent imaging (computed tomography [CT] and/or magnetic resonance imaging [MRI]) should be available and a thorough understanding of the patient's symptoms is mandatory if a procedure is to be undertaken. It is important to know as precisely as possible where the patient's most debilitating pain is, and what worsens or elicits the patient's pain (e.g., weight bearing, sitting, etc.). As patients may have extensive metastatic disease, those most symptomatic areas should be treated first, with other regions being addressed later if required. Unnecessarily treating more extensive areas can put the patient at risk for more complications and potentially turn an effective palliative procedure into one that may worsen the patient's condition.

33.2.2 Technique of Cementoplasty

The exact technique utilized varies considerably from one operator to another, as does the equipment used. A wide variety of different needles, cements, and ablation equipment have been reported in the literature with successful outcomes. Most operators performing cementoplasty already have considerable experience with vertebroplasty and can readily translate these skills to sites outside the spine.

For planning purposes reasonably contemporaneous cross-sectional imaging is required. Ideally, patients should not be coagulopathic and should not have platelet counts below 50,000 in order to minimize bleeding complications. Treatment while the patient has an active infection should also be, whenever possible, avoided. The use of prophylactic antibiotics in many procedures is common and should be employed in cementoplasty in order to minimize the possibility of infection. These procedures can at times be lengthy and uncomfortable for patients. Moreover, comorbidities and narcotic-tolerance can make analgesia difficult. Many operators utilize anesthesiology in order to safely ensure that patients are comfortable, and optimally monitored during the procedure.

Prior to undertaking the procedure, clear goals and reasonable expectations should be established. Areas of greatest stress or weight bearing should be selected to be buttressed and reinforced. Satisfactory outcomes can be achieved without complete filling of the entirety of large lesions, provided the key areas are treated. If cement can also be placed near the interface between tumor and bone, or the interface can be treated with ablation techniques, this can contribute to a good symptomatic outcome. Cementing of undisplaced or minimally displaced fracture sites can provide dramatic improvement in pain.

Although fluoroscopic guidance alone can be utilized with good success, some operators feel more comfortable with CT or cone beam CT guidance. The complex three-dimensional anatomy of the pelvis can make purely fluoroscopic guidance challenging. Combined fluoroscopy with cone beam CT facilitates confirmation of needle placement and also permits real-time evaluation of cement distribution.[3,4,9,10,12]

33.2.3 Assessment of Outcome

Outcomes assessment is patient dependent. Some patients are affected more by pain, others by diminished mobility or side effects of medication. The majority of patients have pain as their primary complaint. Numerous studies have shown that in the majority of treated patients pain significantly diminishes.[10,11,13,14] Ideally pain should be assessed using a visual analog or ordinal scale, providing a quantitative measure of change in symptoms. The center of the lead author of this chapter typically asks the patient what their worst pain is in the week prior to treatment, on the day of treatment, and then will follow up the patient the following day, and one week later with additional assessment and pain queries as required. It is important to manage expectations and patients must realize that it is unlikely that all of their pain will disappear. Most patients are quite satisfied with a significant improvement in their symptoms. Studies have also demonstrated improved mobility and functionality following cementoplasty.[1,15–17] Several authors of this chapter have treated patients who were unable to walk prior to treatment, due to pain on weight bearing, who subsequently became able to ambulate. This can significantly improve the patient's quality of life and ability to participate in their own care.[7,18,–28] Some authors have also examined the reduction in consumption of analgesics.[4,29] Although patients often experience reduction in analgesic consumption it should be remembered that these patients often have multifocal disease, and may continue to require considerable analgesic use for management of symptoms remote from the site of cementoplasty.

33.2.4 Acetabulum/Pelvis

The first site outside the spine where cementoplasty was extensively utilized was the acetabulum. Metastases to the acetabular roof can be highly symptomatic even when quite small due to the weight-bearing stress placed on this site.[4,17] It was quickly noted that these lesions could be treated with small volumes of cement, resulting in dramatic improvement in patient pain and mobility (▶ Fig. 33.2).

Reinforcement of the acetabular roof by placement of a needle from an anterolateral approach allows cement to be injected safely using a route well clear of the femoral neurovascular structures. Continuous fluoroscopic observation during injection of cement can be performed when these procedures are performed under fluoroscopy. If imaging is done under CT guidance or fluoro-CT, frequent CT imaging following injection of small aliquots of cement is done to monitor the cement injection.[14] Any extravasation of cement into the joint or blood vessels can therefore be immediately visualized and the injection terminated.

Some operators have also advocated the use of cannulated screws to supplement the cement injection for lesions of the acetabulum, ilium, and pubic ramus. Screws can be placed quite precisely under imaging guidance and may provide additional structural support, particularly in the presence of large metastatic lesions.[30–32] Although, intuitively, this would seem to be advantageous, as of the writing of this chapter no firm data comparing screw placement with cementoplasty alone is available.

Extrusion of small amounts of cement into surrounding soft tissue extension of the metastases is not usually symptomatic. Although every effort should be made to avoid injection of cement into the joint space, this is often surprisingly well-tolerated by patients. Complications from intra-articular cement injection includes grinding, clicking, and pain from intra-articular loose bodies and rarely chondrolysis.[33]

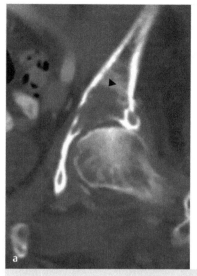 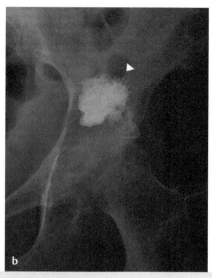 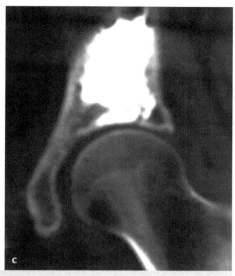

Fig. 33.2 **(a)** Coronal computed tomography (CT) of the left hip of a patient with breast cancer demonstrated a destructive metastasis eroding into the acetabular roof (*black arrowhead*). **(b)** A post-procedural frontal pelvic radiograph demonstrates successful reinforcement by acetabuloplasty (*white arrowhead*). **(c)** A coronal CT of the left hip demonstrates a similar result in a patient with prostate cancer.

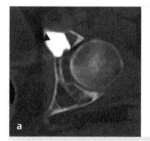 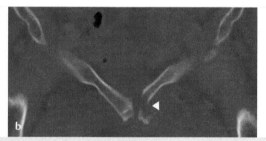 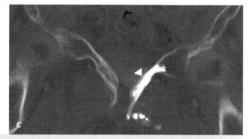

Fig. 33.3 **(a)** Axial post-procedural computed tomography (CT) demonstrates successful deployment of cement into the anterior acetabulum/lateral aspect of the left superior pubic ramus in a patient with a prostate cancer metastasis (*black arrowhead*). **(b)** A pretreatment coronal CT image demonstrates a patient with a painful pathological fracture secondary to osteonecrosis (*white arrowhead*). **(c)** The post-procedure image shows successful cement deployment along the length of the superior pubic ramus, which bridged the fracture (*white arrowhead*).

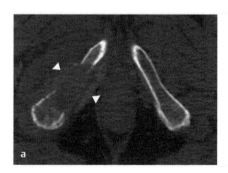 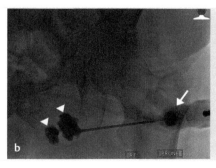

Fig. 33.4 **(a)** An axial computed tomography (CT) demonstrates destruction of the right inferior pubic ramus and ischial tuberosity by a metastatic soft tissue deposit (*white arrowheads*). This was determined clinically to be the source of significant pain for the patient during sitting. **(b)** A posteroanterior fluoroscopic image shows the right ramus and tuberosity successfully reconstructed with cement (*white arrowheads*) via a 13G vertebroplasty needle (*white arrow*).

33.3 Other Sites

Force and stress through the pelvic ring is also transmitted through the pubic body, superior pubic ramus, as well as the portion of the iliac bone adjacent to the sacroiliac joint.[14,34] Fractures, usually undisplaced or minimally displaced, are common at these sites and can respond to injections of small volumes of cement (▶ Fig. 33.3). Although below and outside the kinetic chain of force transmission between lumbar spine and the femora, the inferior pubic rami, including the ischial tuberosity, are important transmitters of compressive force during sitting. They are, therefore, potentially responsive sites

to cementoplasty (▶ Fig. 33.4). In the case of pubic lesions, it can be helpful to decompress the bladder with a urinary catheter prior to the procedure. With large lytic lesions of the ilium, it should be remembered that the lumbar plexus is located nearby anterior to the sacral ala so care must be exercised not to extravasate cement into this area.

At the time of this writing, only modest experience exists with cementoplasty of the long bones. Although cement is extremely good in dealing with compressive forces, cement tends to fracture or shatter with rotational or torque forces, which are typically experienced by long bones, such as the femur.[30] Regardless, reports have appeared which have

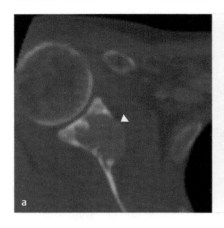
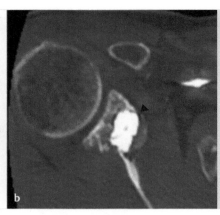

Fig. 33.5 **(a)** Axial CT image demonstrates a lytic metastasis in the neck of the scapula (*white arrowhead*). **(b)** This area of the scapula was treated by cementoplasty (*black arrowhead*).

shown that some patients appear to have significant pain reduction following injection of cement with good clinical outcomes.[1,8,12,15,17,35,36] It would appear that patients with large cortical breaches are poor candidates for treatment. In the proximal femur, an intact calcar in particular may be an important treatment selection criterion.[30] Purely intramedullary metastatic deposits may have a more favorable outcome. The presence of cement within long bones may function as a stress riser in spite of intact overlying cortex, with resultant fractures on additional weight bearing.[17,35,37]

In order to further reinforce the bone and minimize the chance of post-procedural fracturing, other investigators have percutaneously placed thin rods, wires, or guide wires across the tumor site undergoing cementoplasty. Reports of percutaneous placement of multiside large-bore catheters into medullary space of bones, with subsequent injection of bone cement through the catheter, have claimed good clinical results.[37,38] These techniques should be viewed as developmental but may play a valuable role, particularly in patients who are poor candidates for traditional surgical fixation.

Scattered reports of successful cementoplasty of other osseous structures have also appeared in the literature.[18,39,-41] Sternal metastases and fractures can be highly symptomatic but can show significant improvement with injection of small volumes of cement. Similar results have been reported in the clavicle and scapula (▶Fig. 33.5). Particular attention to the nearby neurovascular structures is clearly necessary, emphasizing the importance of using cross-sectional imaging guidance when necessary.

33.4 Complications

As with any percutaneous procedure, both infection and bleeding can occur but are rare.

Pathologic fracture following cementation can occasionally occur in the pelvis, but is more common in the long bones.[2,11,12,39,42-44] Nontarget embolization of cement into the venous system, lungs, joints, and soft tissues can occur, mandating close fluoroscopic monitoring while injecting where ever possible. If injection must be done under CT guidance, injection of small aliquots with frequent imaging must be performed.

Injection of cement into any osseous structure causes embolization of bone marrow elements, and probably tumor into the venous system. This may be a significant consideration

in patients with chronic obstructive lung disease who have limited physiologic pulmonary reserve. Promotion of spread of metastatic disease by embolization of tumor is a theoretical consideration. Clear data on whether cementoplasty promotes spread of malignancy in the clinical setting is not readily available at the present time, but is unlikely to be a significant consideration in those patients who have short life expectancy. The use of accompanying ablative techniques prior to cement injection may diminish the significance of this potential problem.

33.5 Concomitant Use of Ablative Techniques

An expanding body of literature describes the use of combination ablative techniques and cementoplasty in treatment of metastases.[2,29,32,34,42,45-49] The greatest experience at present is with radiofrequency ablation and cryoablation. Ablation provides a theoretical advantage in assisting in the reduction of the volume of viable tumor, compared with what could be achieved with cement injection alone. Ablation of the tumor bone interface prevents further invasion of normal bone. Concomitant ablation of soft tissue extension of the bone metastases can be performed which may be helpful if tumor is causing symptomatic compression or displacement of adjacent nerves, blood vessels, and organs (e.g., bladder, rectum). A theoretical advantage of destroying potentially embolizable tumor on injection of cement has previously been noted above.

Radiofrequency ablation may potentially increase the ease of injection of cement by disrupting the tissue integrity of metastasis. Cryoablation, on the other hand, may impede distribution of cement if the ice ball is incompletely thawed, therefore ensuring complete thawing prior to cement injection is recommended. Impeding the spread of cement in the presence of an ice ball has also been used as a useful tool to guide cement distribution.[50]

33.6 Conclusion

Considerable experience has shown that cementoplasty in the pelvis is a valuable tool in improving patients' symptoms and quality of life in the setting of metastatic disease. Experience outside of the pelvis is limited, but it appears promising that specific clinical situations exist to which cementoplasty is likely helpful. The use of concomitant ablative techniques in selective patients is strongly suggested by the literature.

33.7 Key Points

- Reinforcement of weight- and stress-bearing bone is likely to produce significant patient symptom improvement.
- Significant patient improvement can be achieved with only partial selective treatment in the setting of large metastatic disease and/or extensive deposits.
- Detailed cross-sectional imaging CT +/− MRI is vital in planning the procedure, and the imaging should be recent.
- A detailed understanding of the patient's symptoms is required for tailoring the procedure to be performed, particularly in patients with extensive disease.

References

[1] Feng H, Feng J, Li Z, et al. Percutaneous femoroplasty for the treatment of proximal femoral metastases. Eur J Surg Oncol 2014;40(4):402–405

[2] Kurup AN, Callstrom MR. Ablation of musculoskeletal metastases: pain palliation, fracture risk reduction, and oligometastatic disease. Tech Vasc Interv Radiol 2013;16(4):253–261

[3] Colman MW, Karim SM, Hirsch JA, et al. Percutaneous acetabuloplasty compared with open reconstruction for extensive periacetabular carcinoma metastases. J Arthroplasty 2015;30(9):1586–1591

[4] Gupta AC, Hirsch JA, Chaudhry ZA, et al. Evaluating the safety and effectiveness of percutaneous acetabuloplasty. J Neurointerv Surg 2012;4(2):134–138

[5] Sapkota BH, Hirsch AE, Yoo AJ, et al. Treatment of metastatic carcinoma to the hip with CT-guided percutaneous acetabuloplasty: report of four cases. J Vasc Interv Radiol 2009;20(4):548–552

[6] Zhang J, Yang Z, Wang J, et al. Study of treatment using percutaneous acetabuloplasty and interstitial implantation of (125)I seeds for patients with metastatic periacetabular tumors. World J Surg Oncol 2012;10:250

[7] Hirsch AE, Jha RM, Yoo AJ, et al. The use of vertebral augmentation and external beam radiation therapy in the multimodal management of malignant vertebral compression fractures. Pain Physician 2011;14(5):447–458

[8] Cazzato RL, Buy X, Eker O, Fabre T, Palussiere J. Percutaneous long bone cementoplasty of the limbs: experience with fifty-one non-surgical patients. Eur Radiol 2014;24(12):3059–3068

[9] Cotten A, Demondion X, Boutry N, et al. Therapeutic percutaneous injections in the treatment of malignant acetabular osteolyses. Radiographics 1999;19(3):647–653

[10] Cotten A, Deprez X, Migaud H, Chabanne B, Duquesnoy B, Chastanet P. Malignant acetabular osteolyses: percutaneous injection of acrylic bone cement. Radiology 1995;197(1):307–310

[11] Weill A, Kobaiter H, Chiras J. Acetabulum malignancies: technique and impact on pain of percutaneous injection of acrylic surgical cement. Eur Radiol 1998;8(1):123–129

[12] Wang Z, Zhen Y, Wu C, et al. CT fluoroscopy-guided percutaneous osteoplasty for the treatment of osteolytic lung cancer bone metastases to the spine and pelvis. J Vasc Interv Radiol 2012;23(9):1135–1142

[13] Deschamps F, de Baere T. Cementoplasty of bone metastases. Diagn Interv Imaging 2012;93(9):685–689

[14] Georgy BA. Percutaneous cement augmentations of malignant lesions of the sacrum and pelvis. AJNR Am J Neuroradiol 2009;30(7):1357–1359

[15] Cazzato RL, Palussière J, Buy X, et al. Percutaneous long bone cementoplasty for palliation of malignant lesions of the limbs: a systematic review. Cardiovasc Intervent Radiol 2015;38(6):1563–1572

[16] Guzik G. Treatment of metastatic lesions localized in the acetabulum. J Orthop Surg Res 2016;11(1):54

[17] Iannessi A, Amoretti N, Marcy PY, Sedat J. Percutaneous cementoplasty for the treatment of extraspinal painful bone lesion: a prospective study. Diagn Interv Imaging 2012;93(11):859–870

[18] Kamalian S, Hirsch AE, Growney ML, et al. CT guided percutaneous calcaneoplasty: a case of metastatic intra-articular calcaneus fracture. J Neurointerv Surg 2009;1(2):186–188

[19] Botsa E, Mylona S, Koutsogiannis I, Koundouraki A, Thanos L. CT image guided thermal ablation techniques for palliation of painful bone metastases. Ann Palliat Med 2014;3(2):47–53

[20] Cascella M, Muzio MR, Viscardi D, Cuomo A. Features and role of minimally invasive palliative procedures for pain management in malignant pelvic diseases: a review. Am J Hosp Palliat Care 2017;34(6):524–531

[21] Choi J, Raghavan M. Diagnostic imaging and image-guided therapy of skeletal metastases. Cancer Contr 2012;19(2):102–112

[22] Kurup AN, Morris JM, Schmit GD, et al. Balloon-assisted osteoplasty of periacetabular tumors following percutaneous cryoablation. J Vasc Interv Radiol 2015;26(4):588–594

[23] Ma Y, et al. Percutaneous image-guided ablation in the treatment of osseous metastases from non-small cell lung cancer. Cardiovasc Intervent Radiol 2017

[24] Marcy PY, Palussière J, Descamps B, et al. Percutaneous cementoplasty for pelvic bone metastasis. Support Care Cancer 2000;8(6):500–503

[25] Prologo JD, Passalacqua M, Patel I, Bohnert N, Corn DJ. Image-guided cryoablation for the treatment of painful musculoskeletal metastatic disease: a single-center experience. Skeletal Radiol 2014;43(11):1551–1559

[26] Sun G, Jin P, Liu XW, Li M, Li L. Cementoplasty for managing painful bone metastases outside the spine. Eur Radiol 2014;24(3):731–737

[27] Wallace AN, McWilliams SR, Connolly SE, et al. Percutaneous image-guided cryoablation of musculoskeletal metastases: pain palliation and local tumor control. J Vasc Interv Radiol 2016;27(12):1788–1796

[28] Buy X, Cazzato RL, Catena V, Roubaud G, Kind M, Palussiere J. Techniques de consolidation osseuse guidée par imagerie en oncologie : cimentoplastie et vissage. Bull Cancer 2017;104(5):423–432

[29] Callstrom MR, Dupuy DE, Solomon SB, et al. Percutaneous image-guided cryoablation of painful metastases involving bone: multicenter trial. Cancer 2013;119(5):1033–1041

[30] Deschamps F, de Baere T, Hakime A, et al. Percutaneous osteosynthesis in the pelvis in cancer patients. Eur Radiol 2016;26(6):1631–1639

[31] Pusceddu C, Fancellu A, Ballicu N, Fele RM, Sotgia B, Melis L. CT-guided percutaneous screw fixation plus cementoplasty in the treatment of painful bone metastases with fractures or a high risk of pathological fracture. Skeletal Radiol 2017;46(4):539–545

[32] Hartung MP, Tutton SM, Hohenwalter EJ, King DM, Neilson JC. Safety and efficacy of minimally invasive acetabular stabilization for periacetabular metastatic disease with thermal ablation and augmented screw fixation. J Vasc Interv Radiol 2016;27(5):682–688.e1

[33] Leclair A, Gangi A, Lacaze F, et al. Rapid chondrolysis after an intra-articular leak of bone cement in treatment of a benign acetabular subchondral cyst: an unusual complication of percutaneous injection of acrylic cement. Skeletal Radiol 2000;29(5):275–278

[34] Pusceddu C, Sotgia B, Fele RM, Ballicu N, Melis L. Combined microwave ablation and cementoplasty in patients with painful bone metastases at high risk of fracture. Cardiovasc Intervent Radiol 2016;39(1):74–80

[35] Deschamps F, Farouil G, Hakime A, et al. Cementoplasty of metastases of the proximal femur: is it a safe palliative option? J Vasc Interv Radiol 2012;23(10):1311–1316

[36] Plancarte-Sanchez R, Guajardo-Rosas J, Cerezo-Camacho O, et al. Femoroplasty: a new option for femur metastasis. Pain Pract 2013;13(5):409–415

[37] Liu XW, Jin P, Liu K, et al. Comparison of percutaneous long bone cementoplasty with or without embedding a cement-filled catheter for painful long bone metastases with impending fracture. Eur Radiol 2017;27(1):120–127

[38] He C, Tian Q, Wu CG, Gu Y, Wang T, Li M. Feasibility of percutaneous cementoplasty combined with interventional internal fixation for impending pathologic fracture of the proximal femur. J Vasc Interv Radiol 2014;25(7):1112–1117

[39] Basile A, Giuliano G, Scuderi V, et al. Cementoplasty in the management of painful extraspinal bone metastases: our experience. Radiol Med (Torino) 2008;113(7):1018–1028

[40] Leung OC, Poon WL, Nyaw SF, Luk SH. Percutaneous cementoplasty of osteolytic metastases induces immediate and long-lasting pain relief in oncological patients. Hong Kong Med J 2013;19(4):317–322

[41] Uri IF, Garnon J, Tsoumakidou G, Gangi A. An ice block: a novel technique of successful prevention of cement leakage using an ice ball. Cardiovascular Intervent Radiol 2015;38(2):470–4

[42] Wallace AN, Huang AJ, Vaswani D, Chang RO, Jennings JW. Combination acetabular radiofrequency ablation and cementoplasty using a navigational ra-

diofrequency ablation device and ultrahigh viscosity cement: technical note. Skeletal Radiol 2016;45(3):401–405

[43] Coupal TM, Pennycooke K, Mallinson PI, et al. The hopeless case? Palliative cryoablation and cementoplasty procedures for palliation of large pelvic bone metastases. Pain Physician 2017;20(7):E1053–E1061

[44] Lane MD, Le HB, Lee S, et al. Combination radiofrequency ablation and cementoplasty for palliative treatment of painful neoplastic bone metastasis: experience with 53 treated lesions in 36 patients. Skeletal Radiol 2011;40(1): 25–32

[45] Callstrom MR, Atwell TD, Charboneau JW, et al. Painful metastases involving bone: percutaneous image-guided cryoablation—prospective trial interim analysis. Radiology 2006;241(2):572–580

[46] Callstrom MR, Charboneau JW. Image-guided palliation of painful metastases using percutaneous ablation. Tech Vasc Interv Radiol 2007;10(2): 120–131

[47] Castañeda Rodriguez WR, Callstrom MR. Effective pain palliation and prevention of fracture for axial-loading skeletal metastases using combined cryoablation and cementoplasty. Tech Vasc Interv Radiol 2011;14(3): 160–169

[48] Thacker PG, Callstrom MR, Curry TB, et al. Palliation of painful metastatic disease involving bone with imaging-guided treatment: comparison of patients' immediate response to radiofrequency ablation and cryoablation. AJR Am J Roentgenol 2011;197(2):510–515

[49] Tian QH, Wu CG, Gu YF, He CJ, Li MH, Cheng YD. Combination radiofrequency ablation and percutaneous osteoplasty for palliative treatment of painful extraspinal bone metastasis: a single-center experience. J Vasc Interv Radiol 2014;25(7):1094–1100

[50] Swan JA, Liu DM, Clarkson PW, Munk PL. Cryoablation and cementoplasty of a pathologic fracture in the sternum. Singapore Med J 2013;54(10): e215–e217

34 Treatment of Osteoporosis after Vertebral Augmentation

Amanda Schnell, Sarah Morgan, John W. Amburgy, James Mooney, D. Mitchell Self, and M. R. Chambers

Summary

Osteoporosis, a systemic disorder of altered bone strength, continues to be an under-recognized condition with an immense economic burden and public health impact, despite having a greater associated burden of disability than nearly all types of cancer. As the result of the increasing average age of the population in the United States, the cost of care of osteoporosis is expected to rise significantly to $25.3 billion by 2025. Although diagnosis and treatment results in considerable health care expenditures, the *failure* to diagnose is even more costly. For many patients, the diagnosis of a vertebral compression fracture (VCF) is often the first indication of osteoporosis. It is also an opportunity to provide the patient with appropriate treatment and education about the disease. Patients who experience VCFs are often referred to an osteoporosis specialist following vertebral augmentation. Fracture liaison services (FLSs) are designed to assist with the transition and continuation of osteoporosis care from the inpatient to outpatient setting and are tasked with following and treating patients with osteoporosis and/or osteoporotic fractures. Essential to the success of an FLS or the clinician treating the disease process of osteoporosis after the fragility fracture has been treated is enhanced communication with the health care team providing these treatment services. Using appropriate clinical care pathways based on evidence-based guidelines is also important to ensure the correct approach to treatment. This can be combined with optimal patient education and tracking of patient outcomes in a continued effort to provide the best quality of care.

Keywords: osteoporosis, vertebral compression fracture (VCF), fragility fracture, fracture liaison service, FRAX, bone mineral density, T-score, vertebral fracture assessment, dual-energy X-ray absorptiometry (DXA), trabecular bone score (TBS)

34.1 Introduction

For many patients, the diagnosis of a vertebral compression fracture (VCF) is often the first indication of osteoporosis. It is also an opportunity to provide patients with appropriate treatment and education about the disease.

Osteoporosis, a systemic disorder of altered bone strength, continues to be an under-recognized condition, despite having a greater associated burden of disability (e.g., loss of work days, pain) than all sites of cancer, with the exception of lung cancer. Despite available screening tools, advances in pharmacologic therapy, and widespread education regarding exercise and adequate nutrient intake, the diagnosis and treatment rates of osteoporosis in the United States fall well below standards set by the National Osteoporosis Foundation (NOF) guidelines.[1,2]

The year following an initial fragility fracture (which is defined as any fracture resulting from a fall from standing height or less) holds the greatest risk for subsequent fractures.

One-fifth to nearly one-half of patients experience another fracture within the year after the initial fragility fracture.[3-5] Unfortunately, only one-fourth of patients who sustain a fragility fracture (including a vertebral fracture) are formally diagnosed with osteoporosis within the year, despite the fact that sustaining a fragility fracture is a defining event of osteoporosis[6-8] and only one-fourth of patients who experience an osteoporotic fracture are on pharmacologic osteoporosis therapy at 1 year, putting them at higher risk for additional fractures.[9,10]

34.2 Etiology and Epidemiology

As osteoporosis is a bone disorder characterized by decreased bone strength, it increases the risk of fracture. Bone strength is composed primarily of two components: bone density and bone quality. Bone density is determined by peak bone mass and the rate of subsequent bone loss, and is expressed as grams of mineral per area or volume. Bone quality refers to architecture, turnover, damage accumulation (e.g., micro-fractures) and the degree of mineralization.[11] Osteoporosis results from an imbalance between bone formation and bone loss, with formation being less than loss as well as diminished bone quality. When a failure-inducing force is applied to osteoporotic bone, which can even be normal force on a weakened bone, a fracture occurs.[11]

Osteoporosis occurs in both sexes, but is more often recognized and diagnosed in women following menopause (▶ Fig. 34.1).[11] Both men and women have an age-related decline in bone mineral density (BMD) in midlife due to increased bone resorption as compared to bone formation, though women experience a more rapid bone loss in the early years after menopause.[11] Fractures in men typically occur about a decade later than in women. Peak bone mass is not completed until age 30, after linear bone growth has ceased. Therefore, bone mass attained early in life may be the most important determinant of skeletal health later in life.[11,12]

Peak bone mass may be affected by genetic and lifestyle factors including nutrition (lifetime calcium and vitamin D intake), physical activity, smoking, alcohol, eating disorders, autoimmune diseases, glucocorticoid medications, and endocrine disorders that affect sex steroids.[12] Characteristics associated with low bone mass later in life include female sex, increased age, estrogen deficiency, white race, low weight and body mass index (BMI), and family history of prior fracture.[11] The list of possible secondary causes is lengthy and includes endocrine and metabolic conditions, nutritional or collagen metabolism disorders, and drug side effects. Conditions that may contribute to low bone mass include genetic diseases, hypogonadal states, malabsorption disorders, celiac disease, Crohn disease and gastric bypass, multiple myeloma, malignancy, rheumatologic and autoimmune diseases, end-stage renal disease, and post-organ transplantation status.[13]

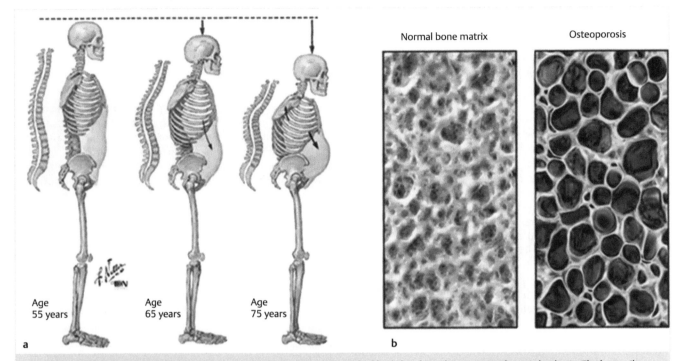

Fig. 34.1 (a) Compression fractures of thoracic vertebrae lead to loss of vertebral body height and progressive thoracic kyphosis. The lower ribs eventually rest on iliac crests, and downward pressure on viscera causes abdominal distention. (Source: Netter 1987. Netter Illustrations reproduced with permission from Icon Learning Systems, a division of MediMedia, USA, Inc. All rights reserved.) (b) Medical illustration showing normal bone (left) with greater thickness of the cancellous bone, less porous bone architecture, and more bridging plates as compared with the osteoporotic bone (right) with less bone, greater porosity, and less bridging plates.

34.3 Economic Burden

Osteoporosis and associated osteoporotic fractures have a profound effect on individual morbidity and mortality and are exceedingly common. The NOF estimates that 10.2 million Americans have osteoporosis and that an additional 43.4 million individuals have low bone mass.

There were an estimated 2 million fractures attributable to osteoporosis in 2005, with 27% of the fractures occurring at vertebral sites.[14] Not only are the fractures quite common, the economic burden and public health impact are immense. It is estimated that over 400,000 hospital admissions, 2.5 million medical office visits, and 180,000 nursing home admissions were related to osteoporotic fractures in 2004.[15] Hospital costs for a single inpatient admission related to vertebral fracture may total approximately $12,000.[16]

Vertebral fractures are roughly twice as common as a hip fracture and are the most common type of osteoporotic fracture. Vertebral insufficiency fractures indicate a high risk for future fractures regardless of whether or not the bone density testing (T-score) meets the threshold for osteoporosis.[14]

Significant costs related to fracture care are incurred by inpatient care, long-term care facilities, and outpatient care.[17] In the year following a fracture, medical and hospitalization costs were 1.6 to 6.2 higher than prefracture costs and 2.2 to 3.5 times higher than those for age-matched controls with costs totaling up to $71,000 for a hip fracture and up to $68,000 for a vertebral fracture.[18] Medicare pays for approximately 80% of these fragility fracture costs.[17] Given the recent prominent increase in the age of the population, the cost of care of osteoporosis is expected to rise to $25.3 billion by 2025.[17] In addition to the medical costs, indirect costs are also prominent, including the price of reduced productivity due to disability and reduced workforce participation, and patients are also at substantial risk of premature death.[15]

Failure to detect clinical osteoporosis when it is present likely contributes to the current lack of awareness of the consequences of the disease by both clinicians and patients. This impacts the reimbursement strategies of payers, influences policy makers in the public health sector by underestimating the number of those at increased fracture risk, and affects the design of clinical trials of new agents to reduce fracture.[19]

34.4 Presentation and Diagnosis

Screening at-risk populations for osteoporosis is essential. In the case of a patient presenting after vertebral augmentation, the diagnosis of osteoporosis is a foregone conclusion, provided the vertebral fracture was a fragility fracture. Many vertebral fractures, however, are silent and often go undiagnosed.

Based on guidelines from the World Health Organization (WHO) and the NOF, the diagnosis of osteoporosis may be made by meeting any one of these criteria: the presence of a fragility fracture in the absence of other metabolic bone disorders or high velocity trauma; a T-score of −2.5 or lower on DXA imaging, even in the absence of a prevalent fracture and in patients with osteopenia and an increased fracture risk, using Fracture Risk Assessment Algorithm (FRAX) country-specific thresholds.[13,14,19,20] (See "Fracture Risk Assessment Algorithm (FRAX below.)

Since approximately 30% of osteoporosis cases in postmenopausal women are believed to be due to a secondary cause, a thorough history, physical exam, and laboratory testing could be performed to identify secondary causes.[1,14,19] Laboratory testing may include:
• Complete blood count (CBC).
• Serum chemistries (calcium, phosphorus, renal, and liver function tests).
• Thyroid-stimulating hormone (TSH).
• 25-Hydroxy vitamin D3 (25(OH)D.
• Intact parathyroid hormone (PTH).
• Serum/urine protein electrophoresis.
• Serum/urine immunofixation electrophoresis.
• Serum-free light chains.
• Tissue transglutaminase antibodies and total IgA.
• Urine calcium/creatinine ratio +/– 24-hour urine for calcium excretion (including urine sodium and creatinine to assess the adequacy of collection).
• Bone turnover markers (BTMs) in select patients:
  – Bone resorption markers: Collagen cross-linked N-telopeptide (NTX), collagen type 1 c-telopeptide (CTX).
  – Anabolic markers: Procollagen 1 propeptide (P1NP), bone-specific alkaline phosphatase (BSAP).

In patients with clinical or biochemical evidence of malabsorption, celiac antibodies should be obtained. Serum and urine protein electrophoresis may be obtained if there is a suspicion for multiple myeloma (e.g., non-PTH-mediated hypercalcemia).[14] Also in select cases, urine-free cortisol, testosterone, follicle-stimulating hormone (FSH), and tryptase levels may be indicated. It should be noted that the 24-hour urine calcium collection must occur after the patient is vitamin D replete and has been on a reasonable calcium intake (1,000–1,200 mg/day) for at least 2 weeks.

34.5 Dual-Energy X-ray Absorptiometry

Dual-energy X-ray absorptiometry (DXA) imaging can provide valuable information in the diagnosis of osteopenia and osteoporosis and in the monitoring of BMD. In general, DXA imaging should be ordered for screening in all women age ≥ 65 years of age, men age ≥ 70, postmenopausal women and men age 50–69 based on risk factor profile, and postmenopausal women and men age ≥ 50 who have had an adult age fracture.[13]

BMD is measured with DXA of the lumbar spine (on the anteroposterior view), femoral neck, and total hip. The distal one-third of the radius should be scanned in individuals with hyperparathyroidism, in those who do not have a valid spine or hip site, or in individuals whose weight exceeds the maximum limit of the table.[20] Area BMD is expressed in g/cm^2 and as a relationship to two norms: the BMD of an age-, sex-, and ethnicity-matched reference population (Z-score) or a young-adult reference population of the same sex (T-score). The difference between the patient's BMD and the mean BMD of the reference population, divided by the standard deviation (SD) of

the reference population, is used to calculate Z- and T-scores.[13] In postmenopausal women and men age 50 and older, the WHO diagnostic T-score criteria are applied. In premenopausal women, men less than 50 years of age, and in children, the ethnic or race-adjusted Z-scores should be used.[21] In premenopausal women and men less than age 50, a Z-score ≤ –2.0 is BMD below the expected range for age and a Z-score > –2.0 is BMD within the expected range for age (see ▶ Fig. 34.2).

The WHO criteria for the diagnosis of osteoporosis based on BMD (T-scores) using DXA measurement are as follows:
• **Normal**: T-score ≥ –1.0 SD.
• **Low bone mass**: –2.5 SD < T-score < –1.0 SD.
• **Osteoporosis**: T-score ≤ –2.5 SD.
• **Severe osteoporosis**: T-score ≤ –2.5 plus one or more fragility fractures.[22]

Along with traditional DXA imaging, other DXA-based tools have been developed to assist the clinician in the evaluation and prediction of risk of fracture for individual patients. These tools include vertebral fracture assessment (VFA), trabecular bone score (TBS), extended femur scans to detect incomplete atypical femoral fractures, vertebral radiographs, and FRAX.

34.6 Vertebral Fracture Assessment

Vertebral fracture assessment (VFA) is a measurement tool that uses lateral images obtained by DXA to identify asymptomatic vertebral fractures. VFA should be performed if the results may alter the decision to treat or not to treat, change the drug selected for treatment, or affect the follow-up of the patient.[23] Three patterns of vertebral deformation have been described in VFA: wedge, biconcave, and crush.[24] Up to 25% of patients over age 60 who are being evaluated for osteoporosis have been found to have vertebral fractures with only 11% of those patients reporting a history of vertebral fracture.[25] Using VFA to identify individuals with asymptomatic vertebral fractures as part of a comprehensive risk assessment may aid in clinical decision-making.[23,26] Detection of vertebral fractures has traditionally relied on standard radiographs of the spine, which are associated with cost and radiation exposure and require a separate visit. Therefore, radiographs are usually not obtained in the standard evaluation of patients with osteoporosis.[25] Using DXA technology, radiation exposure and cost can be lessened, and vertebral anatomic information is available to the physician at the patient's clinic visit.[25]

34.7 Radiographs

In addition to VFA, vertebral imaging with AP, lateral, and in some cases oblique and spot views is indicated in all women age ≥ 70, all men age ≥ 80 if BMD is ≤ –1.0 at the spine, total hip, or femoral neck, in women age 65 to 69 and men age 70 to 79 if BMD T-score is ≤ –1.5 at the spine, total hip, or femoral neck.[13,23] Vertebral imaging is also indicated in postmenopausal women and men age ≥ 50 with the following specific risk factors: low-trauma fracture during adulthood (age 50 and older), historical height loss (difference between the current height and peak height at age 20) of 1.5 inches (4 cm) or

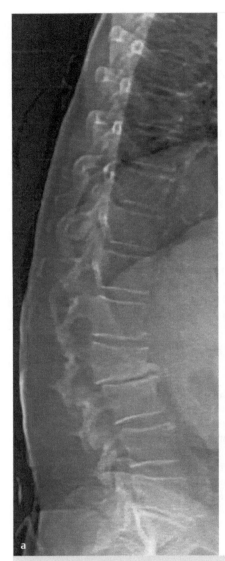
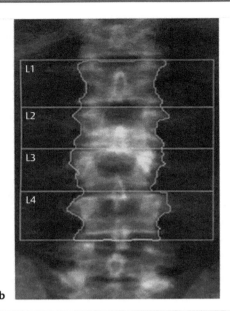

Region	Area (cm²)	BMC (g)	BMD (g/cm²)	T-score	PR (%)	Z-score	AM (%)
L1	13.23	8.64	0.653	-2.5	71	-2.3	72
L2	13.72	10.58	0.771	-2.3	75	-2.1	77
L3	13.89	11.00	0.792	-2.7	73	-2.4	75
L4	15.02	11.84	0.788	-3.0	71	-2.7	72
Total	55.86	42.06	0.753	-2.7	72	-2.4	74

Fig. 34.2 DXA imaging of the lumbar spine including a lateral **(a)** and an anteroposterior view **(b)** and with T- and Z-scores representing the comparison to young healthy adults and matched controls, respectively **(c)**.

more, prospective height loss (difference between the current height and a previously documented height measurement) of 0.8 inches (2 cm) or more, or recent or ongoing long-term glucocorticoid treatment.[13,23]

34.8 Trabecular Bone Score

Trabecular bone score (TBS) is an analytical tool that uses measurements on the lumbar spine DXA to capture information related to trabecular microarchitecture. The TBS decreases with age and reflects qualitative aspects of skeletal structure that complements the quantitative measurement of BMD.[27] Low TBS is consistently associated with an increase in fractures and is partly independent of both clinical risk factors and BMD at the lumbar spine and proximal femur.[28] Therefore, this technique may aid in clinical decision-making regarding the need for pharmacologic therapy or the type of medication used. More studies are needed to determine the optimal clinical use of TBS.

Extended femur scanning by DXA is a screening tool that is used to detect incomplete atypical femur fractures in patients on antiresorptive therapy. Though individuals with atypical femur fractures may present with prodromal groin or thigh pain, others are asymptomatic.[29,30] This tool may be considered in individuals who have previously sustained an atypical femoral fracture, bisphosphonate users who report pain in the hips, groin, or upper legs, and in individuals who have taken antiresorptive therapy for more than five years or have other risk factors for developing an atypical femoral fracture.[29]

34.9 Fracture Risk Assessment Algorithm (FRAX)

FRAX is a risk assessment tool that can be used to estimate the 10-year fracture risk with or without femoral neck BMD. FRAX is a country- and ethnicity-specific fracture risk assessment that

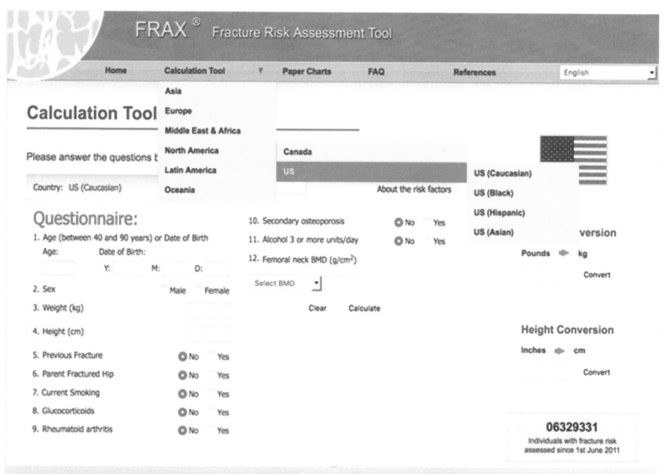

Fig. 34.3 FRAX website. (Reproduced with permission of © Centre for Metabolic Bone Diseases, University of Sheffield, UK.)

combines BMD at the femoral neck (or total hip) with a group of well-validated and weighted clinical risk factors for fracture that are largely independent of BMD.[31] Age and mortality are taken into account, which are unique benefits of this algorithm. Other factors in the algorithm include gender, height, weight, BMI, personal fracture history, parental history of hip fracture, glucocorticoid use, rheumatoid arthritis, and the current use of tobacco and excessive alcohol intake. Treatment is indicated or suggested when the 10-year probability of a major osteoporotic fracture (spine, forearm, hip, or shoulder) is ≥ 20% or the 10-year probability of hip fracture is ≥ 3%. FRAX does have limitations and is most appropriate in patients with low femoral neck BMD. Using FRAX in patients with low BMD at the lumbar spine but a relatively normal BMD at the femoral neck will underestimate fracture risk in these individuals. Furthermore, it may also underestimate fracture risk in patients with recent fractures, multiple osteoporosis-related fractures, and those at increased risk for falling.[13] FRAX (▶ Fig. 34.3) can be accessed at: https://www.sheffield.ac.uk/FRAX/index.aspx.

34.10 Treatment

Treatment of osteoporosis is indicated in any patient with a low velocity fracture or a hip or vertebral fracture (regardless of BMD).[13,20,21,32] Pharmacological osteoporosis therapy should be considered in any patient with a T-score of ≤ −2.5 at the femoral neck, total hip, lumbar spine, or distal one-third of the radius or one with a T-score between −1.0 and −2.5 (osteopenia) and increased fracture risk by FRAX (10-year hip fracture risk of ≥ 3% or a 10-year major osteoporosis-related fracture probability ≥ 20%).[13,20] Pharmacological therapy is also indicated in patients who are at moderate-to-high risk of fracture on glucocorticoid therapy.[33]

34.10.1 Referral

A patient who experiences a fragility fracture is either treated by the physician treating the fracture or the patient may be referred to an osteoporosis specialist following definitive treatment of the fracture. The referral should be prompt, as there is most often a significant risk of additional fracture in the first few months or first year following the incident fracture. The largest vertebral augmentation trial ever published reported a very high rate of additional vertebral fracture of 47.6% during the first year after the initial VCF.[5] Many other patients referred to a specialized osteoporosis center by general medicine specialties may present with an asymptomatic diagnosis of osteoporosis based on DXA imaging. Referral to an osteoporosis specialist is indicated in the following situations:[20]

- A patient with normal BMD who sustains a fracture without major trauma (e.g., a fragility fracture).

- A patient who presents with recurrent fractures or has continued bone loss while on pharmacologic osteoporosis therapy without obvious treatable causes of bone loss.
- When osteoporosis is unexpectedly severe, has unusual features, or less common secondary conditions (e.g., hyperthyroidism, hyperparathyroidism, hypercalciuria, or elevated prolactin) are identified.
- When a patient has a condition that complicates management (e.g., chronic kidney disease: glomerular filtration rate [GFR] < 35, hyperparathyroidism, or malabsorption).

34.10.2 Fracture Liaison Service

In 2011, the International Osteoporosis Foundation (IOF) Committee of Scientific Advisors Fracture Working Group published a report that described a "care gap in secondary prevention" of osteoporosis and called for expansion of existing clinical systems aimed at ensuring appropriate management of patients following fracture.[34] The following year, the American Society of Bone and Mineral Research Task Force report on secondary fracture prevention noted few such systems in place and presented "medical and ethical rationale" for cost-effective interventions to treat and prevent fragility fractures. The authors highlighted strategies and barriers to implementation as well as the "ethical imperatives for providing osteoporosis management … and research questions that remain outstanding."[35]

To facilitate referral of patients seen and treated for hip or vertebral fractures and to minimize the risk of subsequent fractures, a fracture liaison service (FLS) led by a dedicated physician or advanced practice provider coordinator is optimal. FLSs are designed to assist with the transition and continuation of osteoporosis care from the inpatient to outpatient setting—in particular, following treatment of an osteoporotic fracture. Communication with primary care physicians and the health care team as well as tracking of patient care and outcomes is essential to the service. FLS model should include the following key elements:[36]

- Enhanced communication between health care providers.
- Identification of patients diagnosed with a fragility fracture in a health care system.
- Individualized evaluation with fracture risk modification treatment and management by a bone health expert.
- Clinical pathways formulated based on evidence-based guidelines.
- Patient education.
- BMD testing.
- Bone health follow-up and participation in an outcomes registry.

The FLS model has been shown to be cost saving and to promote alignment of the objectives of policy makers, health care professionals, and patients. Successful transformation of care relies upon collaboration among all participants in the multidisciplinary team that cares for fragility fracture patients.[37]

34.10.3 Nonpharmacological Treatment

Pharmacologic therapy and surgical interventions play an integral role in the treatment of osteoporosis, but nonpharmacological treatments are also important and may help prevent future fracture. Most osteoporotic fractures occur due to falls; therefore, clinicians need to assess risk factors and discuss fall prevention measures with patients. Major risk factors of falls include a personal history of falling, muscle weakness, selected medications, abnormal balance, and visual deficits, and dehydration.[38] The Centers for Disease Control and Prevention (CDC) has developed a fall prevention program, named Stopping Elderly Accidents, Deaths & Injuries (STEADI), based on the American and British Geriatrics Societies' clinical guidelines. These recommendations consist of three main elements: screen, assess, and intervene.[39] Patient brochures and questionnaires can easily be implemented into the previsit or clinic visit and accessed at https://www.cdc.gov/steadi/index.html.

Calcium and Vitamin D

Calcium is a building block of bone and is necessary for the development of peak bone mass and maintenance of bone health. Vitamin D plays a key role in the absorption of calcium. Individuals should be advised of the recommended daily dietary intake of calcium and vitamin D as it is a safe and inexpensive way to help reduce fracture risk.[13,40] If adequate dietary intake cannot be achieved, supplementation should be initiated. The Institute of Medicine (IOM) recommends that men age 50 to 70 consume 1,000 mg/day of calcium and that women age 51 and older and men age 71 and older consume 1,200 mg/day of calcium. The NOF recommends adults age 50 and older intake 800 to 1,000 international units (IU) of vitamin D per day. The IOM recommends adults age less than 70 intake 600 IU/day and adults age 71 and older intake 800 IU/day of vitamin D.[41] It should also be kept in mind that vitamin D deficiency is exceedingly common and additional supplementation may be necessary to bring the vitamin D level back to a normal range. Serum 25(OH) D levels should be obtained in patients with osteoporosis or fracture. Serum 1,25(OH)2D should not be measured as it provides no information about vitamin D status and is often normal or elevated due to secondary hyperparathyroidism associated with vitamin D deficiency.[42] There is general agreement that a level of 25(OH)D of < 20 ng/mL is considered to be vitamin D deficiency whereas a level of 25(OH)D of 21 to 29 ng/mL is considered to be insufficient. The goal should be to maintain the level of 25(OH) D at > 30 ng/mL to take full advantage of all the health benefits that vitamin D provides.[42] Levels higher than 70 ng/mL probably provide no additional benefit. There are experts who suggest that there are no detrimental effects of levels of vitamin D higher than 70 ng/mL, but this recommendation is only for short-term use and not intended to be applied for chronic long-term dosing of vitamin D.

Supplementation should be initiated to bring the serum 25(OH) D level optimally between 40 and 50 ng/mL and a maintenance dose continued to maintain this level. Individuals with vitamin D deficiency may be treated with 50,000 IU of vitamin D3 weekly or the equivalent daily dose (7,000 IU vitamin D3) for 8 to 12 weeks to achieve a 25(OH) D level of at least 30 ng/mL but ideally 40 to 50 ng/mL. Replacement should be followed by maintenance dosing of 1,500 to 2,000 IU/day to keep 25(OH) D level between 40 and 50 ng/mL.[40,41]

An alternate dosing regimen that may be used in patients who have had fragility fractures and are being placed on a limited duration of antiosteoporosis medication (i.e., anabolic bone agents) is dosing the vitamin D3 supplementation between 2,000 and 5,000 IUs and giving it along with calcium and the antiosteoporotic medication. In general, 100 IU of vitamin D per day can raise the vitamin D blood test only 1 ng/mL after 2 to 3 months so 1,000 IU per day increases vitamin D blood levels 10 ng/mL and 2,000 IU per day increases vitamin D blood levels 20 ng/mL.[43] This assumed a linear relationship between vitamin D absorption and distribution which is very often not the case and the oral vitamin D bioavailability is dietary and patient dependent. Individuals with poor bowel absorption or an inflamed bowel, or who are obese, can require much more vitamin D3. Given these dosing and absorption factors, an individual who has suffered an osteoporotic fracture can be placed on a dose of vitamin D3 of 2,000 to 5,000 IU daily or 50,000 IU weekly. Based on optimal absorption, this would increase the individual's vitamin D3 levels up to 50 ng/mL. So if the individual is vitamin D deficient, this amount would increase their level up to, or very close to, an optimal level. If they are not vitamin D deficient it would increase it up to levels that, if taken for a limited time period, won't increase the level of vitamin D to harmful levels. Based on risk assessment, a safe upper intake level of 10,000 IU per day in healthy adult has been previously suggested, so a dose of 5,000 IU is thought to be safe for a limited amount of time such as the 18 months to 2-year time period it takes for the treatment with anabolic bone agents.[44,45]

34.10.4 Pharmacological Treatment

As an adjuvant to surgical intervention, pharmacological treatment of osteoporosis reduces risk of future fracture. Current FDA-approved pharmacologic options for osteoporosis treatment are bisphosphonates, calcitonin, estrogen agonists/antagonists, estrogens/hormone replacement therapy, tissue-selective estrogen complexes, parathyroid hormone 1–34 and PTH-rP(teriparatide and abaloparatide), and receptor activator of nuclear factor kappa-B (RANK) ligand inhibitor (denosumab). Commonly used medications for pharmacologic osteoporosis treatment with indications, risks and benefits, efficacy on vertebral or nonvertebral sites, and use in special populations are summarized and listed in ▶ Table 34.1.

Calcitonin is a peptide that is analogous to human calcitonin. It is indicated in use in women who have been postmenopausal for at least 5 years.[13] It has been shown to reduce vertebral fracture occurrence by about 30% in those with prior vertebral fractures, but has not been shown to reduce the risk of nonvertebral fractures.[46,47] It is no longer approved in Europe for treatment of osteoporosis.

Estrogens (including bazedoxifene-conjugated equine estrogen) are FDA approved for the prevention of osteoporosis. The Women's Health Initiative (WHI) found that 5 years of hormone replacement therapy reduced risk of clinical vertebral fractures and hip fractures by 34% and other osteoporotic fractures by 23%.[48] Bazedoxifene-conjugated equine estrogen increased mean lumbar spine BMD at 12 months compared to placebo in women who had been postmenopausal between 1 and 5 years.[49,50] However, drug safety issues exist with hormone replacement therapy, including increased risk of myocardial infarction, stroke, invasive breast cancer, pulmonary emboli, and deep vein thrombosis.[48] Rapid bone loss may also occur when estrogen therapy is discontinued. The FDA now recommends that approved nonestrogen treatment should be carefully considered first if using estrogen solely for prevention of osteoporosis.[13]

Raloxifene is approved by the FDA for both prevention and treatment of osteoporosis in postmenopausal women. It is indicated for reduction in risk of invasive breast cancer in postmenopausal women with osteoporosis and has been shown to reduce risk of vertebral fractures by about 30% in patients with a prior vertebral fracture and by about 55% in patients without

Table 34.1 Medications for the treatment of osteoporosis

Medication	Indication	Vertebral	Nonvertebral	GIOP	Males	Precautions
Calcitonin	Treatment (no longer approved in Europe)	X (limited efficacy)				Nasal congestion
Estrogens	Prevention	X	X			VTE, increased risk of BCA and CVD
Bazedoxifene/Conjugated equine estrogens	Prevention	X	X			VTE, increased risk of BCA and CVD
Raloxifene	Treatment/prevention	X		X		VTE, hot flashes, leg cramps, nausea
Bisphosphonates • Alendronate • Risedronate • Ibandronate • Zolendronic acid	Treatment/prevention Treatment/prevention Treatment/prevention Treatment/prevention	X X X X	X X X	X X X	X X X	Esophagitis, MSK, sx, ONJ, atypical femur fractures IV: acute phase response (after 1st dose), MSK sx, ONJ, atypical femur fx Contraindicated in patients with impaired swallowing, esophageal varices, severe GERD or if unable to sit up for 30 min after administration of medication
Denosumab	Treatment	X	X	X	X	Cellulitis, skin reaction, ONJ, atypical femur fx
Teriparatide/abaloparatide	Treatment	X	X	X	X	Nausea, leg cramps hypercalcemia

Abbreviations: BCA, breast cancer; CVD, cardiovascular disease; GERD, gastro-esophageal reflux disease; MSK, musculoskeletal; ONJ, osteonecrosis of the jaw; VTE, venous thromboembolism.

a prior vertebral fracture over 3 years.[51] Raloxifene increases the risk of venous thromboembolism.

Bisphosphonates are FDA approved for treatment and prevention of osteoporosis in postmenopausal women, men, and for glucocorticoid-induced osteoporosis prevention. Oral bisphosphonates include alendronate, risedronate, and ibandronate. Zolendronic acid is administered as an intravenous infusion. All bisphosphonates have been shown to reduce the risk of vertebral fractures and all but ibandronate have shown to reduce risk of nonvertebral and hip fractures. Alendronate reduced the incidence of vertebral fractures by 48%, ibandronate by 50%, risedronate by 41 to 49%, and zolendronic acid by 70% over 3 years.[52,53,54,55,56] Vitamin D (25-OH) should be obtained before starting bisphosphonate therapy, as symptomatic hypocalcemia can develop in patients with low levels of 25-OH vitamin D who receive concomitant therapy with bisphosphonates.[57] Adverse effects of bisphosphonates include esophagitis (oral administration), an acute phase reaction (IV administration), musculoskeletal symptoms, osteonecrosis of the jaw (ONJ), and atypical femur fracture.[58] It should be emphasized that ONJ is an unusual complication of bisphosphonate therapy and the American Dental Association has published guidelines stating that the benefits of antiresorptive therapy outweigh the low risk of developing ONJ.[59]

Denosumab is a receptor activator of nuclear factor kappa-B (RANK) ligand inhibitor and is FDA approved for the treatment of osteoporosis in postmenopausal women at high risk of fracture and for treatment of glucocorticoid-induced osteoporosis in men and women at high risk of fracture.[60] It may also be used in men and in patients with glucocorticoid-induced osteoporosis. Denosumab has been shown to reduce incidence of vertebral fractures by about 68%, hip fractures by about 40%, and nonvertebral fractures by about 20% over 3 years.[61] Adverse effects include hypocalcemia, increased risk of serious skin infections, rebound effect predisposing to multiple vertebral fractures, ONJ, and atypical femur fractures.[13,57]

Teriparatide and abaloparatide are parathyroid hormone analogs that are FDA approved for the treatment of osteoporosis in postmenopausal women and men at high risk for fracture and for treatment in men and women at high risk of fracture with osteoporosis associated with sustained systemic glucocorticoid therapy.[62] Treatment with teriparatide has been shown to reduce risk of vertebral fractures by about 65% and nonvertebral fragility fractures by about 53% in patients with osteoporosis, after an average of 18 months of therapy.[63] Treatment with abaloparatide has been shown to decrease the risk of vertebral fractures by about 86% and nonvertebral fragility fractures by 43% in osteoporotic patients after an average of 18 months of therapy.[64] In addition to this powerful fracture reduction, the anabolic bone agents can produce a prominent increase in the patients' BMD by approximately 12% after a full course of therapy.[63]

Each of the different classes of antiosteoporotic medications have their own effect on bone turnover with the bisphosphonates and RANK ligand inhibitors slowing bone turnover down sometimes up to 70% in just a few days after starting the medication.[65] The estrogens and estrogen receptor modulator medications have the effect of restoring the bone turnover to premenopausal levels in postmenopausal females, and the anabolic bone agents speed up bone turnover. Bone turnover can be assessed by evaluating the BTMs such as procollagen type 1 N-terminal propeptide (a marker of skeletal bone formation) and carboxy-terminal crosslinking telopeptide of collagen type 1 (a marker of bone resorption). Although it is not necessary to measure BTMs while using antiosteoporotic agents, they can be effective for assessing patient compliance and therapy efficacy. Significant reductions in BTMs are typically seen with antiresorptive therapy and can be associated with fracture reduction whereas significant increases indicate good response to anabolic therapy.[20]

Given the prominent risk reduction in vertebral and nonvertebral fractures, anabolic bone therapy should be the mainstay in treating patients with vertebral fractures. Anabolic agents have been found to reduce the risk of additional vertebral fractures more than any of the antiresorptive medications and are able to produce prominent increases in BMD in a relatively short period of time. Anabolic agents also increase bone turnover which is optimal in patients after having had a major fragility fracture.

It has been suggested that in treatment of naïve patients, initiation of anabolic therapy should be first-line treatment as the substantial BMD increases in the hip and spine are blunted if an antiresorptive agent is given first, followed by the anabolic agent.[66] There is also a risk of rebound effect on patients stopping denosumab if this medication is used first. This rebound effect may result in the occurrence of multiple vertebral fractures and the progressive or transient bone loss can continue in spite of the introduction of an anabolic bone agent, whereas switching from an anabolic bone agent to denosumab results in the continued increase in BMD.[67] Cosman et al concluded in their "Treatment sequence matters" manuscript that the common practice of changing to an anabolic bone agent only after patients have had an inadequate response to antiresorptives is not the optimal utilization of anabolic treatment and may result in transient loss of hip BMD and strength.[66] Given the importance of treatment sequence for clinical outcome optimization for patients who need an anabolic bone agent, this medication should be used instead of an antiresorptive medication to potentially avoid decreasing the efficacy of the anabolic agent.

If anabolic bone agents are used initially and the subsequent medication is an antiresorptive, it has been shown that it is possible to not only continue to increase the BMD but also to propagate the vertebral and nonvertebral fracture reduction.[68] This is important as antiresorptive therapy is optimal to prevent the immediate loss of bone density upon the cessation of the anabolic bone agent. Cosman et al in the ACTIVExtend trial used 2 years of alendronate following 18 months of abaloparatide and found that during the extension the relative risk reduction for vertebral and nonvertebral fractures was maintained, which suggests that the advantageous effects of the anabolic bone agent abaloparatide was still present when following this treatment with alendronate. Additionally, they concluded that there appears to be a cumulative benefit favoring abaloparatide and subsequent alendronate than just alendronate alone.

In addition to improving the clinical outcomes by utilizing the optimal medication treatment sequence, this approach may also improve the cost effectiveness of the therapy. In a Markov cohort model, O'Hanlon et al estimated that during a period of 1.5 years, an anabolic bone agent (abaloparatide) can reduce fractures and provide improvements in quality adjusted life years (QALYs) and produce a cost saving of $17,000,000 per 10,000 patients treated.[69] Some studies have presented data indicating that in postmenopausal women at high risk for fractures, abaloparatide followed by alendronate leads to improved health outcomes by lowering the number of fractures and lower health care costs than using the same medications for treatment but starting with alendronate.[70] The authors measured the lifetime costs and number of fractures and calculated the QALYs and incremental cost-effectiveness ratio (ICER) when treating women 70 years of age with a T-score ≤−3.5.

It should be noted that a black box warning is present on both anabolic bone agents, stating that patients may be at an increased risk of osteosarcoma as there is an increase in osteosarcoma in rats treated with these medications. Despite this, there has been no demonstrable increased rate of osteosarcoma in patients treated with anabolic bone agents for more than a decade and a half. The treatment duration is recommended not to exceed 18 to 24 months and, as mentioned above, follow-up therapy with an antiresorptive agent, usually a bisphosphonate is also advised.[13]

A summary of the American Association of Clinical Endocrinologists/American College of Endocrinology guidelines for treatment of osteoporosis can be found at https://www.aace.com/files/final-algorithm.pdf.

34.11 Treatment of the Osteoporosis by the Physician Treating the Fracture

Although follow-up with an FLS is effective in treating patients after suffering a fragility fracture, the most optimal method of treatment of the underlying osteoporosis is by the provider treating the fracture. Prompt treatment of the decreased BMD is necessary because additional fractures typically occur soon after the incident fracture most commonly in the first year so the sooner the osteoporosis is treated the better.[71] In fact the largest vertebral augmentation trial to date, "Prospective and multicenter evaluation of outcomes for quality of life and activities of daily living for balloon kyphoplasty in the treatment of vertebral compression fractures: the EVOLVE trial", reported that in typical Medicare patients after undergoing kyphoplasty the rate of additional or adjacent-level vertebral fracture was 47.6% in the first year after the fracture.[5] The most optimal way to control prompt treatment of the patient is to discuss the follow-up treatment at the time of the fracture treatment and then commence the antiosteoporotic therapy at the time of the first follow-up. This allows treatment initiation usually at approximately 2 weeks following the initial fracture fixation. Busy practices often hesitate to assume the responsibility of treating the underlying osteoporosis due to concerns that this will create extra work in an already busy practice, but given the fact that treating the underlying disorder can improve the immediate short-term and long-term outcomes of the fracture treatment, this process is essential for those practices that are interested in a sustainable and ideal treatment regimen. ▶Table 34.2

Table 34.2 Follow-up after vertebral augmentation

1. Follow-up visit—2 weeks (CPT 99213)
2. Nurse Injection Training of Patient (CPT 96372)
3. DXA scan (CPT Code 77080 and 76077 if VFA is performed)
4. Home Health Dispatched with physical therapy focus on lumbar extension training and core muscle strengthening. Injection training is reviewed (Code G0180)
5. Follow-up visit—1 year (CPT 99213)
6. DXA scan (CPT Code 77080 and 76077 if VFA is performed)
7. Follow-up visit—2 year (CPT 99213)
8. DXA scan (CPT Code 77080 and 76077 if VFA is performed)
9. Follow-up of osteoporosis treatment with injection of maintenance medication (CPT 96372) or with initiation of noninjectable antiresorptive medication

outlines a streamlined follow-up that may be incorporated for treating osteoporosis after the patient's first vertebral fragility fracture. This involves obtaining typical preoperative laboratory assessment including a complete blood count (CBC) and complete blood chemistry (i.e., Chem-20). Provided the laboratory values including the patients renal function, calcium level, and alkaline phosphatase are normal and there was no suspicion of additional pathologic process on the imaging evaluation (i.e., metastatic disease or multiple myeloma detected on the imaging studies) or the biopsy obtained during fracture fixation, the treatment may proceed as outlined in ▶Table 34.2. The patient receives injection training at the time of the first visit as anabolic agents are both currently only available in an injectable form and these agents are used in the vast majority of patient with fragility fractures. The DXA scan is used not to diagnose osteoporosis (which is already apparent from the clinical history of a low-velocity injury producing a fracture) but performed mostly to monitor the patients' BMD response to therapy. We have found that home health involvement is helpful in furthering the patient understanding of the treatment goals and in continuing the education of how to use the injectable medication and why this is being prescribed. The DXA is repeated at the first follow-up visit and an increase of 2 to 5 percent is expected when compared to the initial DXA scan. If this is not present, the patient is sent for a full secondary osteoporosis workup involving the laboratory tests mentioned previously in this chapter. The DXA is repeated at year 2 and the results of the anabolic therapy are discussed with the patient. The discussion at this time also involves placing the patient on an antiresorptive medication such as alendronate or denosumab and the patient is then sent back to their primary care physician for continuation of care. This follow-up has been shown to be a contributor to significantly better results in terms of improving patients' pain and increasing their function when treating patients with VCFs. The combination of treating the fracture and the underlying disorder was shown to produce statistically significantly better results than simply treating the VCF alone.[5]

34.12 Conclusion

Osteoporosis is an underappreciated bone disorder that has tremendous impact on individuals and public health. Diagnosis and treatment result in considerable health care expenditures. More important are the costs of *failure* to diagnose. The number of patients at risk for fractures is markedly underestimated. Without education and awareness, the diagnosis will remain elusive, and decreasing reimbursement strategies for this diagnostic process has become antagonistic to patient's wellbeing and the economic burden. Early diagnosis is key and screening tools are becoming more advanced to detect and predict future fracture risk. The most important strategy to treat patients with osteoporosis is to diagnose and treat the underlying disorder after the patient's first fragility fracture. Pharmacologic therapy can slow bone loss, increase BMD, and even increase bone mass, leading to prevention of fractures. There are many organizations dedicated to recognizing and treating osteoporosis. The American Society of Bone and Mineral Research Task Force very appropriately entitled their report on secondary fracture prevention, "Making the first fracture the last fracture." Postfracture initiation of treatment and follow-up is improved by collaborative care models such as an FLS involving primary, critical care and emergency physicians, radiologists, surgeons, and osteoporosis specialists.[9] FLSs that assist with the transition and continuation of osteoporosis care from the inpatient to outpatient setting are becoming more widespread to assist with this process, but are not currently available in all centers.[72–74] The most expeditious and possibly the most optimal way to treat the patients' underlying disorder is by the surgeons and interventionalists who initially treated the patient's fragility fracture. These providers, who may first encounter these patients in the hospital as the result of a fracture, should be knowledgeable in the basic principles of diagnosis and management of osteoporosis and discuss the treatment of the underlying diagnosis of osteoporosis with the patient. Evidence indicates that additional fractures happen in close temporal proximity to the incident fracture and that treating the underlying disorder along with the fragility fracture produces significantly better results than just treating the fracture itself. Therefore, prompt initiation of treatment preferably by the physician who treated the initial fracture should produce the best results possible.

34.13 Useful Websites

- **National Osteoporosis Foundation**
  - https://www.nof.org
- **National Osteogenesis Imperfecta Foundation**
  - http://www.oif.org/
- **American Association of Clinical Endocrinologists**
  - https://www.aace.com
  - https://www.aace.com/files/<wbr />final-algorithm.pdf
  - https://www.aace.com/files/<wbr />postmenopausal-guidelines.pdf
- **American College of Rheumatology**
  - https://www.rheumatology.org
- **American Society for Bone and Mineral Research**
  - http://www.asbmr.org
  - http://www.asbmr.org/asbmr-task-force-reports
- **Centers for Disease Control**
  - https://www.cdc.gov/steadi/index.html
- **American Orthopaedic Association: Own the Bone**
  - https://www.ownthebone.org
  - https://www.aoassn.org/aoaimis/OTB
- **National Bone Health Alliance**
  - https://www.nbha.org/

References

[1] Saag K, Morgan S, Clines G. Diagnosis and Management of Osteoporosis. 2nd ed. West Islip, NY: Professional Communications, Inc.; 2017

[2] Elliot-Gibson V, Bogoch ER, Jamal SA, Beaton DE. Practice patterns in the diagnosis and treatment of osteoporosis after a fragility fracture: a systematic review. Osteoporos Int 2004;15(10):767–778

[3] Lindsay R, Silverman SL, Cooper C, et al. Risk of new vertebral fracture in the year following a fracture. JAMA 2001;285(3):320–323

[4] Curtis JR, Arora T, Matthews RS, et al. Is withholding osteoporosis medication after fracture sometimes rational? A comparison of the risk for second fracture versus death. J Am Med Dir Assoc 2010;11(8):584–591

[5] Beall DP, Chambers MF, Thomas SM, et al. Prospective and multicenter evaluation of outcomes for quality of life and activities of daily living for balloon kyphoplasty in the treatment of vertebral compression fractures: the EVOLVE trial. J Neurosurg 2018;0:1–11

[6] Follin SL, Black JN, McDermott MT. Lack of diagnosis and treatment of osteoporosis in men and women after hip fracture. Pharmacotherapy 2003;23(2):190–198

[7] Aboyoussef M, Vierkoetter KR. Underdiagnosis and under-treatment of osteoporosis following fragility fracture. Hawaii Med J 2007;66(7):185–187

[8] Weaver J, Sajjan S, Lewiecki EM, Harris ST, Marvos P. Prevalence and cost of subsequent fractures among U.S. patients with an incident fracture. J Manag Care Spec Pharm 2017;23(4):461–471

[9] Solomon DH, Johnston SS, Boytsov NN, McMorrow D, Lane JM, Krohn KD. Osteoporosis medication use after hip fracture in U.S. patients between 2002 and 2011. J Bone Miner Res 2014;29(9):1929–1937

[10] Kanis JA, Johnell O, De Laet C, et al. A meta-analysis of previous fracture and subsequent fracture risk. Bone 2004;35(2):375–382

[11] NIH Consensus Development Panel on Osteoporosis Prevention, Diagnosis, and Therapy, March 7–29, 2000: highlights of the conference. South Med J 2001;94(6):569–573

[12] Heaney RP, Abrams S, Dawson-Hughes B, et al. Peak bone mass. Osteoporos Int 2000;11(12):985–1009

[13] Cosman F, de Beur SJ, LeBoff MS, et al; National Osteoporosis Foundation. Clinician's guide to prevention and treatment of osteoporosis. Osteoporos Int 2014;25(10):2359–2381

[14] Kanis JA; WHO Study Group. Assessment of fracture risk and its application to screening for postmenopausal osteoporosis: synopsis of a WHO report. Osteoporos Int 1994;4(6):368–381

[15] Office of the Surgeon G. Reports of the Surgeon General. In: Bone Health and Osteoporosis: A Report of the Surgeon General. Rockville, MD: Office of the Surgeon General (US); 2004

[16] Weycker D, Li X, Barron R, Bornheimer R, Chandler D. Hospitalizations for osteoporosis-related fractures: economic costs and clinical outcomes. Bone Rep 2016;5:186–191

[17] Burge R, Dawson-Hughes B, Solomon DH, Wong JB, King A, Tosteson A. Incidence and economic burden of osteoporosis-related fractures in the United States, 2005–2025. J Bone Miner Res 2007;22(3):465–475

[18] Budhia S, Mikyas Y, Tang M, Badamgarav E. Osteoporotic fractures: a systematic review of U.S. healthcare costs and resource utilization. Pharmacoeconomics 2012;30(2):147–170

[19] Siris ES, Adler R, Bilezikian J, et al. The clinical diagnosis of osteoporosis: a position statement from the National Bone Health Alliance Working Group. Osteoporos Int 2014;25(5):1439–1443

[20] Camacho PM, Petak SM, Binkley N, et al. American Association of Clinical Endocrinologists and American College of Endocrinology clinical practice guidelines for the diagnosis and treatment of postmenopausal osteoporosis: executive summary. Endocr Pract 2016;22(9):1111–1118

[21] Kanis JA, Melton LJ III, Christiansen C, Johnston CC, Khaltaev N. The diagnosis of osteoporosis. J Bone Miner Res 1994;9(8):1137–1141

[22] Assessment of fracture risk and its application to screening for postmenopausal osteoporosis. Report of a WHO Study Group. World Health Organ Tech Rep Ser 1994;843:1–129

[23] Lewiecki EM, Laster AJ. Clinical review: clinical applications of vertebral fracture assessment by dual-energy x-ray absorptiometry. J Clin Endocrinol Metab 2006;91(11):4215–4222

[24] Genant HK, Jergas M. Assessment of prevalent and incident vertebral fractures in osteoporosis research. Osteoporos Int 2003;14(Suppl 3):S43–S55

[25] Vokes TJ, Dixon LB, Favus MJ. Clinical utility of dual-energy vertebral assessment (DVA). Osteoporos Int 2003;14(11):871–878

[26] Cosman F, Krege JH, Looker AC, et al. Spine fracture prevalence in a nationally representative sample of US women and men aged ≥40 years: results from

the National Health and Nutrition Examination Survey (NHANES) 2013–2014. Osteoporos Int 2017;28(6):1857–1866

[27] Silva BC, Leslie WD, Resch H, et al. Trabecular bone score: a noninvasive analytical method based upon the DXA image. J Bone Miner Res 2014;29(3):518–530

[28] Harvey NC, Glüer CC, Binkley N, et al. Trabecular bone score (TBS) as a new complementary approach for osteoporosis evaluation in clinical practice. Bone 2015;78:216–224

[29] van de Laarschot DM, Smits AA, Buitendijk SK, Stegenga MT, Zillikens MC. Screening for atypical femur fractures using extended femur scans by DXA. J Bone Miner Res 2017;32(8):1632–1639

[30] La Rocca Vieira R, Rosenberg ZS, Allison MB, Im SA, Babb J, Peck V. Frequency of incomplete atypical femoral fractures in asymptomatic patients on long-term bisphosphonate therapy. AJR Am J Roentgenol 2012;198(5):1144–1151

[31] Kanis JA, Harvey NC, Johansson H, Odén A, Leslie WD, McCloskey EV. FRAX update. J Clin Densitom 2017;20(3):360–367

[32] Melton LJ III, Chrischilles EA, Cooper C, Lane AW, Riggs BL. How many women have osteoporosis? JBMR Anniversary Classic. JBMR, Volume 7, Number 9, 1992. J Bone Miner Res 2005;20(5):886–892

[33] Buckley L, Guyatt G, Fink HA, et al. American College of Rheumatology guideline for the prevention and treatment of glucocorticoid-induced osteoporosis. Arthritis Care Res (Hoboken) 2017;69(8):1095–1110

[34] Marsh D, Akesson K, Beaton DE, et al; IOF CSA Fracture Working Group. Coordinator-based systems for secondary prevention in fragility fracture patients. Osteoporos Int 2011;22(7):2051–2065

[35] Eisman JA, Bogoch ER, Dell R, et al; ASBMR Task Force on Secondary Fracture Prevention. Making the first fracture the last fracture: ASBMR task force report on secondary fracture prevention. J Bone Miner Res 2012;27(10):2039–2046

[36] Aizer J, Bolster MB. Fracture liaison services: promoting enhanced bone health care. Curr Rheumatol Rep 2014;16(11):455

[37] Javaid MK, Kyer C, Mitchell PJ, et al; IOF Fracture Working Group. EXCO. Effective secondary fracture prevention: implementation of a global benchmarking of clinical quality using the IOF Capture the Fracture Best Practice Framework tool. Osteoporos Int 2015;26(11):2573–2578

[38] Guideline for the prevention of falls in older persons. American Geriatrics Society, British Geriatrics Society, and American Academy of Orthopaedic Surgeons Panel on Falls Prevention. J Am Geriatr Soc 2001;49(5):664–672

[39] Prevention CfDCa. Algorithm for Fall Risk Screening, Assessment, and Intervention. 2017

[40] Larsen ER, Mosekilde L, Foldspang A. Vitamin D and calcium supplementation prevents osteoporotic fractures in elderly community dwelling residents: a pragmatic population-based 3-year intervention study. J Bone Miner Res 2004;19(3):370–378

[41] Institute of Medicine (US) Committee to Review Dietary Reference Intakes for Vitamin D and Calcium. Ross AC, Taylor CL, Yaktine AL, et al., eds. In. Dietary Reference Intakes for Calcium and Vitamin D. Washington, DC: National Academies Press; 2011

[42] Holick MF. Vitamin D status: measurement, interpretation, and clinical application. Ann Epidemiol 2009;19(2):73–78

[43] Moyad MA. Vitamin D: a rapid review. Dermatol Nurs 2009;21(1):25–30, 55

[44] Hathcock JN, Shao A, Vieth R, Heaney R. Risk assessment for vitamin D. Am J Clin Nutr 2007;85(1):6–18

[45] Ross AC, Taylor CL, Yaktine AL, Del Valle HB. Dietary Reference Intakes for Calcium and Vitamin D. Washington, DC: National Academies Press; 2011

[46] Chesnut CH III, Silverman S, Andriano K, et al; PROOF Study Group. A randomized trial of nasal spray salmon calcitonin in postmenopausal women with established osteoporosis: the prevent recurrence of osteoporotic fractures study. Am J Med 2000;109(4):267–276

[47] Binkley N, Bolognese M, Sidorowicz-Bialynicka A, et al; Oral Calcitonin in Postmenopausal Osteoporosis (ORACAL) Investigators. A phase 3 trial of the efficacy and safety of oral recombinant calcitonin: the Oral Calcitonin in Postmenopausal Osteoporosis (ORACAL) trial. J Bone Miner Res 2012;27(8):1821–1829

[48] Rossouw JE, Anderson GL, Prentice RL, et al; Writing Group for the Women's Health Initiative Investigators. Risks and benefits of estrogen plus progestin in healthy postmenopausal women: principal results From the Women's Health Initiative randomized controlled trial. JAMA 2002;288(3):321–333

[49] Gennari L, Merlotti D, De Paola V, Martini G, Nuti R. Bazedoxifene for the prevention of postmenopausal osteoporosis. Ther Clin Risk Manag 2008;4(6):1229–1242

[50] Pinkerton JV, Pickar JH, Racketa J, Mirkin S. Bazedoxifene/conjugated estrogens for menopausal symptom treatment and osteoporosis prevention. Climacteric 2012;15(5):411–418

[51] Ettinger B, Black DM, Mitlak BH, et al; Multiple Outcomes of Raloxifene Evaluation (MORE) Investigators. Reduction of vertebral fracture risk in postmenopausal women with osteoporosis treated with raloxifene: results from a 3-year randomized clinical trial. JAMA 1999;282(7):637–645

[52] Cummings SR, Black DM, Thompson DE, et al. Effect of alendronate on risk of fracture in women with low bone density but without vertebral fractures: results from the Fracture Intervention Trial. JAMA 1998;280(24):2077–2082

[53] Harris ST, Watts NB, Genant HK, et al; Vertebral Efficacy With Risedronate Therapy (VERT) Study Group. Effects of risedronate treatment on vertebral and nonvertebral fractures in women with postmenopausal osteoporosis: a randomized controlled trial. JAMA 1999;282(14):1344–1352

[54] Reginster J, Minne HW, Sorensen OH, et al; Vertebral Efficacy with Risedronate Therapy (VERT) Study Group. Randomized trial of the effects of risedronate on vertebral fractures in women with established postmenopausal osteoporosis. Osteoporos Int 2000;11(1):83–91

[55] Chesnut CH III, Skag A, Christiansen C, et al; Oral Ibandronate Osteoporosis Vertebral Fracture Trial in North America and Europe (BONE). Effects of oral ibandronate administered daily or intermittently on fracture risk in postmenopausal osteoporosis. J Bone Miner Res 2004;19(8):1241–1249

[56] Black DM, Delmas PD, Eastell R, et al; HORIZON Pivotal Fracture Trial. Once-yearly zoledronic acid for treatment of postmenopausal osteoporosis. N Engl J Med 2007;356(18):1809–1822

[57] Black DM, Rosen CJ. Postmenopausal osteoporosis. N Engl J Med 2016;374(21):2096–2097

[58] Favus MJ. Bisphosphonates for osteoporosis. N Engl J Med 2010;363(21):2027–2035

[59] Hellstein JW, Adler RA, Edwards B, et al; American Dental Association Council on Scientific Affairs Expert Panel on Antiresorptive Agents. Managing the care of patients receiving antiresorptive therapy for prevention and treatment of osteoporosis: executive summary of recommendations from the American Dental Association Council on Scientific Affairs. J Am Dent Assoc 2011;142(11):1243–1251

[60] Prolia (denosumab). Thousand Oaks, CA: Amgen Inc; 2018

[61] Cummings SR, San Martin J, McClung MR, et al; FREEDOM Trial. Denosumab for prevention of fractures in postmenopausal women with osteoporosis. N Engl J Med 2009;361(8):756–765

[62] Saag KG, Shane E, Boonen S, et al. Teriparatide or alendronate in glucocorticoid-induced osteoporosis. N Engl J Med 2007;357(20):2028–2039

[63] Neer RM, Arnaud CD, Zanchetta JR, et al. Effect of parathyroid hormone (1-34) on fractures and bone mineral density in postmenopausal women with osteoporosis. N Engl J Med 2001;344(19):1434–1441

[64] Miller PD, Hattersley G, Riis BJ, et al; ACTIVE Study Investigators. Effect of abaloparatide vs placebo on new vertebral fractures in postmenopausal women with osteoporosis: a randomized clinical trial. JAMA 2016;316(7):722–733

[65] Binkley N, Silverman SL, Simonelli C, et al. Monthly ibandronate suppresses serum CTX-I within 3 days and maintains a monthly fluctuating pattern of suppression. Osteoporos Int 2009;20(9):1595–1601

[66] Cosman F, Nieves JW, Dempster DW. Treatment sequence matters: anabolic and antiresorptive therapy for osteoporosis. J Bone Miner Res 2017;32(2):198–202

[67] Leder BZ, Tsai JN, Uihlein AV, et al. Denosumab and teriparatide transitions in postmenopausal osteoporosis (the DATA-Switch study): extension of a randomised controlled trial. Lancet 2015;386(9999):1147–1155

[68] Cosman F, Miller PD, Williams GC, et al. Eighteen months of treatment with subcutaneous abaloparatide followed by 6 months of treatment with alendronate in postmenopausal women with osteoporosis: results of the ACTIVExtend trial. Mayo Clin Proc 2017;92(2):200–210

[69] O'Hanlon CE, Parthan A, Kruse M, et al. A model for assessing the clinical and economic benefits of bone-forming agents for reducing fractures in postmenopausal women at high, near-term risk of osteoporotic fracture. Clin Ther 2017;39(7):1276–1290

[70] Nexus AMCP. Maastricht University, the Netherlands, Radius Health, Inc., MA, Cedar-Sinai Medical Center and UCLA School of Medicine, Los-Angeles, CA, University of Liège, Belgium; AMCP—Academy of Managed Care Pharmacy; 2018

[71] van Geel TA, van Helden S, Geusens PP, Winkens B, Dinant GJ. Clinical subsequent fractures cluster in time after first fractures. Ann Rheum Dis 2009;68(1):99–102

[72] Fraser M, McLellan AR. A fracture liaison service for patients with osteoporotic fractures. Prof Nurse 2004;19(5):286–290

[73] Wright SA, McNally C, Beringer T, Marsh D, Finch MB. Osteoporosis fracture liaison experience: the Belfast experience. Rheumatol Int 2005;25(6):489–490

[74] Charalambous CP, Mosey C, Johnstone E, et al. Improving osteoporosis assessment in the fracture clinic. Ann R Coll Surg Engl 2009;91(7):596–598

Chapter 35

Miscellaneous Tips by the Masters of Vertebral Augmentation

35.1 If You Aim at Height Restoration, Mind the Access!

Alessandro Cianfoni

Some of the original intended advantages of balloon kyphoplasty (BKP) were to achieve height restoration and spinal realignment in patients with vertebral fractures, but BKP has inconsistently shown to be able to obtain significant fracture reduction.[1] Up to one-third of BKP-treated cases show no appreciable height restoration, either because the balloons expand in trajectories that produce inefficient internal fracture distraction or due to the loss of previously restored height and kyphotic realignment after balloon deflation.[2]

Newer percutaneous devices have been introduced to achieve fracture reduction and kyphosis correction and are used along with vertebral cement augmentation. Two of these systems, vertebral body stents (VBS; DePuy Synthes-Johnson & Johnson) and SpineJack (Vexim-Stryker), offer the possibility to perform a kyphoplasty with an internal framework that consists of rigid devices that produce internal vertebral body distraction. The devices expand in a different manner than balloons that expand spherically and centrifugally. These devices expand in a predictable manner and in a way that exerts a strong predetermined craniocaudal distraction force perpendicular to the major fracture axis.[3–7]

In order to allow the device to perform its craniocaudal distraction force and obtain the most efficient fracture reduction and height restoration, the axis of insertion of the device in the vertebral body is of paramount, yet sometimes underestimated, importance.

While the transpedicular access used to perform vertebroplasty and BKP aims at the safe zones at and around the pedicle to stay as far as possible from the medial pedicular cortical boundaries, in kyphoplasty with structural implants the pedicular access should be adapted in order to obtain a device placement inside the vertebral body along an axis parallel to the anticipated alignment of the original prefracture end plates (►Fig. 35.1). When only one end plate is fractured and deformed, the axis of device insertion can be parallel to the intact end plate. The distraction performed perpendicular to this axis approximates the original prefracture shape of the vertebral body and allows the device to achieve maximum expansion and fracture reduction (►Fig. 35.2 and ►Fig. 35.3). A different axis of insertion of the device causes the distraction force to be incident with an angle that is nonperpendicular to one or both end plates, thereby resulting in less efficient fracture reduction and increases the risk of iatrogenic end plate disruption that can limit the device expansion to a lesser degree of height restoration than is optimal.

It is not always easy to obtain insertion of the device along the desired axis. The most frequently injured portion of the vertebral body in compression fractures is the superior end plate, often creating an unfavorable access angle between pedicles and superior end plate. In such cases, the transpedicular access is performed through the most caudal aspect of the pedicle and then advanced just tangentially underneath the superior end plate (►Fig. 35.1).

Accessing the caudal part of the pedicle poses some technical challenges:
- During the trocar docking into the cortex of the posterior elements, the trocar tends to slide caudally and poses the risk of inadvertently entering the neural foramen.
- The caudal aspect of the pedicle is often smaller than the cranial part; attention should be made not to violate the medial pedicular cortex that protects the central canal, and the inferior cortex that protects the neural foramen (►Fig. 35.1).

We suggest the use of a beveled tip low-profile (12- to 14-gauge) trocar to perform the initial access so as to be able to dock and steer along the optimal access path. This will provide the maximum control and precision placement of the trocar, especially while sliding under a fractured end plate. The initial access is then followed by insertion of larger access trocar via using k-wire exchange. The larger trocar is then able to accommodate the placement of the distraction devices (►Fig. 35.2).

When the access is correct, the expansion of the distraction device can occur in an optimally craniocaudal orientation within the vertebral body, thereby maximizing the chances of full vertebral body height restoration and kyphosis correction (►Fig. 35.2 and ►Fig. 35.3).

If you are aiming at fracture reduction, to restore the prefracture vertebral body height in order to optimize pain relief, physiological biomechanics, and to prevent more fractures of adjacent and distant vertebral bodies, **mind the access!**

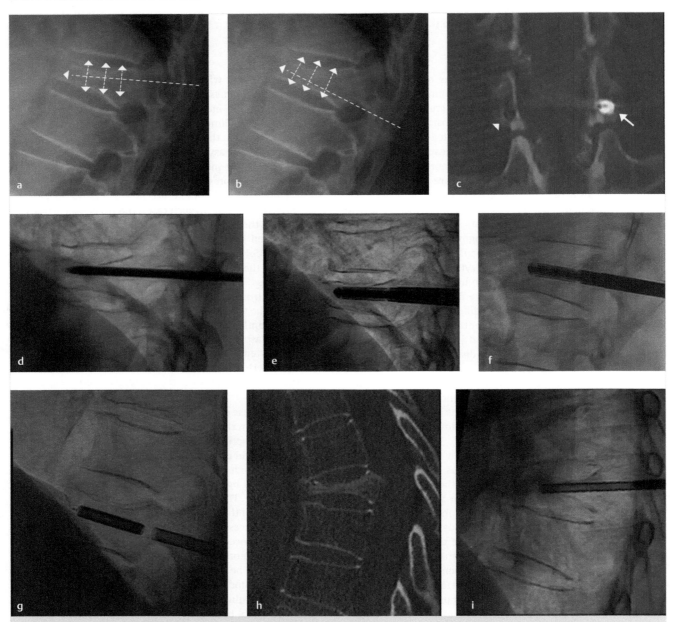

Fig. 35.1 Examples of pedicular accesses to achieve height restoration. In (a) and (b) schematic drawings on lateral X-ray views of the thoracolumbar junction represent two axes of transpedicular access to the wedged vertebral body of T12. The superior end plate is more deformed than the inferior end plate. (a) A standard access (*dashed long arrow*) in the center of the pedicle that could be easily performed and used for a vertebroplasty. If used to insert a distraction device to achieve height restoration, the perpendicular forces (*small arrows*) exerted by the device would have an incident angle on both end plates that would prevent efficient height restoration. (b) The *long dashed arrow* represents a more correct axis to insert and operate a distraction device. The access is along the caudal aspect of the pedicle with the *small arrows* predicting how the device would exert fracture reduction and more efficiently reconstitute vertebral body height. (c) A postprocedure coronal multiplanar reconstructed CT image showing the hole left by the trocar in the inferior portion of the pedicle on the right (*arrowhead*) and the pedicular screw on the left (*arrow*). (d–g) Four examples of transpedicular access along the inferior portion of the pedicle, to insert the distraction devices (12-gauge trocar in **d**, Spinejack in **e** and **f**, vertebral body stents [VBS] in **g**), along the correct axis, parallel to the intact inferior end plate. (h) A sagittal multiplanar reconstructed CT image of a midthoracic vertebra plana and (i) its corresponding intraprocedural fluoroscopic image showing access to the vertebral body between the collapsed end plates (cannula shown in **i**).

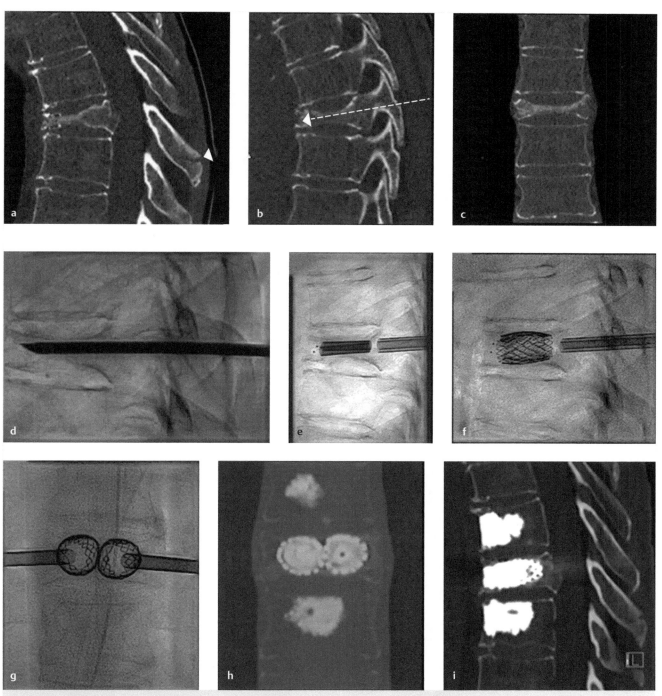

Fig. 35.2 Height restoration in a vertebra plana with vertebral body stents (VBS). **(a–c)** Multiplanar reconstructed CT images of a T8 vertebral compression fracture with vertebra plana deformity. **(a)** Midsagittal image showing the focal kyphosis due to the collapse of the vertebral body and a fracture of the spinous process (*arrowhead*). **(b)** It is important to look at the sagittal image through the pedicles to study the angle between the pedicles and the fractured superior end plate that influences the axis of the pedicular access (*dashed arrow*). **(c)** Coronal image showing the prominent collapse of the end plates. In the cases with prominent central collapse of the vertebral body, a more anteroposterior trocar approach, lateral to midline, will be favored. **(d)** The beveled tip trocar is inserted through the caudal aspect of the pedicle and precisely steered and advanced between the end plates. The trocar is then exchanged over a k-wire with a larger access cannula that allows the insertion of the balloon-mounted VBS **(e)**. **(f, g)** The balloons are inflated and the VBS deployed. After cement augmentation, **(h, i)** the postprocedure CT images show the fracture reduction, with significant height restoration and kyphosis correction.

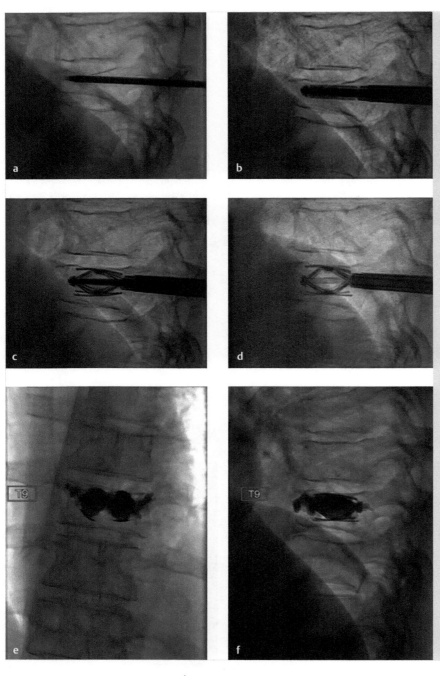

Fig. 35.3 Height restoration with Spinejack. Lateral fluoroscopic images show a posttraumatic T9 compression fracture, with more than 50% vertebral body height loss. Both end plates are fractured and deformed, but their alignment is nearly parallel. The beveled tip trocar in (**a**) is placed along an axis parallel to both end plates. The trocar is placed along the caudal portion of the pedicle and sliding just underneath the superior end plate. This access allows insertion of the Spinejack distraction devices parallel to the expected prefracture end plate alignment (shown in **b**) that allows a craniocaudal distraction of the Spinejack leading to efficient fracture reduction and height restoration (**c, d**). Cement augmentation completes the procedure, as shown on postoperative (**e**) anteroposterior and (**f**) lateral fluoroscopic images.

References

[1] Beall D, Lorio MP, Yun BM, Runa MJ, Ong KL, Warner CB. Review of vertebral augmentation: an updated meta-analysis of the effectiveness. Int J Spine Surg 2018;12(3):295–321

[2] Disch AC, Schmoelz W. Cement augmentation in a thoracolumbar fracture model: reduction and stability after balloon kyphoplasty versus vertebral body stenting. Spine 2014;39(19):E1147–E1153

[3] Rotter R, Martin H, Fuerderer S, et al. Vertebral body stenting: a new method for vertebral augmentation versus kyphoplasty. Eur Spine J 2010;19(6):916–923

[4] Diel P, Röder C, Perler G, et al. Radiographic and safety details of vertebral body stenting: results from a multicenter chart review. BMC Musculoskelet Disord 2013;14:233

[5] Wang D, Zheng S, Liu A, et al. The role of minimally invasive vertebral body stent on reduction of the deflation effect after kyphoplasty: a biomechanical study. Spine 2018;43(6):E341–E347

[6] Noriega D, Krüger A, Ardura F, et al. Clinical outcome after the use of a new craniocaudal expandable implant for vertebral compression fracture treatment: one year results from a prospective multicentric study. BioMed Res Int 2015;2015:927813

[7] Noriega D, Maestretti G, Renaud C, et al. Clinical performance and safety of 108 SpineJack implantations: 1-year results of a prospective multicentre single-arm registry study. BioMed Res Int 2015; 2015:173872

35.2 Pearls of Vertebroplasty and Kyphoplasty

Deborah H. Tracy

There are several important pearls in accomplishing an accurate needle placement and an optimal fill, and good post-op outcomes when performing kyphoplasty or vertebroplasty. These techniques include using last image hold, utilizing a bevel needle for maximum needle steering capability when driving the access needle, magnifying the image if visualization is difficult, and dressing the wound site with steri-strips, which can be left on for 5 days.

The fluoroscopic last-minute hold allows the provider to save the last image on the screen (▶Fig. 35.4). For example, if you save the anteroposterior (AP) view as you reach the medial

cortex, then rotate to the lateral view and it shows the access needle is not in the vertebral body, the AP image information displayed can be used to determine if there is enough room medial to the pedicle to advance. Additionally, the last image hold can display the lateral view before injecting cement to see densities already present prior to cement injection, for example, a calcified aorta or a radiopaque material within the colon will be visually documented prior to injection so as not to confuse these densities with cement extravasation. Collimation of the X-ray beam will decrease scatter by decreasing the number of electrons passing through the X-ray tube and will also improve the image (▶Fig. 35.5, ▶Fig. 35.6, and ▶Fig. 35.7).

When high-grade fractures require precise trajectories, use a bevel needle to drive the access to the vertebral body. The bevel point up will drive the needle tip upward, bevel point down will drive the needle tip downward, bevel point medial will drive the needle tip toward the center, and bevel point lateral will drive the needle tip lateral (▶Fig. 35.8 and ▶Fig. 35.9). This is especially helpful when you need room to pass by the medial wall of the pedicle if you are close to the medial cortex.

Leaving a transparent film dressing on the wound will allow the patient's caretaker to monitor for bleeding, swelling, and infection while maintaining a sterile environment under the transparent film dressing (▶Fig. 35.10).

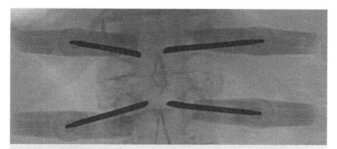

Fig. 35.4 Anteroposterior view of the thoracolumbar junction showing bilateral vertebral augmentation needles placed via a transpedicular approach and the good-quality image obtained by using the last image hold.

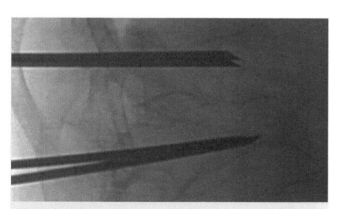

Fig. 35.5 Lateral view of the thoracolumbar junction showing vertebral augmentation needles placed into the T12 and L1 vertebral bodies. This image was obtained by using live fluoroscopy.

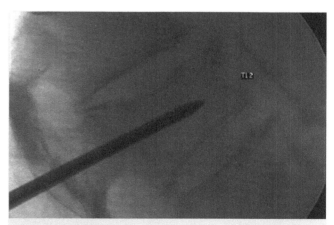

Fig. 35.6 Lateral fluoroscopic view showing two needles in the L1 vertebral body and calcification in the aorta as captured with the last image hold function.

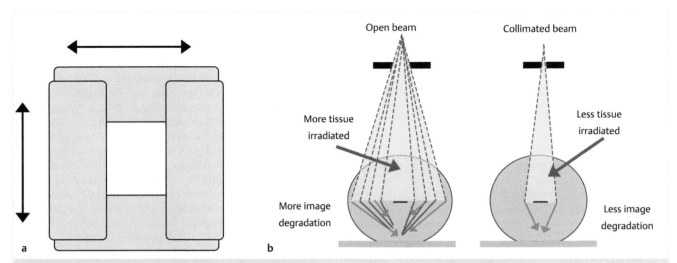

Fig. 35.7 The collimator consists of shutters that move to provide a geometric limitation to the X-ray field and can be either circular or rectangular in shape (**a**). The collimation serves to limit the amount of radiation to the patient and this also produces less X-ray scatter and associated image degradation (**b**).

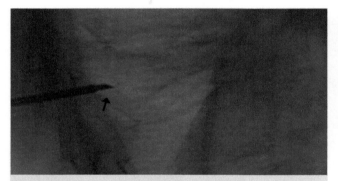

Fig. 35.8 Lateral X-ray view of the thoracolumbar junction shows the needle entering the vertebral body with the bevel tip (*black arrow*) directed down. The needle tip will then move in a downward trajectory.

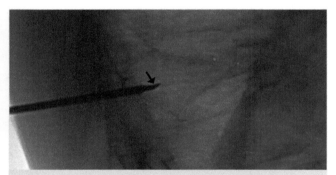

Fig. 35.9 Lateral X-ray view of the thoracolumbar junction shows the needle entering the vertebral body with the bevel tip (*black arrow*) directed up. The needle tip will then move in an upward trajectory.

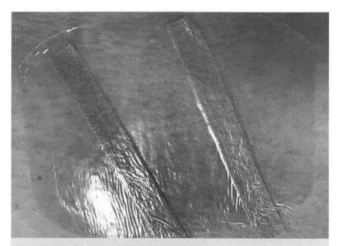

Fig. 35.10 Photograph of the patient's lumbar kyphoplasty wound with Steri-strips and a film dressing in place.

35.3 Excellence is a Habit

Derrick D. Wagoner

> *"We are what we repeatedly do. Excellence, then, is not an act, but a habit."*
>
> –Will Durant

We have the privilege of offering a treatment to patients that nearly immediately alleviates the agony they are experiencing and simultaneously restores the functionality lost secondary to their ailment. We must remember to put the patient first. Time and again, patients are not offered interventional treatment for vertebral fractures given that many fractures do not require treatment. This is true. There are many vertebral fractures that are not terribly painful and do not limit a patient's function. The question concerning whether a fracture requires treatment is centered on one question. How much pain is the patient in? If the patient is in severe pain, their functionality is sure to be diminished. Waiting to see if your patient will either spontaneously "heal" or remain bedbound in a back brace, potentially developing pneumonia in the next 4 to 6 weeks, should not be contemplated. The benefits of the treatment far outweigh the risks.

35.4 Osteonecrosis of the Spine (Kümmel–Verneuil Disease)

Stephan Becker

Osteonecrosis (ON), vascular necrosis, pseudarthrosis, and Kümmel's spondylitis[1-12] are descriptions of severe complications of a vertebral osteoporotic fracture (VOF). It has been discussed that disruption of anterior perforating vessels results in pseudarthrosis of the vertebra; hence, ON is mostly located at the anterior aspect of the vertebra (▶ Fig. 35.11). In addition to a VOF, malignancy, infection, radiation therapy, liver cirrhosis, alcoholism, steroid treatments, sarcoidosis, hemoglobinopathies such as sickle cell anemia, Cushing's syndrome, Gaucher's syndrome, and dysbarism after diving accidents can also lead to ON.[1,4,10-12] Nevertheless, osteoporosis and a fracture are by far the main causes for developing ON. This pathology bears typical changes on X-ray and MR imaging.[13-17] On X-ray or CT, we typically find an intravertebral cleft, also described as a "gas sign" demonstrating fluid and/or gas in the vertebral body.[14,17] On MRI, we find fluid or gas in the vertebral body, which can be seen as a dark or bright zones on T1 and T2/short tau inversion recovery (STIR) depending on what is present within the cleft.[6,8,14,17]

In typical cases of ON, no bone healing occurs, and the risk of severe kyphosis and compression of the dorsal neural structures increases massively. This disease may be missed if only standing X-rays are performed; therefore, it is indicated to perform a prone or supine X-ray, which can help in making the appropriate diagnosis.

Nonsurgical treatment is not indicated to avoid plegic complications. In the past, vertebroplasty and balloon kyphoplasty (BKP) have been performed. Both techniques have led to severe bone resorption, collapse, and cement dislocation with ON, but this is seen more commonly with BKP (▶ Fig. 35.12). It is known that cement filling after BKP and all other bone displacement vertebral augmentation procedures lead to stress shielding of the vertebra and increased resorption in the portions of the vertebral body not affected by the fracture, so it is thought that BKP and other procedures like it should be avoided in ON.[18-21] Stress-shielding phenomena have not been found in vertebroplasty.[18,19]

In order to achieve a good cement fill and interdigitation, vertebroplasty in cases of ON should be performed by experienced practitioners. New bone-preserving kyphoplasty procedures using implants such as the Kiva implant or the SpineJack have, so far, not resulted in cement dislocation and might be indicated to achieve good stabilization of the vertebral body without increased stress shielding and an increased risk of cement dislocation (▶ Fig. 35.13).

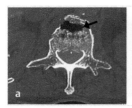
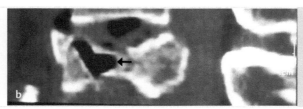

Fig. 35.11 Axial **(a)** and sagittal reconstruction **(b)** images from a CT scan in a patient with a T12 vertebral compression fractures show evidence of osteonecrosis with gas (*black arrows*) present within the anterior portion of the vertebral body. This is a typical location for the intravertebral gas.

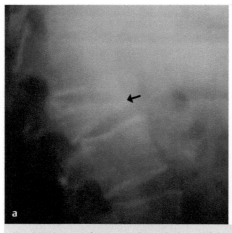
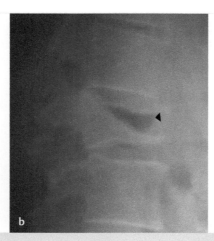
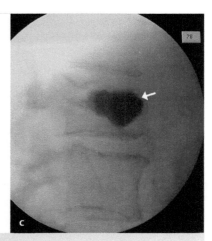

Fig. 35.12 Lateral X-rays (a, b) and a lateral fluoroscopic image (c) in a 72-year-old man show a vertebral compression fracture that is severely collapsed when the patient is in a standing position (*black arrow* in a) that reduces and fills with air (*black arrowhead* in b). After vertebral augmentation, there is a normal cement fill within the vertebral cleft (*white arrow* in c).

(Continued)

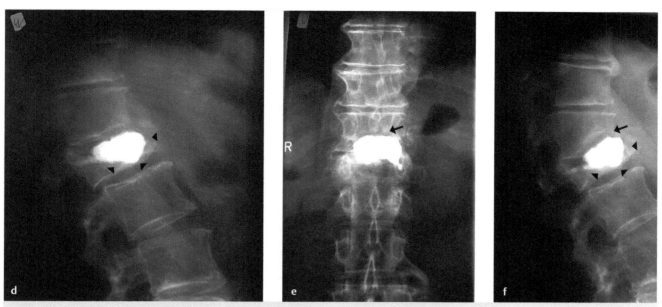

Fig. 35.12 (*Continued*) Six weeks after vertebral augmentation, there has been bone resorption around the cement (*black arrowheads* in **d**) and 10 weeks after augmentation, there is further bone resorption (*black arrowheads* in **f**) along with a now clearly defined adjacent-level vertebral fracture of D11 (*black arrows* in **e** and **f**).

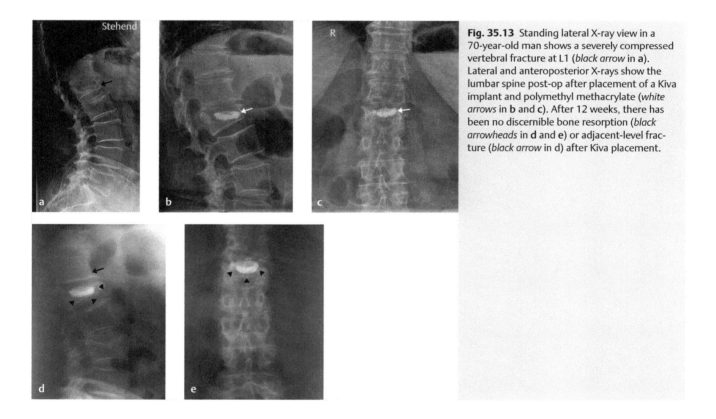

Fig. 35.13 Standing lateral X-ray view in a 70-year-old man shows a severely compressed vertebral fracture at L1 (*black arrow* in **a**). Lateral and anteroposterior X-rays show the lumbar spine post-op after placement of a Kiva implant and polymethyl methacrylate (*white arrows* in **b** and **c**). After 12 weeks, there has been no discernible bone resorption (*black arrowheads* in **d** and **e**) or adjacent-level fracture (*black arrow* in **d**) after Kiva placement.

References

[1] Chou LH, Knight RQ. Idiopathic avascular necrosis of a vertebral body. Case report and literature review. Spine 1997;22(16):1928–1932

[2] Hasegawa K, Homma T, Uchiyama S, Takahashi H. Vertebral pseudarthrosis in the osteoporotic spine. Spine 1998;23(20):2201–2206

[3] Huy MD, Jensen ME, Marx WF, Kallmes DF. Percutaneous vertebroplasty in vertebral osteonecrosis (Kümmell's spondylitis). Neurosurg Focus 1999;7(1):e2

[4] Ito M, Motomiya M, Abumi K, et al. Vertebral osteonecrosis associated with sarcoidosis. Case report. J Neurosurg Spine 2005;2(2):222–225

[5] Jang JS, Kim DY, Lee SH. Efficacy of percutaneous vertebroplasty in the treatment of intravertebral pseudarthrosis associated with noninfected avascular necrosis of the vertebral body. Spine 2003;28(14):1588–1592

[6] Maheshwari PR, Nagar AM, Prasad SS, Shah JR, Patkar DP. Avascular necrosis of spine: a rare appearance. Spine 2004;29(6):E119–E122

[7] Murakami H, Kawahara N, Gabata T, Nambu K, Tomita K. Vertebral body osteonecrosis without vertebral collapse. Spine 2003;28(16):E323–E328

[8] Van Eenenaam DP, el-Khoury GY. Delayed post-traumatic vertebral collapse (Kummell's disease): case report with serial radiographs, computed tomographic scans, and bone scans. Spine 1993;18(9):1236–1241

[9] Young WF, Brown D, Kendler A, Clements D. Delayed post-traumatic osteonecrosis of a vertebral body (Kummell's disease). Acta Orthop Belg 2002;68(1):13–19

[10] Allen BL Jr, Jinkins WJ III. Vertebral osteonecrosis associated with pancreatitis in a child. A case report. J Bone Joint Surg Am 1978;60(7):985–987

[11] Brower AC, Downey EF Jr. Kümmell disease: report of a case with serial radiographs. Radiology 1981;141(2):363–364

[12] Hutter CD. Dysbaric osteonecrosis: a reassessment and hypothesis. Med Hypotheses 2000;54(4):585–590

[13] Lieberman IH, Dudeney S, Reinhardt MK, Bell G. Initial outcome and efficacy of "kyphoplasty" in the treatment of painful osteoporotic vertebral compression fractures. Spine 2001;26(14):1631–1638

[14] Maldague BE, Noel HM, Malghem JJ. The intravertebral vacuum cleft: a sign of ischemic vertebral collapse. Radiology 1978;129(1):23–29

[15] Van Bockel SR, Mindelzun RE. Gas in the psoas muscle secondary to an intravertebral vacuum cleft: CT characteristics. J Comput Assist Tomogr 1987;11(5):913–915

[16] Bhalla S, Reinus WR. The linear intravertebral vacuum: a sign of benign vertebral collapse. AJR Am J Roentgenol 1998;170(6):1563–1569

[17] McKiernan F, Faciszewski T. Intravertebral clefts in osteoporotic vertebral compression fractures. Arthritis Rheum 2003;48(5):1414–1419

[18] Becker S. The impact of cement stiffness, bone density and filling volume after balloon kyphoplasty and the risk of stress shielding on adjacent vertebral fractures. Osteoporos Int 2010;21(Suppl 1):118–119

[19] Dabirrahmani D, Becker S, Hogg M, Appleyard R, Baroud G, Gillies M. Mechanical variables affecting balloon kyphoplasty outcome: a finite element study. Comput Methods Biomech Biomed Engin 2012;15(3):211–220

[20] Krüger A, Oberkircher L, Kratz M, Baroud G, Becker S, Ruchholtz S. Cement interdigitation and bone-cement interface after augmenting fractured vertebrae: a cadaveric study. Int J Spine Surg 2012;6(1):115–123

[21] Rohlmann A, Boustani HN, Bergmann G, Zander T. A probabilistic finite element analysis of the stresses in the augmented vertebral body after vertebroplasty. Eur Spine J 2010;19(9):1585–1595

35.5 Cement Augmentation

Majid Khan

Percutaneous vertebroplasty (PVP) is widely used in the management of osteoporotic vertebral compression fractures (VCFs), but there are reported cases where a patient's symptoms show partial response with change in the nature of pain. Upon referral to our institution, we revisited the imaging on such cases and found in some cases to have either too little cement deposition or, more frequently, uneven cement distribution only on one side of the treated vertebrae.

The author has found in his practice that a salvage procedure after failure of an improperly used technique can be quite beneficial to some patients and can help prevent open surgical intervention. Proper patient selection using both clinical and imaging findings is critical and it should be remembered that all patients may not be suited for repeat vertebroplasty.

PVP may be done using a unipedicular or bipedicular approach for cement injection with straight or curved needles. Regardless of needle type, the cement should be placed in the midline with adequate and uniform cement deposition. In certain cases with improperly performed techniques, we do see patients with uneven cement distribution or a small amount of cement within the vertebral body. Injection using a bipedicular technique tends to deliver a more uniform cement distribution more so than a unipedicular technique. When such vertebroplasty cases are deemed failure of treatment, performing repeat salvage cement augmentation can be considered the first choice prior to open surgery, especially for patients in whom the unipedicular approach was initially used.

Bone cement is introduced via the pedicle on the side of the vertebral body with the least amount of cement for cement delivery into the nonfilled portion of the previously partially filled vertebral body. This will give rise to a more uniform cement distribution and will help in filling any previously unfilled fracture clefts. For patients in whom a bipedicular approach was initially used, repeat vertebroplasty is technically more difficult, but usually the pedicle size is sufficient enough so a repeat augmentation can still be performed. At times, a small pedicle may necessitate the use of a small gauge access cannula and delivery port in order to properly access the vertebral body. At higher levels in the spine, especially in the thoracic spine, a parapedicular approach can be used.

The author's clinical practice is primarily focused around treatment of pathological osteolytic compression fractures with all types of cases including metastatic disease with a complete breach of the vertebral cortices including the posterior vertebral body wall.

Cement filling of pathologically fractured vertebral body is very different from filling an osteoporotic VCF as benign fractures usually have a fill pattern that is homogeneous where a cement ball is seen to form at the point of injection, which grows in size as more cement is injected and is ultimately seen to fill the anterior and middle portions of the vertebral body as the injection is observed under constant fluoroscopic imaging. In severe osteolytic pathologically fractured vertebra, the initial cement injection shows cement spreading toward channels of least resistance and can be seen darting toward the breached posterior cortex. If this happens, the operator may have to stop the injection as extravasation into the spinal canal can lead to neurologic injury and the result of limiting the amount of cement can sometimes produce inadequate stabilization of the vertebral body.

35.5.1 Pearls

Inject contrast into the vertebral body before cement delivery to get a good idea about channels of least resistance. Based on what is seen on the injection of contrast, the tip of the delivery port can be extended more anteriorly or into another location within the vertebral body. If another appropriate location cannot be accessed with the initial straight needle, a curved needle can be used for delivery of cement to a different location.

After cement is seen extending into the posterior third of the vertebral body or noted to abut the breached cortex of any vertebral wall, the author usually waits for 2 to 3 minutes, which lets the cement to harden a bit and this hardened cement can serve as a barrier to unwanted cement extension. This technique can help more cement to be deposited into appropriate areas within the vertebral body.

35.6 Tips and Techniques of Vertebral Augmentation

Thomas Guido Andreshak and Edward Yoon

35.6.1 Cementing Tips after Prior Vertebral Augmentation

During vertebroplasty or vertebral augmentation in patients with compression fractures, inadequate cement fill will lead to fracture extension, collapse, or result in nonunion clefts. Using slow and low-pressure cement injection with thick cement is key to a successful cement fill. The bone filling cannula needs to be placed in the middle of the cement ball and it is imperative to obtain stability of the vertebral fracture by adding cement to the fracture clefts and the load-bearing portion of the vertebral body between the pedicles.

When reaugmenting a previous vertebroplasty or vertebral augmentation, an en face view may be used to visualize the pedicle outline and the upper vertebral margins. A transpedicular or parapedicular approach can be utilized to reaccess the vertebral body. Kambin's triangle offers access to the superior end plate in order to obtain a sufficiently medial trajectory of the cannula and to avoid the neural canal and the nerve root. The use of a smaller (10- to 11-gauge) cannula is recommended for revision augmentation. The operator needs to be certain that there are no new subjacent fractures and if there is no significant postprocedural pain relief, continued fracture due to an unfilled cleft, collapse of the vertebral body, or fracture around the cement needs to be suspected. Upright lateral X-rays can be used to visualize significant vertebral body collapse and any positional change of height. A computed tomography (CT) scan can also demonstrate vacuum clefts and fissures. Magnetic resonance (MR) imaging or bone scan can also be used to assess for postoperative complications if these are suspected. CT may also be used and can be used

to assess the adequacy of the cement fill in regard to filling the fracture clefts and stabilizing the overall structure of the vertebral body.

35.6.2 Kyphoplasty and Revision of L3 Pedicle Screw after Posttraumatic Screw Displacement

A 78-year-old woman with past medical history of primary osteoporosis and frequent falls as well as loss of balance due to spinal stenosis and scoliosis had a L3–S1 spinal fusion 4 weeks prior to a fall (▶Fig. 35.14). The patient presented with new and increasing back pain different in nature from the surgical pain and proximal to the incision. A lateral radiograph demonstrated osteoporotic vertebral compression fractures of L2 and L3 with the left L3 pedicle screw dehiscent superiorly into the L2–L3 intervertebral disk (▶Fig. 35.15). Sagittal short tau inversion recovery (STIR) and postcontrast T1-weighted MR images demonstrated vertebral body linear signal abnormalities typical of that of a vertebral fracture of L2 and an end plate fracture of L3 (▶Fig. 35.16).

A decision was made to perform a balloon kyphoplasty of L2 to treat the vertebral compression fracture above the construct and at L3 to treat the vertebral fracture as well as to restabilize the dehiscent hardware (▶Fig. 35.17). A drill was directed through the left L3 pedicle away from the superior end plate and a balloon tamp was then placed in the center of the left side of the vertebral body (▶Fig. 35.18) The balloon tamp was inflated and a right-sided one-step introducer was also placed via a parapedicular approach (▶Fig. 35.19).

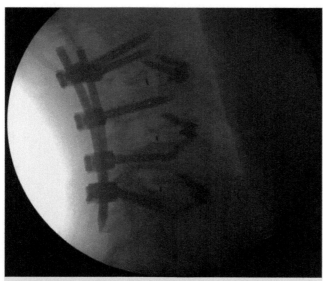

Fig. 35.14 Lateral radiograph demonstrating spinal fusion with pedicle screw and rod augmentation and interbody fusions from L3-S1 without complications.

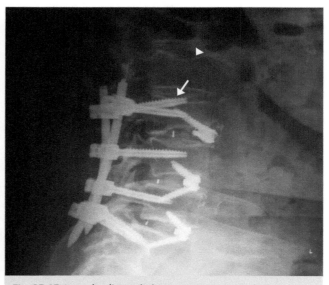

Fig. 35.15 Lateral radiograph demonstrating osteoporotic vertebral compression fractures of L2 (*white arrowhead*) and L3 with the L3 pedicle screw dehiscent superiorly into the L2-L3 intervertebral disk space (*white arrow*).

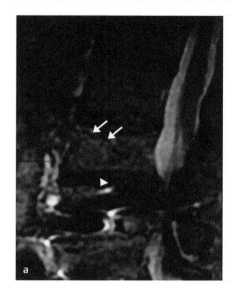
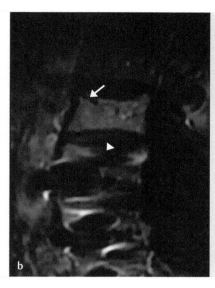

Fig. 35.16 Sagittal short tau inversion recovery (STIR) (**a**) and post contrast T1-weighted (**b**) sagittal images demonstrating a linear signal abnormality within the L2 vertebral body (*white arrows* in a and b) and a superior endplate deformity of L3 (*white arrowheads* in a and b) indicative of vertebral compression fractures of L2 and L3.

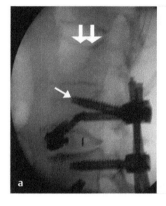
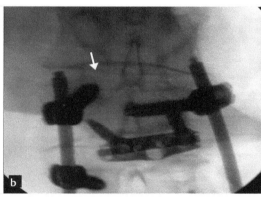

Fig. 35.17 Intraoperative lateral (**a**) and anteroposterior (**b**) fluoroscopic images demonstrating an L2 compression fracture (*thick white arrows* in a) and a compression fracture of L3 with the pedicle screw protruding into the L2-3 disk space (*thin white arrows* in a and b).

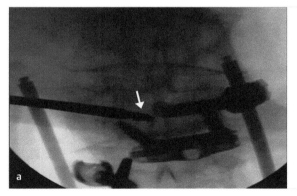
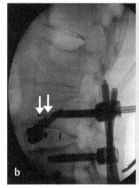

Fig. 35.18 Anteroposterior (**a**) fluoroscopic image showing a drill (*white arrow*) being directed through the left L3 pedicle and away from the superior endplate. Lateral (**b**) fluoroscopic image demonstrates a balloon tamp being placed in the center of the left side of the vertebral body (*white arrows* in **b**).

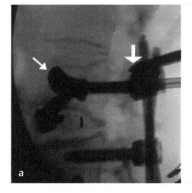
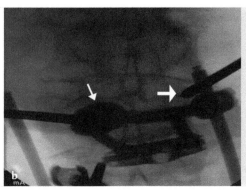

Fig. 35.19 Lateral (**a**) and anteroposterior (**b**) fluoroscopic images showing the balloon inflated creating a bone void (*thin white arrows* in a and b). A right sided one-step introducer was also placed via a para-pedicular approach (*thick white arrows* in a and b).

A drill was then advanced through the introducer into the center of the vertebral body, adjacent to the inflated left-sided balloon (▸Fig. 35.20). Attention was then turned to the L2 vertebral body with bilateral transpedicular right and left balloon tamps placed and inflated. The right-sided L3 drill was placed without a balloon following the drill placement due to the risk of balloon rupture if it came in contact with the contralateral pedicle screw (▸Fig. 35.21). Polymethyl methacrylate injection was then performed at the L2 and L3 levels with cement filling the voids (▸Fig. 35.22). Final images demonstrated no leakage or extravasation of cement (▸Fig. 35.23).

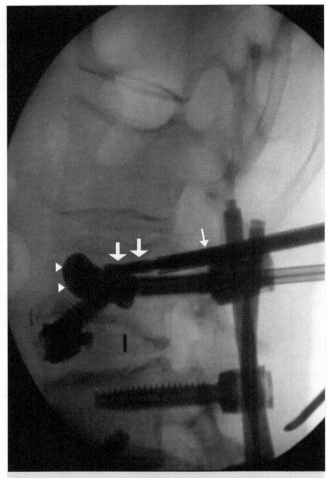

Fig. 35.20 Lateral fluoroscopic images demonstrate a drill (*thick white arrows*) being advanced through the para-pedicular introducer (*thin white arrow*) and into the vertebral body. The inflated left sided balloon is also seen (*white arrowheads*).

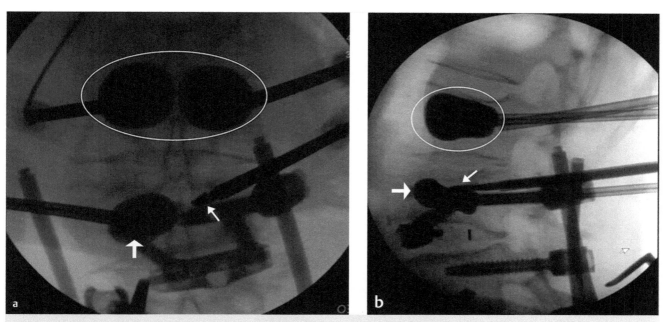

Fig. 35.21 Anteroposterior (**a**) and lateral (**b**) fluoroscopic images demonstrate right and left balloon tamps inflated at the level of L2 (*circles*). The right sided L3 drill (*thin white arrows* in **a** and **b**) was initially placed but no balloon was used at this location due to the risk of balloon rupture if it inflated against the contralateral pedicle screw.

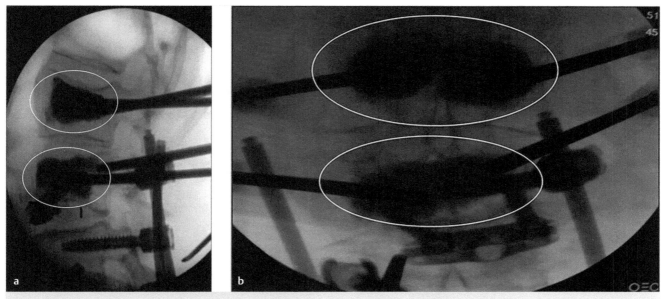

Fig. 35.22 Lateral (**a**) and anteroposterior (**b**) fluoroscopic images show cement filling the voids of L2 and L3 (area within the *white circles*).

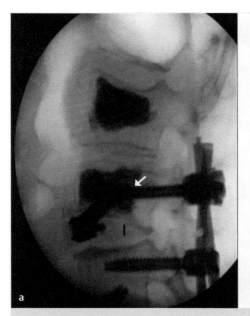
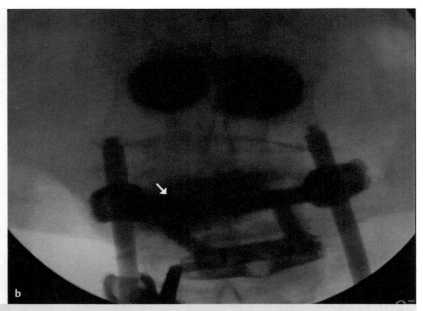

Fig. 35.23 Final images at the end of the procedure showing no leakage or extravasation of cement and optimal placement of the left L3 pedicle screw (*white arrows* in **a** and **b**).

35.6.3 Treating Recurring Fractures after Vertebroplasty

A 74-year-old woman with primary osteoporosis and super-imposed secondary osteoporosis due to oral steroids presents with postprocedure pain in the lumbar region. The patient had prior vertebroplasty of T6 in 2012 and a subsequent vertebroplasty at T11 (►Fig. 35.24) with balloon kyphoplasty of L2 in 2013. Further depression of L2 superior end plate with minimal cement volume was seen (►Fig. 35.25). A decision was made to reaugment the L2 vertebral body using a drill, an inflatable bone tamp (IBT), a bone curet, and hydroxyapatite cement (►Fig. 35.25, ►Fig. 35.26, ►Fig. 35.27, ►Fig. 35.28).

A unilateral parapedicular approach was used to gain access to the superior aspect of the vertebral body at the site of the recurring collapse (►Fig. 35.25). A drill was used to gain access to the site of collapse (►Fig. 35.26) superior to preexisting cement and inferior to the collapsed superior end plate. A curet was inserted toward the superior and anterior portion of the

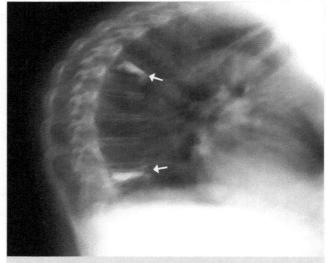

Fig. 35.24 Lateral radiograph demonstrates vertebroplasties of T6 and T12 (*white arrows*).

central vertebral body for the purpose of directing the balloon expansion to the correct position (▶Fig. 35.27). Then the balloon was expanded at the superior aspect of the anterior and central vertebral body in the location previously treated by the curet (▶Fig. 35.28). The cement filled the void created and

supported the superior end plate of L2 (▶Fig. 35.29). In addition, kyphoplasty of the L1 vertebral body was also performed due to the fracture, which was only seen on the MRI (▶Fig. 35.29). The patient reported a 90% pain relief and was discharged from the hospital the next day.

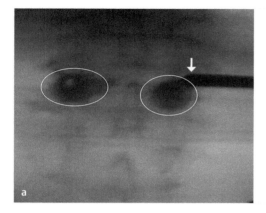
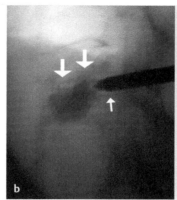

Fig. 35.25 (a) Anteroposterior and (b) lateral fluoroscopic views demonstrating reaugmentation needle (*thin white arrows*) access of the vertebral body with cement from prior augmentation at L2s (*circles* in **a**). There is minimal cement volume with recurring collapse (*thick white arrows* in **b**).

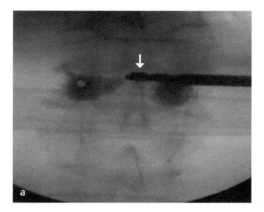
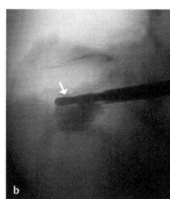

Fig. 35.26 (a) Anteroposterior and (b) lateral fluoroscopic views demonstrating a parapedicular approach using drill (*white arrows* in **a** and **b**) at the superior aspect of the cement just inferior to the collapse of the superior end plate of L2.

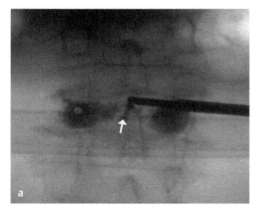
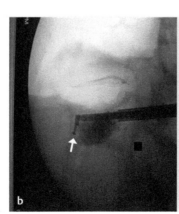

Fig. 35.27 (a) Anteroposterior and (b) lateral fluoroscopic views demonstrating a curet (*white arrows* in **a** and **b**) inserted toward the central and anterior portion of the superior vertebral body for the purpose of directing the balloon expansion to the correct position.

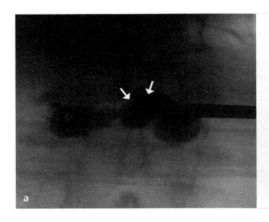
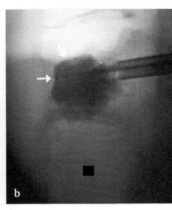

Fig. 35.28 (a) Anteroposterior and (b) lateral fluoroscopic views show the balloon expanded at the superior and anterior aspect of the central vertebral body (*white arrows* in a and b) in the location previously treated by the curet.

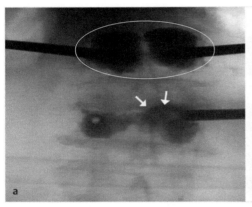
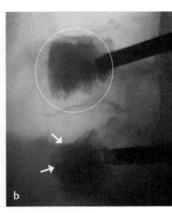

Fig. 35.29 (a) Anteroposterior and (b) lateral fluoroscopic views demonstrate the cement filling the previously created void (*white arrows* in a and b). A balloon kyphoplasty was also performed at the L1 level (*circles* in a and b) due to a fracture that was only seen on MRI.

35.6.4 Allowing for Access to Pedicle Screw Placement after Vertebral Augmentation

There are occasions where pedicle screws may need to be placed in the vertebral body after vertebral augmentation. In cases of lumbar spondylolisthesis and spinal stenosis, a decompression and fusion surgery may need to be performed at a later time. At junctional levels after fusion, it is common to need surgical decompression and fusion around previous levels of augmentation. Patients with osteoporosis may fracture around pedicle screws requiring revision. Regardless of the many reasons, it is optimal to be able to easily access a previous vertebral level that has undergone vertebral augmentation.

The technique of preserving the accessibility for pedicle screw placement uses a 4.2-mm (8-gauge) needle that allows one to use almost any spinal instrumentation system to fill the access hole with a 5.5-mm screw once the needle is removed from its position within the cement mass (▶Fig. 35.30). The technique involves initially placing the needles with an approach identical

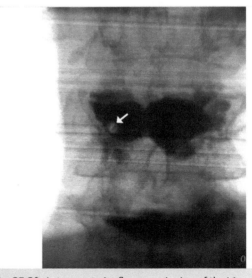

Fig. 35.30 Anteroposterior fluoroscopic view of the L1 vertebral body showing a circular hole in the bone cement (*white arrow*).

to that of pedicle screw placement. The needle placement is a bilateral transpedicular placement with the screws as parallel to the end plates as possible. Once the needles are placed and the vertebral augmentation is performed, the needles are left at least halfway into the vertebral body until the cement has sufficiently hardened. After the needles are removed, the needle tracks remain within the cement (▶Fig. 35.31 and ▶Fig. 35.32). This will allow for recannulation with a K-wire at a later time. The pedicle screw is then placed over the K-wire and screwed into an optimal position. This technique avoids the use of fenestrated screws, which can be difficult to use and allow for proximal junctional levels to be stabilized with hardware. Access to the vertebral body through the cement channel is typically preserved from months to years after the vertebral augmentation procedure.

35.6.5 Tips and Techniques of Vertebral Augmentation

A 76-year-old man status postposterior lumbar fusion 2 months prior presented with lower back pain. A vertebral compression fracture was seen in the L2 vertebral body at the superior portion of the pedicle screw and rod construct with 25% compression of the L2 vertebral body in both the coronal and sagittal planes (▶Fig. 35.33). A cleft with partial reduction was also seen on sagittal STIR MR images (▶Fig. 35.34).

A size 3 IBT was selected after an en face view demonstrated that the inferior pedicle was sufficiently open to access the vertebral body (▶Fig. 35.35). A left-sided inferior transpedicular approach allowed for best positioning of the drill (▶Fig. 35.36), and a curet was used in aiding the appropriate balloon expansion by disrupting the bone preventing this expansion (▶Fig. 35.37). After the curettage, a balloon was placed into the vertebral body to support and reduce the fracture (▶Fig. 35.38). The left side was cemented well, but there was still inadequate cement placement with a unilateral approach (▶Fig. 35.39). Therefore, the right side was also cannulated with a similar technique. A drill was used to transverse to the cement bolus to ensure best position of the two cement mantles (▶Fig. 35.40). Subsequently, a balloon was used to create a void for the contralateral cement placement on the right with the cement filling the void and supporting the end plate/screw–bone junction (▶Fig. 35.41 and ▶Fig. 35.42).

The patient reported immediate pain relief with improved mobility and stopped using his walker. The patient was then able to care for the spouse who had recent surgery. Medical treatment using an anabolic bone agent for his underlying osteoporosis was also prescribed.

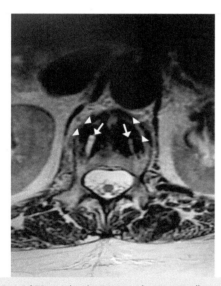

Fig. 35.31 Axial T2-weighted MR image showing needle tracks (*white arrows*) within the bilateral cement masses (*white arrowheads*).

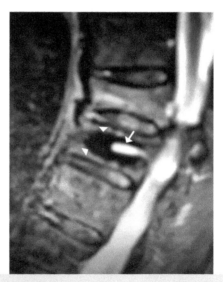

Fig. 35.32 Sagittal short tau inversion recovery (STIR) MR image demonstrating a fluid-filled track (*white arrow*) within the cement mass (*white arrowheads*).

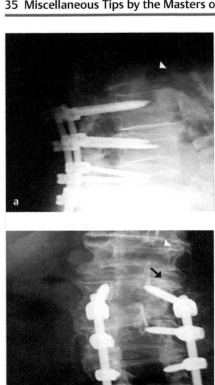
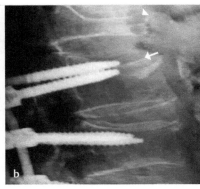
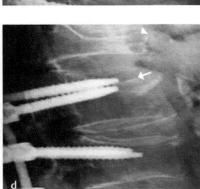

Fig. 35.33 Radiographs demonstrating 2-month postoperative lateral X-rays **(a)** and current films **(b)** with back pain onset. Pathologic vertebral fracture is seen with 25% compression (*white arrows* in **b** and **d**). Note coronal (*black arrow* in **c**) and sagittal (*white arrows* in **b** and **d**). A chronic L1 fracture is also noted (*white arrowheads*).

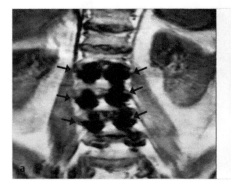
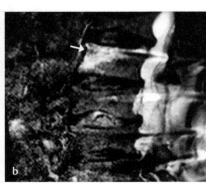

Fig. 35.34 **(a)** Coronal T1-weighted and **(b)** sagittal short tau inversion recovery (STIR) images demonstrating the pedicle screw and rod construct (*black arrows* in **a**) as well as the fracture cleft (*white arrow* in **b**) and partial reduction with supine positioning for MRI compared to upright lateral X-rays.

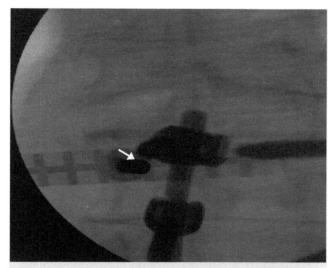

Fig. 35.35 Enface view demonstrating vertebral augmentation needle access of the inferior portion of the pedicle just inferior to the existing pedicle screw (*white arrow*). This portion of the pedicle was seen to be open to percutaneous needle access.

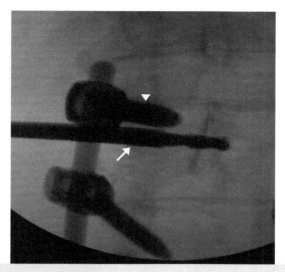

Fig. 35.36 Anteroposterior fluoroscopic image showing an inferior transpedicular approach with the drill (*white arrow*) passing inferior to the pedicle screw (*white arrowhead*) and into the center of the vertebral body.

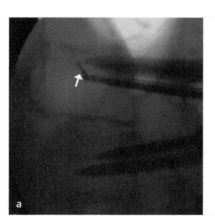

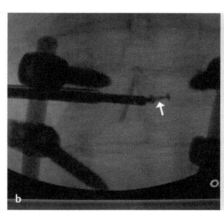

Fig. 35.37 (a) Lateral and (b) anteroposterior fluoroscopic views show a curet (*white arrows* in a and b) inserted toward the anterior and contralateral vertebral body for the purpose of directing the balloon expansion to the correct position.

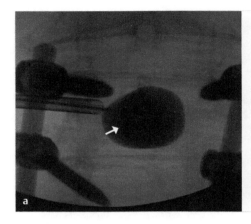 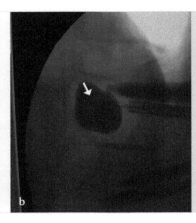

Fig. 35.38 **(a)** Anteroposterior and **(b)** lateral fluoroscopic views show the balloon expanded concentrically in midportion of the vertebral body (*white arrows* in **a** and **b**) and in the regions previously treated by the curet.

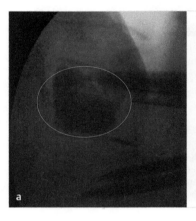 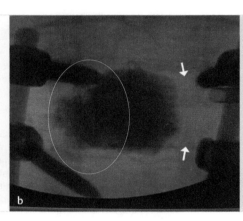

Fig. 35.39 **(a)** Lateral and **(b)** anteroposterior fluoroscopic views show cement in the mid to anterior portion of the vertebral body (*area within the white circle* in **a**) and that on the left side is cemented well (*area within the white oval* in **b**), but there is still inadequate cement on the right side with a left-side unipedicular approach (*white arrows* in **b**).

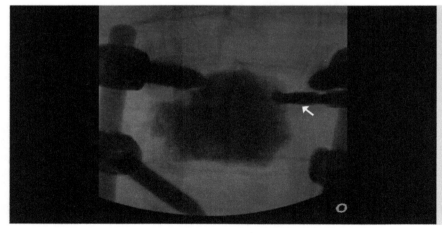

Fig. 35.40 Anteroposterior fluoroscopic images showing a drill (*white arrow*) traversing to the cement bolus using a similar approach on the right as was done previously on the left to access the right side of the vertebral body in preparation for deployment of the balloon.

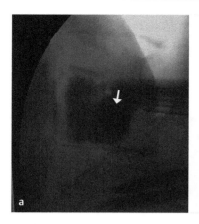
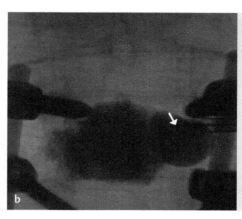

Fig. 35.41 (a) Lateral and (b) anteroposterior fluoroscopic views show an inflated balloon (*white arrows* in **a** and **b**) that is creating a void for the contralateral cement injection.

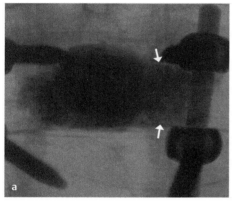
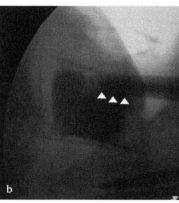

Fig. 35.42 (a) Anteroposterior and (b) lateral fluoroscopic views show the cement filling the void (*white arrows* in **a**) and supporting the end plate and screw–bone junction (*white arrowheads* in **b**).

35.7 Radiofrequency Ablation and Vertebral Implant Augmentation in a Patient with Lytic Metastatic Disease

Bassem Georgy

A 63-year-old man presented with back pain from metastatic lung disease to the spine. Multiple lesions were seen throughout the thoracolumbar spine and the preoperative computed tomography (CT) examination showed relatively well-defined lytic lesions at the T12 and L1 levels. The T12 lesion involved the left half of the vertebra and the L1 lesion involved the anterior two-thirds of the vertebral body (▶Fig. 35.43, ▶Fig. 35.44, ▶Fig. 35.45). The patient had severe pain to closed-fist percussion at the thoracolumbar junction level on physical examination. Vertebral augmentation was requested for stabilization and pain control. Due to the focal nature of the disease, a radiofrequency ablation of the lesions was first performed using the STAR ablation device (Merit Medical, South Jordan, UT, United States). Ablation was performed using a unipedicular access on both levels for average of 8 minutes at each level (▶Fig. 35.44). The access cannula was then exchanged over a Kirschner wire and a Kiva implant (Benvenue Medical, San Jose, CA, United States) was deployed in the center of the ablated lesions (▶Fig. 35.45a, b). Postprocedure CT images show well-placed implants in the center of the lesions with minimal amount of cement injected and no leakage (▶Fig. 35.46a–d).

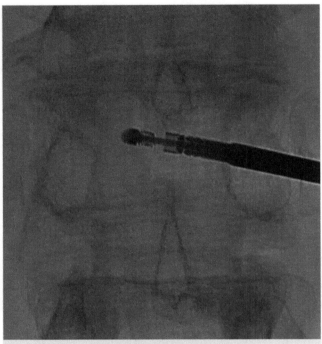

Fig. 35.44 Anteroposterior fluoroscopic image shows a radiofrequency ablation device placed via a unilateral transpedicular right sided approach.

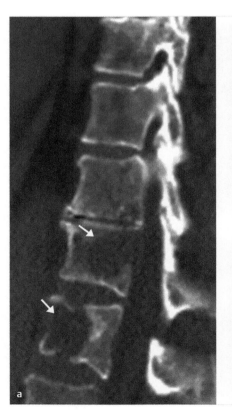
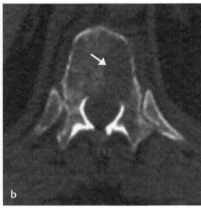
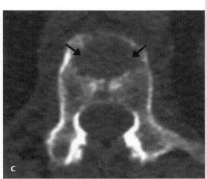

Fig. 35.43 Sagittal computed tomography (CT) reconstruction (a) shows lytic metastases involving the T12 and L1 vertebral bodies (*white arrows* in **a**). Axial CT images also the lytic lesions that involve the left vertebral body of T12 (*white arrow* in **b**) and the anterior portion of the L1 vertebral body (*black arrows* in **c**).

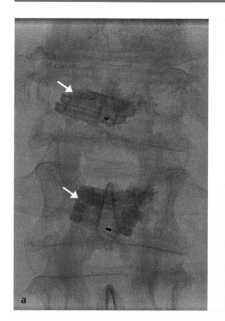 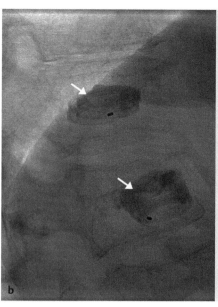

Fig. 35.45 Anteroposterior (**a**) and lateral (**b**) fluoroscopic images show Kiva implants in the T12 and L1 vertebral bodies (*white arrows* in **a** and **b**).

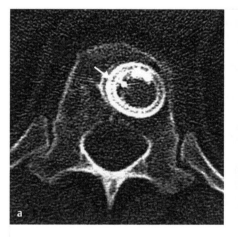 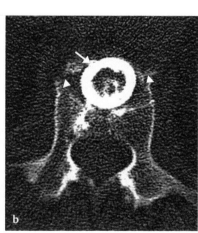

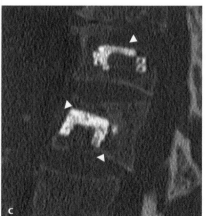 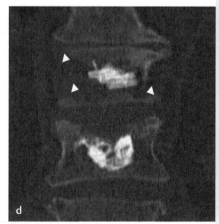

Fig. 35.46 Axial (**a** and **b**) CT images along with sagittal (**c**) and coronal (**d**) CT reconstruction images show Kiva implants and bone cement (*white arrows*) within the lytic metastatic foci (*white arrowheads*).

35.8 Vertebral Hemangioma Causing Congestive Myelopathy Despite Absence of Angiographically Evident Arteriovenous Shunting

John D. Barr and Marco C. Pinho

A 70-year-old man presented with a 2-month history of progressive lower extremity motor and sensory loss, inability to ambulate, and incontinence. Outside magnetic resonance (MR) imaging demonstrated abnormally increased T2 spinal cord signal intensity (SI) and multiple flow voids surrounding the distal spinal cord, as well as a large vertebral hemangioma at T10 (▶Fig. 35.47a, b). Imaging was suboptimal due to the patient's very large body habitus (body mass index [BMI] 50). Complete spinal angiography did not demonstrate a dural arteriovenous (AV) fistula, as had been expected. Hypervascularity of the T10 hemangioma without AV shunting was noted (▶Fig. 35.48).

Dynamic contrast-enhanced MR angiography (MRA) performed the following day demonstrated early epidural venous plexus enhancement at the T10 level immediately preceding filling of abnormally dilated perimedullary veins (▶Fig. 35.49). Despite the absence of angiographically identified AV shunting, the MRA suggested that the large T10 hemangioma was the probable cause of AV shunting and spinal venous hypertension.

Embolization of the T10 hemangioma was done by a percutaneous transpedicular injection of 5.5 mL of Onyx 34 (Medtronic, Dublin, Ireland). This was performed under general anesthesia. Onyx embolization was selected rather than polymethyl methacrylate (PMMA) with consideration that any possible future surgical treatment might be complicated by the presence of the PMMA. Immediate pre-embolization bilateral

T10 intercostal artery arteriograms and a percutaneous direct vertebrogram (▶Fig. 35.50) again revealed only vertebral hypervascularity with no AV shunting. Postembolization images and arteriograms confirmed extensive vertebral embolization with Onyx and minimal remaining hypervascularity (▶Fig. 35.51a, b); additional transarterial embolization was therefore felt to be unnecessary. Almost immediately upon awakening from general anesthesia, the patient reported improved lower extremity sensation. His symptoms significantly improved over the next month with recovery of limited ambulation and improved urinary continence.

Approximately 2 months after embolization, the patient began to experience worsening of his symptoms with regression to his pretreatment level by month 4. Repeat MR imaging and MRA again demonstrated persistent abnormal spinal cord SI, multiple flow voids, early T10-level epidural plexus enhancement, and dilated perimedullary veins. Successful transarterial embolization of the hemangioma via bilateral injections of the T10 intercostal arteries with a total of 4-mL Onyx 34 was performed (▶Fig. 35.52a, b); this was more difficult than usual because the Onyx already in place impaired visualization of the newly injected Onyx. Immediate pre-embolization bilateral T9–T11 intercostal artery arteriograms had again revealed only T10 vertebral hypervascularity with no AV shunting. The patient continued to decline neurologically with regression to paraplegia and incontinence, as well as worsening of the spinal cord swelling and edema on MR imaging. Open surgical

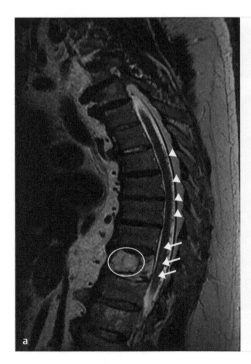
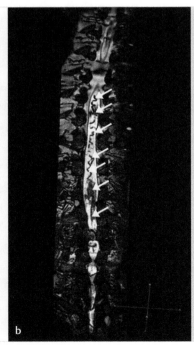

Fig. 35.47 Pretreatment T2-weighted sagittal MR imaging examination **(a)** shows increased distal spinal cord signal intensity (*white arrows* in **a**), extensive surrounding flow voids (*white arrowheads*), and a large T10 hemangioma (*white circle*). Curved coronal reformat **(b)** of balanced steady-state free precession (balanced fast field echo) better depicts the extensive network of tortuous, engorged veins (*white arrows* in **b**).

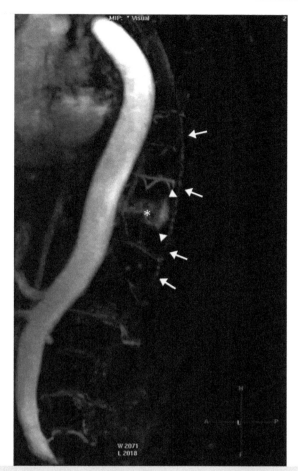

Fig. 35.48 Late arterial phase of sagittal contrast-enhanced MRA shows enlarged T10 intercostal arteries and hypervascularity of the T10 hemangioma (*asterisk*). Dynamic sequences showed early filling of the epidural venous plexus at T10 (*arrowheads*) and subsequent filling of perimedullary veins (*long arrows*).

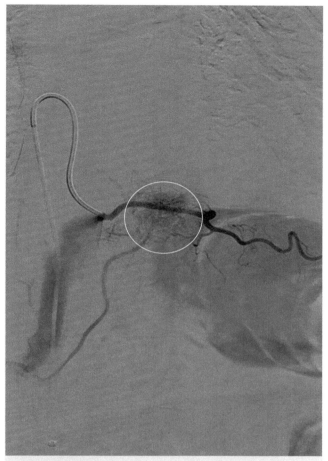

Fig. 35.49 Selective left T10 intercostal arteriography (anteroposterior view) revealed only hypervascularity of the hemangioma (*vessels within the white circle*) without arteriovenous shunting.

corpectomy to definitively eliminate the residual AV shunting was deemed infeasible due to the very high risk posed by the patient's large body habitus.

Approximately 1 year later, the patient began to experience severe radiating mid-abdominal pain consistent with a T10 dermatomal distribution. His neurological status was otherwise unchanged. Repeat MR imaging and MRA demonstrated significant worsening of the spinal cord edema, now extending superiorly to the level of T3–T4 (▶Fig. 35.53a, b), and newly developed areas of patchy abnormal postcontrast enhancement along the lower thoracic spinal cord, permeated by nonenhancing necrotic foci, consistent with venous infarcts, complicating the chronic congestive myelopathy. Definitive elimination of the apparently persistent AV shunting was felt to be necessary to prevent progressive myelopathy with upper extremity impairment and, possibly, to relieve the new-onset radicular pain. Open surgical corpectomy was again deemed to have unacceptable risks.

Treatment options including radiofrequency (RF) ablation, RF ablation combined with PMMA augmentation, and stereotactic radiosurgery were considered. The latency period associated with radiosurgery was considered a negative factor, given the patient's ongoing severe pain. Given that two embolization treatments had failed to adequately eliminate the AV shunting, we felt that RF ablation combined with PMMA augmentation would have the highest probability of success. We recognized, however, that visualization of PMMA during injection would be difficult and have increased risk of leakage into the spinal canal or neural foramen with the large amount of Onyx already in place. This increased risk was balanced by the fact that the patient had essentially already lost spinal cord function at and below the target level. The primary treatment goal was to prevent progressive ascending myelopathy. PMMA injection under CT guidance or cone beam CT was considered to allow more precise PMMA placement, but use of these modalities was precluded by the patient's large body habitus.

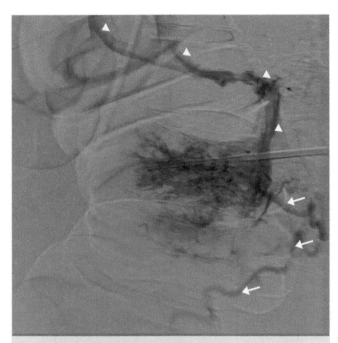

Fig. 35.50 A T10 vertebrogram (lateral view) showed only epidural (*white arrow*) and central venous (*white arrowheads*) drainage from the hemangioma.

Seventeen months after initial treatment, the patient underwent T10 RF ablation under general anesthesia using the OsteoCool system (Medtronic, Dublin, Ireland). Immediately prior to the ablation, a vertebrogram was performed with no AV shunting demonstrated. After ablation, a total of 7 mL of PMMA was deliberately injected until very minimal filing of the epidural plexus was noted (▶Fig. 35.54a, b). The treatment goal was to devascularize and disconnect the hemangioma from the epidural plexus to the greatest extent possible.

The patient's pain resolved almost immediately after the RF ablation and augmentation procedure. His neurological status has remained otherwise stable. MR imaging and MRA performed 5 months after the last procedure demonstrated resolution of the spinal cord edema, swelling, and enhancement, with development of atrophy and myelomalacia in the lower thoracic cord (corresponding to the location of the venous infarct), and only very minimal persistent AV shunting (▶Fig. 35.55a, b). This case is notable for the lack of AV shunting demonstrable by conventional catheter-based spinal angiography as well as by a direct vertebrogram. Although such shunting was evidenced by the abnormal intradural flow voids on MR imaging and dynamic MRA, no other cause for the dilated perimedullary veins was identified. That such apparently subtle AV shunting caused severe spinal cord venous hypertension was confirmed by the positive treatment responses following the first and third interventions and the near complete resolution of imaging abnormalities after the final intervention.

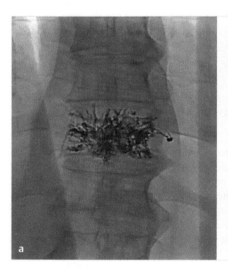

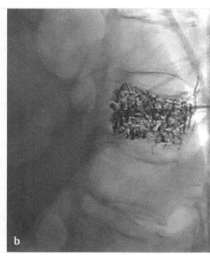

Fig. 35.51 Postpercutaneous embolization radiographs, posteroanterior **(a)** and lateral **(b)** views, show extensive permeation of the hemangioma with Onyx.

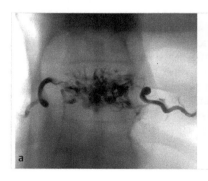

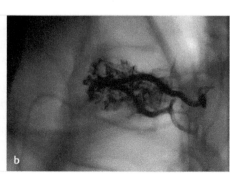

Fig. 35.52 Postarterial embolization radiographs, posteroanterior **(a)** and lateral **(b)** views, show further permeation of the hemangioma with additional Onyx.

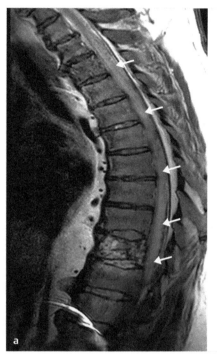 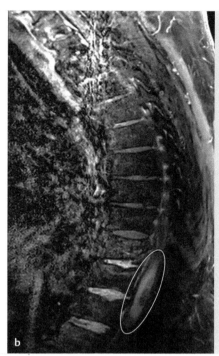

Fig. 35.53 One year postarterial embolization MR imaging examination. A T2-weighted image in the sagittal plane **(a)** shows abnormally increased spinal cord signal intensity and swelling now extending to the upper thoracic level (*white arrows*). Postcontrast T1-weighted image **(b)** demonstrates areas of marked abnormal postcontrast enhancement in the conus (*area within the white oval*), with irregular hypoenhancing foci, consistent with venous infarction.

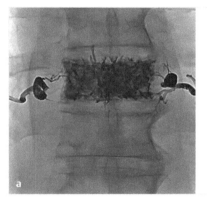 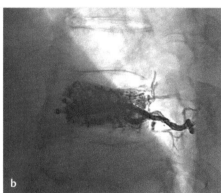

Fig. 35.54 Postradiofrequency ablation and augmentation radiographs, **(a)** posteroanterior and **(b)** lateral views, show extensive permeation of the hemangioma with polymethyl methacrylate and Onyx.

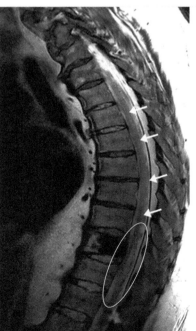 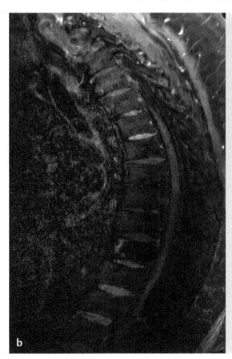

Fig. 35.55 Sagittal T2-weighted **(a)** and T1-weighted contrast-enhanced **(a)** MR images obtained 5 months after the final procedure demonstrated marked improvement of cord edema, swelling, and enhancement (*white arrows* in **a**), with development of atrophy and myelomalacia in the lower thoracic cord (*area within the white oval*). Dynamic MRA **(b)** showed only very minimal persistent arteriovenous shunting.

35.9 Vertebral Augmentation Devices in the Treatment of Traumatic Vertebral Fractures

Stefano Marcia

Vertebral trauma is a common condition that can give rise to both major and minor complications. Multiple classifications have been published in the past trying to establish stable and unstable fractures and surgical and nonsurgical fractures (see Chapter 2).[1–4] Traumatic vertebral fractures can be defined as stable or unstable relative to the disruption of three or four columns. Although multiple classification systems exist within the literature, Magerl's classification is the most commonly used and considers the type of injury to be divided into compression, rotation, and distraction injuries with multiple subtypes. There is increasing severity from A to C, and within each group, the severity usually increases within the subgroups from 0.1 to 0.2 to 0.3. All these pathomorphologies are supported by a mechanism of injury, which is responsible for the extent of the injury. The type of injury with its groups and subgroups is also able to suggest the treatment modality.

The management of traumatic spine fracture patients is well known and has been defined by many protocols (Chapter 2).[5–8] An important factor is the presence or absence of associated clinical neurological symptoms such as myelopathy, motor deficit, and bladder or bowel dysfunction. The injury characteristic can be further defined by using diagnostic imaging resources such as X-ray, MRI, multidetector computed tomography (MDCT), or both MRI/MDCT, but treatment philosophies and strategies still differ significantly.

Magerl A1 type vertebral compression fractures (VCFs) represent the main indication for percutaneous vertebroplasty (PVP), percutaneous balloon kyphoplasty (BKP), or vertebral augmentation (VA), but these types of fractures can also be treated with orthotic devices, bed rest, as well as medical and/or physical therapy at least for 3 to 6 months. This nonsurgical management (NSM) is only marginally effective and cannot always mitigate the possibility of the VCF worsening with additional collapse and worsening of the kyphotic deformity. It should also be considered that orthotic bracing will also cause other problems such as cardiorespiratory diseases, sleep disorders, and gastrointestinal motility reduction.

Fracture types A1 and A2 (except for A2.3) are regarded as stable, while burst fractures and fractures involving the posterior wall, especially the higher rated A3.3 fractures that lack sufficient anterior column support, are designated as unstable. Flexion–distraction injuries as seen in the B1- to B3-type fractures are unstable. The highest degree of instability is seen in type C fractures, which are characterized by a rotational component. NSM is feasible in types A1, A2, and some lower rated A3 fractures. In these patients, axial alignment and bracing are done during an emergency department or hospital stay with subsequent mobilization and ambulation under the supervision of a physical therapist. Surgical intervention with secondary anterior vertebral replacement might be needed in A2.3 pincer fractures. Burst fractures (A3) are characterized by their incapability to withstand anterior load, which designates these fractures as unstable injuries. In A3 fractures, there is a high rate of unseen posterior injury, which, if present, can be an indication for posterior instrumentation.

According to AO principles (anatomic reduction: fracture reduction and fixation to restore functional anatomical relationships; stable fixation: stability by rigid fixation or splinting, as the specific type of the fracture and the injury requires; maintaining good blood supply: preservation of the blood supply to soft tissue and bone by careful handling and gentle reduction techniques; early mobilization: early and safe mobilization of the fractured part and the patient) and as an evolution and alternative to BKP, VA mechanical devices were introduced in last few years.[9,10] These devices were developed to maximize long-term vertebral height restoration and to restore as much of the original anatomic alignment as possible. Clinical experience has demonstrated that one of the limitations of BKP was a loss of restored height after balloon deflation due to vertebral elastic recoil[11] along with difficulty in treating A2 fractures because the vertebral split fractures were difficult to treat with the balloon that expanded centrifugally. Thanks to the capacity of certain implant VA devices to restore the physiologic vertebral height and to obtain a more homogeneous distribution of the cement with a better axial resistance to load, this treatment certainly has the capability of treating patients with more complex A2 and A3 fractures as well as the patient with less damaged Magerl A1 fractures. Due to the capacity of some VA devices to produce ligamentotaxis, the more complex burst fractures may be better reduced and the fracture fragments pulled together and stabilized. The most commonly used VA systems on the market are the following: Osseofix (Alphatec Spine Inc, Carlsbad, CA, United States), a titanium self-expandable mesh cage, Vertebral Body Stenting (VBS; Synthes, Soletta, Switzerland), a titanium balloon-expandable stent, Tektona (SpineArt, Geneva, Switzerland), a vertebral remodeling system, and the SpineJack (Vexim, Balma, France), a titanium endovertebral jack.

These procedures can be performed in an operating room equipped with a C arm or in an angiography room. Usually local anesthesia, moderate sedation, or deep sedation is used, but some surgeons prefer the use of general anaesthesia.[9]

All these implants require the same bipedicular approach, with the access cannulas inserted using the anteroposterior (AP) view or the oblique view and then advanced in the AP projection to the medial aspect of the pedicle. The medial margin of the pedicle as seen in the AP view is a very important anatomical landmark to check to make sure the needle is in the posterior portion of the vertebral body in the lateral view before advancing it farther into the vertebral body.

The OsseoFix[12,13,17] mesh cage implant uses two Kirschner's wires that are inserted into the access cannulas, followed by removal of the cannulas and insertion of the drill into the anterior third of the vertebral body. An implant delivery system helps insert the two titanium mesh cages. A mechanical actuation system is used to deploy the expandable cages in a controlled manner. The size of the cage is selected according to preoperative planning from preoperative CT scans. Cement injection is then performed by means of dedicated bone fillers. Although the conventional OsseoFix implant is used with cement, some authors described the implant of the mesh cages without PMMA injection.[13]

The VBS[14,15,17] device represents an evolution of BKP, having a balloon-expandable CoCrWNi alloy stent that can be delivered with balloon inflation.[14,15] Through the working cannula, a metallic drill can be used to access the anterior portion of the vertebral body and create a channel for the placement of the metallic implant. The drill is then removed and the mechanical system is inserted. The systems are connected and, under fluoroscopic guidance, the balloon is inflated and the stent is expanded. After implant deployment, the PMMA is injected into the cavity created by the balloon and the expanded stent. The cement can be injected through a slow injection system such as a bone filler or through 1-mL syringe. A high-viscosity cement is typically used to help prevent extravasation.

The introduction of the Tektona device requires the same bipedicular approach. After the inner cannula is removed, a blunt wire is introduced. Once the wire is in place, a metallic drill, preassembled with a working cannula, is used over the wire to access the anterior portion of the vertebral body. The drill is then disconnected from the working cannula and removed, and the Vertebral Fracture Reducer (VFR) mechanical system is then inserted through the working cannula. After VFR insertion, the expansion of the lamella can be performed by squeezing the handle. Fluoroscopic guidance is used to check the position of the lamella and the proper expansion until the desired fracture reduction is attained. Once the desired expansion has been achieved, the VFR instrument is removed, leaving the working cannula in place. The PMMA is then prepared and injected into the cavity. The bone cement is mixed with a dedicated mixing device and then injected through a cement filler under continuous fluoroscopic guidance. The bone fillers and the working cannulas are then removed.

The concept of the SpineJack[15–17] implant is different from the other VA systems in that there is a craniocaudal expansion of the device (instead of a spherical expansion that is seen in most other devices). This allows forces to be applied only on the vertebral end plates in a way that optimizes height restoration. Reduction of the bone fragments is also seen with this height restoration due to the ligamentotaxis that occurs with fracture reduction. After the trocar access needles are placed, a Kirschner wire is inserted. A manual cannulated reamer is then used to create the pathway for the template. The procedure is then repeated through the contralateral pedicle. The implants are then placed into the vertebral body and expanded with manual rotation of a multifunctional handle. The expansion of the implant produces fracture reduction and height restoration and provides mechanical support to the fractured vertebral body. Once the implants are delivered, the bone cement can be injected through dedicated bone fillers under fluoroscopic guidance (▶Fig. 35.56 and ▶Fig. 35.57). After all these procedures, the patients are kept for 2 to 3 hours in the hospital for clinical monitoring and then discharged.

All of the various devices available on the market have their own characteristics and method of reducing VCFs. Although most of these are effective in producing fracture reduction and stabilization of the vertebral body, the SpineJack seems to be the most suitable in the treatment of traumatic fractures, even A2 or A3 fractures as a standalone without any other posterior instrumentation.[17]

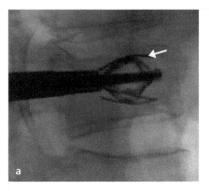
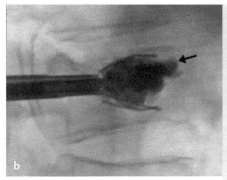
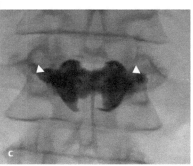
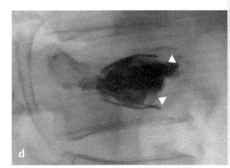

Fig. 35.56 Treatment of traumatic A3.3 fracture of L1 with the SpineJack device. The SpineJack is placed into the vertebral body and expanded (*white arrow* in **a**). Cement is then injected (*black arrow* in **b**) and the cannulas are removed, leaving an expanded SpineJack and cement (*white arrowheads* in **c** and **d**).

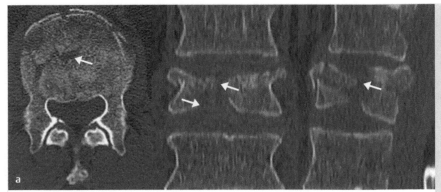

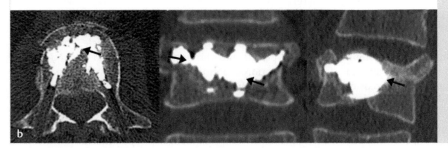

Fig. 35.57 Computed tomography exam taken before (**a**) and after (**b**) SpineJack placement. A Magerl A3.3 fracture is seen to have prominent comminution of the fracture (*white arrows* in **a**) and loss of vertebral body height. After placement of the SpineJack and injection of cement, the fracture fragments appear stable (*black arrows* in **b**) and the vertebral height restored.

References

[1] Magerl F, Aebi M, Gertzbein SD, Harms J, Nazarian S. A comprehensive classification of thoracic and lumbar injuries. Eur Spine J 1994;3(4):184–201

[2] Vaccaro AR, Lehman RA Jr, Hurlbert RJ, et al. A new classification of thoracolumbar injuries: the importance of injury morphology, the integrity of the posterior ligamentous complex, and neurologic status. Spine 2005;30(20):2325–2333

[3] Denis F. The three column spine and its significance in the classification of acute thoracolumbar spinal injuries. Spine 1983;8(8):817–831

[4] Vaccaro AR, Oner C, Kepler CK, et al; AOSpine Spinal Cord Injury & Trauma Knowledge Forum. AOSpine thoracolumbar spine injury classification system: fracture description, neurological status, and key modifiers. Spine 2013;38(23):2028–2037

[5] Zhang L, Zou J, Gan M, Shi J, Li J, Yang H. Treatment of thoracolumbar burst fractures: short-segment pedicle instrumentation versus kyphoplasty. Acta Orthop Belg 2013;79(6):718–725

[6] Yi L, Jingping B, Gele J, Baoleri X, Taixiang W. Operative versus non-operative treatment for thoracolumbar burst fractures without neurological deficit. Cochrane Database Syst Rev 2006(4):CD005079

[7] Fuentes S, Blondel B, Metellus P, Gaudart J, Adetchessi T, Dufour H. Percutaneous kyphoplasty and pedicle screw fixation for the management of thoraco-lumbar burst fractures. Eur Spine J 2010;19(8):1281–1287

[8] Verlaan JJ, Dhert WJA, Oner FC. Intervertebral disc viability after burst fractures of the thoracic and lumbar spine treated with pedicle screw fixation and direct end-plate restoration. Spine J 2013;13(3):217–221

[9] Muto M, Marcia S, Guarnieri G, Pereira V. Assisted techniques for vertebral cementoplasty: why should we do it? Eur J Radiol 2015;84(5):783–788

[10] Filippiadis DK, Marcia S, Ryan A, et al. New implant-based technologies in the spine. Cardiovasc Intervent Radiol 2018;41(10):1463–1473

[11] Verlaan JJ, van de Kraats EB, Oner FC, van Walsum T, Niessen WJ, Dhert WJ. Bone displacement and the role of longitudinal ligaments during balloon vertebroplasty in traumatic thoracolumbar fractures. Spine 2005;30(16):1832–1839

[12] Ender SA, Wetterau E, Ender M, Kühn JP, Merk HR, Kayser R. Percutaneous stabilization system Osseofix for treatment of osteoporotic vertebral compression fractures: clinical and radiological results after 12 months. PLoS One 2013;8(6):e65119

[13] Eschler A, Ender SA, Ulmar B, Herlyn P, Mittlmeier T, Gradl G. Cementless fixation of osteoporotic VCFs using titanium mesh implants (OsseoFix): preliminary results. BioMed Res Int 2014;2014:853897

[14] Hartmann F, Griese M, Dietz SO, Kuhn S, Rommens PM, Gercek E. Two-year results of vertebral body stenting for the treatment of traumatic incomplete burst fractures. Minim Invasive Ther Allied Technol 2015;24(3):161–166

[15] Kruger A, Oberkircher L, Figiel J, et al. Height restoration of osteoporotic vertebral compression fractures using different intravertebral reduction devices: a cadaveric study. Spine J 2015;15(5):1092–1098

[16] Noriega D, Maestretti G, Renaud C, et al. Clinical performance and safety of 108 spinejack implantations: 1-year results of a prospective multicentre single-arm registry study. BioMed Res Int 2015;2015:173872

[17] Vanni D, Galzio R, Kazakova A, et al. Third-generation percutaneous vertebral augmentation systems. J Spine Surg 2016;2(1):13–20

35.10 Vertebral Augmentation: Tips and Tricks

Wayne J. Olan

As we enter a new era in vertebral augmentation with fixation with the release of the SpineJack device from Stryker in the fall of 2018, the use of this product and being facile with the subtleties of its indications and performance will help maximize the benefit to both the operator and the patient and will ensure maximum clinical benefit when using this device.[1]

To maximize the benefit and the reduction with SpineJack, we are using a simple technique to make certain we take full advantage of the lifting power and reducing force of the device. Just prior to elevating the SpineJack, we take an anteroposterior (AP) image to the vertebral body with both SpineJacks in place and a wide enough field of view so we can see the bottom of the handles that hold the implant. Confirming that the base of the handles are parallel to the inferior end plates of the treating vertebral body assures the operator that when the device opens it will open perpendicular to the end plates and will contribute maximally to the most effective end plate elevation and subsequent vertebral body reduction. Remember, AP to the patient does not always mean AP to the vertebral body.

Reference

[1] A Prospective, Multicenter, Randomized, Comparative Clinical Study to Compare the Safety and Effectiveness of Two Vertebral Compression Fracture (VCF) Reduction Techniques: The SpineJack and the KyphX Xpander Inflatable Bone Tamp. The U.S. National Library of Medicine and Clinical Trials.gov Web site. https://clinicaltrials.gov/ct2/show/NCT02461810. Published May 1, 2018. Accessed October 31, 2018

35.11 Dorsal Root Ganglion Stimulation to Treat Persistent Radicular Pain after Compression Fracture

Timothy Deer

Dorsal root ganglion (DRG) stimulation was first reported in its current form in 2011 in a pilot study of 10 patients with chronic nerve pain. In recent years, this therapy has been approved for widespread use in the United States, Europe, and Australia for focal neuropathic pain. In the current literature, the use of DRG stimulation has not been reported to treat persistent nerve pain after vertebral fracture and subsequent kyphoplasty.

The patient was a 53-year-old woman who suffered a traumatic fracture of the L1 vertebrae during a rollover accident. The patient was treated successfully with vertebral augmentation kyphoplasty of the fracture that involved the vertebral body and had no obvious damage to the posterior elements or to the adjacent neural elements, but immediately postprocedure she developed severe burning bilateral foot pain. The MR imaging examination showed no compression or retropulsion, but the pain persisted and she eventually failed injections, physical therapy, anticonvulsants, and opioid therapy. She was subsequently referred to an interventional pain physician for neuromodulation.

The patient underwent bilateral S1 DRG stimulation under general anesthesia with neuromonitoring (▶Fig. 35.58). The trial resulted in 85% relief at day 10, and subsequently the patient underwent a permanent implant. At the 6-month follow-up, both the L1 area and her foot pain were well controlled, and the patient was back to full employment with no oral medications. This case shows potential solutions to postprocedure nerve irritation after the fracture is adequately stabilized, but the postoperative course is complicated by neuropathic pain.

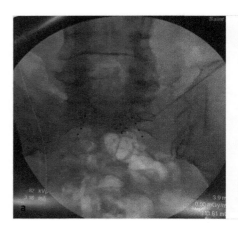 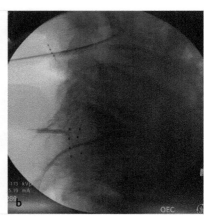

Fig. 35.58 (a, b) Bilateral S1 DRG stimulation under general anesthesia with neuromonitoring.

35.12 Vertebral Augmentation Tips and Tricks of the Trade
Neal H. Shonnard

35.12.1 Thermally Accelerated Cement

Cement augmentation of vertebral compression fractures utilizes polymethyl methacrylate (PMMA) or bone cement. The cement cures and solidifies through a polymerization process that produces an exothermic reaction. Applying heat (▶Fig. 35.59) of approximately 120°F for 10 to 20 seconds to the cement immediately after mixing accelerates the polymerization process, increasing the viscosity of the cement. A thicker cement allows for better control over the distribution of the cement and lessens the frequency of cement leakage outside the vertebral body. Cement injection may be performed immediately after the cement is heated in a water bath and is observed closely under lateral fluoroscopic visualization.

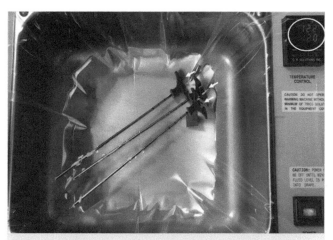

Fig. 35.59 Hot bath at 120°F (*white circle*) to enhance cement viscosity. The bone fillers with cement (*white arrows*) are placed in the water bath for 10 to 15 seconds.

35.12.2 Unipedicular Approach for Bilateral Cementation

A standard unilateral approach may be done through the ipsilateral pedicle or via a parapedicular approach. The introducer needle is placed into the vertebral body and then the drill is and inserted and angled to reach the midline in the anterior portion of the vertebral body (▶Fig. 35.60a, b). The curet is then introduced after removal of the drill (▶Fig. 35.61a), and is deployed toward the contralateral pedicle (▶Fig. 35.61b, c). The curet is pulled dorsally from the anterior vertebral body to the posterior third of the vertebral body (▶Fig. 35.62a, b). This technique is repeated while angling the curet toward the contralateral portion of the vertebral body until the curet reaches the location of the opposite pedicle on the anteroposterior view (▶Fig. 35.61c). The subsequent expansion of the balloon (▶Fig. 35.63a, b) will tend to conform to the location of the previous curettage and the cement will also flow into the cavities created by the curet and balloon (▶Fig. 35.64a, b).

35.12.3 Avoiding Wrong Level Surgery

A reliable intraoperative X-ray technique for establishing the intended level of treatment utilizes a 14-gauge needle placed at the L2 level. The lumbar levels are counted proximally from the pelvis, using a 14-gauge needle at the pedicle of L2 as a reference point. The fluoroscopy is moved proximally to count the distal thoracic vertebral levels until the intended level(s) is reached (▶Fig. 35.65a, b). This technique is very helpful to identify nondisplaced mid- and proximal thoracic vertebral fractures and to avoid wrong level surgery.

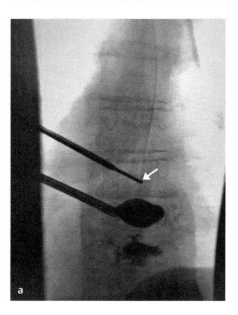
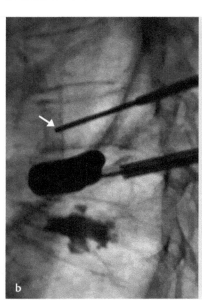

Fig. 35.60 (a) Anteroposterior and (b) lateral fluoroscopic views of the mid-thoracic spine shows the drill angled to reach the midline (*white arrow* in a) in the anterior portion of the vertebral body (*white arrow* in b).

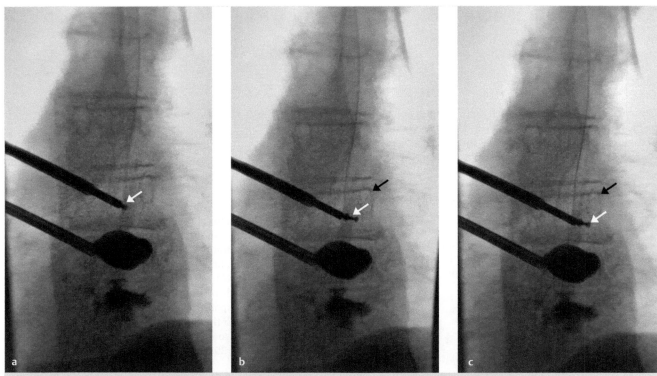

Fig. 35.61 Anteroposterior fluoroscopic views of the mid-thoracic spine shows the curet is then introduced after removal of the drill (*white arrow* in **a**), and is deployed toward the contralateral pedicle (*white arrows* in **b** and **c**; pedicle shown by *black arrows* in **b** and **c**).

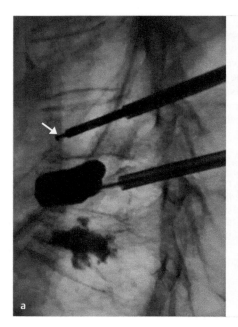
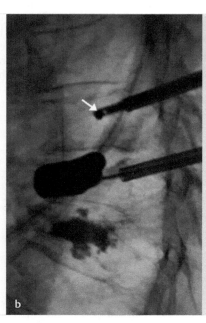

Fig. 35.62 Lateral fluoroscopic views of the mid-thoracic spine shows the curet is pulled dorsally from the anterior vertebral body to the posterior third of the vertebral body (*white arrows* in **a** and **b**).

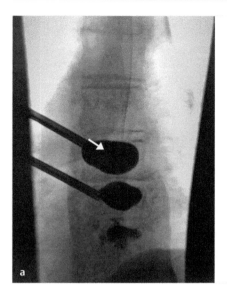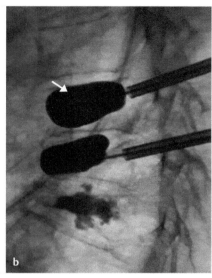

Fig. 35.63 (a) Anteroposterior and (b) lateral fluoroscopic views of the mid-thoracic spine show the expansion of the balloon (*white arrows* in **a** and **b**) in the location of the previous curettage.

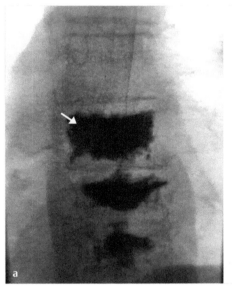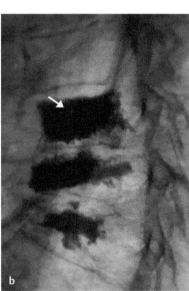

Fig. 35.64 (a) Anteroposterior and (b) lateral fluoroscopic views of the mid-thoracic spine show adequate cement fill in the location of the cavities created by the curet and balloon (*white arrows* in **a** and **b**).

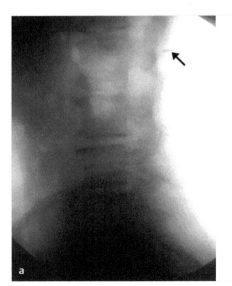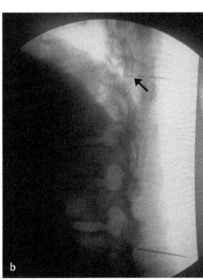

Fig. 35.65 Lateral fluoroscopic views of the lumbar spine (a) and the thoracolumbar junction (b) shows a 14-gauge needle just posterior to the pedicle at L2 (*black arrow* in **a**). A second needle is placed at the target level just posterior to T10 (*black arrow* in **b**).

35.13 Treatment of a Thoracic Vertebral Compression Fracture with Vertebra Plana

J. Dana Dunleavy

Included is a case of a thoracic vertebra plana. Interestingly, this underscores the importance of treating patients with compression fractures promptly since the fracture continued to progress in the interval between identification of the fracture and treatment.

Many practices do not treat thoracic compression fractures (and have even spread false information that lumbar augmentation provides clinical benefit but thoracic augmentation has no benefit) and do not treat vertebra plana or burst fractures because it is "unsafe." The facts behind both of the above scenarios is that they are more technically challenging but just as important and just as helpful to treat and optimal results are very achievable and safe with proper planning and technique (▶ Fig. 35.66, ▶ Fig. 35.67, ▶ Fig. 35.68, ▶ Fig. 35.69, and ▶ Fig. 35.70).

Pedicles are shorter and narrower and have a greater craniocaudal angulation in the thoracic spine as compared with the lumbar spine and therefore access needs to be more cranial than the planned level of augmentation. In the provided case, we used a Merit directional osteotome (Merit Medical Systems, Inc, South Jordan, UT) to gain intrapedicular access while curving the cannula within the markedly compressed fracture.

This allowed for an excellent cement fill without any extravasation of cement into the disk space. Many surgeons expect and allow cement within the disk space because it is assumed to be unavoidable with a thoracic vertebra plana. This case shows, however, that you can get excellent height restoration and cement fill with improved stabilization without extravasating cement into the intervertebral disk.

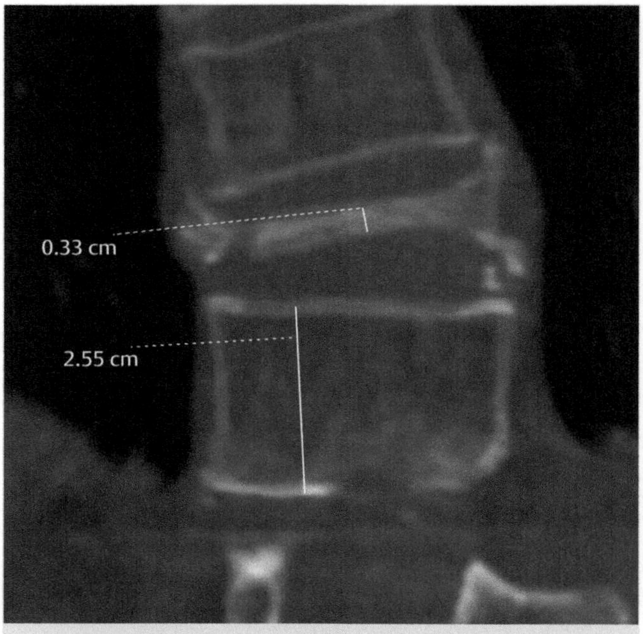

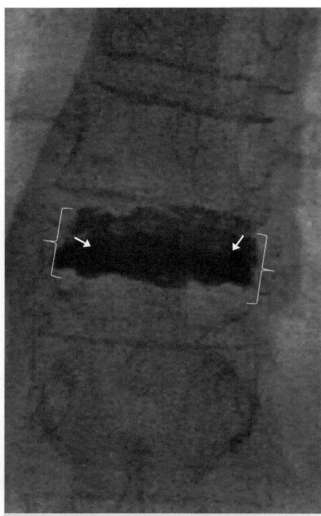

Fig. 35.67 Anteroposterior fluoroscopic image obtained at the conclusion of the procedure shows excellent height restoration (*white brackets*) and cement fill (*white arrows*) within the treated severe fracture, without any cement extravasation into the vertebral plexus, intervertebral disks, or epidural space.

0.33 cm

2.55 cm

Fig. 35.66 Cone beam CT obtained in the angiography suite (coronal plane) demonstrates the fractured thoracic vertebral body measuring only 3 mm in thickness, while the adjacent vertebral body measures 26 mm, a factor of 8.7 times different.

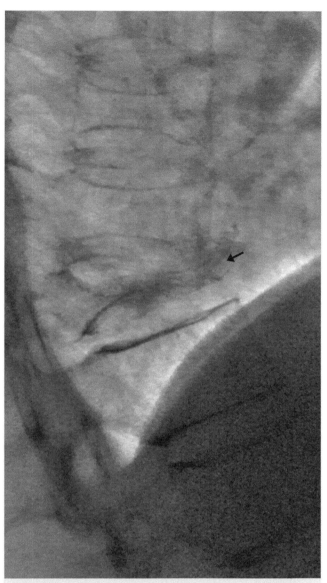

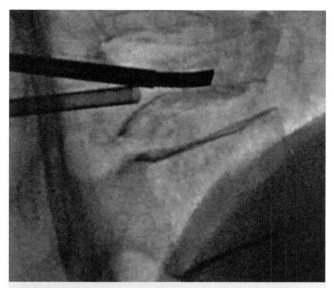

Fig. 35.69 Although unipedicular treatment is feasible, bipedicular technique was utilized here to maximize cement fill within the severely compressed fracture.

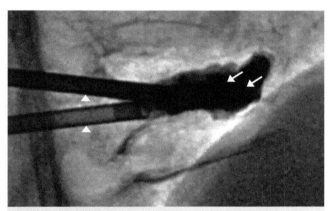

Fig. 35.70 Lateral fluoroscopic image showing cement within the vertebral body (*white arrows*) having been delivered through both cannulas (*white arrowheads*). If administering cement one cannula at a time, keep inner needle within the osteointroducer needle to avoid cement crossing midline and entering the contralateral cannula, which could otherwise harden within the contralateral cannula and prohibit treatment through that side.

Fig. 35.68 Lateral intraprocedure fluoroscopic image demonstrates the small target due to severe vertebral body compression (*black arrow*).

35.14 Vertebroplasty of a Myelomatous C3 Vertebral Body through an Anterolateral Route

Bassam Hamze and Jean-Denis Laredo

Vertebroplasty has taken an important place in the treatment of multiple myeloma of the spine.[1] Cervical vertebroplasty, however, is relatively uncommon and is usually performed through an anterolateral route.[2]

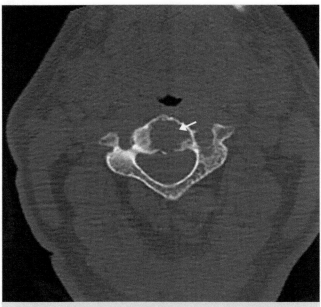

Fig. 35.71 Axial CT image of the C3 vertebral body shows C3 vertebral body osteolysis (*white arrow*).

35.14.1 Case Report

A 63-year-old man was consulted for persistent cervical pain. Plain film radiographs showed an ill-defined osteolysis of the C3 vertebral body. Blood and bone marrow samples demonstrated multiple myeloma. A computed tomography (CT) scan (▶Fig. 35.71) and a magnetic resonance (MR) imaging examination showed advanced destruction of the vertebral body cancellous bone with relative preservation of the cortical bone. The posterior vertebral body cortex was grossly preserved and there was no epidural extension of tumor.

A vertebroplasty to treat this lesion was decided after a multidisciplinary consultation. It was performed under general anesthesia and using fluoroscopic guidance. The patient was placed in the decubitus position with the head in neutral position. Arms were pulled downward to facilitate C3 lateral fluoroscopic viewing. The carotid artery and jugular vein were moved apart with manual pressure and an 11-gauge × 100-mm-long trocar (Kensington, Coaxial Bone Biopsy Kit, Merit Medical, Jordan, UT) was advanced through an anterolateral ascending approach between the carotid artery–jugular vein bundle and the tracheoesophageal anatomy. The C3 vertebral body was reached close to the midline under anteroposterior fluoroscopy and a cannula was advanced into the vertebral body under lateral fluoroscopic visualization. A total of. 2.5 mL of polymethyl methacrylate (PMMA; Vertecem V+ DePuy Synthes) was then slowly injected into the vertebral body under lateral fluoroscopic control (▶Fig. 35.72a, b).

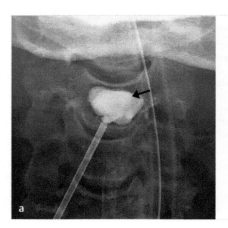
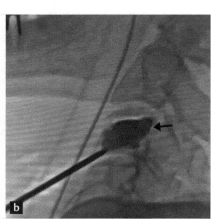

Fig. 35.72 (a) Anteroposterior and (b) lateral fluoroscopic images show PMMA cement filling C3 vertebral body (*black arrows* in **a** and **b**).

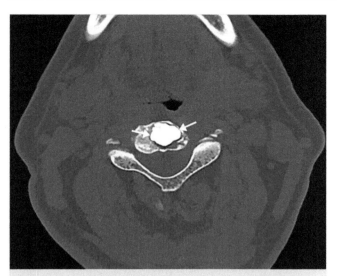

Fig. 35.73 Axial CT image of the C3 vertebral body shows PMMA within the region of osteolysis (*white arrows*).

A postoperative CT scan showed no cement extravasation (▶Fig. 35.73). The patient was standing up 6 hours after the intervention. The following days were uneventful and his neck pain decreased from 80/100 mm preoperatively to 20/100 mm postoperatively.

References

[1] McDonald RJ, Trout AT, Gray LA, Dispenzieri A, Thielen KR, Kallmes DF. Vertebroplasty in multiple myeloma: outcomes in a large patient series. AJNR Am J Neuroradiol 2008;29(4):642–648

[2] Pflugmacher R, Schleicher P, Schröder RJ, Melcher I, Klostermann CK. Maintained pain reduction in five patients with multiple myeloma 12 months after treatment of the involved cervical vertebrae with vertebroplasty. Acta Radiol 2006;47(8):823–829

35.15 Refracture after Kyphoplasty

James R. Webb

Occasionally, a patient will have partial relief of pain after vertebral augmentation kyphoplasty that is relieved with the injection of additional polymethyl methacrylate (PMMA). The scenario of insufficient fracture stabilization is seen more common in severely compressed fractures such as vertebra plana deformities or comminuted Magerl A-type fractures. In general, this is because pain is caused by macroscopic/microscopic trabecular motion and there was not enough PMMA reaching enough fracture lines to adequately stabilize the vertebral body and relieve pain. Most of the time that is due to caution taken during the injection of the cement and not predictable. The key determinant of whether the patient is refractured or if the fracture was inadequately stabilized is whether the patient ever converted to a negative closed-fist percussion exam (CFPE) after treatment. If not and this examination maneuver still elicits pain, the author would consider these to be an active nonunion rather than a recurrent fracture.

A more common scenario is a refracture in patients who were asymptomatic after an initial kyphoplasty at the incident level. This can occur days or years after the primary procedure. The most definitive way to document refracture is conversion from a positive to a negative CFPE at that level during the postprocedure follow-up. Then, at some point, the patient may develop a new fracture at the previously treated level that is now once again CFPE positive. The author makes a point to document CFPE status at all levels, T1–L5, at each visit. This helps document not only the timing and age of the fracture, but also the progress on those patients with multiple CFPE positive levels and multiple fractures that have to be treated at different times.

A refracture should be addressed in the same way as a primary fracture. Kyphoplasty is effective in recurrent fractures after patients have failed additional conservative care. Sometimes there is only enough room in the vertebral body to perform vertebroplasty, but preprocedure planning CT is often helpful for analyzing the existing cement pattern and in finding an appropriate needle approach. Cross-sectional imaging can be helpful for identifying residual marrow areas with less PMMA. These are usually the places that correlate with residual fractures that cause pain. Outside of this, the imaging diagnosis is problematic as there are no definitive criteria to assist in identifying recurrent vertebral fractures at the incident level.

Vertebral refractures are rarely demonstrated on plain films as additional collapse. Paraspinal short tau inversion recovery (STIR) edema or edema within the vertebral body out of proportion with what is expected is probably the single most helpful imaging finding to confirm the refracture. Increased STIR signal and increased radiotracer uptake on nuclear medicine bone scan are both common after kyphoplasty and are generally considered normal following vertebral augmentation. As such, it is imperative that the treating clinician (1) understands the limitations of imaging for diagnosis of refracture and (2) is comfortable in diagnosing fracture by clinical history and physical examination alone.

In the author's experience, it is uncommon to see obvious definitive fracture findings such as a low T1 fracture line, a fluid-filled instability cleft, or a prominent increased STIR signal when compared to a prior study, but these findings are occasionally seen and should be looked for on the diagnostic imaging study.

The figures demonstrate a typical case of a woman in her sixth decade of life with secondary osteoporosis due mainly to chronic selective serotonin reuptake inhibitor (SSRI) use and hypothyroidism. She had a T score of –1.5 and was found to have six mild height loss vertebral compression fractures at the time of her initial presentation. After treatment, she presented with recurrent pain to closed-fist percussion at T5 and T9 and complained of pain that she rated as a 10 out of 10 on the pain scale. She then underwent revision kyphoplasty and noted improvement in her pain by 4 days postrevision with her pain level remaining at a 2 out of 10 on the 1-month postrevision follow-up and a 1 out of 10 4 months later. Her first kyphoplasty was done 5 years earlier at T9 and her second kyphoplasty was done 7 months earlier at the T5 level (▶Fig. 35.74 and ▶Fig. 35.75).

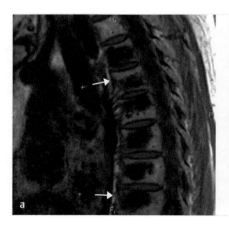 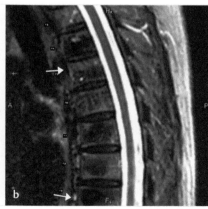

Fig. 35.74 (a) A sagittal T1-weighted MR image shows the absence of any specific low T1 fracture lines at T5 and T9 (*white arrows*). (b) Sagittal short tau inversion recovery (STIR) MR image shows nonspecific increased STIR at all previously treated levels (*white arrows* in b showing nonspecific increased marrow and paraspinal signal). For example, the increased STIR signal at T5 in the marrow is no greater than at T6 or the other treated levels.

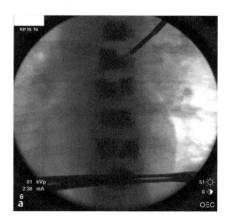 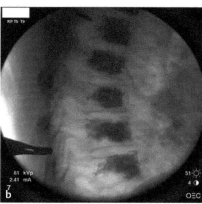

Fig. 35.75 (a) Anteroposterior fluoroscopic image shows markers over T5 and T9 corresponding to the locations of the patient's pain that was elicited with a closed-fist percussion exam. These areas were chosen to retreat during the revision kyphoplasty. (b) Lateral fluoroscopic image shows thoracic vertebral bodies that appear to be adequately filled with polymethyl methacrylate making the point that vertebral refractures often occur in vertebrae that appear to be adequately treated.

35.16 The Tripod Approach for Treating Vertebral Compression Fractures

Michael J. DePalma

A reasonable treatment plan for a nonhealing osteoporotic vertebral compression fracture (VCF) is what we refer to as the tripod approach consisting of (1) percutaneous fracture stabilization, (2) treatment of the underlying metabolic bone disorder, and (3) exercise training for appropriate and adaptive posture and body mechanics. Percutaneous augmentation of a persistently painful VCF can reduce morbidity and mortality and can be performed by direct injection of bone cement[1–3] or bone glue[4] or by void creation before cementation.[2,5] A variety of fracture augmentation devices are readily available and each is associated with claims of success. Which fracture repair option to utilize, however, may be less critical to determining the success of the treatment than proper patient selection.

Asymptomatic VCFs have been observed despite extensive bone edema as seen on the MR imaging examination.[6] Emerging reports have also demonstrated that the facet joints at the segmental level of the VCF can serve as the source of back pain in patients with quiescent or nonpainful VCFs.[1,7] Therefore, despite morphologic abnormalities on MR imaging, a VCF may not be the reason for the patient's back pain. The presence of a VCF as seen on MR imaging or computed tomography (CT) must be supported by the clinician's physical examination. Pain production upon percussion with a closed fist over the putatively painful VCF and pain provocation by assuming the supine position is sensitive and specific in the detection of painful VCFs.[8]

Merely stabilizing the VCF itself is insufficient to adequately treat the fracture and minimize risk of recurrent VCFs. Within the first initial year after an osteoporotic VCF, just 25% of affected patients are prescribed pharmacologic agents for the treatment of their underlying bone disorder.[9] After medication is started, patient adherence varies and can dwindle to one out of four patients within 6 to 12 months after drug initiation.[10–12] Osteoporotic patients who have been treated with a bisphosphonate for at least 5 years experience VCF rates similar to that of their nontreated counterparts.[13] Pharmacologic treatment with abaloparatide or teriparatide, unless contraindicated, combined with proper amounts of vitamin D and calcium supplementation, helps stimulate bone healing and reduce the onset of new fractures by 65 to 86%.[14,15] Hormonal deficiency such as reduced testosterone in elderly men may lead to osteopenia or osteoporosis and must be addressed as well. This comprehensive approach helps reduce the risk for developing an additional VCF as well as to directly address and treat the underlying reason for the patients' osteoporotic fracture.

Kyphotic posture contributes to further kyphosis, leading to an increased risk of additional VCFs.[16] A successful strategy to reduce kyphotic deformity may be multifaceted addressing fracture reduction both by optimizing vertebral body height and by improving postural maintenance. The patient's posture, neuromuscular conditioning, and degenerative intervertebral disk disease are implicated in the dynamic relationship between routine activities and fracture risk.[17–19] With aging, there is an involutional loss of functional muscle motor units that reduces an individual's postural control, contributing to their kyphosis.[19] A 2-year, structured back extension exercise program has been shown to reduce the incidence of VCFs and increase bone mineral density in healthy, postmenopausal women, up to 8 years after cessation of the program.[16] Likewise, exercise training after VCF augmentation reduces the number of additional VCFs.[20] Although intuitive, the objective evidence also suggests that extension-based exercise helps maintain bone mineral density and prevent baseline and additional VCFs probably due to improved posture and spine stabilization.

References

[1] Alvarez L, Alcaraz M, Pérez-Higueras A, et al. Percutaneous vertebroplasty: functional improvement in patients with osteoporotic compression fractures. Spine 2006;31(10):1113–1118

[2] Taylor RS, Taylor RJ, Fritzell P. Balloon kyphoplasty and vertebroplasty for vertebral compression fractures: a comparative systematic review of efficacy and safety. Spine 2006;31(23):2747–2755

[3] Hulme PA, Krebs J, Ferguson SJ, Berlemann U. Vertebroplasty and kyphoplasty: a systematic review of 69 clinical studies. Spine 2006;31(17):1983–2001

[4] Linovitz R, Westerlund E, Peppers T, et al. An evaluation of the safety and efficacy of an alternative material to polymethylmethacrylate bone cement for vertebral augmentation. White Paper; 2010

[5] Wardlaw D, Cummings SR, Van Meirhaeghe J, et al. Efficacy and safety of balloon kyphoplasty compared with non-surgical care for vertebral compression fracture (FREE): a randomised controlled trial. Lancet 2009;373(9668):1016–1024

[6] McKiernan FE. The broadening spectrum of osteoporotic vertebral fracture. Skeletal Radiol 2009;38(4):303–308

[7] Bogduk N. The pain of Vertebral Compression Fractures Can Be in the Posterior Elements. ISIS 16th Annual Scientific Meeting, Las Vegas, NV; 2008:201–202

[8] Langdon J, Way A, Heaton S, Bernard J, Molloy S. Vertebral compression fractures--new clinical signs to aid diagnosis. Ann R Coll Surg Engl 2010;92(2):163–166

[9] Andrade SE, Majumdar SR, Chan KA, et al. Low frequency of treatment of osteoporosis among postmenopausal women following a fracture. Arch Intern Med 2003;163(17):2052–2057

[10] McCombs JS, Thiebaud P, McLaughlin-Miley C, Shi J. Compliance with drug therapies for the treatment and prevention of osteoporosis. Maturitas 2004;48(3):271–287

[11] Tosteson ANA, Grove MR, Hammond CS, et al. Early discontinuation of treatment for osteoporosis. Am J Med 2003;115(3):209–216

[12] Segal E, Tamir A, Ish-Shalom S. Compliance of osteoporotic patients with different treatment regimens. Isr Med Assoc J 2003;5(12):859–862

[13] Liberman UA, Weiss SR, Bröll J, et al; The Alendronate Phase III Osteoporosis Treatment Study Group. Effect of oral alendronate on bone mineral density and the incidence of fractures in postmenopausal osteoporosis. N Engl J Med 1995;333(22):1437–1443

[14] Miller PD, Hattersley G, Riis BJ, et al; ACTIVE Study Investigators. Effect of abaloparatide vs placebo on new vertebral fractures in postmenopausal women with osteoporosis: a randomized clinical trial. JAMA 2016;316(7):722–733

[15] Neer RM, Arnaud CD, Zanchetta JR, et al. Effect of parathyroid hormone (1–34) on fractures and bone mineral density in postmenopausal women with osteoporosis. N Engl J Med 2001;344(19):1434–1441

[16] Kayanja MM, Togawa D, Lieberman IH. Biomechanical changes after the augmentation of experimental osteoporotic vertebral compression fractures in the cadaveric thoracic spine. Spine J 2005;5(1):55–63

[17] Sinaki M, Itoi E, Wahner HW, et al. Stronger back muscles reduce the incidence of vertebral fractures: a prospective 10 year follow-up of postmenopausal women. Bone 2002;30(6):836–841

[18] Pollintine P, Dolan P, Tobias JH, Adams MA. Intervertebral disc degeneration can lead to "stress-shielding" of the anterior vertebral body: a cause of osteoporotic vertebral fracture? Spine 2004;29(7):774–782

[19] McComas AJ, Fawcett PR, Campbell MJ, Sica RE. Electrophysiological estimation of the number of motor units within a human muscle. J Neurol Neurosurg Psychiatry 1971;34(2):121–131

[20] Huntoon EA, Schmidt CK, Sinaki M. Significantly fewer refractures after vertebroplasty in patients who engage in back-extensor-strengthening exercises. Mayo Clin Proc 2008;83(1):54–57